**The Maudsley Practice
Guidelines for Physical
Health Conditions in
Psychiatry**

THE MAUDSLEY GUIDELINES

Other books in the *Maudsley Prescribing Guidelines* series include:

The Maudsley Prescribing Guidelines in Psychiatry, 14th edition (coming in 2021) David M. Taylor, Thomas R.E. Barnes, Allan H. Young.

The Maudsley Guidelines on Advanced Prescribing in Psychosis Paul Morrison, David M. Taylor, Phillip McGuire.

The Maudsley Practice Guidelines for Physical Health Conditions in Psychiatry

David M. Taylor BSc, MSc, PhD, FCMHP, FFRPS, FRPharmS, FRCP (Edin)

Director of Pharmacy and Pathology, Maudsley Hospital;
and Professor of Psychopharmacology, King's College, London, UK

Fiona Gaughran MD, FRCP(I), FRCP (Lon), FRCP (Edin), FRCPsych, FHEA

Lead Consultant Psychiatrist, National Psychosis Service (Bethlem Royal Hospital);
Director of Research and Development, South London and Maudsley NHS Foundation Trust;
Reader in Psychopharmacology and Physical Health, King's College, London, UK

Toby Pillinger MA (Oxon), BM BCh, MRCP, PhD

Academic Clinical Fellow, South London and Maudsley NHS Foundation Trust
and the Institute of Psychiatry, Psychology and Neuroscience, Kings College, London, UK

WILEY Blackwell

Registered Offices
John Wiley & Sons, Inc., 111 River Street, Hoboken, NJ 07030, USA
John Wiley & Sons Ltd, The Atrium, Southern Gate, Chichester, West Sussex, PO19 8SQ, UK

Editorial Office
111 River Street, Hoboken, NJ 07030, USA

For details of our global editorial offices, customer services, and more information about Wiley products visit us at www.wiley.com.

Wiley also publishes its books in a variety of electronic formats and by print-on-demand. Some content that appears in standard print versions of this book may not be available in other formats.

Library of Congress Cataloging-in-Publication Data

Names: David M. Taylor, 1963– editor. | Gaughran, Fiona, editor. | Pillinger, Toby, editor.
Title: The Maudsley practice guidelines for physical health conditions in psychiatry / [edited by] David M. Taylor, Fiona Gaughran, Toby Pillinger.
Description: Hoboken, NJ : John Wiley & Sons, Inc., 2021. | Includes index.
Identifiers: LCCN 2020025468 (print) | LCCN 2020025469 (ebook) | ISBN 9781119554202 (paperback) | ISBN 9781119554219 (adobe pdf) | ISBN 9781119554240 (epub)
Subjects: MESH: Mental Disorders–complications | Patient Care–methods | Diagnostic Techniques and Procedures | Referral and Consultation | Evidence-Based Practice | Practice Guideline
Classification: LCC RC454 (print) | LCC RC454 (ebook) | NLM WM 140 | DDC 616.89–dc23
LC record available at https://lccn.loc.gov/2020025468
LC ebook record available at https://lccn.loc.gov/2020025469

Cover Design: Wiley
Cover Image: © SciePro/Shutterstock

Set in 10/12pt Sabon by SPi Global, Pondicherry, India

SKY10074878_050924

For Aloysius, welcome to the world.

Contents

Preface

It is well documented that people with severe mental illness have elevated mortality rates compared with the general population, with physical health conditions the predominant cause. There are several potential mechanisms underlying this mortality gap. First, lifestyle factors such as poor diet, reduced exercise levels, and higher rates of smoking play a role. Second, psychiatric medications are associated with physical side effects, and can contribute to progressive impairment of multiple organ systems. Third, individuals with serious mental illness are less likely to present to a general practitioner or medical hospital with a physical complaint, thereby allowing conditions to progress without treatment. Fourth, when physical conditions are identified while under the care of psychiatric services, practitioners may lack the knowledge and confidence to act.

This, the first edition of *The Maudsley Practice Guidelines for Physical Health Conditions in Psychiatry*, aims to bridge the gap between psychiatric and physical health services which are usually geographically and organisationally separate. A key objective is to enhance the clinical confidence of psychiatric practitioners by providing these individuals with a practical and evidence-based 'toolkit' with which to assess, investigate, and potentially initiate treatment for common physical health conditions seen in patients with serious mental illness. It is hoped that co-working relationships between psychiatrists and general practitioners, physicians, and surgeons alike will be enhanced owing to improved quality of referrals. Furthermore, it is anticipated that the standard of clinical care delivered to patients with serious mental illness will improve by expediting appropriate investigation and management of physical comorbidity. Finally, we hope that the patient–practitioner relationship will be enhanced as psychiatric patients become aware that both body and mind are being considered as part of their holistic care.

The Maudsley Practice Guidelines for Physical Health Conditions in Psychiatry consists of 89 chapters, covering 14 different organ systems, alongside emergency presentations. Although *The Guidelines* are predominantly based on UK practice, we have made efforts to acknowledge the anticipated international readership, and as such have also included references to psychiatric and medical drugs not currently licensed in the UK. However, the reader should be aware that no guideline can take into account every drug available across the world, so omissions are inevitable.

This text may be seen as a sister volume to the *The Maudsley Prescribing Guidelines in Psychiatry*. Like that book, the *The Maudsley Practice Guidelines for Physical Health Conditions in Psychiatry* is the product of a group of local and international experts; we are indebted to the 125 individuals from across medicine, surgery, and psychiatry who have contributed. At present, the world's attention is centred on the COVID-19 pandemic and never has there been a greater need for clinicians from across specialties to work together for the greater good of patients. We hope that *The Maudsley Practice Guidelines for Physical Health Conditions in Psychiatry* will go some way to facilitate this, not only in the current climate but for years to come.

Toby Pillinger
London, UK
September 2020

Abbreviations

ABPM	ambulatory blood pressure monitoring
ACE	angiotensin-converting enzyme
ACOS	asthma–COPD overlap syndrome
ACS	acute coronary syndrome
ADH	antidiuretic hormone
ADR	adverse drug reaction
AE	autoimmune encephalitis
AED	antiepileptic drug
AF	atrial fibrillation
AFB	acid-fast bacilli
AKI	acute kidney injury
ALP	alkaline phosphatase
ALT	alanine aminotransferase
ANC	absolute neutrophil count
ARB	angiotensin II receptor blocker
ART	antiretroviral therapy
ASPD	advanced sleep phase disorder
AST	aspartate aminotransferase
ATT	antitubercular treatment
AUR	acute urinary retention
BEN	benign ethnic neutropenia
BMI	body mass index
BNP	brain natriuretic peptide
BP	blood pressure
BPH	benign prostatic hyperplasia
CAP	community-acquired pneumonia
CBT	cognitive-behavioural therapy
CI	confidence interval
CIM	clozapine-induced myocarditis
CKD	chronic kidney disease
CLD	chronic liver disease

CNS	central nervous system
COPD	chronic obstructive pulmonary disease
COVID-19	coronavirus disease 2019
CPAP	continuous positive airway pressure
CRP	C-reactive protein
CSF	cerebrospinal fluid
CT	computed tomography
CVD	cardiovascular disease
DAA	direct-acting antiviral
DEXA	dual-energy X-ray absorptiometry
DI	diabetes insipidus
DKA	diabetic ketoacidosis
DRE	digital rectal examination
DSPD	delayed sleep phase disorder
DVT	deep vein thrombosis
ECT	electroconvulsive therapy
EDS	excessive daytime sleepiness
eGFR	estimated glomerular filtration rate
EPSE	extrapyramidal side effect
ESC	European Society of Cardiology
ESR	erythrocyte sedimentation rate
ESRF	end-stage renal failure
FBC	full blood count
FDA	Food and Drug Administration
FEV_1	forced expiratory volume in 1 s
FVC	forced vital capacity
GABA	gamma-aminobutyric acid
GCS	Glasgow Coma Scale
GGT	gamma-glutamyltransferase
GORD	gastro-oesophageal reflux disease
HAD	HIV-associated dementia
HAND	HIV-associated neurocognitive disorders
HAP	hospital-acquired pneumonia
HBPM	home blood pressure monitoring
HBV	hepatitis B virus
HCG	human chorionic gonadotrophin
HCV	hepatitis C virus
HDL	high-density lipoprotein
HHS	hyperosmolar hyperglycaemic state
HMOD	hypertension-mediated organ damage
HRT	hormone replacement therapy
HSV	herpes simplex virus
ICD	implantable cardioverter-defibrillator
ICP	intracranial pressure

ICU	intensive care unit
IGRA	interferon gamma release assay
INR	international normalised ratio
IOP	intraocular pressure
IUD	intrauterine device
LARC	long-acting reversible contraceptive
LBBB	left bundle branch block
LDL	low-density lipoprotein
LFT	liver function test
LLQ	left lower quadrant
LMWH	low-molecular-weight heparin
LOS	lower oesophageal sphincter
LP	lumbar puncture
LUQ	left upper quadrant
LVH	left ventricular hypertrophy
MAOI	monoamine oxidase inhibitor
MCV	mean corpuscular volume
MDD	major depressive disorder
MOH	major obstetric haemorrhage
MRI	magnetic resonance imaging
MRSA	methicillin-resistant *Staphylococcus aureus*
MSU	mid-stream urine
NAFLD	non-alcoholic fatty liver disease
NICE	National Institute for Health and Care Excellence
NMDA	N-methyl-D-aspartate
NMS	neuroleptic malignant syndrome
NNRTI	non-nucleoside reverse transcriptase inhibitor
NRT	nicotine replacement therapy
NSAID	non-steroidal anti-inflammatory drug
NSTEMI	non-ST-segment elevation myocardial infarction
OD	odds ratio
OGTT	oral glucose tolerance test
OIC	opioid-induced constipation
OSA	obstructive sleep apnoea
PA	physical activity
PAMORA	peripherally acting μ-opioid receptor antagonist
PCI	percutaneous coronary intervention
PCR	polymerase chain reaction
PE	pulmonary embolism
PEF	peak expiratory flow
PEFR	peak expiratory flow rate
PEP	post-exposure prophylaxis
PHAP	psychiatric hospital-acquired pneumonia
PID	pelvic inflammatory disease

PLMS	periodic limb movements in sleep
PLWHIV	people living with HIV
PNES	psychogenic non-epileptic seizures
POI	premature ovarian insufficiency
PPI	proton-pump inhibitor
PPS	psychogenic pseudosyncope
PUD	peptic ulcer disease
PwE	people with epilepsy
RAPD	relative afferent pupillary defect
RID	relative infant dose
RLS	restless leg syndrome
RR	relative risk
RUQ	right upper quadrant
SARS-CoV-2	severe acute respiratory syndrome coronavirus 2
SD	sexual dysfunction
SIADH	syndrome of inappropriate antidiuretic hormone secretion
SJS	Stevens–Johnson syndrome
SLE	systemic lupus erythematosus
SMI	serious mental illness
SNRI	serotonin/noradrenaline reuptake inhibitor
SPECT	single photon emission computed tomography
SSRI	selective serotonin reuptake inhibitor
STEMI	ST-segment elevation myocardial infarction
STI	sexually transmitted infection
SVT	supraventricular tachycardia
TD	tardive dyskinesia
T2DM	type 2 diabetes mellitus
TEN	toxic epidermal necrolysis
TFT	thyroid function test
TIA	transient ischaemic attack
TIBC	total iron-binding capacity
TLE	temporal lobe epilepsy
TLOC	transient loss of consciousness
TNF	tumour necrosis factor
TRH	thyrotropin releasing hormone
TSH	thyroid stimulating hormone
UA	unstable angina
ULN	upper limit of normal
UPSI	unprotected sexual intercourse
UTI	urinary tract infection
VGKC	voltage-gated potassium channel
VT	ventricular tachycardia
VTE	venous thromboembolism
WHO	World Health Organization

Part 1

Cardiology

Chapter 1

Tachycardia

Guy Hindley, Eromona Whiskey, Nicholas Gall

In adults, tachycardia is defined as a heart rate faster than 100 beats per minute (bpm). This may represent a normal physiological response, a sign of systemic illness, or primary cardiac pathology [1]. There are several possible cardiac rhythms associated with tachycardia. Identifying the underlying rhythm is central to the diagnostic process and directs management. Classifying these rhythms according to the width of the QRS complex and the regularity of the rhythm (as seen on an ECG) helps to simplify this process (Table 1.1) [2].

SINUS TACHYCARDIA

Sinus tachycardia is the most commonly encountered rhythm disturbance. In the majority of cases, this is an appropriate physiological response mediated by the sympathetic nervous system to an identifiable cause, which may be benign or pathological (Box 1.1) [3]. In the context of mental health, sinus tachycardia may be experienced during episodes of agitation, anxiety or panic. Sympathomimetic and anticholinergic drugs are also important causes to consider, including clozapine which causes a transient sinus tachycardia in 25% of patients, usually limited to the first six weeks of treatment [4]. Among pathological causes, people with serious mental illness (SMI) are at higher risk of sepsis [5] and pulmonary embolism [5,6], while sinus tachycardia is also associated with clozapine-induced myocarditis [7], neuroleptic malignant syndrome, and serotonin syndrome [8]. Hyperthyroidism and, more rarely, phaeochromocytoma may present with both psychiatric symptoms and sinus tachycardia [9,10]. The reader is directed to other chapters for detailed information on sepsis (Chapter 72), venous thromboembolism (Chapter 18), myocarditis (Chapter 8), neuroleptic malignant syndrome (Chapter 85), serotonin syndrome (Chapter 86), and hyperthyroidism (Chapter 79).

The Maudsley Practice Guidelines for Physical Health Conditions in Psychiatry, First Edition.
David M. Taylor, Fiona Gaughran, and Toby Pillinger.
© 2021 John Wiley & Sons Ltd. Published 2021 by John Wiley & Sons Ltd.

Table 1.1 Differential diagnosis of tachycardia according to the length of the QRS complex and regularity of rhythm [2].

	Narrow QRS (≤120 ms)	Broad QRS (>120 ms)

Regular	Sinus tachycardia
	Supraventricular tachycardia
	Atrioventricular re-entrant
	  tachycardia (AVRT)
	Atrioventricular nodal re-entrant
	  tachycardia (AVNRT)
	Atrial flutter (with regular
	  atrioventricular block)
	Focal atrial tachycardia
		Monomorphic ventricular tachycardia (VT)
		Any regular narrow-complex tachycardia with aberrant conduction
		(e.g. bundle branch block/accessory pathway)

Irregular	Atrial fibrillation (AF) Atrial flutter with varying atrioventricular block Multifocal atrial tachycardia	Torsade de pointes Polymorphic VT Ventricular fibrillation AF with aberrant conduction (bundle branch block/accessory pathway)

ATRIAL FIBRILLATION

Atrial fibrillation (AF) is the second most prevalent rhythm disturbance, occurring in 0.4–1% of adults [11]. Risk increases significantly with age [11]. Alcohol and stimulant use, hyperthyroidism, heart failure, hypertension, and chronic lung disease are associated with AF, all of which are more prevalent in patients with SMI (Table 1.2) [12]. AF can cause acute cardiac decompensation presenting as pulmonary oedema or myocardial ischaemia (see Chapters 67 and 68), as well as longer-term complications such as thromboembolic disease (e.g. stroke; see Chapter 82) [13].

SUPRAVENTRICULAR TACHYCARDIA

Conventionally, supraventricular tachycardia (SVT) refers to any tachycardia other than AF that originates above the level of the ventricles, i.e. involving the atria, the atrioventricular node, or the bundle of His [2]. Atrioventricular nodal re-entrant tachycardia (AVNRT), atrioventricular re-entrant tachycardia (AVRT), atrial flutter, and focal atrial tachycardia are the most common forms of SVT and each is associated with its own distinct pathophysiology and management [14]. Among people with SMI, alcohol and stimulant use may precipitate SVT (see Box 1.1) [15]. Ischaemic heart disease is also an important risk factor [16], the incidence of which is higher in people with SMI [17]. Among the general population, SVT rates are higher in women and those older than 65, although in the absence of ischaemic heart disease, SVT tends to present in younger people with a mean age of 37 [16].

Box 1.1 Common or important causes of tachycardia: those associated with serious mental illness are highlighted in italic

Sinus tachycardia

Emotional/physical arousal: anxiety/panic/agitation
Pain
Circulatory compromise:
  Sepsis
  Pulmonary embolism
  Hypovolaemia including haemorrhage
Heart failure
Myocardial ischaemia
Anaemia
Hyperthyroidism
Electrolyte disturbance (hypokalaemia, hypomagnesaemia)
Pregnancy
Postural orthostatic tachycardia syndrome
Inappropriate sinus tachycardia
Orthostatic intolerance
Alcohol/opiate/benzodiazepine withdrawal
Serotonin syndrome
Neuroleptic malignant syndrome
Drugs:
  Salbutamol
  Caffeine
  Cocaine
  Amphetamine
  Cannabis
  Clozapine
  Tricyclic antidepressants
  Carbamazepine
  Methylphenidate

Supraventricular tachycardia [2,15,16]

Wolff–Parkinson–White syndrome (AVRT)
Electrolyte disturbances (hypokalaemia/hyperkalaemia, hypomagnesaemia)
Ischaemic heart disease
Drugs:
  Alcohol
  Cocaine
  Amphetamine
  Caffeine

Atrial fibrillation [12]

Older age
Sepsis
Pulmonary embolism
Heart failure
Valvular heart disease
Hypertension

Chronic lung disease and lung cancer
Hyperthyroidism
Electrolyte disturbance (hypokalaemia, hypomagnesaemia)
Drugs:
    Atropine
    Alcohol
    Caffeine
    Cocaine
    Amphetamine

Ventricular tachycardia [23–26]

Myocardial infarction
Cardiomyopathy
Structural heart disease
Electrolyte disturbances (hypokalaemia/hyperkalaemia, hypomagnesaemia)
Prolonged QTc interval (congenital or acquired)
Brugada syndrome (phenotype associated with antipsychotics)
Eating disorders
Drugs:
    Cocaine
    Amphetamines
    Tricyclic antidepressants
    QTc prolonging medication including antipsychotics (see Chapter 3)
    Digoxin

VENTRICULAR TACHYCARDIA

Ventricular tachycardia (VT) is less common but is associated with high mortality and is the leading cause of sudden cardiac death [18]. The majority of cases are experienced in the context of structural heart disease, myocardial infarction or cardiomyopathy (both ischaemic and non-ischaemic) [19]. Although a specific association between VT and SMI has not been investigated, sudden cardiac death is significantly more prevalent in the psychiatric population and particularly among those taking antipsychotic medication and people with eating disorders [20,21]. Torsades de pointes (TdP), an irregular polymorphic VT, is of particular relevance due to its association with many antipsychotics and other psychotropic medications that prolong the QT interval (see Chapter 3). Despite this, TdP is still relatively rare, with an annual incidence of 0.16% in general hospital inpatients [22].

DIAGNOSTIC PRINCIPLES

History

1 Define cardiac symptoms.
    a Palpitations (Box 1.2): if these are paroxysmal (i.e. intermittent), ask the patient to tap out the rhythm; this may provide information on the rate and the regularity of

---

> **Box 1.2** Clinical assessment of paroxysmal palpitations
>
> - Palpitations are defined as the abnormal sensation of one's own heartbeat.
> - They may be associated with tachyarrhythmias but can also be experienced during other abnormal cardiac rhythms such as ectopic beats or bradyarrhythmias (see Chapter 1.2) [28].
> - Common causes include anxiety and somatisation (31%), paroxysmal atrial fibrillation (16%), and paroxysmal supraventricular tachycardia (10%) [29].
> - Although psychiatric symptoms are an important risk factor for a non-cardiac cause of palpitations, 13% of such patients have an underlying cardiac abnormality and so further investigation may be warranted in the presence of other cardiac symptoms or red flag features [30].

---

the heartbeat during the palpitations (if irregularly irregular, strongly suggestive of paroxysmal AF).

  b Symptoms of haemodynamic compromise, e.g. chest pain, shortness of breath, syncope/presyncope.

  c Symptoms of heart failure, e.g. orthopnoea (shortness of breath on lying flat), paroxysmal nocturnal dyspnoea (sensation of shortness of breath that wakes a patient from their sleep), swollen ankles.

  d Symptoms of myocardial infarction (assessment of chest pain including character, site, and radiation; nausea/vomiting, sweating).

2 Determine possible precipitants including exercise, stress, drugs, or alcohol.

3 Symptoms suggestive of systemic illness.

  a Sepsis: fever, rigors, presyncope/syncope, confusion, symptoms related to infective source.

  b Dehydration/hypovolaemia: recent evidence of volume loss (diarrhoea/vomiting, reduced oral intake, blood loss).

  c Hyperthyroidism: weight loss despite increased appetite, oligomenorrhoea, emotional lability, heat intolerance.

  d Anxiety/panic: paraesthesia, breathlessness, association with psychosocial stressors.

4 Medication history including any new medications or recent dose changes/withdrawal, paying particular attention to any sympathomimetic or anticholinergic drugs (e.g. clozapine).

5 Past medical history, including:

  a ischaemic, structural, or valvular heart disease or heart failure

  b chronic lung disease (e.g. chronic obstructive pulmonary disease/obstructive sleep apnoea)

  c thyroid disease

  d diabetes mellitus

  e previous tachyarrhythmias

  f eating disorder (purging behaviour may be associated with electrolyte disturbance)

  g panic attacks/anxiety.

6   Family history of sudden cardiac death/unexplained death under 40 or tachyarrhythmias [27].
7   Social history including alcohol and tobacco use, illicit substance use, and consumption of caffeinated drinks (see Chapter 46).
8   Perform a mental state examination, exploring for any psychiatric symptoms that may be associated with autonomic activation, e.g. panic, anxiety, or fear in the context of delusional beliefs or hallucinatory experiences.

Examination

1   In an emergency (e.g. the unconscious patient), resuscitate using the ABCDE approach and refer to emergency medical services.
2   Observations: heart rate, blood pressure, temperature, respiratory rate, oxygen saturations.
3   In stable patients, perform a cardiovascular examination paying particular attention to the following.
    a   Inspection: dyspnoea, raised jugular venous pressure, swollen ankles (evidence of heart failure).
    b   Palpation: examine pulse for rate, rhythm, character, and volume.
    c   Auscultation: murmurs (valvular heart disease), S3/S4 (heart failure), pulse deficit (additional heartbeats that do not correspond to a palpable pulse are a sign of AF), chest (pulmonary oedema).
    d   Palpation for sacral and pedal oedema (heart failure).
4   Focused examination if underlying cause suspected, as in the following examples.
    a   If infection is suspected, focused examination for potential sources (e.g. chest).
    b   If hyperthyroidism suspected: fine tremor, sweaty palms, exophthalmos/lid lag, palpate for goitre (see Chapter 12 for focused examination).
5   Lying and standing blood pressure may elicit postural drop in blood pressure indicative of haemodynamic compromise.

Investigations

1   ECG (see Box 1.3 for descriptions of ECGs for common or important tachyarrhythmias with examples).
2   Bloods:
    a   full blood count (anaemia, high/low neutrophil count)
    b   renal function (hypovolaemia, hypokalaemia/hyperkalaemia)
    c   bone profile (hypomagnesaemia, hypocalcaemia)
    d   C-reactive protein (infection)
    e   thyroid function (hyperthyroidism)
    f   antipsychotic levels (toxicity)
    g   troponin (if suspecting an ischaemic event or myocarditis)
    h   D-dimer (see Chapter 18 to guide use of this test)
    i   brain natriuretic peptide (heart failure)
    j HbA_{1c} (diabetes mellitus)
    k   blood sugar (diabetic ketoacidosis/hyperosmolar hyperglycaemic state).

Box 1.3 ECG characteristics of different tachyarrhythmias [32]

- Sinus tachycardia: P waves preceding every QRS complex, QRS complex following every P wave.

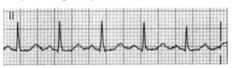

- Atrial fibrillation: irregularly irregular rhythm without P waves

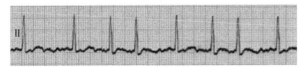

- Atrial flutter: saw-tooth pattern reflecting atrial contractions at 300 bpm best seen in leads II, III and aVF. Usually narrow QRS complexes at 150 bpm (2 , 1 AV node conduction, as shown here).

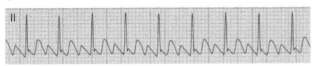

- Supraventricular tachycardia (atrioventricular re-entrant tachycardia or atrioventricular nodal re-entry tachycardia): regular tachycardia 140–300 bpm. Narrow QRS complexes (unless aberrant conduction). ST depression and T-wave inversion possible even in the absence of coronary artery disease.

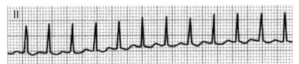

- Wolff–Parkinson–White in sinus rhythm: short PR interval <120 ms. Delta wave: slowly rising QRS complex. QRS prolongation >110 ms. ST-segment and T-wave changes.

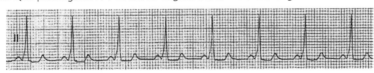

- Monomorphic ventricular tachycardia: regular rhythm, very broad QRS complexes (>160 ms) typically in the elderly or those with structural heart disease.

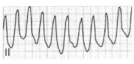

- Torsade de pointes: variable QRS complexes which 'twist' around isoelectric line.aVL

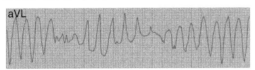

3 Urine toxicology (cocaine, amphetamines, cannabis).
4 Urine dipstick (urinary tract infection, ketonuria, glycosuria).
5 Chest X-ray (cardiomegaly, pulmonary oedema, pneumonia, lung cancer).

Specialist investigations

1 Echocardiogram (valvular heart disease, systolic/diastolic dysfunction, structural heart disease).
2 A 24-hour ECG (paroxysmal tachyarrhythmias, e.g. paroxysmal AF, SVTs) for symptomatic episodes that occur less than 24 hours apart, or suspected asymptomatic episodes.
3 Consider use of an event recorder if symptomatic episodes more than 24 hours apart and referral to cardiology [31].

MANAGEMENT

Sinus tachycardia

The management of sinus tachycardia depends entirely on the underlying cause. Indeed, since sinus tachycardia may represent a physiological response, attempts to slow the heart rate in this context may result in hypotension [33].

- If a specific cause is identified, management should focus on treatment of the underlying condition.
- In psychiatric inpatients, if agitation or panic is suspected but alternative diagnoses cannot initially be discounted (e.g. evolving infection), then increasing frequency of observations and clinical reviews may be indicated, even if only temporarily [8].
- The presence of red flag symptoms including persistent chest pain, syncope, hypotension, pyrexia, tachypnoea or hypoxia may necessitate transfer to the accident and emergency department (A&E) for further investigation, higher levels of monitoring, and acute management [28].

Clozapine-induced sinus tachycardia

Clozapine-induced sinus tachycardia is very common in the early stages of treatment but is usually benign and may be dose related. For asymptomatic patients without signs of myocarditis (e.g. fever, chest pain), clozapine-induced sinus tachycardia in the early stages of treatment can generally be managed conservatively with monitoring of clozapine levels, appropriate dose modification, and reassurance and daily observations [34]. If symptomatic, then rate control with beta-blockers such as bisoprolol (starting oral dose 1.25–2.5 mg once daily, titrate to response) may be used as first-line medical therapy, although the evidence base for beta-blockade in the context of clozapine use is limited [35], and may be associated with side effects such as fatigue, weight gain, postural hypotension and, in men, impotence. If beta-blockers are contraindicated or not tolerated, ivabradine can be considered (5–7.5 mg, oral, twice daily) [36,37]. Seek advice from a cardiologist if first-line treatment fails, as untreated tachycardia has been associated with cardiomyopathy [38]. Evidence is currently lacking to support the treatment of asymptomatic clozapine-induced tachycardia, and therefore management should weigh the risks of rate-control medication against the potential risk of long-term tachycardia (i.e. cardiomyopathy). If pharmacological rate control is not pursued, ongoing monitoring of these patients is recommended, with consideration of annual echocardiograms to screen for cardiomyopathy, and where appropriate discussion with cardiology.

Atrial fibrillation

Guidelines published by the National Institute for Health and Care Excellence (NICE), the European Cardiac Society and the American College of Cardiology provide comprehensive algorithmic approaches to the management of AF. A brief summary is provided here, and readers are encouraged to consult the complete guidelines (accessed at https://pathways.nice.org.uk/pathways/atrial-fibrillation, https://www.escardio.org/ Guidelines and https://www.acc.org/guidelines) [13]. General principles involve offering symptomatic patients rate control (e.g. a beta-blocker) and anticoagulation if the risk of thromboembolism is high (CHA_2DS_2VASc score ≥2; Table 1.2) but not outweighed by the risk of major bleeding (calculated using the HAS-BLED score; Table 1.3) [39,40]. Choice of anticoagulant should be made after a joint discussion of risks and benefits between doctor and patient. Options include warfarin or a direct oral

Table 1.2 CHA_2DS_2VASc score to assess risk of thromboembolic event in atrial fibrillation and need for anticoagulation [39].

Risk criteria	Score
Congestive heart failure	1
Hypertension	1
Female sex	1
Age: 65–74	1
≥75	2
Diabetes	1
Stroke/TIA/thromboembolism	2
Vascular disease	1

Score = 0: anticoagulation not indicated

Score = 1: consider anticoagulation in men

Score ≥2: anticoagulate if it outweighs risk of bleeding

TIA, transient ischaemic attack.

Table 1.3 HAS-BLED score determines risk of major bleeding for people with atrial fibrillation[a] [40].

Risk criteria	Score
Hypertension: uncontrolled, >160 mmHg systolic	1
Renal disease: dialysis, transplant, Cr >200 μmol/L	1
Liver disease: cirrhosis or bilirubin more than twice normal and AST/ALT/AP more than three times normal	1
Stroke history: prior major bleeding or predisposition to bleeding	1
Labile INR: unstable/high INRs, time in therapeutic range <60%	1
Age >65 years	1
Medication: aspirin, clopidogrel, NSAIDs	1
Alcohol: eight or more drinks per week	1
Score ≤0–1: low risk, consider anticoagulation	
Score = 2: moderate risk, consider anticoagulation	
Score ≥2: high risk, consider alternatives	

[a] HAS-BLED score does not relate directly to CHA_2DS_2VASc score and cannot be compared quantitatively.
ALT, alanine aminotransferase; AP, alkaline phosphatase; AST, aspartate aminotransferase; Cr, creatinine; INR, international normalised ratio; NSAIDs, non-steroidal anti-inflammatory drugs.

anticoagulant (e.g. apixaban, dabigatran, rivaroxaban, and edoxaban). Referral to cardiology is recommended if anticoagulation is contraindicated. Anticoagulation, rate control, and symptoms should be reviewed at least annually alongside an assessment of cardiovascular risk and potential complications such as heart failure. Referral to cardiology is indicated if pharmacological or electrical cardioversion is being considered.

Supraventricular tachycardia

Persistent new-onset SVT requires *immediate transfer* to A&E due to risk of haemodynamic compromise [2]. Non-pharmacological interventions such as the Valsalva manoeuvre or carotid sinus massage can be attempted and immediate transfer to hospital can be avoided for people with known SVT who revert to sinus rhythm.

Further acute management may involve intravenous adenosine administration, synchronised cardioversion or intravenous antiarrhythmics such as diltiazem or beta-blockers [14]. Long-term management should be directed by a cardiologist. Lifestyle advice on alcohol, caffeine, and illicit drug use as potential precipitants should be offered, as well as strict control of general cardiac risk factors (e.g. smoking cessation) [2].

Broad-complex tachycardia

Any broad-complex tachycardia should be managed as VT until proven otherwise [28,29,41]. For psychiatric inpatients or people in the community, this is likely to

---

Box 1.4 Driving and working advice for patients with arrhythmia in the UK

In the UK, if the arrhythmia has caused or is likely to cause incapacity (e.g. syncope or VT), the patient should be advised to stop driving until:

- a satisfactory diagnosis is found
- the symptoms are controlled for at least 4 weeks (Group 1 entitlement: motor car or motorcycle) or 3 months (Group 2 entitlement: lorries, buses or HGVs) [42].

Note that guidelines differ somewhat internationally [43]. Please refer to local guidelines if not UK-based.
   If the patient is working in potentially dangerous occupations (at height or with heavy machinery), they should be advised to:

- stop working until the condition is controlled
- notify their occupational health department if applicable [29].

---

require urgent transfer to A&E where further investigations and initial treatment can be enacted in a monitored environment, although immediate resuscitation will be required using the ABCDE approach if the patient loses cardiac output (see Chapter 70) [28,29,41]. Sinus tachycardia or AF in a patient with known bundle-branch block are the most likely exceptions to this rule. However, if in doubt, referral to emergency services is recommended given the high mortality associated with VT [28,29,41].

Advice from the UK government regarding driving and working for patients with arrhythmia is shown in Box 1.4. We advise reviewing the guidance at source as it is updated monthly (https://www.gov.uk/guidance/cardiovascular-disorders-assessing-fitness-to-drive).

When to refer to a specialist

Urgent transfer to A&E is indicated for the following conditions [28,29,41].

- Any tachycardia with 'red flag' features:
  - haemodynamic instability
  - significant breathlessness
  - chest pain
  - syncope or near syncope
  - family history of sudden cardiac death under 40
  - symptoms precipitated by exercise.
- Suspected VT.
- Persistent SVT.
- AF with evidence of serious complication (e.g. stroke or heart failure).
- Evidence of concurrent illness that necessitates admission (e.g. sepsis).

What information to include in a referral to a specialist

Referral to a specialist should include any positive findings and salient negative findings from the history, examination and investigations (summarized in Box 1.5). Where possible, include all relevant ECGs. In emergency situations, it may be possible to send scanned ECGs via secure email. Also include contact details of the patient's mental healthcare team/support network, and if the appointment should be sent to anyone in addition to the patient. Finally, provide details of any reasonable adjustments needed for the patient (e.g. time or duration of appointment, carer/support worker in attendance).

Box 1.5 Diagnostic summary for the tachycardic patient

History

- Define cardiac symptoms
- Determine possible precipitants
- Assessment of palpitations (if paroxysmal)
- Screen for symptoms of systemic illness
- Past medical and psychiatric history: any cardiac disease, hypertension, diabetes, thyroid disease, chronic lung disease, anxiety, panic
- Medication history
- Drug and alcohol history
- Family history of sudden cardiac death

Examination

- ABCDE assessment
- Cardiovascular examination
- Focused examination if systemic illness suspected

Investigations

- ECG
- Bloods
- Urine dipstick
- Consider echocardiogram or 24-hour tape

References

1. Kumar P, Clark ML, Feather A (eds). *Kumar and Clark's Clinical Medicine*, 9th edn. London: Elsevier, 2017.
2. Katritsis DG, Boriani G, Cosio FG, et al. European Heart Rhythm Association (EHRA) consensus document on the management of supraventricular arrhythmias, endorsed by Heart Rhythm Society (HRS), Asia-Pacific Heart Rhythm Society (APHRS), and Sociedad Latinoamericana de Estimulación Cardiaca y Electrofisiologia (SOLAECE). *Europace* 2017;19(3):465–511.
3. Yusuf S, Camm AJ. The sinus tachycardias. *Nat Clin Pract Cardiovasc Med* 2005;2:44–52.
4. Lieberman JA. Maximizing clozapine therapy: managing side effects. *J Clin Psychiatry* 1998;59(Suppl 3):38–43.
5. Khaykin E, Ford DE, Pronovost PJ, et al. National estimates of adverse events during nonpsychiatric hospitalizations for persons with schizophrenia. *Gen Hosp Psychiatry* 2010;32(4):419–425.
6. Hsu W-Y, Lane H-Y, Lin C-L, Kao C-H. A population-based cohort study on deep vein thrombosis and pulmonary embolism among schizophrenia patients. *Schizophr Res* 2015;162(1):248–252.

7. Swart LE, Koster K, Torn M, et al. Clozapine-induced myocarditis. *Schizophr Res* 2016;174(1):161–164.

8. Perry PJ, Wilborn CA. Serotonin syndrome vs neuroleptic malignant syndrome: a contrast of causes, diagnoses, and management. *Ann Clin Psychiatry* 2012;24(2):155–162.

9. Ross DS, Burch HB, Cooper DS, et al. 2016 American Thyroid Association guidelines for diagnosis and management of hyperthyroidism and other causes of thyrotoxicosis. *Thyroid* 2016;26(10):1343–1421.

10. Lenders JWM, Eisenhofer G, Mannelli M, Pacak K. Phaeochromocytoma. *Lancet* 2005;366(9486):665–675.

11. Go AS, Hylek EM, Phillips KA, et al. Prevalence of diagnosed atrial fibrillation in adults. National implications for rhythm management and stroke prevention: the AnTicoagulation and Risk Factors In Atrial Fibrillation (ATRIA) Study. *JAMA* 2001;285(18):2370–2375.

12. Munger TM, Wu L-Q, Shen WK. Atrial fibrillation. *J Biomed Res* 2014;28(1):1–17.

13. National Institute for Health and Care Excellence. *Atrial Fibrillation: Management.* Clinical Guideline CG180. London: NICE, 2014. Available at https://www.nice.org.uk/guidance/cg180

14. Page RL, Joglar JA, Caldwell MA, et al. Guideline for the management of adult patients with supraventricular tachycardia. *J Am Coll Cardiol* 2016;67(13):e27–e115.

15. Medi C, Kalman JM, Freedman SB. Supraventricular tachycardia. *Med J Aust* 2009;190(5):255–260.

16. Orejarena LA, Vidaillet H, DeStefano F, et al. Paroxysmal supraventricular tachycardia in the general population. *J Am Coll Cardiol* 1998;31(1):150–157.

17. Laursen TM, Wahlbeck K, Hällgren J, et al. Life expectancy and death by diseases of the circulatory system in patients with bipolar disorder or schizophrenia in the Nordic countries. *PLoS One* 2013;8(6):e67133.

18. de Luna AB, Coumel P, Leclercq JF. Ambulatory sudden cardiac death: mechanisms of production of fatal arrhythmia on the basis of data from 157 cases. *Am Heart J* 1989;117(1):151–159.

19. Lo R, Chia KKM, Hsia HH. Ventricular tachycardia in ischemic heart disease. *Card Electrophysiol Clin* 2017;9(1):25–46.

20. Koponen H, Alaräisänen A, Saari K, et al. Schizophrenia and sudden cardiac death: a review. *Nord J Psychiatry* 2008;62(5):342–345.

21. Jones ME, Campbell G, Patel D, et al. Risk of mortality (including sudden cardiac death) and major cardiovascular events in users of olanzapine and other antipsychotics: a study with the General Practice Research Database. *Cardiovasc Psychiatry Neurol* 2013;2013:647476.

22. Vandael E, Vandenberk B, Vandenberghe J, et al. Incidence of torsade de pointes in a tertiary hospital population. *Int J Cardiol* 2017;243:511–515.

23. Al-Khatib SM, Stevenson WG, Ackerman MJ, et al. 2017 AHA/ACC/HRS guideline for management of patients with ventricular arrhythmias and the prevention of sudden cardiac death: a report of the American College of Cardiology/American Heart Association Task Force on Clinical Practice Guidelines and the Heart Rhythm Society. *Heart Rhythm* 2018;15(10):e73–e189.

24. Polcwiartek C, Kragholm K, Schjerning O, et al. Cardiovascular safety of antipsychotics: a clinical overview. *Expert Opin Drug Saf* 2016;15(5):679–688.

25. Isner JM, Roberts W, Heymsfield S, Yager J. Anorexia nervosa and sudden death. *Ann Intern Med* 1985;102(1):49–52.

26. Facchini M, Sala L, Malfatto G, et al. Low-K⁺ dependent QT prolongation and risk for ventricular arrhythmia in anorexia nervosa. *Int J Cardiol* 2006;106(2):170–176.

27. Behr ER, Casey A, Sheppard M, et al. Sudden arrhythmic death syndrome: a national survey of sudden unexplained cardiac death. *Heart* 2007;93(5):601–605.

28. Wexler RK, Pleister A, Raman S V. Palpitations: evaluation in the primary care setting. *Am Fam Physician* 2017;96(12):784–789.

29. Wolff A, Cowan C. 10 steps before your refer for palpitations. *Br J Cardiol* 2009;16(4):182–186.

30. Barsky AJ, Cleary PD, Coeytaux RR, Ruskin JN. The clinical course of palpitations in medical outpatients. *Arch Intern Med* 1996;2(5):66.

31. Kinlay S, Leitch JW, Neil A, Chapman BL, Hardy DB, Fletcher PJ. Cardiac event recorders yield more diagnoses and are more cost-effective than 48-hour Holter monitoring in patients with palpitations: a controlled clinical trial. *Ann Intern Med* 1995;155(16):1782–1788.

32. Life in the Fastlane. https://litfl.com/ (accessed 2 February 2019).

33. Pitcher D, Nolan J. Peri-arrest arrhythmias. https://www.resus.org.uk/resuscitation-guidelines/peri-arrest-arrhythmias

34. Taylor DM, Barnes TRE, Young AH. *The Maudsley Prescribing Guidelines in Psychiatry*, 13th edn. Chichester: Wiley Blackwell, 2018.

35. Lally J, Docherty MJ, MacCabe JH. Pharmacological interventions for clozapine-induced sinus tachycardia. *Cochrane Database Syst Rev* 2016;(6):CD011566.

36. Das P, Kuppuswamy PS, Rai A, Bostwick JM. Verapamil for the treatment of clozapine-induced persistent sinus tachycardia in a patient with schizophrenia: a case report and literature review. *Psychosomatics* 2014;55(2):194–195.

37. Lally J, Brook J, Dixon T, et al. Ivabradine, a novel treatment for clozapine-induced sinus tachycardia: a case series. *Ther Adv Psychopharmacol* 2014;4(3):117–122.

38. Shinbane JS, Wood MA, Jensen DN, et al. Tachycardia-induced cardiomyopathy: a review of animal models and clinical studies. *J Am Coll Cardiol* 1997;29(4):709–715.

39. Lip GY, Frison L, Halperin JL, Lane DA. Identifying patients at high risk for stroke despite anticoagulation: a comparison of contemporary stroke risk stratification schemes in an anticoagulated atrial fibrillation cohort. *Stroke* 2010;41(12):2731–2738.

40. Pisters R, Lane DA, Nieuwlaat R, et al. A novel user-friendly score (HAS-BLED) to assess 1-year risk of major bleeding in patients with atrial fibrillation: the Euro Heart Survey. *Chest* 2010;138(5):1093–1100.

41. Raviele A, Giada F, Bergfeldt L, et al. Management of patients with palpitations: a position paper from the European Heart Rhythm Association. *Europace* 2011;13(7):920–934.

42. UK Driver and Vehicle Licensing Agency. *Assessing Fitness To Drive: A Guide for Medical Professionals.* https://www.gov.uk/government/publications/assessing-fitness-to-drive-a-guide-for-medical-professionals

43. Banning AS, Ng GA. Driving and arrhythmia: a review of scientific basis for international guidelines. *Eur Heart J* 2012;34(3):236–244.

Bradycardia

Eleanor Croft, Nicholas Gall

Sinus bradycardia is defined as sinus rhythm at a rate of less than 60 beats per minute (bpm) [1] (Figure 2.1). However, sinus bradycardia is 'normal' for many young adults (particularly those who exercise regularly), some elderly patients [2], or during sleep (when rates may transiently drop to as low as 30 bpm). Therefore, in clinical practice it is usually more pragmatic to categorise the bradycardic patient as either symptomatic/asymptomatic and appropriate/inappropriate for the circumstance, which will then guide appropriate assessment and management. Symptoms may be subtle, with some patients noticing only fatigue; however, other patients may present with light-headedness or collapse (see Chapter 4) [3,4]. Although asymptomatic bradycardia may be a benign presentation reflecting normal physiology, it could signpost serious underlying pathology, and therefore a low threshold for further investigation or at least discussion with cardiology is recommended.

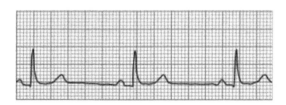

Figure 2.1 Sinus bradycardia, rate 50 bpm, as measured from lead II of the ECG.

The Maudsley Practice Guidelines for Physical Health Conditions in Psychiatry, First Edition.
David M. Taylor, Fiona Gaughran, and Toby Pillinger.
© 2021 John Wiley & Sons Ltd. Published 2021 by John Wiley & Sons Ltd.

CHAPTER 2

Common causes of bradycardia in the general and psychiatric population are documented in Table 2.1. These can be divided into intrinsic disorders of the heart (e.g. ischaemic heart disease), systemic conditions (e.g. hypothyroidism), or extrinsic insults (e.g. medication) [5]. In the psychiatric patient population, bradycardia may be seen in the context of electrolyte imbalance or reduced body mass index (BMI) in those with eating disorders [6,7], neglect, alcohol dependence [8], as a consequence of psychiatric medication such as lithium [9] or chronic selective serotonin reuptake inhibitor (SSRI) treatment [10,11], or in association with physical health conditions that have neuropsychiatric sequelae (e.g. hypothyroidism) [12].

Table 2.1 Causes of bradycardia in the general and psychiatric population.

General and psychiatric population	Special consideration in psychiatric population
Intrinsic disorders of the heart	
Sinoatrial node dysfunction ('sick sinus syndrome'): associated with age due to fibrotic/degenerative destruction of the sinus node and surrounding nerves [3–5]	N/A
Acute myocardial infarction (seen in up to 25% of patients) [3–5]	
Genetic mutations associated with sinoatrial node dysfunction (e.g. *HCN4* and *SCN5A*) [13]	
Systemic conditions	
Low BMI [5,6]	Low BMI and electrolyte imbalance may be present in those with eating disorders [5,6] or alcohol dependence [7]
Hypothyroidism [4,5]	
Hypothermia [4,5]	
Infection, e.g. Lyme disease, *Legionella*, malaria [3–5]	See Potassium derangement (Chapter 33), Acute kidney injury (Chapter 73), Chronic kidney disease (Chapter 34), and Alcohol and physical health (Chapter 24)
Obstructive sleep apnoea (see Chapter 49) [14]	
Exaggerated vagal activity (e.g. following coughing, micturition, or vomiting; see Chapter 4) [4,5]	
Increased intracranial pressure following head injury [4,5]	
Electrolyte disturbance [4,5]	
Medication	
Drugs that potentiate parasympathetic activity, e.g. acetylcholinesterase inhibitors [15]	Lithium, both as a direct side effect or related to associated thyroid dysfunction [3,17]
Drugs that inhibit sympathetic activity, e.g. beta-blockers, methyldopa [3–5]	SSRIs, e.g. fluoxetine [9,10], citalopram [18]
Opioids and sedatives, e.g. benzodiazepines [4,16]	Individual case reports of antipsychotics, e.g. olanzapine [19]
Digoxin [3–5]	Several drugs may cause bradycardia in overdose (see https://www.toxbase.org/)
Calcium channel blockers (e.g. diltiazem) [3–5]	
Ivabradine [4]	
Amiodarone [4]	

BMI, body mass index; SSRI, selective serotonin reuptake inhibitor.

DIAGNOSIS

Bradycardia can represent a medical emergency. If there is evidence of haemodynamic compromise (e.g. low blood pressure, shortness of breath, or chest pain), then resuscitation and transfer to emergency services should be performed (see Chapter 70). In the absence of haemodynamic compromise, an approach to assessing a patient with bradycardia is described in the following sections and summarised in Box 2.1.

Box 2.1 Summary approach to assessment, investigation, and management of bradycardia

History

- Symptoms typical of bradycardia, symptoms of ischaemic heart disease
- Risk factors for bradycardia from past medical history
- Psychiatric history (e.g. eating disorder)
- Medication history (medical and psychiatric)
- Family history of arrhythmia or sudden cardiac death
- Social history (alcohol consumption)

Examination

- If any concerns regarding haemodynamic stability, transfer to emergency services
- Check heart rate, blood pressure, temperature, oxygen saturation
- Calculate BMI
- Cardiac and respiratory examination for evidence of ischaemic heart disease and heart failure
- Consider thyroid examination if appropriate

Investigation

- ECG: confirm sinus bradycardia, rule out heart block
- Bloods: electrolytes, thyroid function, and if appropriate cardiac enzymes, BNP, drug levels (e.g. lithium)

Management

- Asymptomatic patients may need no further investigation or treatment
- Address underlying reversible causes
- If possible, rationalise medication
- If medication rationalisation is not possible or there is intrinsic cardiac disease, patient may require permanent pacing so refer to cardiology

---

History

Elicit symptoms

In most patients, sinus bradycardia will be asymptomatic. However, symptoms may emerge if bradycardia progresses to the extent of cerebral hypoperfusion, or in the context of comorbidity that may be exacerbated by the compromised cardiac output of bradycardia (e.g. in patients with ischaemic heart disease, bradycardia may result in angina). Specific symptoms that may be reported include:

- dizziness and light-headedness (presyncope)
- syncope (see Chapter 4 for comprehensive syncope history)
- chest pain, shortness of breath
- fatigue
- reduced exercise tolerance.

Identify risk factors

- Advanced age.
- Ischaemic heart disease and associated risk factors (e.g. smoking, diabetes mellitus, hypercholesterolaemia).
- Past medical history: thyroid disease (see Chapter 12), obstructive sleep apnoea (see Chapter 49), recent infection.
- Previous cardiac surgery.
- Family history of cardiac disease, unexplained collapse, atrial fibrillation, or sudden cardiac death.
- Eating disorder.
- Alcohol abuse.

Medication history

As described in Table 2.1. Note any recent medication changes, including dose changes.

Social history

- Alcohol use.
- Recreational drug use.

Examination

General inspection and observations

- Body habitus (calculate BMI) and nutritional status.
- Evidence of systemic disease (e.g. hypothyroidism).
- Heart rate, blood pressure, oxygen saturation, temperature.

Physical examination

- Cardiac and respiratory examination: examine for evidence of heart failure.
- If appropriate, consider a thyroid examination (see Chapter 12).

Investigations

ECG

ECG is used to confirm the presence of sinus bradycardia. ECG can also be used to exclude other causes of bradyarrythmia such as atrioventricular block, which can be defined as follows.

- First-degree heart block:
  - defined as a PR interval >200 ms
  - QRS can be narrow or wide depending on the site of the block.
- Second-degree heart block:
  - Mobitz type I (Wenckebach): progressively increasing PR interval until a P wave does not conduct (the QRS is absent); the PR interval is then shorter again.
  - Mobitz type II: there is no change to the PR interval, but some P waves are not conducted through to the ventricles (the QRS is absent); the QRS complex is usually broad in this circumstance.
- Third-degree (complete heart block): P waves fail to conduct from the atria to the ventricles and, as such, P waves and QRS complexes are not associated.

Blood tests

- Electrolytes (sodium, potassium, calcium, and magnesium).
- Cardiac enzymes (troponin) if there are ECG changes suggestive of ischaemia or if the history is in keeping with a cardiac event.
- Brain natriuretic peptide (BNP) if there is evidence of heart failure.
- Thyroid function.
- If appropriate, consider checking lithium and digoxin levels.

Specialist investigations

- Echocardiography may be considered if there is suspicion of underlying structural cardiac disease.
- 24/48-hour ECG monitoring may be considered if there is suspicion of paroxysmal bradyarrythmia (see Chapter 4).

MANAGEMENT AND WHEN TO REFER TO A SPECIALIST

Asymptomatic patients with sinus bradycardia do not necessarily require either intervention or treatment.

Addressing an underlying reversible cause may be sufficient to treat symptomatic bradycardia, for example electrolyte disturbance or hypothyroidism. Rationalisation of medication may also be indicated. In the case of psychiatric medications such as lithium, a multidisciplinary approach involving input from psychiatry, cardiology, and of course the patient to determine the best therapeutic approach is advised (i.e. weighing up the risks and benefits of continuing lithium treatment).

In the case of intrinsic disease of the heart (e.g. sick sinus syndrome) or if a causative medication cannot be stopped, then a permanent pacemaker may be indicated, and referral to cardiology should be made.

References

1. Spodick DH, Raju P, Bishop RL, Rifkin RD. Operational definition of normal sinus heart rate. *Am J Cardiol* 1992;69(14):1245–1246.
2. Agruss NS, Rosin EY, Adolph RJ, Fowler NO. Significance of chronic sinus bradycardia in elderly patients. *Circulation* 1972;46(5):924–930.
3. Katritsis DG, Gersh BJ, Camm AJ. Bradyarrhythmias. In: *Clinical Cardiology: Current Practice Guidelines*. Oxford: Oxford University Press, 2013:537–557.
4. Olshansky B, Saha S, Gopinathannair R. Bradycardia. *BMJ Best Practice*. https://bestpractice.bmj.com/topics/en-gb/832. Last updated: January 2020.
5. Mangrum JM, DiMarco JP. The evaluation and management of bradycardia. *N Engl J Med* 2000;342(10):703–709.
6. Miller K, Grinspoon SK, Ciampa J, et al. Medical findings in outpatients with anorexia nervosa. *Arch Intern Med* 2005;165(5):561–566.
7. Misra M, Aggarwal A, Miller K, et al. Effects of anorexia nervosa on clinical, hematologic, biochemical and bone density parameters in community-dwelling adolescent girls. *Pediatrics* 2004;114(6):1574–1583.
8. Vamvakas S. Teschner M, Bahner U, Heidland A. Alcohol abuse: potential role in electrolyte disturbances and kidney diseases. *Clin Nephrol* 1998;49(4):205–213.
9. Rosenqvist M, Bergfeldt L, Aili H, Mathé AA. Sinus node dysfunction during long term lithium treatment. *Br Heart J* 1993;70:371–375.
10. Pacher P, Ungvari Z, Kecskemeti V, Furst S. Review of cardiovascular effects of fluoxetine, a selective serotonin reuptake inhibitor, compared to tricyclic antidepressants. *Curr Med Chem* 1998;5(5):381–390.
11. Enemark B. The importance of ECG monitoring in antidepressant treatment. *Nordic J Psychiatry* 1993;47:57–65.
12. Vaidya B, Pearce SH. Management of hypothyroidism in adults. *BMJ* 2008;337:a801.
13. Nof E, Glikson M, Antzelevitch C. Genetics and sinus node dysfunction. *J Atr Fibrillation* 2009;1(6):151.
14. Zwillich C, Devlin T, White D, et al. Bradycardia during sleep apnea. Characteristics and mechanism. *J Clin Invest* 1982;69(6):1286–1292.
15. Hernandez RK, Farwell W, Cantor MD, Lawler EV. Cholinesterase inibitors and incidence of bradycardia in patients with dementia in the Veterans Affairs New England Healthcare System. *J Am Geriatr Soc* 2009;57(11):1997–2003.
16. Chen A, Ashburn MA. Cardiac effects of opioid therapy. *Pain Med* 2015;16(Suppl 1):S27–S31.
17. Lazarus JH. Lithium and thyroid. *Best Pract Res Clin Endocrinol Metab* 2009;23(6):723–733.
18. Rasmussen S, Overø KF, Tanghø P. Cardiac safety of citalopram: prospective trials and retrospective analyses. *J Clin Psychopharmacol* 1999;19(5):407–415.
19. Lee TW, Tsai SJ, Hwang JP. Severe cardiovascular side effects of olanzapine in an elderly patient: case report. *Int J Psychiatry Med* 2003;33(4):399–401.

QT Interval Prolongation

Guy Hindley, Nicholas Gall

Prolongation of the corrected QT interval (QTc) is an independent risk factor for torsade de points (TdP), a potentially fatal ventricular tachyarrhythmia, and sudden cardiac-related death (SCD) (see Box 3.1). Definitions of QTc prolongation for men and women vary in the literature, often described as more than 440 ms for men and more than 470 ms for women [1]. However, the risk of TdP increases with increasing QTc, and the clearest evidence of an association is apparent when QTc is greater than 500 ms (for both men and women) [2].

QTc prolongation can be inherited or acquired. Inherited forms are rare (1 in 3000 to 1 in 5000) and predominantly caused by mutations in genes encoding sodium, potassium, and calcium channels present in the myocardium [5]. Acquired QTc prolongation is particularly common among people with serious mental illness (SMI), with prevalence estimated as high as 8% among psychiatric inpatients [6].

Box 3.1 Understanding and measuring the QTc interval

- The QT interval measures the time between the start of ventricular depolarisation and the end of ventricular repolarisation.
- This is represented on an ECG by the beginning of the Q wave to the end of the T wave. QT intervals vary significantly between different ECG leads [3] and most normal reference ranges are based on measurements from lead II [4].
- Since QT varies with the length of the cardiac cycle, it is corrected for heart rate, most commonly using Bazett's formula: $QTc = QT/\sqrt{RR}$, where QT is the interval in seconds and RR is cardiac cycle in seconds.

The Maudsley Practice Guidelines for Physical Health Conditions in Psychiatry, First Edition.
David M. Taylor, Fiona Gaughran, and Toby Pillinger.
© 2021 John Wiley & Sons Ltd. Published 2021 by John Wiley & Sons Ltd.

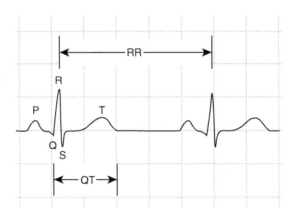

- Most ECG machines will calculate the QTc automatically. However, it may measure the RR or QT interval incorrectly, so it is important to check this.
- Bear in mind that Bazett's formula may over-correct if the patient is tachycardic and under-correct if bradycardic.
- Alternatives to the Bazett formula exist for when patients present with tachycardia or bradycardia, e.g. the Fridericia, Hodges, and Framingham corrections. If there are uncertainties regarding QTc calculation, discuss with cardiology.

Medication is the most frequently identified contributing factor to acquired QTc prolongation [7]. Table 3.1 provides an overview of the effects of commonly prescribed psychotropic medications on the QTc interval, while Box 3.2 lists some commonly encountered non-psychotropic drugs associated with QTc prolongation. The association between QTc prolongation and antipsychotics is particularly well characterised and their use is associated with increased rates of sudden cardiac death [8–11]. Risk is increased when given parenterally or in overdose [12,13]. Indeed, all antipsychotics given intravenously are considered to be high risk for TdP, and combinations of antipsychotics also confer increased risk. The effect of drugs on QTc interval is usually plasma level-dependent [14], and therefore high doses and combination with cytochrome P450 inhibitors (e.g. fluvoxamine, fluoxetine, and paroxetine) may be causative [11].

For a comprehensive list of medications that increase the QTc and that is updated on a regular basis, please refer to crediblemeds.org or the CredibleMeds mobile phone application [12].

Despite the clear risk of certain medication regimens in prolonging the QTc interval, it is rare for medication to be the only identified risk factor in cases of TdP [15,16]. Furthermore, the association between risk of QTc prolongation and risk of TdP is unclear for several psychotropics. It is therefore important to consider other physiological causes [7], summarised in Box 3.3 [17]. For example, in patients with anorexia nervosa, QTc alterations may be influenced by not only medication but also electrolyte abnormalities and bradycardia [18,19]. Cardiovascular disease (CVD) is also associated with QTc prolongation, and this should be considered in the psychiatric population, especially considering the increased rates of CVD in this group [20].

Table 3.1 Effects of psychotropic medication on QTc [17].

Class	No known effect	Low effect	Moderate effect	High effect	Unknown effect
Antipsychotics [17]	Brexpiprazole Cariprazine Lurasidone	Aripiprazole Asenapine Clozapine Flupentixol Fluphenazine Loxapine Olanzapine Paliperidone Perphenazine Prochlorperazine Risperidone Sulpiride	Amisulpride Chlorpromazine Haloperidol Iloperidone Levomepromazine Melperone Quetiapine Ziprasidone	Any intravenous antipsychotic Pimozide Sertindole Any drug or combination of drugs used in doses exceeding recommended maximum	Pipotiazine Trifluoperazine Zuclopenthixol
Antidepressants [21–23]	Paroxetine[a] Fluvoxamine[a] Sertraline[a]	Fluoxetine[a] Venlafaxine Bupropion Duloxetine Mirtazapine Amitriptyline Trazodone	Citalopram Escitalopram Clomipramine Trimipramine Nortriptyline Imipramine		
Others [24–33]	Carbamazepine Valproate Lamotrigine Benzodiazepines Gabapentin Pregabalin	Buprenorphine Lithium Promethazine Memantine Galantamine	Methadone (especially >100 mg/day)		

[a] P450 inhibitor and so may prolong QTc if prescribed in combination with another QTc-prolonging drug.
High effect indicates significant average QTc prolongation at therapeutic doses (usually >20 ms).
Moderate effect indicates moderate average QTc prolongation at therapeutic doses (10–20 ms).
Low effect indicates severe QTc prolongation only in overdose or small average increases (<10 ms).
No effect indicates no known QTc prolongation at therapeutic doses or in overdose.

Box 3.2 Common non-psychotropic drugs associated with QTc prolongation [12]

Cardiac

Amiodarone
Dronedarone
Flecainide
Quinidine
Sotalol

Antibiotics

Azithromycin
Ciprofloxacin
Clarithromycin
Erythromycin

Other antimicrobials

Fluconazole
Chloroquine

Other drugs

Domperidone
Ondansetron
Terfenadine
Ciclosporin
Tacrolimus
Tramadol
Bendroflumethiazide/loop diuretics (hypokalaemia)

Box 3.3 Non-pharmacological causes of acquired QTc prolongation: factors relevant to individuals with SMI are highlighted in italic [17,34,35]

Inherited

Long QT syndrome

Electrolyte abnormalities

Hypokalaemia
Hypomagnesaemia
Hypocalcaemia

Cardiac causes

Arrhythmia
Bradycardia
Ischaemic heart disease (left ventricular hypertrophy, heart failure)
Hypertension

Metabolic/endocrine

Thyroid disease (hypothyroidism/hyperthyroidism)
High body mass index
Diabetes
Hypercholesterolaemia

Other medical

Liver failure
Renal failure
Intracerebral haemorrhage

Psychiatric

Anorexia nervosa

Others

Extreme physical exertion
Smoking
Extremes of age
Female gender

PRESCRIBING QTC-PROLONGING MEDICATION

There is a lack of high-quality evidence and consensus over the prescription and monitoring of QTc-prolonging medication [17,36–38]. The list that follows describes six key considerations when prescribing [37]. The reader is also directed to the review by Brouillette and Nattel [39] which provides an algorithmic approach to minimising the risk of drug-induced QTc prolongation.

1 Avoid using QTc-prolonging medication where possible [38].
2 Avoid polypharmacy with other QTc-prolonging drugs as the effect is likely additive [15].
3 Use the lowest effective dose and avoid drugs that have significant metabolic interactions as QTc prolongation is likely dose-dependent [14,17].
4 Assess cardiac risk (personal history, family history, cardiac symptoms, cardiovascular risk factors) before commencing any drug with a possible risk of QTc prolongation or arrhythmia (moderate or high risk in Table 3.1).
5 Consider ECG screening prior to commencing any QTc-prolonging medication and repeat once steady state has been achieved or in the presence of cardiovascular risk factors [37]. The National Institute for Health and Care Excellence (NICE) recommendations for ECG screening prior to initiating antipsychotic therapy are summarised in Box 3.4 [40].
6 Consider consulting a cardiologist before commencing any QTc-prolonging drug in the presence of cardiovascular risk factors or symptoms suggestive of arrhythmia [40].

> **Box 3.4** NICE guidelines for ECG screening during antipsychotic treatment [40]
>
> A screening ECG should be offered to patients before starting any antipsychotic medication known to cause QTc prolongation if:
>
> - specified in the drug's summary of product characteristics
> - a specific cardiovascular risk factor is identified during history or physical examination (e.g. hypertension)
> - personal history of cardiovascular disease
> - patient is an inpatient/on admission.
>
> Consider repeating the ECG once the therapeutic dose has been reached and yearly thereafter.

DIAGNOSTIC PRINCIPLES

The RISQ-PATH risk score for QTc prolongation provides a system for predicting QTc prolongation, and can be used to guide the intensity of QTc monitoring that should be offered patients [41].

QTc prolongation should be suspected in any individual presenting with symptoms suggestive of arrhythmia (e.g. palpitations or unexplained collapse), particularly if taking antipsychotics or any other QTc-prolonging medication. The diagnosis may also be made on a screening ECG or as an incidental finding in the absence of any preceding symptoms [42].

A detailed clinical assessment is still essential following diagnosis in order to:

- screen for symptoms suggestive of arrhythmia
- identify pharmacological and physiological causes
- elicit other cardiovascular risk factors for TdP or sudden cardiac death.

History

1 Relevant cardiac symptoms, including palpitations, syncope, dizziness/light-headedness (to be distinguished from vertigo), chest pain, shortness of breath.
2 History suggestive of electrolyte disturbance, such as diarrhoea, vomiting, malnutrition, and eating disorder.
3 Cardiovascular risk factors, including personal history and family history of CVD, smoking, obesity, diabetes mellitus, hypertension, and hypercholesterolaemia.
4 History of significant cardiac event, such as syncope, ventricular tachyarrhythmia, TdP, cardiac arrest, unexplained falls/car crashes.
5 Other relevant past medical history (see Table 3.1):
   a liver failure
   b renal failure
   c hyperthyroidism/hypothyroidism.
6 Detailed drug history (see Box 3.2), including possible deliberate or accidental overdose.
7 Family history of sudden cardiac death/unexplained death especially under 40 or long QT syndrome.
8 Social history: smoking history, alcohol and substance use.

Examination

1 Full cardiovascular examination paying special attention to the following.
   a Inspection: high or low BMI, peripheral oedema, raised jugular venous pressure (heart failure).
   b Palpation: pulse (regularity plus rate).
   c Auscultation: murmurs or added sounds (heart failure/left ventricular hypertrophy), pulmonary oedema.
   d Palpation for pedal/sacral oedema (heart failure, renal failure).
2 Lying and standing blood pressure if history of presyncope/syncope.

Investigations

1 Bloods:
   a full blood count
   b urea and electrolytes (renal failure, hypokalaemia, hypomagnesaemia, hypocalcaemia)
   c liver function tests (liver failure)
   d lipid profile (hypercholesterolaemia)
   e thyroid function tests (hyperthyroidism/hypothyroidism)
   f antipsychotic plasma levels (toxicity)
   g brain natriuretic peptide (BNP, if history suggestive of heart failure).
2 ECG [43]
   a Ischaemia: ST depression/elevation, T-wave inversion, pathological Q waves.
   b Left ventricular hypertrophy (LVH): left axis deviation, increased amplitude R waves in V4–V6 plus deep S waves in V1–V3. If LVH is suspected, refer patient for transthoracic echocardiogram.
   c Hypokalaemia: PR prolongation, T-wave flattening and inversion, ST depression, U waves.
   d QTc interval (see Box 3.1).
3 Consider requesting an echocardiogram if history or examination is suggestive of heart failure, ischaemia or structural heart disease (following consultation with cardiology).
4 Consider 24-hour ECG monitoring if history suggestive of arrhythmia (consult cardiologist).

MANAGEMENT

High-quality evidence for the management of acquired QTc prolongation is lacking [37,44]. A history of significant cardiac events, such as syncope or tachyarrhythmias or severe prolongation greater than 500 ms, may necessitate emergency medical attention and management should be led by a cardiologist [17,37]. Table 3.2 describes the management of acquired QTc prolongation, while Box 3.5 summarises a general approach to QTc prolongation. For the management of tachyarrhythmias please refer to Chapter 1.

Table 3.2 The management of acquired QTc prolongation [17,37,44].

QTc interval	Action	Discuss with cardiologist/senior medic
440–500 ms (men) or 470–500 ms (women)	Consider dose reduction of presumed causative medication, or switch to alternative treatment with reduced risk Address non-pharmacological risk factors Repeat ECG in 1–2 weeks	Immediately if associated with unexplained cardiac symptoms *or* clinically unable to reduce/stop QTc-prolonging drug
>500 ms *or* increase of >60 ms	Stop QTc-prolonging medication and switch to lower-risk alternative (see Table 3.1) Address non-pharmacological risk factors Repeat ECG in 1–2 weeks or earlier	Immediately

---

Box 3.5 Approach to QTc prolongation

Prescribing, screening, and monitoring

- Avoid QTc prolonging medication if possible
- Use lowest effective dose
- Avoid polypharmacy
- Assess cardiovascular risk and consider need for screening ECG
- Consult cardiologist if in doubt

Assessment

- Screen for symptoms of arrhythmia
- Identify pharmacological and non-pharmacological causes
- Assess cardiovascular risk
- Bloods plus ECG (with or without 24-hour tape/echocardiogram)

Management

- Consider stopping or reducing dose of offending drugs
- Address non-pharmacological risk factors
- Monitor proactively
- Refer to cardiologist if:
  - >500 ms or >60 ms increase
  - associated with history suggestive of arrhythmia
  - prior cardiac event
  - unable to stop or reduce medication

Initial management

Rationalising medication

1 Any decision regarding a change in medication needs to weigh up the risk of continuing treatment (i.e. the risk of QTc prolongation) against the risk of medication change (i.e. the risk of deterioration in mental state).

2 Where possible, stop or reduce the dose of the QTc-prolonging medication, particularly when QTc is greater than 500 ms.
3 Consider changing to treatment with lower risk of QTc prolongation.
4 When in doubt, discussion with cardiology is recommended [37].

Addressing non-pharmacological risk factors (likely to be performed by medical practitioners rather than psychiatrists)

1 Replace electrolytes [37].
2 Optimise management of cardiovascular risk (hypertension, hypercholesterolaemia, hyperlipidaemia, diabetes, smoking cessation, lifestyle advice) [37].
3 Optimise management of other relevant medical conditions (e.g. thyroid disease and heart failure) [44].

Monitoring QTc interval

1 Repeat ECG in one to two weeks of any significant dose change [37].
2 Monitoring every six months to one year thereafter [17,45].

When to refer to a specialist

Immediate referral to a cardiologist is indicated if:

- QTc >500 ms or change in QTc >60 ms since commencing QTc-prolonging drug
- new unexplained cardiac symptoms plus QTc >440 ms (men) or QTc >470 ms (women)
- history suggestive of arrhythmia (see Chapters 1, 2 and 70).

Consider discussion with cardiology if planning to initiate QTc-prolonging medication in a patient with:

- cardiovascular disease
- other significant non-pharmacological risk factors
- already prescribed a QTc-prolonging medication.

Information to include in a referral to cardiology

A comprehensive handover to a specialist should include, where possible, the history, examination, and investigation findings described in the preceding sections. In the scenario where a psychiatric medication is prescribed that may be responsible for QTc prolongation, explain the rationale behind its prescription, and the potential risks of stopping its prescription (this may aid a risk–benefit decision regarding continuation of a given treatment). Also include the contact details of the patient's mental health-care team/support network and clarify if the appointment should be sent to anyone in addition to the patient. Finally, document any reasonable adjustments needed for the patient, for example time or duration of appointment, carer/support worker in attendance.

CHAPTER 3

Further management your patient may be offered by cardiology

Treatment of inherited QTc prolongation and high-risk cases of acquired QTc prolongation should be initiated and monitored by a cardiologist.

1 Persistently prolonged acquired QTc may indicate the need for genetic testing and family screening [46].
2 Beta-blockers may be considered in severe or refractory cases or if associated with significant cardiac events, although they do not shorten the QTc interval and randomised controlled trials are lacking. Meta-analysis of observational studies has demonstrated a mortality benefit for beta-blockade in congenital long QT syndrome [47]. However, they may be not be effective for acquired QTc prolongation and may in fact increase risk [48].
3 Implantable cardioverter-defibrillators (ICDs) may be considered in patients who [49]:
   a remain symptomatic despite beta-blocker therapy
   b have a history of cardiac arrest
   c present with QTc >550 msec
   d are unable to be prescribed beta blockers.
4 Left cervicothoracic sympathectomy is a procedure which denervates the heart from its sympathetic input. This may be considered if an ICD is contraindicated or if an individual requires multiple ICD shocks [50].

References

1. Botstein P. Is QT interval prolongation harmful? A regulatory perspective. *Am J Cardiol* 1993;72:50B–52B.
2. Bednar MM, Harrigan EP, Anziano RJ, et al. The QT interval. *Prog Cardiovasc Dis* 2001;43(5 Suppl 1):1–45.
3. Cowan JC, Yusoff K, Moore M, et al. Importance of lead selection in QT interval measurement. *Am J Cardiol* 1988;61(1):83–87.
4. Lepeschkin E, Surawicz B. The measurement of the QT interval of the electrocardiogram. *Circulation* 1952;6(3):378–388.
5. Goldenberg I, Moss AJ. Long QT syndrome. *J Am Coll Cardiol* 2008;51(24):2291–2300.
6. Reilly JG, Ayis SA, Ferrier IN, et al. QTc-interval abnormalities and psychotropic drug therapy in psychiatric patients. *Lancet* 2000;355(9209):1048–1052.
7. Van Noord C, Eijgelsheim M, Stricker BHC. Drug- and non-drug-associated QT interval prolongation. *Br J Clin Pharmacol* 2010; 70(1):16–23.
8. Jones ME, Campbell G, Patel D, et al. Risk of mortality (including sudden cardiac death) and major cardiovascular events in users of olanzapine and other antipsychotics: a study with the General Practice Research Database. *Cardiovasc Psychiatry Neurol* 2013;2013:647476.
9. Liperoti R, Gambassi G, Lapane KL, et al. Conventional and atypical antipsychotics and the risk of hospitalization for ventricular arrhythmias or cardiac arrest. *Arch Intern Med* 2005;165(6):696–701.
10. Hennessy S, Bilker WB, Knauss JS, et al. Cardiac arrest and ventricular arrhythmia in patients taking antipsychotic drugs: cohort study using administrative data. *BMJ* 2002;325(7372):1070.
11. Barbui C, Bighelli I, Carrà G, et al. Antipsychotic dose mediates the association between polypharmacy and corrected QT interval. *PLoS One* 2016;11(2):e0148212.
12. crediblemeds.org. https://www.crediblemeds.org (accessed 30 January 2019).
13. Beach SR, Celano CM, Noseworthy PA, et al. QTc prolongation, torsades de pointes, and psychotropic medications. *Psychosomatics* 2013;54(1):1–13.
14. Gupta A, Lawrence AT, Krishnan K, et al. Current concepts in the mechanisms and management of drug-induced QT prolongation and torsade de pointes. *Am Heart J* 2007;153(6):891–899.
15. Hasnain M, Vieweg WVR. QTc interval prolongation and torsade de pointes associated with second-generation antipsychotics and antidepressants: a comprehensive review. *CNS Drugs* 2014;28(10):887–920.
16. Zeltser D, Justo D, Halkin A, et al. Torsade de pointes due to noncardiac drugs: most patients have easily identifiable risk factors. *Medicine (Baltimore)* 2003;82(4):282–290.
17. Taylor DM, Barnes TRE, Young AH. *The Maudsley Prescribing Guidelines in Psychiatry*, 13th edn. Chichester: Wiley Blackwell, 2018.

18. Westmoreland P, Krantz MJ, Mehler PS. Medical complications of anorexia nervosa and bulimia. *Am J Med* 2016;129(1):30–37.

19. Isner JM, Roberts W, Heymsfield S, Yager J. Anorexia nervosa and sudden death. *Ann Intern Med* 1985;102(1):49–52.

20. De Hert M, Correll CU, Bobes J, et al. Physical illness in patients with severe mental disorders. I. Prevalence, impact of medications and disparities in health care. *World Psychiatry* 2011;10(1):52–77.

21. Funk KA, Bostwick JR. A comparison of the risk of QT prolongation among SSRIs. *Ann Pharmacother* 2013;47(10):1330–1341.

22. Jasiak NM, Bostwick JR. Risk of QT/QTc prolongation among newer non-SSRI antidepressants. *Ann Pharmacother* 2014;48(12):1620–1628.

23. van Noord C, Straus SMJM, Sturkenboom MCJM, et al. Psychotropic drugs associated with corrected QT interval prolongation. *J Clin Psychopharmacol* 2009;29(1):9–15.

24. Wang D, Wu Y, Wang A, et al. Electrocardiogram changes of donepezil administration in elderly patients with ischemic heart disease. *Cardiol Res Pract* 2018;2018:9141320.

25. Wedam EF, Bigelow GE, Johnson RE, et al. QT-interval effects of methadone, levomethadyl, and buprenorphine in a randomized trial. *Arch Intern Med* 2007;167(22):2469–2475.

26. Mujtaba S, Romero J, Taub CC. Methadone, QTc prolongation and torsades de pointes: current concepts, management and a hidden twist in the tale? *J Cardiovasc Dis Res* 2013;4(4):229–235.

27. Mehta N, Vannozzi R. Lithium-induced electrocardiographic changes: a complete review. *Clin Cardiol* 2017;40(12):1363–1367.

28. Owczuk R, Twardowski P, Dylczyk-Sommer A, et al. Influence of promethazine on cardiac repolarisation: a double-blind, midazolam-controlled study. *Anaesthesia* 2009;64(6):609–614.

29. Saetre E, Abdelnoor M, Amlie JP, et al. Cardiac function and antiepileptic drug treatment in the elderly: a comparison between lamotrigine and sustained-release carbamazepine. *Epilepsia* 2009;50(8):1841–1849.

30. Venkatraman N, O'Neil D, Hall AP. Life-threatening overdose with lamotrigine, citalopram, and chlorpheniramine. *J Postgrad Med* 2008;54(4):316–317.

31. Apfelbaum JD, Caravati EM, Kerns II WP, et al. Cardiovascular effects of carbamazepine toxicity. *Ann Emerg Med* 1995;25(5):631–635.

32. Kurt E, Emul M, Ozbulut O, et al. Is valproate promising in cardiac fatal arrhythmias? Comparison of P- and Q-wave dispersion in bipolar affective patients on valproate or lithium–valproate maintenance therapy with healthy controls. *J Psychopharmacol* 2008;23(3):328–333.

33. Acciavatti T, Martinotti G, Corbo M, et al. Psychotropic drugs and ventricular repolarisation: the effects on QT interval, T-peak to T-end interval and QT dispersion. *J Psychopharmacol* 2017;31(4):453–460.

34. Vandael E, Vandenberk B, Vandenberghe J, et al. Risk factors for QTc-prolongation: systematic review of the evidence. *Int J Clin Pharm* 2017;39(1):16–25.

35. Popescu D, Laza C, Mergeani A, et al. Lead electrocardiogram changes after supratentorial intracerebral hemorrhage. *Maedica (Buchar)* 2012;7(4):290–294.

36. Shah AA, Aftab A, Coverdale J. QTc prolongation with antipsychotics: is routine ECG monitoring recommended? *J Psychiatr Pract* 2014;20(3):196–206.

37. Fanoe S, Kristensen D, Fink-Jensen A, et al. Risk of arrhythmia induced by psychotropic medications: a proposal for clinical management. *Eur Heart J* 2014;35(20):1306–1315.

38. Zolezzi M, Cheung L. A literature-based algorithm for the assessment, management, and monitoring of drug-induced QTc prolongation in the psychiatric population. *Neuropsychiatr Dis Treat* 2018;15:105–114.

39. Brouillette J, Nattel S. A practical approach to avoiding cardiovascular adverse effects of psychoactive medications. *Can J Cardiol* 2017;33(12):1577–1586.

40. National Institute for Health and Care Excellence. *Psychosis and Schizophrenia in Adults: Prevention and Management.* Clinical Guideline CG178. London: NICE, 2014. Available at https://www.nice.org.uk/guidance/cg178

41. Vandael E, Vandenberk B, Vandenberghe J, et al. Development of a risk score for QTc-prolongation: the RISQ-PATH study. *Int J Clin Pharm* 2017;39(2):424–432.

42. Mahmud R, Gray A, Nabeebaccus A, Whyte MB. Incidence and outcomes of long QTc in acute medical admissions. *Int J Clin Pract* 2018;72(11):e13250.

43. Life in the Fastlane. https://litfl.com/ (accessed 2 February 2019).

44. Aktas MK, Daubert JP. Long QT syndrome. *BMJ Best Practice.* https://bestpractice.bmj.com/topics/en-gb/829. Lasr updated: January 2018.

45. Krantz MJ. QTc interval screening in methadone treatment. *Ann Intern Med* 2009;150(6):387–395.

46. Giudicessi JR, Wilde AAM, Ackerman MJ. The genetic architecture of long QT syndrome: a critical reappraisal. *Trends Cardiovasc Med* 2018;28(7):453–464.

47. Ahn J, Kim HJ, Choi J-I, et al. Effectiveness of beta-blockers depending on the genotype of congenital long-QT syndrome: a meta-analysis. *PLoS One* 2017;12(10):e0185680.

48. Barra S, Agarwal S, Begley D, Providência R. Post-acute management of the acquired long QT syndrome. *Postgrad Med J* 2014;90(1064):348–358.

49. Schwartz PJ, Spazzolini C, Priori SG, et al. Who are the long-QT syndrome patients who receive an implantable cardioverter-defibrillator and what happens to them? Data from the European Long-QT Syndrome Implantable Cardioverter-Defibrillator (LQTS ICD) Registry. *Circulation* 2010;122(13):1272–1282.

50. Schneider HE, Steinmetz M, Krause U, et al. Left cardiac sympathetic denervation for the management of life-threatening ventricular tachyarrhythmias in young patients with catecholaminergic polymorphic ventricular tachycardia and long QT syndrome. *Clin Res Cardiol* 2013;102(1):33–42.

CHAPTER 3

Chapter 4

Syncope

Luke Vano, Nicholas Gall

Syncope is defined as a transient loss of consciousness (TLOC) secondary to reduction in blood flow to the brain (i.e. cerbral hypoperfusion) [1]. It is rapid in onset, rarely lasts longer than two minutes, and recovery is spontaneous. Longer periods of unconsciousness are unlikely to be secondary to syncope or syncope alone (e.g. syncope resulting in head injury may result in a longer period of loss of consciousness).

Syncope is one of multiple causes of TLOC that also include seizure, intoxication, metabolic disturbance (e.g. hypoglycaemia or adrenal insufficiency*), and trauma [2]. As such, after consciousness is regained, a clinician must first differentiate syncope from other precipitants of TLOC, before then determining cause of syncope, which are similarly numerous.

CAUSES OF SYNCOPE

- *Cardiac syncope* describes loss of consciousness secondary to reduced cardiac output. Common causes include arrhythmia (see Chapters 1–3 and 70) and structural heart disease (e.g. aortic stenosis and hypertrophic cardiomyopathy).
- *Reflex/neurally mediated syncope* is the result of altered autonomic regulation of postural tone resulting in inappropriate bradycardia and/or vasodilation. Types of reflex syncope include vasovagal syncope, carotid sinus syncope, and micturition syncope.

---

* Patients with adrenal insufficiency (Addison's disease) present with non-specific symptoms including postural hypotension and syncope, abdominal pain, nausea, vomiting, fatigue, weakness, and confusion. Adrenal insufficiency is a medical emergency, and as such the patient should be reviewed in the accident and emergency department.

The Maudsley Practice Guidelines for Physical Health Conditions in Psychiatry, First Edition.
David M. Taylor, Fiona Gaughran, and Toby Pillinger.
© 2021 John Wiley & Sons Ltd. Published 2021 by John Wiley & Sons Ltd.

■ *Orthostatic syncope* is caused by reduced cerebral perfusion on standing (see Chapter 6). Common causes include prescribed medication, volume loss, autonomic failure, and heart disease.

SYNCOPE AND SERIOUS MENTAL ILLNESS

Compared with the general population, people with mental illness are at higher risk of syncopal episodes [3,4]. Orthostatic hypotension can be a consequence of some psychiatric treatment (see Chapter 6) [5] and may follow intravascular volume depletion in anorexia nervosa [6]. Some psychotropic medications prolong the QTc interval and predispose to torsades de pointes (see Chapter 4), thus increasing risk of cardiac syncope [7]. Those with a diagnosis of somatisation disorder are at increased risk of vasovagal syncope [8].

Psychogenic pseudosyncope (PPS) describes the appearance of TLOC in the absence of true loss of consciousness [9]. PPS is often secondary to conversion disorder, hypothesised to represent the physical manifestation of internal stressors [9]. Risk factors for PPS include being young, female, and having a comorbid psychiatric diagnosis [10,11]. People with conversion disorder are also more likely to experience psychogenic nonepileptic seizures (see Chapter 53) [12]. Cataplexy is a rare cause of TLOC, in which patients briefly lose voluntary muscle control and have associated rapid eye movement sleep. This typically occurs when people with narcolepsy experience a strong emotional reaction. There is some evidence of a link between narcolepsy–cataplexy and schizophrenia [13].

DIAGNOSTIC PRINCIPLES

The following sections are based on the UK National Institute for Health and Care Excellence (NICE) guidelines for assessing TLOC and syncope [14]. This guidance assumes recovery from the episode of unconsciousness. In the acute setting, the patient should be managed as per the ABCDE approach (see Chapter 78 on an approach to the unconscious patient) and, based on clinical judgement, a decision should be made regarding whether the patient requires immediate transfer to emergency services.

History

1 Ask the patient about the circumstances surrounding loss of consciousness. Ideally questions should also be directed at anyone who witnessed the event.
   a What was the patient doing at the time? Did the patient fall to the floor and/or sustain injuries? Syncope during exercise suggests a cardiac arrhythmia (whereas syncope after exercise is more likely to be vasovagal).
   b Was the event in association with a change in posture (e.g. on standing)?
   c Was there a clear provoking factor (e.g. pain)?

d Did the patient experience any presyncopal symptoms (e.g. light-headedness, palpitations, sweating)?

e What did the patient look like during the episode (e.g. change in skin colour)?

f Were there any associated symptoms that may indicate cardiac pathology (e.g. chest pain)?

g Were there any associated symptoms that might indicate seizure activity (e.g. limb-jerking during the episode, tongue biting)?

h Was recovery rapid or was there a period of confusion after the event?

i Was there any history of recent bleeding (e.g. melaena)? (See Chapter 20.)

2 Past medical history:

a previous syncopal episodes, including number and frequency

b cardiac history, if pacemaker/implantable cardioverter defibrillator *in situ*.

3 Medication history: any recent changes to medication or dose.

4 Family history, including history of cardiac disease, sudden cardiac death, or unexplained sudden death of a family member aged <40 years.

5 Social history, recording smoking status, alcohol and substance use.

Examination

1 Vital signs, including heart rate, blood pressure (lying and standing; see Chapter 6), and oxygen saturations.

2 General inspection: pallor (anaemia, blood loss), decreased skin turgor (plasma volume depletion), presence of pacemaker.

3 Cardiac examination: pulse rate and rhythm, evidence of heart failure, murmurs.

4 Neurological examination: focal neurology that may suggest vascular event (see Chapter 82).

5 Gastrointestinal examination: for evidence of an intra-abdominal bleed (rigid tender abdomen, abnormal rectal examination).

Investigations

1 ECG is needed in all patients. Examine for:

a bradycardia

b ventricular arrhythmia

c prolonged QTc

d Brugada sign (coved ST elevation >2 mm in more than one of V1–V3 followed by negative T wave)

e ventricular pre-excitation of Wolff–Parkinson–White syndrome (short PR interval and delta wave)

f T-wave inversion (ischaemia or cardiomyopathy)

g pathological Q waves (myocardial infarction)

h atrial arrythmia

i paced rhythm.

2 Capillary glucose (hypoglycaemia; see Chapter 74).

CHAPTER 4

3 Further investigations may be indicated if other specific causes of TLOC are suspected, such as the following.

a Full blood count to assess for anaemia.

b Urea and electrolytes (including magnesium and calcium) to assess for dehydration or electrolyte imbalance which may accompany metabolic disturbance (e.g. hyponatraemia and hyperkalaemia of Addison's disease) or cause cardiac arrythmia.

c Creatine kinase (if patient obtunded).

d Troponin if there are concerns regarding an acute coronary event (see Chapter 69).

e EEG should not be ordered unless epilepsy is suspected (i.e. based on a high pretest probability) and following discussion with neurology.

4 Other investigations may be requested by specialist care (e.g. cardiology).

a If structural heart disease is suspected (e.g. hypertrophic obstructive myopathy), perform echocardiogram.

b Exercise testing, if the syncope is exercise-induced.

c If Brugada syndrome is suspected, an ajmaline study is performed, coordinated by an inherited cardiac conditions clinic.

d Tilt test if recurrent vasovagal syncope is suspected with associated detrimental impact on quality of life and/or representing high risk of injury (assessing if syncope is associated with severe cardioinhibitory response, usually asystole).

e If carotid sinus syncope is suspected, or in unexplained syncope in patients aged >60, perform carotid sinus massage (only in a controlled environment, with ECG recording, with resuscitation equipment to hand as long as there is no carotid stenosis >50% or recent stroke/transient ischaemic attack).

f Ambulatory ECG if suspected cardiac arrhythmia (or if syncope unexplained):

　i Holter monitoring if episodes occurring several times a week

　ii external event recording if episodes occurring every one to two weeks

　iii implantable event recorder if episodes occurring less than every two weeks.

DIAGNOSIS AND MANAGEMENT

Where diagnosis is unclear, a referral to a specialist syncope clinic may be indicated, or where such services do not exist, cardiology. A diagnosis of uncomplicated vasovagal syncope (a faint) may be made if there are no features of an alternative diagnosis, and the events are associated with the '3 Ps': posture (prolonged standing, prevented by sitting down), provoking factors (e.g. pain), and prodromal symptoms (presyncope: sweating, light-headedness). Similarly, a diagnosis of situational syncope may be made if there are no features of an alternative diagnosis and there is a clear situational precipitant (e.g. micturition). For both uncomplicated and situational syncope, if there are no safety concerns then no further immediate management is required. Patients should be provided with information regarding their diagnosis and strategies to avoid syncopal episodes (e.g. to sit/lie down when presyncopal symptoms emerge).

Orthostatic syncope has a typical history and on testing of lying/standing blood pressure, postural hypotension should be observed. Postural hypotension has several potential causes (see Chapter 6), and medication represents a major differential. In such patients a medication review and where appropriate rationalisation may be required.

Any suspicion of cardiac syncope should prompt referral to cardiology, urgently in the case of syncope associated with exercise. Suspect seizures if any of the following features are present: tongue biting, unusual posturing, prolonged rhythmic limb jerking (this can briefly accompany syncopal episodes), loss of bowel or bladder control, postictal phase, prodromal déjà vu or jamais vu [14]. These patients will require a referral to neurology (see Chapter 53).

Patients should be provided with advice about driving in the context of syncopal episodes. Advise all people who are waiting for a specialist assessment that they must not drive. Those from the UK are directed to the Driver and Vehicle Licensing Agency (DVLA) website for the latest guidance [15].

References

1. Brignole M, Moya A, de Lange FJ, et al. 2018 ESC guidelines for the diagnosis and management of syncope. *Eur Heart J* 2018;39(21):1883–1948.
2. Soteriades ES, Evans JC, Larson MG, et al. Incidence and prognosis of syncope. *N Engl J Med* 2002;347(12):878–885.
3. Kouakam C, Lacroix D, Klug D, et al. Prevalence and prognostic significance of psychiatric disorders in patients evaluated for recurrent unexplained syncope. *Am J Cardiol* 2002;89(5):530–535.
4. Kapoor WN, Fortunato M, Hanusa BH, Schulberg HC. Psychiatric Illnesses in patients with syncope. *Am J Med* 1995;99(5):505–512.
5. Gugger JJ. Antipsychotic pharmacotherapy and orthostatic hypotension: identification and management. *CNS Drugs* 2011;25(8):659–671.
6. Sachs KV, Harnke B, Mehler PS, Krantz MJ. Cardiovascular complications of anorexia nervosa: a systematic review. *Int J Eat Disord* 2016;49(3):238–248.
7. Akhondzadeh S, Mojtahedzadeh V, Mirsepassi GR, et al. Diazoxide in the treatment of schizophrenia: novel application of potassium channel openers in the treatment of schizophrenia. *J Clin Pharm Ther* 2002;27(6):453–459.
8. Alhuzaimi A, Aljohar A, Alhadi AN, et al. Psychiatric traits in patients with vasovagal and unexplained syncope. *Int J Gen Med* 2018;11:99–104.
9. Raj V, Rowe AA, Fleisch SB, et al. Psychogenic pseudosyncope: diagnosis and management. *Auton Neurosci* 2014;184:66–72.
10. Iglesias JF, Graf D, Forclaz A, et al. Stepwise evaluation of unexplained syncope in a large ambulatory population. *Pacing Clin Electrophysiol* 2009;32(Suppl 1):S202–S206.
11. Wiener Z, Shapiro NI, Chiu DT, Grossman SA. The prevalence of psychiatric disease in emergency department patients with unexplained syncope. *Intern Emerg Med* 2013;8(5):427–430.
12. Gelauff J, Stone J, Edwards M, Carson A. The prognosis of functional (psychogenic) motor symptoms: a systematic review. *J Neurol Neurosurg Psychiatry* 2014;85(2):220–226.
13. Sansa G, Gavalda A, Gaig C, et al. Exploring the presence of narcolepsy in patients with schizophrenia. *BMC Psychiatry* 2016;16:177.
14. Alphs L, Bossie CA, Fu DJ, et al. Onset and persistence of efficacy by symptom domain with long-acting injectable paliperidone palmitate in patients with schizophrenia. *Expert Opin Pharmacother* 2014;15(7):1029–1042.
15. Driver and Vehicle Licensing Agency (DVLA). Neurological disorders: assessing fitness to drive. https://www.gov.uk/guidance/neurological-disorders-assessing-fitness-to-drive. Last updated: 4 March 2020.

CHAPTER 4

Hypertension

Luke Vano, Toby Pillinger, J. Kennedy Cruickshank

Previous American and current European guidelines define hypertension as a systolic blood pressure (BP) above 140 mmHg or a diastolic pressure exceeding 90 mmHg [1,2], while recent American guidelines are more aggressive, defining hypertension as systolic BP above 130 mmHg and diastolic BP above 80 mmHg [3]. Irrespective of definitions, the higher a patient's BP, the greater the risk of hypertensive-associated complications, including [4,5] myocardial infarction, stroke, left ventricular hypertrophy (LVH), heart failure, chronic kidney disease, and cognitive decline [6,7]. Moreover, all-cause mortality increases with worsening BP control [2]. Globally, hypertension has a prevalence of over 25% [2,5]. Patients with serious mental illness (SMI) are 12% more likely to be hypertensive compared with the general population [8–11], and are more likely to have hypertension untreated [12]. (Readers are referred to Chapter 71 on hypertensive crisis if the patient's BP is ≥180/≥110 mmHg.)

Essential hypertension describes raised BP when no direct cause can be identified, which occurs in approximately 90% of cases [13]. Risk factors for essential hypertension are described in Box 5.1 [13]. Secondary hypertension describes increased BP in the setting of a causative comorbidity or drug (Box 5.2) [14]. Many of the risks for both primary and secondary hypertension are shared between the general population and those with SMI. However, lifestyle factors such as reduced levels of physical activity, poor diet, and increased rates of metabolic syndrome and smoking increase the likelihood of essential hypertension in people with SMI [11,15–17]. Also, certain antidepressants and catecholaminergic medications (see Box 5.2) have been shown to worsen hypertension [18–22], thereby increasing the risk of secondary hypertension in this group.

Box 5.1 Common risk factors for essential hypertension [1–7,13]

Past medical history

- Diabetes mellitus
- Obstructive sleep apnoea
- Dyslipidaemia

Modifiable (lifestyle) risk factors

- Obesity
- Aerobic exercise less than three times a week
- Alcohol
- Salt intake over 5 g daily [2]
- Low fruit and vegetable intake
- Stimulants (e.g. caffeine, nicotine)

Non-modifiable risk factors

- Age
- Family history of hypertension or cardiovascular disease
- Black ethnicity

Box 5.2 Causes of secondary hypertension in the general and psychiatric patient population [1–7,13,18–23]

Medication

- Non-steroidal anti-inflammatory drugs
- Corticosteroids
- Anabolic steroids
- Ciclosporin and tacrolimus
- Erythropoietin
- Oral contraceptives, particularly oestrogen-containing agents
- Decongestants (e.g. phenylephrine)
- Tricyclic antidepressants (e.g. amitriptyline)
- Serotonin/noradrenaline reuptake inhibitors (e.g. venlafaxine)
- Monoamine oxidase inhibitors (e.g. selegiline)
- Catecholaminergic medications (e.g. methylphenidate, bupropion)
- Atypical antipsychotics

Renal disease

- Glomerulonephritis
- Polyarteritis nodosa
- Systemic sclerosis
- Polycystic kidney disease
- Renovascular disease (renal artery stenosis)

Endocrine disease

- Conn's syndrome
- Cushing's syndrome
- Phaeochromocytoma
- Hypothyroidism/hyperthyroidism
- Acromegaly
- Hyperparathyroidism

Lifestyle factors

- Stimulants (e.g. cocaine, amphetamines)
- Excessive liquorice ingestion

DIAGNOSTIC PRINCIPLES

History, examination, and investigations are performed to look for secondary causes of hypertension, assess for related risk factors, and to identify hypertension-mediated organ damage (HMOD). HMOD include any established cardiovascular disease (CVD), renal disease, advanced retinopathy, and LVH on ECG or echocardiogram.

History

1 Hypertension, unless severe, is usually asymptomatic. However, headaches, neurological symptoms, visual symptoms, and nose bleeds may herald a hypertensive emergency (see Chapter 71). Secondary causes of hypertension (see Box 5.2) may have characteristic presenting complaints depending on the underlying cause, for example weight loss, palpitations, excessive sweating, and disturbed sleep in hyperthyroidism.
2 Past medical history (Box 5.2).
3 Medication history (Box 5.2).
4 Family history of hypertension or CVD.
5 Social history, including smoking, alcohol, and substance misuse history.

Examination

1 Blood pressure measurement (Box 5.3). Ambulatory BP monitoring (ABPM) and home BP monitoring (HBPM) measurements have been shown to be a greater predictor of HMOD and CVD outcomes than office readings [24,25]. They can and therefore should be used, where possible, in clinical practice. ABPM involves the use of a wearable cuff for 24 hours that automatically takes BP measurements every 15–60 minutes throughout the day, usually hourly at night (which does disturb sleep and BP measurement in some people) [26], whilst HBPM involves the patient taking their own BP using an automated device four times a day for at least 4 days [26]. The average of these measurements is then used to calculate an average BP value.

> **Box 5.3** Blood pressure measurement technique
>
> If this is the patient's first measurement, then both arms should be tested. If there is a significant difference in readings, then the arm providing the highest value should be used for future measurements. This difference in measurements is usually due to atheromatous vascular disease.
>
> When performing office BP measurements, automated and manual BP methods may be used, though the manual technique is required if the patient has an active arrhythmia (e.g. atrial fibrillation). Ensure the patient has been seated in a relaxed environment for five minutes prior to measurement. An appropriately sized cuff should be used and placed around the arm at the level of the patient's heart. After three measurements have been taken, with ideally one minute between each, the average of the final two readings should be calculated and used as the recorded value. If there is a discrepancy of over 10 mmHg, then further measurements should be taken.

2 Measure height and weight and calculate body mass index (BMI).
3 Physical examination may be indicated to examine for signs of end-organ damage secondary to hypertension. This will include cardiovascular (left ventricular heave of hypertrophy, raised jugular venous pressure, ankle oedema), respiratory (pulmonary oedema), and neurological (focal signs secondary to stroke) examination, including (if possible) ophthalmoscopy to examine for hypertensive retinopathy.

Investigations

1 ECG: examine for LVH or evidence of previous myocardial infarction.
2 Urinalysis: proteinuria, haematuria, glycosuria.
3 Bloods: urea and electrolytes, fasting blood glucose and HbA_{1c}, lipid levels, liver function tests, bone profile.
4 Consider sending a urine sample to quantify proteinuria (albumin/creatinine ratio).
5 Echocardiogram may be considered to further assess for LVH.

DIAGNOSIS

Hypertension is most often diagnosed on routine testing. No other investigations are needed for the diagnosis, unless there is reason to believe a secondary cause is present (see section on when to refer to a specialist). The algorithm in Figure 5.1 details how to diagnose hypertension as per National Institute for Health and Care Excellence (NICE) guidelines [26]. Management is determined by the degree of hypertension (in mmHg based on clinic readings: stage 1, 140–159/90–99; stage 2, 160–179/100–109; severe, ≥180/≥110), the age of the patient, comorbidities, and the presence of end-organ damage.

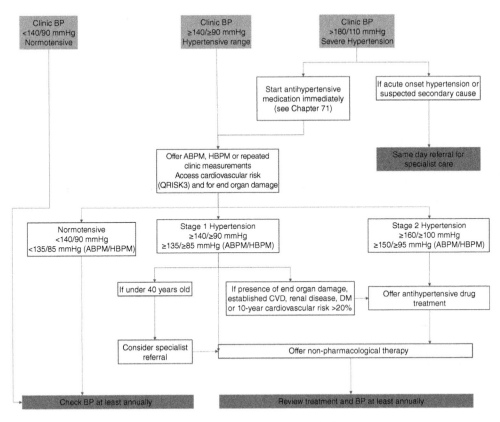

Figure 5.1 Criteria for diagnosis of hypertension. ABPM, ambulatory blood pressure monitoring; HBPM, home blood pressure monitoring; CVD, cardiovascular disease; DM, diabetes mellitus.

MANAGEMENT

Non-pharmacological therapy

Lifestyle advice should be provided to all hypertensive patients, including:

- salt restriction (5 g/day) [2]
- Dietary Approaches to Stop Hypertension (DASH) diet [3,27] with emphasis on low-fat proteins, whole grains, low sodium, five servings of fruit and five servings of vegetables daily [27]
- smoking cessation (see Chapter 46)
- weight loss (see Chapter 14)
- increase levels of exercise (see Chapter 10) [28]
- reducing alcohol consumption.

CHAPTER 5

Consider rationalising psychiatric medication

Serotonin/noradrenaline reuptake inhibitors [18,20], tricyclic antidepressants [19], and monoamine oxidase inhibitors may contribute to hypertension; in patients prescribed these medications, switching to a selective serotonin reuptake inhibitor, which as a class has been shown to have at most only a very slight effect on BP, may be considered [18,19]. Sertraline is considered safe in patients with ischaemic heart disease [29].

Pharmacological therapy

There is robust evidence that pharmacological management of hypertension is associated with significant reduction in CVD and improves mortality rates [30]. For example, compared with placebo, pharmacological antihypertensive therapy in the general population reduces the risk of heart failure, stroke and myocardial infarction by 20–50% [30]. Figure 5.1 defines when pharmacological treatment should be offered. Please note that American guidelines recommend that BP is treated if >130/>80 mmHg [3].

Target readings

- Aim for a target clinic BP below 140/90 mmHg in people aged under 80 years, or those of any age with diabetes mellitus, with treated hypertension.
- Aim for a target clinic BP below 150/90 mmHg in people aged 80 years and over with treated hypertension.

Prescribing algorithm

When prescribing antihypertensives, start at a low dose and titrate as necessary. Follow the algorithm in Figure 5.2 to guide additional treatment [26].

Angiotensin-converting enzyme inhibitors and angiotensin II receptor blockers

Angiotensin-converting enzyme (ACE) inhibitors and angiotensin II receptor blockers (ARBs) act therapeutically by reducing levels of circulating angiotensin II or its action at angiotensin receptors. This relaxes blood vessels and reduces fluid retention, resulting in a fall in BP. An example prescription for an ACE inhibitor is ramipril at a starting dose of 2.5 mg once daily (oral), increasing to 10 mg total, starting twice-daily dosing when the total dose reaches 5 mg. If an ACE inhibitor is not tolerated (ACE inhibitors can be associated with development of a cough), then switch to an ARB, for example losartan 50 mg once daily (oral) up to a maximum dose of 100 mg daily. Do not prescribe an ACE inhibitor and ARB in combination. Start with half the dose if elderly, if using a diuretic, or in the presence of chronic kidney disease. Do not start ACE inhibitors or ARBs without specialist advice if estimated glomerular filtration rate (eGFR) is below 30 mL/min per 1.73 m². Urea and electrolytes should be checked prior to initiation, at week 1 and at week 4, and also after each titration, every 1–2 weeks. ACE inhibitors reduce lithium clearance, and therefore plasma lithium levels should be checked following initiation.

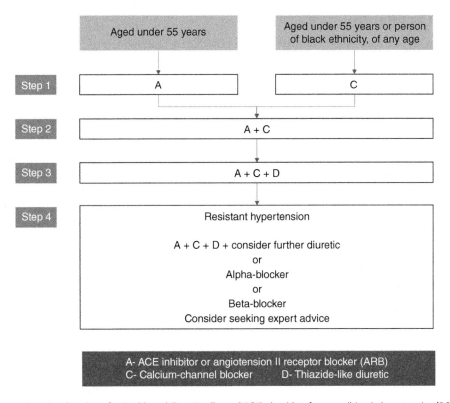

Figure 5.2 National Institute for Health and Care Excellence (NICE) algorithm for prescribing in hypertension [26].

Calcium channel blockers

Calcium channel blockers act on arterial vascular smooth muscle to relax blood vessels, resulting in a fall in BP. An example prescription for a calcium channel blocker is amlodipine starting at a dose of 5 mg daily (oral), increasing to 10 mg daily, as required. The most common side effect is ankle swelling.

Thiazide-like diuretics

Thiazide diuretics work by inhibiting reabsorption of sodium and chloride ions in the distal convoluted tubules in the kidneys thereby causing diuresis, reducing intravascular volume, and by association BP. An example prescription is indapamide 2.5 mg once daily (1.5 mg if SR preparation), taken in the morning. Higher doses are rarely required. Urea and electrolytes are required prior to and during treatment owing to risk of hypokalaemia and/or hyponatraemia. Thiazide diuretics can dramatically increase plasma lithium levels: use together with caution and check lithium levels.

CHAPTER 5

When to refer to a specialist

If the patient has a blood pressure ≥180/≥110 mmHg and evidence of end-organ damage, please refer to Chapter 71. In case of hypertensive emergency, the patient may need to be seen immediately by emergency/acute medical services.

It is important to refer to a specialist, ideally a specialist hypertension clinic, if there is any suspicion of a secondary cause (including patients aged under 40 with BP ≥160/≥100 mmHg). If specialist hypertension clinics are not available, then discuss with cardiology or endocrinology colleagues to clarify to whom a referral should be made. Patients with treatment-resistant hypertension (i.e. poorly controlled BP despite adherence to three antihypertensives of different classes) or those with sudden onset of hypertension should also be referred.

When writing a referral letter to secondary care, it is important to include the following information: a detailed history of any symptoms that may indicate a secondary cause of hypertension, past medical history, current medication along with allergy status, a brief social history and any findings from clinical examination, remembering to include information on previous BP readings and treatment. Ensure that the patient's psychiatric history is included in the letter.

References

1. James PA, Oparil S, Carter BL, et al. 2014 evidence-based guideline for the management of high blood pressure in adults: report from the panel members appointed to the Eighth Joint National Committee (JNC 8). *JAMA* 2014;311(5):507–520.
2. Williams B, Mancia G, Spiering W, et al. 2018 ESC/ESH guidelines for the management of arterial hypertension. *Eur Heart J* 2018;39(33):3021–3104.
3. Whelton PK, Carey RM, Aronow WS, et al. 2017 ACC/AHA/AAPA/ABC/ACPM/AGS/APhA/ASH/ASPC/NMA/PCNA guideline for the prevention, detection, evaluation, and management of high blood pressure in adults: executive summary. A report of the American College of Cardiology/American Heart Association Task Force on Clinical Practice Guidelines. *Hypertension* 2018;71(6):1269–1324.
4. Lewington S, Clarke R, Qizilbash N, et al. Age-specific relevance of usual blood pressure to vascular mortality: a meta-analysis of individual data for one million adults in 61 prospective studies. *Lancet* 2002;360(9349):1903–1913.
5. Kearney PM, Whelton M, Reynolds K, et al. Global burden of hypertension: analysis of worldwide data. *Lancet* 2005;365(9455):217–223.
6. Arboix A. Cardiovascular risk factors for acute stroke: risk profiles in the different subtypes of ischemic stroke. *World J Clin Cases* 2015;3(5):418–429.
7. Rahimi K, Emdin CA, MacMahon S. The epidemiology of blood pressure and its worldwide management. *Circ Res* 2015;116(6):925–936.
8. Carroll D, Phillips AC, Gale CR, Batty GD. Generalized anxiety and major depressive disorders, their comorbidity and hypertension in middle-aged men. *Psychosom Med* 2010;72(1):16–19.
9. Leboyer M, Soreca I, Scott J, et al. Can bipolar disorder be viewed as a multi-system inflammatory disease? *J Affect Disord* 2012;141(1):1–10.
10. Goff DC, Sullivan LM, McEvoy JP, et al. A comparison of ten-year cardiac risk estimates in schizophrenia patients from the CATIE study and matched controls. *Schizophr Res* 2005;80(1):45–53.
11. Vancampfort D, Stubbs B, Mitchell AJ, et al. Risk of metabolic syndrome and its components in people with schizophrenia and related psychotic disorders, bipolar disorder and major depressive disorder: a systematic review and meta-analysis. *World Psychiatry* 2015;14(3):339–347.
12. Nasrallah HA, Meyer JM, Goff DC, et al. Low rates of treatment for hypertension, dyslipidemia and diabetes in schizophrenia: data from the CATIE schizophrenia trial sample at baseline. *Schizophr Res* 2006;86(1–3):15–22.
13. Bolivar JJ. Essential hypertension: an approach to its etiology and neurogenic pathophysiology. *Int J Hypertens* 2013;2013:547809.
14. Charles L, Triscott J, Dobbs B. Secondary hypertension: discovering the underlying cause. *Am Fam Physician* 2017;96(7):453–461.
15. Vancampfort D, Probst M, Knapen J, et al. Associations between sedentary behaviour and metabolic parameters in patients with schizophrenia. *Psychiatry Res* 2012;200(2–3):73–78.
16. Bly MJ, Taylor SF, Dalack G, et al. Metabolic syndrome in bipolar disorder and schizophrenia: dietary and lifestyle factors compared to the general population. *Bipolar Disord* 2014;16(3):277–288.
17. Dickerson F, Stallings CR, Origoni AE, et al. Cigarette smoking among persons with schizophrenia or bipolar disorder in routine clinical settings, 1999–2011. *Psychiatr Serv* 2013;64(1):44–50.

18. Licht CM, de Geus EJ, Seldenrijk A, et al. Depression is associated with decreased blood pressure, but antidepressant use increases the risk for hypertension. *Hypertension* 2009;53(4):631–638.

19. Zhong Z, Wang L, Wen X, et al. A meta-analysis of effects of selective serotonin reuptake inhibitors on blood pressure in depression treatment: outcomes from placebo and serotonin and noradrenaline reuptake inhibitor controlled trials. *Neuropsychiatr Dis Treat* 2017;13:2781–2796.

20. Thase ME. Effects of venlafaxine on blood pressure: a meta-analysis of original data from 3744 depressed patients. *J Clin Psychiatry* 1998;59(10):502–508.

21. Yamada M, Yasuhara H. Clinical pharmacology of MAO inhibitors: safety and future. *Neurotoxicology* 2004;25(1–2):215–221.

22. Wilens TE, Hammerness PG, Biederman J, et al. Blood pressure changes associated with medication treatment of adults with attention-deficit/hyperactivity disorder. *J Clin Psychiatry* 2005;66(2):253–259.

23. De Hert M, Dekker JM, Wood D, et al. Cardiovascular disease and diabetes in people with severe mental illness: position statement from the European Psychiatric Association (EPA), supported by the European Association for the Study of Diabetes (EASD) and the European Society of Cardiology (ESC). *Eur Psychiatry* 2009;24(6):412–424.

24. Banegas JR, Ruilope LM, de la Sierra A, et al. Relationship between clinic and ambulatory blood-pressure measurements and mortality. *N Engl J Med* 2018;378:1509–1520.

25. Sega R, Facchetti R, Bombelli M, et al. Prognostic value of ambulatory and home blood pressures compared with office blood pressure in the general population: follow-up results from the Pressioni Arteriose Monitorate e Loro Associazioni (PAMELA) study. *Circulation* 2005;111:1777–1783.

26. National Institute for Health and Care Excellence. *Hypertension in Adults: Diagnosis and Management*. NICE Guideline NG136. London: NICE, 2019. https://www.nice.org.uk/guidance/ng136

27. Sacks FM, Svetkey LP, Vollmer WM, et al. Effects on blood pressure of reduced dietary sodium and the Dietary Approaches to Stop Hypertension (DASH) diet. DASH-Sodium Collaborative Research Group. *N Engl J Med* 2001;344(1):3–10.

28. Whelton SP, Chin A, Xin X, He J. Effect of aerobic exercise on blood pressure: a meta-analysis of randomized, controlled trials. *Ann Intern Med* 2002;136(7):493–503.

29. Glassman AH, O'Connor CM, Califf RM, et al. Sertraline treatment of major depression in patients with acute MI or unstable angina. *JAMA* 2002;288(6):701–709.

30. Blood Pressure Lowering Treatment Trialists Collaboration, Turnbull F, Neal B, Ninomiya T, et al. Effects of different regimens to lower blood pressure on major cardiovascular events in older and younger adults: meta-analysis of randomised trials. *BMJ* 2008;336(7653):1121–1123.

CHAPTER 5

Postural Hypotension

Toby Pillinger, Ian Osborne, Thomas Ernst,
J. Kennedy Cruickshank

Postural (orthostatic) hypotension is defined as a fall in systolic blood pressure of at least 20 mmHg or diastolic pressure of at least 10 mmHg within two to five minutes of standing after a five-minute period lying flat [1]. Postural hypotension has several causes, including impairment in autonomic reflexes (which may occur naturally with ageing), medication or depletion in intravascular volume. Common causes in the general population, and specifically in an individual with serious mental illness (SMI), are summarised in Table 6.1.

Specific considerations for psychiatric patients include a psychiatric medication review, as well as a drug and alcohol history (Box 6.1). Eating disorders may be associated with volume loss secondary to vomiting/diarrhoea in the context of diuretic, laxative or emetic use. Neurodegenerative diseases with psychiatric sequelae may be associated with inherent autonomic disturbance, or involve treatment with medications which impact autonomic function. Higher rates of type 2 diabetes mellitus in psychiatric patients should lead to consideration of autonomic neuropathy. Other conditions that present with both psychiatric symptomatology and autonomic instability include vitamin deficiencies (e.g. B_{12}/folate), thyroid disease, renal failure/uraemia, porphyria, and infection (e.g. syphilis and HIV). In old-age psychiatry, the impact of ageing is important to consider; the prevalence of postural hypotension in those aged over 65 is 18% [2].

The Maudsley Practice Guidelines for Physical Health Conditions in Psychiatry, First Edition.
David M. Taylor, Fiona Gaughran, and Toby Pillinger.

Table 6.1 Common causes of postural hypotension in the general and psychiatric patient population.

	General population	Individual with SMI
Medication	Alpha-adrenergic antagonists (mainly used for high blood pressure/enlarged prostate, e.g. doxazosin) α_2-Agonists (e.g. clonidine, lofexidine) Antihypertensives (e.g. amlodipine) Anti-parkinsonian drugs (e.g. levodopa) Beta-blockers (e.g. bisoprolol) Diuretics (e.g. furosemide) Muscle relaxants (e.g. baclofen) Opioids Phosphodiesterase inhibitors (e.g. sildenafil) Vasodilators (e.g. isosorbide mononitrate)	Antidepressants (see Table 6.2) Antipsychotics Anti-parkinsonian drugs (e.g. levodopa) Diuretics/laxative abuse (eating disorders) Opioids
Volume loss	Vomiting/diarrhoea Fever Fluid restriction Anaemia Adrenal insufficiency Thyroid disease	Vomiting/diarrhoea (eating disorders) Dehydration (poor self-care, catatonia) Thyroid disease
Autonomic failure	Neurodegenerative disease (e.g. Parkinson's disease, dementia with Lewy bodies, multiple system atrophy) Neuropathies (e.g. diabetes, alcohol, amyloid, sarcoid, B_{12}/folate deficiency, infection, renal failure, porphyria, paraneoplastic, autoimmune, familial)	Neurodegenerative disease (e.g. Parkinson's disease and dementia with Lewy bodies) Neuropathies (e.g. diabetes mellitus, alcohol, B_{12}/folate deficiency, porphyria, syphilis, and HIV)
Heart disease	Heart failure Valve disease Cardiomyopathy Myocarditis Cardiomyopathy Arrhythmia	Myocarditis/cardiomyopathy secondary to psychotropic medication Ischaemic cardiomyopathy
	Ageing Alcohol Sympathicotonic orthostatic hypotension refers to orthostatic hypotension seen in individuals with excessive sympathetic discharge. This can be due to chronic stress from any cause. A rare but important medical cause includes phaeochromocytoma [3]	

Box 6.1 Diagnostic summary for postural hypotension

History

- Define symptoms
- Define symptoms suggestive of neuropathy/autonomic dysfunction
- Exclude volume loss (e.g. diarrhoea)
- Past medical history: diabetes, heart disease, malignancy, rheumatological and autoimmune disorders, renal failure
- Medication history
- Drug and alcohol history
- Family history of similar presentation

Examination

- Lying and standing blood pressure
- Neurologial examination
- Cardiovascular examination

Investigations

- Bloods
- ECG
- Urine dip

DIAGNOSTIC PRINCIPLES

History

1 Symptoms of postural hypotension are a consequence of cerebral hypoperfusion, and include dizziness/light-headedness, visual disturbances (e.g. blurring), and potentially (but rarely) syncope (see Chapter 4). Dizziness should be distinguished from vertigo, i.e. the illusion of movement, most commonly a spinning sensation. Symptoms typically occur on standing but may also arise following a meal (more commonly in the elderly), on exertion, or following prolonged standing.
2 Medication history, specifically asking if there has been a recent change in medication (see Table 6.1).
3 Recent evidence of volume loss (diarrhoea/vomiting/infection).
4 Associated symptoms that may point towards a peripheral neuropathy or autonomic dysfunction, e.g. constipation, erectile dysfunction, urinary incontinence, abnormal sweating.
5 Family history of similar symptoms, suggestive of familial neuropathy.
6 Past medical history, including screening for malignancy, heart disease, diabetes mellitus, autoimmune disease, renal failure, amyloid, sarcoid, and porphyria.
7 Social history, including a quantification of alcohol intake.

Examination

1 Lying/sitting and standing blood pressure. Blood pressure should be taken manually with a stethoscope (oscillometric devices can take a prolonged period of time to inflate, during which the postural episode may already have settled).
2 Neurological examination, specifically examining for evidence of Parkinsonism, ataxia (as a consequence of alcohol abuse/multiple system atrophy), peripheral neuropathy, autonomic dysfunction (e.g. pupillary changes, sweating abnormalities).
3 Cardiovascular examination (evidence of heart failure, valve disease).

CHAPTER 6

Investigations

1 Bloods:
   (a) full blood count (evidence of pernicious anaemia)
   (b) renal function (renal failure, uraemia or dehydration)
   (c) liver function (alcohol abuse)
   (d) bone profile/calcium (hypercalcaemia is osmotic diuretic which will contribute to hypovolaemia)
   (e) glucose and HbA_{1c} levels (diabetic neuropathy)
   (f) thyroid function
   (g) B_{12}/folate levels
   (h) autoimmune screen
   (i) infection screen (syphilis, HIV)
   (j) brain natriuretic peptide levels if there are clinical features suggestive of heart failure
   (k) morning cortisol* (adrenal insufficiency).
2 ECG to examine for cardiac disease.
3 Urine dip for glucose and proteinuria (diabetes mellitus).
4 In selected cases with features of strong sympathetic excess, consider 24-hour urine metanephrines.

MANAGEMENT

Up to one-third of patients in the general population with postural hypotension may have no identifiable cause [4]. In the psychiatric patient population, psychotropic medications are potentially responsible, and rationalising pharmacotherapy may be key to providing symptomatic relief.

Rationalising psychiatric and non-psychiatric medication

Several antidepressants and antipsychotics cause postural hypotension, although the risk profile is diverse (Tables 6.2 and 6.3). In patients who are well established on an efficacious antipsychotic or antidepressant regimen and where there is a reluctance to change medication, consider dose reduction. Rationalisation of hypnotic use should also be considered. With general medical advice, rationalisation of non-psychiatric medication may also be indicated; for example, in the case of benign prostatic hypertrophy, switching doxazosin to tamsulosin, or for hypertension, switching non-dihydropridine calcium channel blockers to dihydropyridines (e.g. amlodipine).

---

* Indicated if there are concerns regarding adrenal insufficiency (i.e. if the patient is 'Addisonian'). These patients present with non-specific symptoms including postural hypotension, abdominal pain, nausea, vomiting, fatigue, weakness, and confusion. If there are acute concerns about Addison's, patients should be seen and reviewed in the accident and emergency department.

Table 6.2 Approximate relative hypotensive severity of antidepressants.

Antidepressant	Hypotension
Tricyclics	
Amitriptyline	+++
Clomipramine	+++
Dosulepin	+++
Doxepin	++
Imipramine	+++
Lofepramine	+
Nortriptyline	++
Trimipramine	+++
Monoamine oxidase inhibitors (MAOIs)	
Isocarboxazid	+++
Phenelzine	+++
Tranylcypromine	+++
Reversible inhibitor of monoamine oxidase A (RIMA)	
Moclobemide	−
Selective serotonin reuptake inhibitors (SSRIs)	
Citalopram	−
Escitalopram	−
Fluoxetine	−
Fluvoxamine	−
Paroxetine	−
Sertraline	−
Vortioxetine[a]	+
Other antidepressants	
Agomelatine	−
Duloxetine[b]	−
Mianserin	−
Mirtazapine	+
Reboxetine[b]	−
Trazodone	+
Venlafaxine[b]	−

[a] Vortioxetine classed as an SSRI for convenience here; it has several other pharmacological effects.
[b] Usually increase blood pressure.
+++, high incidence/severity; ++, moderate; +, low; −, very low.

CHAPTER 6

Table 6.3 Approximate relative hypotensive severity of antipsychotics.

Antipsychotic	Hypotension
Amisulpride	–
Aripiprazole	–
Asenapine	–
Benperidol	+
Brexpiprazole	–
Cariprazine	–
Chlorpromazine	+++
Clozapine	+++
Flupentixol	+
Fluphenazine	+
Haloperidol	+
Iloperidone	+
Loxapine	++
Lurasidone	–
Olanzapine	+
Paliperidone	++
Perphenazine	+
Pimozide	+
Pipotiazine	++
Promazine	++
Quetiapine	++
Risperidone	++
Sertindole	+++
Sulpiride	–
Trifluoperazine	+
Ziprasidone	+
Zuclopenthixol	+

+++, high incidence/severity; ++, moderate; +, low; –, very low.

Non-pharmacological therapy

1 Lifestyle modification.
   (a) Sitting up slowly in stages from supine to standing.
   (b) Maintain hydration.

(c) Increased salt and water intake: a target daily ingestion of 1.5–3 L of water and 6–10 g of sodium has been recommended [5–8].

(d) Meal modification may be suggested if there is a clear postprandial association with hypotensive episodes. Advice includes reducing meal size, reducing alcohol intake with meals, and increasing water intake with meals.

2 Anti-embolism elastic stockings that extend to the waist reduce peripheral blood pooling [9]. These are contraindicated in patients with peripheral vascular disease; if unsure, measurement of ankle–brachial pressure index should be sought first. Ensure regular foot inspection in patients with peripheral neuropathy.

3 Physical manoeuvres, e.g. isometric handgrip when standing [10].

4 Mild to moderate exercise and evidence-based stress reduction programmes (e.g. mindfulness-based stress reduction, Tai Chi) are recommended in individuals with identified high stress burden.

Pharmacological therapy

Use of medication specifically targeting symptoms of postural hypotension should be accompanied by regular blood pressure monitoring by the patient at home.

1 Fludrocortisone is a synthetic mineralocorticoid that may be considered for patients whose postural hypotension does not respond to lifestyle modification [11]. Three randomised controlled trials examining use of fludrocortisone for postural hypotension have provided conflicting outcomes [11–13], with two demonstrating improvement [11,12] and one no benefit [13], although the studies investigated diverse populations (diabetic neuropathy [11], Parkinson's disease [12], and chronic fatigue syndrome [13]) with small numbers of participants and potentially subtherapeutic fludrocortisone doses. Fludrocortisone works primarily to increase extracellular volume and thereby blood pressure. The dose of fludrocortisone starts at 100 µg daily in the morning, with an incremental increase in dose (if necessary) by 100 µg every week, to a maximum dose of 400 µg daily. Monitor for peripheral oedema (leg swelling), hypertension, and hypokalaemia (low potassium). Because fludrocortisone is a steroid, if it is taken for more than 3 weeks the dose should be gradually reduced when it is stopped. People taking fludrocortisone should carry a steroid treatment card. This card should always be carried with them and shown to anyone who treats them.

2 If the patient remains symptomatic or does not tolerate fludrocortisone, a sympathomimetic agent such as midodrine (a selective α_1 agonist) can be added/substituted [14–16]. Midodrine increases arterial resistance thereby increasing blood pressure. It does not cross the blood–brain barrier, which means the sympathomimetic side effects that can accompany the use of adrenergic agents (e.g. anxiety and tachycardia) do not occur. The dose should be increased from 2.5 mg three times daily up to 10 mg three times daily at weekly intervals. Midodrine should not be used in patients with heart disease, urinary retention or uncontrolled hypertension. Monitor for hypertension, urinary retention, gastro-oesophageal reflux, and pruritis. Midodrine should be given at or just before rising in the morning, a further dose 4 hours after the first, and a further dose 4 hours after the second dose. Avoid a dose of midodrine within 4 hours of going to bed.

CHAPTER 6

3 There is evidence for the use of pyridostigmine [17], non-steroidal anti-inflammatories [18], caffeine [19], and erythropoietin [20] as adjunctive agents in patients who remain symptomatic with the above regimen.

4 In the case of clozapine-associated postural hypotension, reduce dose or slow down rate of increase. Increase fluid intake as described in the section on non-pharmacological therapy. Alongside fludrocortisone, there is evidence for the use of moclobemide (a reversible monoamine oxidase inhibitor, 150 mg three times daily) given together with one measure (12 g) of Bovril up to three times daily [21].

When to refer to a specialist

Postural hypotension can usually be managed in primary care, although referral to a medical subspecialty may be appropriate if investigations demonstrate an underlying condition, for example heart disease requiring a cardiology opinion. Frequent falls or persistent symptomatic orthostatic hypotension despite adhering to the advice in this chapter would warrant referral to a specialist 'falls prevention' clinic.

References

1. Freeman R, Wieling W, Axelrod FB, et al. Consensus statement on the definition of orthostatic hypotension, neurally mediated syncope and the postural tachycardia syndrome. *Clin Auton Res* 2011;21(2):69–72.
2. Rutan GH, Hermanson B, Bild DE, et al. Orthostatic hypotension in older adults. The Cardiovascular Health Study. CHS Collaborative Research Group. *Hypertension* 1992;19(6 Pt 1):508–519.
3. Schatz IJ. Orthostatic hypotension. I. Functional and neurogenic causes. *Arch Intern Med* 1984;144(4):773–777.
4. Sathyapalan T, Aye MM, Atkin SL. Postural hypotension. *BMJ* 2011;342:d3128.
5. Nwazue VC, Raj SR. Confounders of vasovagal syncope: orthostatic hypotension. *Cardiol Clin* 2013;31(1):89–100.
6. Fedorowski A, Melander O. Syndromes of orthostatic intolerance: a hidden danger. *J Intern Med* 2013;273(4):322–335.
7. Shibao C, Lipsitz LA, Biaggioni I. ASH position paper: evaluation and treatment of orthostatic hypotension. *J Clin Hypertens (Greenwich)* 2013;15(3):147–153.
8. Lanier JB, Mote MB, Clay EC. Evaluation and management of orthostatic hypotension. *Am Fam Physician* 2011;84(5):527–536.
9. Henry R, Rowe J, O'Mahony D. Haemodynamic analysis of efficacy of compression hosiery in elderly fallers with orthostatic hypotension. *Lancet* 1999;354(9172):45–46.
10. Clarke DA, Medow MS, Taneja I, et al. Initial orthostatic hypotension in the young is attenuated by static handgrip. *J Pediatr* 2010;156(6):1019–1022.e1.
11. Campbell IW, Ewing DJ, Clarke BF. 9-Alpha-fluorohydrocortisone in the treatment of postural hypotension in diabetic autonomic neuropathy. *Diabetes* 1975;24(4):381–384.
12. Schoffer KL, Henderson RD, O'Maley K, O'Sullivan JD. Nonpharmacological treatment, fludrocortisone, and domperidone for orthostatic hypotension in Parkinson's disease. *Mov Disord* 2007;22(11):1543–1549.
13. Rowe PC, Calkins H, DeBusk K, et al. Fludrocortisone acetate to treat neurally mediated hypotension in chronic fatigue syndrome: a randomized controlled trial. *JAMA* 2001;285(1):52–59.
14. Izcovich A, Gonzalez Malla C, Manzotti M, et al. Midodrine for orthostatic hypotension and recurrent reflex syncope: a systematic review. *Neurology* 2014;83(13):1170–1177.
15. Jankovic J, Gilden JL, Hiner BC, et al. Neurogenic orthostatic hypotension: a double-blind, placebo-controlled study with midodrine. *Am J Med* 1993;95(1):38–48.
16. Low PA, Gilden JL, Freeman R, et al. Efficacy of midodrine vs placebo in neurogenic orthostatic hypotension. A randomized, double-blind multicenter study. *JAMA* 1997;277(13):1046–1051.
17. Singer W, Sandroni P, Opfer-Gehrking TL, et al. Pyridostigmine treatment trial in neurogenic orthostatic hypotension. *Arch Neurol* 2006;63(4):513–518.
18. Kochar MS, Itskovitz HD. Treatment of idiopathic orthostatic hypotension (Shy–Drager syndrome) with indomethacin. *Lancet* 1978;i(8072):1011–1014.
19. Onrot J, Goldberg MR, Biaggioni I, et al. Hemodynamic and humoral effects of caffeine in autonomic failure. Therapeutic implications for postprandial hypotension. *N Engl J Med* 1985;313(9):549–554.
20. Hoeldtke RD, Streeten DH. Treatment of orthostatic hypotension with erythropoietin. *N Engl J Med* 1993;329(9):611–615.
21. Taylor D, Reveley A, Faivre F. Clozapine-induced hypotension treated with moclobemide and Bovril. *Br J Psychiatry* 1995;167(3):409–410.

Chapter 7

Peripheral Oedema
Thomas Whitehurst, Theresa McDonagh

Fluid accumulation in the interstitial compartment is termed oedema. This chapter discusses only palpable oedema found in distal dependent areas, i.e. *peripheral oedema*. In ambulant patients, peripheral oedema accumulates mostly in the lower limbs, but also occasionally in the distal upper limbs and, in bedbound patients, the sacrum.

Oedema occurs when the rate at which fluid filters from the capillaries is greater than the rate at which it is drained by the lymphatic system or reabsorbed into the capillaries [1]. Causes of oedema divide into those effecting an increase in capillary filtration, and those that decrease lymphatic drainage. Capillary filtration is dependent on several factors. Firstly, increased capillary pressure increases filtration. This may occur in association with right ventricular failure, deep vein thrombosis (DVT) or use of vasodilators. Furthermore, capillary permeability increases in inflamed areas, thereby increasing filtration. Finally, reduced capillary osmotic pressure, a common consequence of low albumin in association with malnutrition, nephrotic syndrome or liver disease, can also lead to oedema [1]. In developed countries, reductions in lymphatic drainage are mainly due to infiltration/compression by cancer, or secondary to cancer treatments such as lymphadenectomy or radiotherapy. However, worldwide, the most common cause is infection, with filariasis accounting for most cases [2].

Special considerations in the psychiatric population fall into three categories. Firstly, some psychotropic medications cause oedema directly (Table 7.1 and Box 7.1). Secondly, some may increase the risk of systemic illnesses that cause oedema. For example, the complications of lithium include hypothyroidism and renal disease, both of which can cause peripheral oedema. Thirdly, subsets of the psychiatric population may be at increased risk of systemic illness independent of medication effects, for example malnutrition occurring in severe depression or anorexia may lead to hypoalbuminaemia and oedema. A degree of interaction between these categories is also possible, as illustrated by the example of an acutely unwell person with a diagnosis of schizoaffective disorder

The Maudsley Practice Guidelines for Physical Health Conditions in Psychiatry, First Edition.
David M. Taylor, Fiona Gaughran, and Toby Pillinger.
© 2021 John Wiley & Sons Ltd. Published 2021 by John Wiley & Sons Ltd.

who is prescribed sodium valproate. Sodium valproate can cause acute bilateral oedema, which is reversible upon discontinuation, perhaps mediated by the effect of γ-aminobutyric acid (GABA) on capillary permeability [3]. Alternatively, valproate can induce hepatotoxicity, manifesting as peripheral oedema, jaundice, and ascites [4]. Furthermore, heart failure is more common in schizoaffective disorder (indeed it is more common in patients with serious mental illness in general) [5,6] and may present with shortness of breath on exertion and peripheral oedema [7].

DIAGNOSTIC PRINCIPLES

A clinical approach to assessment of peripheral oedema should first aim to rule out acute or life-threatening causes (e.g. DVT; see Chapter 18), followed by a systematic assessment aiming to examine for drug-induced or other causative systemic/localised conditions. Figure 7.1 presents an algorithmic approach to assessing a patient with peripheral oedema.

History

History of presenting complaint

1   Enquire as to the site, whether bilateral, unilateral or asymmetric. Bilateral oedema generally implies a systemic cause, whereas unilateral oedema suggests local venous obstruction, infection or lymphatic blockage. Swelling of the lower limb, sparing the feet and arising at puberty, is characteristic of lipoedema, mostly found in young women [27].

2   Define speed of onset and course of the swelling, and whether it is intermittent or persistent. Oedema developing over less than three days is generally considered acute, and chronic if developing over more than three days.

3   Enquire as to associated pain, redness or loss of function.

4   Enquire if there is a history of injury. Excluding DVT, the commonest cause of unilateral leg swelling is muscle strain or tear [82].

5   Enquire if there are any risk factors for DVT, including recent paralysis, immobility, orthopaedic surgery, pregnancy or malignancy (see Chapter 18).

6   Enquire if dietary intake has recently reduced significantly.

7   Enquire as to any symptoms suggestive of specific organ failure.

   a   Heart: reduced exercise tolerance and fatigue, progressing to orthopnoea, shortness of breath at rest, and peripheral oedema.

   b   Liver: jaundice, right upper quadrant pain, abdominal swelling, pale stools, bleeding (see Chapter 23).

   c   Kidney: reduced urine output, confusion, muscle weakness (see Chapters 34 and 73).

   d   Thyroid: intolerance to heat, hair loss, weight gain (see Chapter 12).

8   Foreign travel: other than long-haul flights increasing risk of DVT, travel to sub-Saharan Africa or Southeast Asia will increase risk of filariasis.

Table 7.1 Common causes of oedema in the general and psychiatric population.

	General population	Individuals with serious mental illness (SMI)
Systemic illness	Heart disease	Those with SMI are at increased risk of heart failure and death from coronary heart disease [5–7]. Antipsychotic use may underlie part of this increased risk, either through direct cardiotoxicity or by exacerbation of metabolic risk factors [10,11]. Myocarditis is more common in those taking clozapine (see Chapter 8) [12]. Abuse of alcohol, nicotine, and stimulants is more common in SMI [13] and increases risk of heart disease [14–16]
	Liver disease	Higher rates of chronic liver disease are observed in schizophrenia [17]. SMI is associated with higher rates of substance misuse, including alcoholism. There are higher rates of blood-borne viruses in those with schizophrenia and substance use disorders [18,19]. Deliberate overdose of commonly available medications often has a primary pathological effect on the liver, e.g. paracetamol
	Kidney disease	Kidney disease is a recognised adverse effect of lithium treatment [20] (see Chapter 34 for more information)
	Thyroid disease	Thyroid disease is increased with the use of first-generation antipsychotics [21]. Second-generation antipsychotics seem to have less propensity to cause hypothyroidism [22]. Prevalence of lithium-induced hypothyroidism is around 15% in women, around threefold the rate in men [23,24] (see Chapter 12 for more information
	Malnutrition/malabsorption	Starvation occurs in anorexia nervosa, catatonia, and severe depression. Malabsorption and malnutrition may occur in the context of alcohol abuse or excessive use of laxatives
	Obstructive sleep apnoea (OSA) may lead to oedema secondary to pulmonary hypertension [25]	OSA is more common in SMI compared to the general population [26] (see Chapter 49)
Medication	Antihypertensive drugs (especially calcium channel blockers and vasodilators, but also beta-blockers), steroids, hormone replacement (e.g. oestrogens, testosterone), non-steroidal anti-inflammatory drugs (NSAIDs), antidiabetics (e.g. glitazones) [8,27]	See Box 7.1

CHAPTER 7

(continued)

Table 7.1 (Continued)

	General population	Individuals with serious mental illness (SMI)
Deep vein thrombosis	Cancer, thrombotic disorder, inflammatory or infectious condition, obesity, pregnancy, hormone replacement or combined oral contraceptives, paralysis, dehydration	Meta-analysis has found that antipsychotic medication is a risk factor for DVT, especially in the elderly and those prescribed atypical antipsychotics, in particular clozapine [28]. Immobility in catatonia or depressive stupor, or secondary to seclusion and restraint, is associated with DVT [29,30] (see Chapter 18)
Cellulitis	Immunocompromise, injury or cut, diabetes, chronic skin conditions (e.g. eczema), obesity, intravenous drug use	Increased risk of bacterial infection in schizophrenia [31] Intravenous drug use is more common in SMI [32] Uncontrolled HIV infection is more common in SMI [33] Clozapine may reduce immune response, thereby increasing vulnerability to infection [34]
Trauma or muscle strain	History of injury or assault, competitive sport, high BMI, older age [35,36]	High psychiatric distress is a risk factor for musculoskeletal problems [37]
Chronic venous insufficiency	Hypertension, obesity, older age, family history, smoking, phlebitis, venous thromboembolism, standing occupation, possibly female sex [38]	Many risk factors, including smoking, hypertension and obesity, are more common in SMI [39–41]
Lymphoedema (oedema caused by blockage of lymphatic drainage)	Either primary (inherited) or secondary. Most often due to cancer, radiotherapy or lymphadenectomy. In developing world, helminth infection (filariasis) is most important cause	While cancer is no more common in SMI, those with SMI have lower cancer survival rates, likely due to later presentation with more advanced disease [42,43]. Therefore, infiltration of tumours into lymph nodes and vessels may be more likely. Cancer patients with SMI may be less likely to receive surgery or radiotherapy [43]. Repeated application of ligatures or tourniquets in those who self-harm can produce lymphoedema [44,45]
Complex regional pain syndrome	Initiated by trauma or immobility (usually a fracture in the upper limb). More common in elderly females	There is contradictory evidence as to whether this syndrome is more common in any particular psychiatric or psychological condition, although it is possible that anxiety, depression, and somatisation are associated [46]
Lipoedema	Genetic, possibly X-linked condition, arising in puberty, almost always in females. Distinguishable from obesity by pain and discomfort in affected areas, as well as ease of bruising. Diet and exercise have no effect on swelling [47]	
Physiological states	Peripheral oedema occurs in almost half of all healthy pregnancies, and is a non-specific sign of pre-eclampsia, although the latter can be investigated with a urine dipstick, testing renal function, and blood pressure monitoring (see Chapter 62) [48,49] Oedema is a well-described element of the premenstrual syndrome, although the most common sites are the breasts, upper arms, abdomen, and pelvis [50]	

Box 7.1 Psychiatric medication and risk of peripheral oedema

Antipsychotics

- Over half of a study of 49 outpatients taking olanzapine had oedema, although found with lower frequency in clinical trials (3%) [51]. There are case reports for quetiapine [52], risperidone [53], ziprasidone [54], paliperidone [55], clozapine [56], and amisulpiride [57]. A recent systematic review of self-limiting oedema associated with atypical antipsychotics reported such reactions had a mean onset in the fifth decade, were more common in females and usually occurred in the first four weeks of treatment [58]. There were more case reports for olanzapine, risperidone, and quetiapine than other atypicals.
- Pimavanserin, used for the treatment of Parkinson's psychosis, caused oedema in 7% of patients in phase III clinical trials (vs. 3% for placebo) [59].
- Antidepressants (monamine oxidase inhibitors): phenelzine (up to 10%) [60] and rasagiline (7% vs. 4% in placebo group) [61] are the most likely to cause oedema. Tranylcypromine [62] and isocarboxazid [63] have been found to cause oedema, albeit less frequently [64].
- Prescribing information for most selective serotonin reuptake inhibitors lists peripheral oedema as an 'infrequent side effect' (0.1–1% of patients), and oedema is not a common side effect of tricyclics [65–68].
- Trazodone [69] and venlafaxine [70] both have several cases reported.
- Mirtazapine has at least four cases reported as well as having oedema listed as a possible side effect in product literature, with an incidence of about 1% greater than placebo [71–73].
- Oedema occurs in bupropion treatment at a rate above 1% [74].
- Duloxetine was less likely to cause peripheral oedema than placebo in a large trial [75].

Mood stabilisers

- Sodium valproate [3], carbamazepine [76] and, very rarely, lamotrigine [77] can cause self-limiting peripheral oedema.
- Oedema in a patient treated with lithium should prompt assessment for systemic disease, particularly renal, cardiac and thyroid [78].

Others

- Pregabalin and gabapentin caused oedema in 5–15% of patients in clinical trials [64,79,80].
- Peripheral oedema is a recognised side effect of granulocyte colony-stimulating factor (GCSF), which may be used to increase neutrophil count during clozapine treatment (see Chapter 16) [81].

Past medical history

Record any history of systemic conditions that may predispose an individual to peripheral oedema, especially cardiac, kidney or liver disease (see Table 7.1). As already described, important risk factors for DVT include active cancer, cancer treated in the last six weeks, or previous history of DVT.

Medication history

See Table 7.1 and Box 7.1.

Family history

Thrombotic disorders, cancer, and familial lymphoedema.

CHAPTER 7

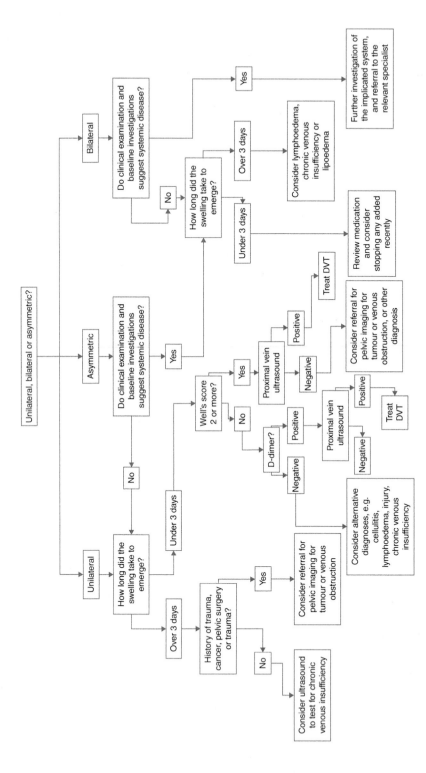

Figure 7.1 Algorithmic diagnostic approach to peripheral oedema. Source: adapted from diagrams in Trayes et al. [8] to reflect National Institute for Health and Care Excellence (NICE) guidelines on investigation for venous thrombosis [9].

Social history

1 Intravenous drug use is associated with both lymphatic blockage and chronic venous insufficiency, as well as systemic disease [83].
2 Quantify alcohol and nicotine use.

Examination

1 Basic observations: heart rate, blood pressure, respiratory rate, oxygen saturations, and temperature.
2 Measure weight and calculate body mass index (BMI).
3 Note whether the oedema is bilateral, unilateral or asymmetric.
4 Extent (to ankle, calf, thigh or entire leg) which may help assessment of progression of oedema over time.
5 Pitting or non-pitting (i.e. leaving no indentation when removing a finger after five seconds of pressure). Non-pitting oedema is associated with lymphoedema, although early lymphoedema may still exhibit pitting [84]. *Checking for pitting oedema may be uncomfortable for the patient, and therefore give warning prior to performing this assessment.*
6 Measure the circumference of the calves 10 cm below the tibial tuberosity. A difference of more than 3 cm between the two measurements is considered significantly asymmetric.
7 Skin changes: in cellulitis, skin may be red, hot, and tender; in chronic venous insufficiency, there is hardening, pigmentation, ulcers or prominent superficial veins; in pretibial myxoedema, thick, dry, 'orange peel' skin.
8 Dilated superficial veins or tenderness along the deep veins.
9 Note whether you can pinch and lift the skin over the dorsum of the second toe (negative Stemmer's sign). Positive Stemmer's sign is associated with lymphoedema.
10 Palpate for lymph nodes.
11 If leg oedema is present, check the arms and sacrum.
12 Cardiovascular and respiratory examination: signs of heart failure may include 'gallop' rhythm on auscultation, raised jugular venous pressure, and basal crackles on auscultation of the chest (pulmonary oedema).
13 Abdominal examination: ascites, jaundice, spider naevi, ascites or hepatomegaly in liver failure.
14 Examine the neck for signs of thyroid disease, and eyes for proptosis (see Chapter 12 for full thyroid examination).
15 Perform a general examination/inspection looking for skin folds indicating rapid weight loss, pallor in the conjunctiva or nails indicating malnutrition or anaemia, clubbing, palmar erythema, and evidence of intravenous injection.

If there is unilateral leg swelling, based on history and examination, calculate the revised Wells score for suspected DVT [9] (see Chapter 18).

CHAPTER 7

Investigations

Bloods

1 Full blood count.
2 Urea and electrolytes.
3 Liver function tests.
4 C-reactive protein.
5 If DVT suspected but Well's score is less than 2, send for a D-dimer [85] (see Chapter 18).
6 Thyroid function tests (if indicated by above assessment).
7 B-type natriuretic peptide (BNP) or N-terminal pro-hormone BNP (NTproBNP) if heart failure is suspected.
8 Addition of troponin if there is suspicion of acute heart failure.
9 Mid-stream urine dipstick to test for protein (renal disease).
10 ECG and chest X-ray may be useful if cardiac disease and/or pulmonary oedema is suspected.

For bilateral oedema, further investigation depends on history, examination, and initial investigation results. Where these indicate acute involvement of a particular organ system, refer to the relevant chapters (Chapter 73 for acute kidney injury, Chapter 23 for deranged liver function tests, Chapter 68 for shortness of breath, and Chapter 69 for acute coronary syndrome), and involve the relevant medical specialist. When initial assessment does not suggest systemic disease, lipoedema or chronic venous insufficiency, review medication. Calculating a Naranjo score may be helpful, by determining the likelihood of an adverse drug reaction (e.g. oedema) indeed being secondary to a drug [86].

In acute-onset unilateral oedema, proximal leg vein ultrasound is recommended if DVT is expected [9] (refer to Chapter 18 for further information). In unilateral oedema occurring over a longer time period, also consider pelvic imaging to exclude lymphatic obstruction and venous Doppler to assess for venous insufficiency [8].

MANAGEMENT

For peripheral oedema associated with chronic kidney disease, liver disease, and thyroid disease, the reader is directed to Chapters 34, 23 and 12, respectively. In the case of acute onset of heart failure with shortness of breath, transfer immediately to an emergency unit as immediate supportive care is necessary for these patients. A specialist heart failure multidisciplinary team should diagnose chronic heart failure, with first-line treatments including angiotensin-converting enzyme (ACE) inhibitors and beta-blockers, and diuretic therapy recommended to treat oedema [87].

The general approach to the treatment of peripheral oedema is the slow removal of excess fluid using diuretic therapy [88]. Daily weights and fluid input–output charts are used to monitor treatment progress. For heart failure and renal disease, the suggested rate of removal is between 1 and 3 l per day. In cirrhotic patients, removal of oedema from ascites at a rate of over 500 ml daily may lead to intravascular volume depletion, as peritoneal capillaries cannot absorb ascites any faster [89].

Thiazide diuretics, such as bendroflumethiazide and indapamide, reduce renal excretion of lithium, increasing serum lithium concentrations, and as such should be avoided in these patients [20]. Loop diuretics such as furosemide seem to have less effect on lithium concentration. The effect of diuretic treatment on lithium concentration is apparent in the first month [20]. Caution is advised in the use of lithium in heart failure. ACE inhibitors reduce lithium clearance, and plasma lithium levels should therefore be checked following initiation.

Diuretics all have the potential to cause electrolyte imbalance, which can exacerbate QTc prolongation if co-prescribed with other causative agents (see Chapter 3). Diuretics are also associated with orthostatic hypotension, exacerbating the effects of agents such as clozapine and olanzapine (see Chapter 6) [90].

Those with oedema secondary to chronic venous insufficiency should be referred to a vascular surgery service, where the mainstays of treatment are leg elevation, exercise to build calf strength, and compression stockings. Novel venoactive drugs may be of use [88,91,92]. Cellulitis may be managed in primary care with antibiotics, provided there are no signs of sepsis (see Chapter 72).

The prognosis is poor for lymphoedema, with progressive impairment likely [84,93]. Complex decongestive therapy performed by trained physiotherapists combines specialised massage techniques and compressive bandages to reduce swelling [84]. General measures such as limb elevation, keeping to a healthy weight, patient education, and psychosocial support may improve quality of life [94]. Diuretic therapy, once the diagnosis of lymphoedema is confirmed, is of little benefit and may cause harm (e.g. via electrolyte imbalance) [84].

References

1. Mortimer PS, Levick JR. Chronic peripheral oedema: the critical role of the lymphatic system. *Clin Med* 2004;4(5):448–453.
2. Joshi P. Epidemiology of lymphatic filariasis. In: Tyagi BK (ed.) *Lymphatic Filariasis*. Singapore: Springer, 2018:1–14.
3. Lin S-T, Chen C-S, Yen C-F, et al. Valproate-related peripheral oedema: a manageable but probably neglected condition. *Int J Neuropsychopharmacol* 2009;12(7):991–993.
4. Powell-Jackson P, Tredger J, Williams R. Hepatotoxicity to sodium valproate: a review. *Gut* 1984;25(6):673–681.
5. Bobes J, Arango C, Aranda P, et al. Cardiovascular and metabolic risk in outpatients with schizoaffective disorder treated with antipsychotics: results from the CLAMORS study. *Eur Psychiatry* 2012;27(4):267–274.
6. Correll CU, Solmi M, Veronese N, et al. Prevalence, incidence and mortality from cardiovascular disease in patients with pooled and specific severe mental illness: a large-scale meta-analysis of 3,211,768 patients and 113,383,368 controls. *World Psychiatry* 2017;16(2):163–180.
7. Curkendall SM, Mo J, Glasser DB, et al. Cardiovascular disease in patients with schizophrenia in Saskatchewan, Canada. *J Clin Psychiatry* 2004;65(5):715–720.
8. Trayes KP, Studdiford JS, Pickle S, Tully AS. Edema: diagnosis and management. *Am Fam Physician* 2013;88(2):102–110.
9. National Institute for Health and Care Excellence. *Venous Thromboembolic Diseases: Diagnosis, Management and Thrombophilia Testing*. Clinical Guideline CG144. London: NICE, 2012. Available at https://www.nice.org.uk/guidance/cg144/chapter/Recommendations#diagnosis-2 (accessed 3 May 2019).
10. Correll CU, Detraux J, De Lepeleire J, De Hert M. Effects of antipsychotics, antidepressants and mood stabilizers on risk for physical diseases in people with schizophrenia, depression and bipolar disorder. *World Psychiatry* 2015;14(2):119–136.
11. Vancampfort D, Correll CU, Galling B, et al. Diabetes mellitus in people with schizophrenia, bipolar disorder and major depressive disorder: a systematic review and large scale meta-analysis. *World Psychiatry* 2016;15(2):166–174.
12. Bellissima BL, Tingle MD, Cicović A, et al. A systematic review of clozapine-induced myocarditis. *Int J Cardiol* 2018;259:122–129.
13. Sara GE, Burgess PM, Malhi GS, et al. Stimulant and other substance use disorders in schizophrenia: prevalence, correlates and impacts in a population sample. *Aust N Z J Psychiatry* 2014;48(11):1036–1047.

CHAPTER 7

14. Peng S, French W, Pelikan P. Direct cocaine cardiotoxicity demonstrated by endomyocardial biopsy. *Arch Pathol Lab Med* 1989;113(8):842–845.
15. Karch S, Billingham M. The pathology and etiology of cocaine-induced heart disease. *Arch Pathol Lab Med* 1988;112(3):225–230.
16. Darke S, Kaye S, McKetin R, Duflou J. Major physical and psychological harms of methamphetamine use. *Drug Alcohol Rev* 2008;27(3):253–262.
17. Gabilondo A, Alonso-Moran E, Nuño-Solinis R, et al. Comorbidities with chronic physical conditions and gender profiles of illness in schizophrenia. Results from PREST, a new health dataset. *J Psychosom Res* 2017;93:102–109.
18. Bauer-Staeb C, Jörgensen L, Lewis G, et al. Prevalence and risk factors for HIV, hepatitis B, and hepatitis C in people with severe mental illness: a total population study of Sweden. *Lancet Psychiatry* 2017;4(9):685–693.
19. Hughes E, Bassi S, Gilbody S, et al. Prevalence of HIV, hepatitis B, and hepatitis C in people with severe mental illness: a systematic review and meta-analysis. *Lancet Psychiatry* 2016;3(1):40–48.
20. Taylor DM, Barnes TR, Young AH. *The Maudsley Prescribing Guidelines in Psychiatry*, 13th edn. Chichester: Wiley Blackwell, 2018.
21. Vedal TSJ, Steen NE, Birkeland KI, et al. Free thyroxine and thyroid-stimulating hormone in severe mental disorders: A naturalistic study with focus on antipsychotic medication. *J Psychiatr Res* 2018;106:74–81.
22. Khalil RB, Richa S. Thyroid adverse effects of psychotropic drugs: a review. *Clin Neuropharmacol* 2011;34(6):248–255.
23. Kirov G, Tredget J, John R, et al. A cross-sectional and a prospective study of thyroid disorders in lithium-treated patients. *J Affect Disord* 2005;87(2–3):313–317.
24. Johnston AM, Eagles JM. Lithium-associated clinical hypothyroidism: prevalence and risk factors. *Br J Psychiatry* 1999;175(4):336–339.
25. Blankfield RP, Hudgel DW, Tapolyai AA, Zyzanski SJ. Bilateral leg edema, obesity, pulmonary hypertension, and obstructive sleep apnea. *Arch Intern Med* 2000;160(15):2357–2362.
26. Stubbs B, Vancampfort D, Veronese N, et al. The prevalence and predictors of obstructive sleep apnea in major depressive disorder, bipolar disorder and schizophrenia: a systematic review and meta-analysis. *J Affect Disord* 2016;197:259–267.
27. Cho S, Atwood JE. Peripheral edema. *Am J Med* 2002;113(7):580–586.
28. Parker C, Coupland C, Hippisley-Cox J. Antipsychotic drugs and risk of venous thromboembolism: nested case-control study. *BMJ* 2010;341:c4245.
29. Morioka H, Nagatomo I, Yamada K, et al. Deep venous thrombosis of the leg due to psychiatric stupor. *Psychiatry Clin Neurosci* 1997;51(5):323–326.
30. De Hert M, Einfinger G, Scherpenberg E, et al. The prevention of deep venous thrombosis in physically restrained patients with schizophrenia. *Int J Clin Pract* 2010;64(8):1109–1115.
31. Pankiewicz-Dulacz M, Stenager E, Chen M, Stenager E. Incidence rates and risk of hospital registered infections among schizophrenia patients before and after onset of illness: a population-based nationwide register study. *J Clin Med* 2018;7(12):E485.
32. Gottesman II, Groome CS. HIV/AIDS risks as a consequence of schizophrenia. *Schizophr Bull* 1997;23(4):675–684.
33. Helleberg M, Pedersen MG, Pedersen CB, et al. Associations between HIV and schizophrenia and their effect on HIV treatment outcomes: a nationwide population-based cohort study in Denmark. *Lancet HIV* 2015;2(8):e344–e350.
34. Ponsford M, Castle D, Tahir T, et al. Clozapine is associated with secondary antibody deficiency. *Br J Psychiatry* 2019;214(2):83–89.
35. Toohey LA, Drew MK, Cook JL, et al. Is subsequent lower limb injury associated with previous injury? A systematic review and meta-analysis. *Br J Sports Med* 2017;51(23):1670–1678.
36. Heir T, Eide G. Age, body composition, aerobic fitness and health condition as risk factors for musculoskeletal injuries in conscripts. *Scand J Med Sci Sports* 1996;6(4):222–227.
37. Manninen P, Heliövaara M, Riihimäki H, Mäkelä P. Does psychological distress predict disability? *Int J Epidemiol* 1997;26(5):1063–1070.
38. Beebe-Dimmer JL, Pfeifer JR, Engle JS, Schottenfeld D. The epidemiology of chronic venous insufficiency and varicose veins. *Ann Epidemiol* 2005;15(3):175–184.
39. Holt RI, Peveler RC. Obesity, serious mental illness and antipsychotic drugs. *Diabetes Obes Metab* 2009;11(7):665–679.
40. McClave AK, McKnight-Eily LR, Davis SP, Dube SR. Smoking characteristics of adults with selected lifetime mental illnesses: results from the 2007 National Health Interview Survey. *Am J Public Health* 2010;100(12):2464–2472.
41. Patten SB, Williams JV, Lavorato DH, et al. Major depression as a risk factor for high blood pressure: epidemiologic evidence from a national longitudinal study. *Psychosom Med* 2009;71(3):273–279.
42. Kisely S, Crowe E, Lawrence D. Cancer-related mortality in people with mental illness. *JAMA Psychiatry* 2013;70(2):209–217.
43. Dalton SO, Suppli NP, Ewertz M, et al. Impact of schizophrenia and related disorders on mortality from breast cancer: a population-based cohort study in Denmark, 1995–2011. *Breast* 2018;40:170–176.
44. Matthews W, Wallis D. Patterns of self-inflicted injury. *Trauma* 2002;4(1):17–20.
45. Nwaejike N, Archbold H, Wilson DS. Factitious lymphoedema as a psychiatric condition mimicking reflex sympathetic dystrophy: a case report. *J Med Case Rep* 2008;2(1):216.
46. Borchers A, Gershwin ME. Complex regional pain syndrome: a comprehensive and critical review. *Autoimmun Rev* 2014;13(3):242–265.
47. Child AH, Gordon KD, Sharpe P, et al. Lipedema: an inherited condition. *Am J Med Genet A* 2010;152(4):970–976.
48. Thomson A, Hytten F, Billewicz W. The epidemiology of oedema during pregnancy. *J Obstet Gynaecol Br Commonw* 1967;74(1):1–10.
49. Robertson E. The natural history of oedema during pregnancy. *J Obstet Gynaecol Br Commonw* 1971;78(6):520–529.
50. Tacani PM, de Oliveira Ribeiro D, Guimarães BEB, et al. Characterization of symptoms and edema distribution in premenstrual syndrome. *Int J Womens Health* 2015;7:297–303.
51. Ng B, Postlethwaite A, Rollnik J. Peripheral oedema in patients taking olanzapine. *Int Clin Psychopharmacol* 2003;18(1):57–59.

52. Rozzini L, Ghianda D, Chilovi BV, et al. Peripheral oedema related to quetiapine therapy. *Drugs Aging* 2005;22(2):183–184.

53. Tamam L, Ozpoyraz N, Unal M. Oedema associated with risperidone. *Clin Drug Invest* 2002;22(6):411–414.

54. Ku H-L, Su T-P, Chou Y-H. Ziprasidone-associated pedal edema in the treatment of schizophrenia. *Prog Neuropsychopharmacol Biol Psychiatry* 2006;30(5):963–964.

55. Cicek E, Cicek IE, Uguz F. Bilateral pretibial edema associated with paliperidone palmitate long-acting injectable: a case report. *Clin Psychopharmacol Neurosci* 2017;15(2):184–186.

56. Durst R, Raskin S, Katz G, et al. Pedal edema associated with clozapine use. *Israel Med Assoc J* 2000;2(6):485–486.

57. Chen C-K, Chou Y-H. Amisulpride-associated pedal edema. *Eur Psychiatry* 2004;19(7):454–455.

58. Umar MU, Abdullahi AT. Self-limiting atypical antipsychotics-induced edema: clinical cases and systematic review. *Indian J Psychol Med* 2016;38(3):182–188.

59. Cummings J, Isaacson S, Mills R, et al. Pimavanserin for patients with Parkinson's disease psychosis: a randomised, placebo-controlled phase 3 trial. *Lancet* 2014;383(9916):533–540.

60. Middlefell R, Frost I, Egan G, Eaton H. A report on the effects of phenelzine (Nardil), a monoamine oxidase inhibitor, in depressed patients. *J Ment Sci* 1960;106(445):1533–1538.

61. Mylan Pharmaceuticals Inc. Rasagiline tablets, for oral use. Full prescribing information. https://www.accessdata.fda.gov/drugsatfda_docs/label/2017/201971Orig1s000lbl.pdf (accessed 17 May 2019).

62. Atkinson RM, Ditman KS. Tranylcypromine: a review. *Clin Pharmacol Ther* 1965;6(5):631–655.

63. Zisook S. Side effects of isocarboxazid. *J Clin Psychiatry* 1984;45(7 Pt 2):53–58.

64. Freeman R, Durso-DeCruz E, Emir B. Efficacy, safety, and tolerability of pregabalin treatment for painful diabetic peripheral neuropathy: findings from seven randomized, controlled trials across a range of doses. *Diabetes Care* 2008;31(7):1448–1454.

65. Trindade E, Menon D, Topfer L-A, Coloma C. Adverse effects associated with selective serotonin reuptake inhibitors and tricyclic antidepressants: a meta-analysis. *Can Med Assoc J* 1998;159(10):1245–1252.

66. Forest Pharmaceuticals Limited. Celexa (citalopram hydrobromide) tablets/oral solution. Package insert. https://www.accessdata.fda.gov/drugsatfda_docs/label/2009/020822s037,021046s015lbl.pdf (accessed 21 May 2019).

67. Forest Pharmaceuticals Limited. Lexapro (escitalopram oxalate). Package insert. https://www.accessdata.fda.gov/drugsatfda_docs/label/2009/021323s032,021365s023lbl.pdf (accessed 21 May 2019).

68. Pfizer Inc. Zoloft (sertraline hydrochloride). Package insert. https://www.accessdata.fda.gov/drugsatfda_docs/label/2009/019839s070,020990s032lbl.pdf (accessed 21 May 2019).

69. Barrnett J, Frances A, Kocsis J, et al. Peripheral edema associated with trazodone: a report of ten cases. *J Clin Psychopharmacol* 1985;5(3):161–164.

70. Ballon JS, Schulman MC. Venlafaxine and the rapid development of anasarca. *J Clin Psychopharmacol* 2006;26(1):97–98.

71. Kutscher EC, Lund BC, Hartman BA. Peripheral edema associated with mirtazapine. *Ann Pharmacother* 2001;35(11):1494–1495.

72. Saddichha S. Mirtazapine associated tender pitting pedal oedema. *Aust N Z J Psychiatry* 2014;48(5):487.

73. Lai FYX, Shankar K, Ritz S. Mirtazapine-associated peripheral oedema. *Aust N Z J Psychiatry* 2016;50(11):1108.

74. Hebert S. Bupropion (Zyban®, sustained-release tablets): reported adverse reactions. *Can Med Assoc J* 1999;160(7):1050–1051.

75. Wernicke J, Lledo A, Raskin J, et al. An evaluation of the cardiovascular safety profile of duloxetine. *Drug Saf* 2007;30(5):437–455.

76. Novartis Pharmaceuticals Corporation. Tegretol (carbamazepine). Package insert. https://www.accessdata.fda.gov/drugsatfda_docs/label/2009/016608s101,018281s048lbl.pdf (accessed 21 May 2019).

77. GlaxoSmithKline. Lamictal (lamotrigine). Prescribing information. https://www.accessdata.fda.gov/drugsatfda_docs/label/2009/020241s037s038,020764s030s031lbl.pdf (accessed 21 May 2019).

78. Gitlin M. Lithium side effects and toxicity: prevalence and management strategies. *Int J Bipolar Disord* 2016;4(1):27.

79. Pfizer Inc. Lyrica (pregabalin). Prescribing information. https://www.accessdata.fda.gov/drugsatfda_docs/label/2011/021446s026,022488s005lbl.pdf (accessed 21 May 2019).

80. Moore RA, Wiffen PJ, Derry S, Rice AS. Gabapentin for chronic neuropathic pain and fibromyalgia in adults. *Cochrane Database Syst Rev* 2014;(4):CD007938.

81. Rechner I, Brito-Babapulle F, Fielden J. Systemic capillary leak syndrome after granulocyte colony-stimulating factor (G-CSF). *Hematol J* 2003;4(1):54–56.

82. Smith CC. Clincial manifestations and evaluation of edema in adults. https://www.uptodate.com/contents/clinical-manifestations-and-evaluation-of-edema-in-adults.

83. Del Giudice P. Cutaneous complications of intravenous drug abuse. *Br J Dermatol* 2004;150(1):1–10.

84. Executive Committee. The diagnosis and treatment of peripheral lymphedema: 2016 consensus document of the International Society of Lymphology. *Lymphology* 2016;49(4):170–184.

85. Wells PS, Anderson DR, Rodger M, et al. Evaluation of D-dimer in the diagnosis of suspected deep-vein thrombosis. *N Engl J Med* 2003;349(13):1227–1235.

86. Naranjo CA, Busto U, Sellers EM, et al. A method for estimating the probability of adverse drug reactions. *Clin Pharmacol Ther* 1981;30(2):239–245.

87. National Institute for Health and Care Excellence. *Chronic Heart Failure in Adults: Diagnosis and Management.* NICE Guideline NG106. London: NICE, 2018. Available at https://www.nice.org.uk/guidance/ng106 (accessed 28 May 2019).

88. Sterns RH. General principles of the treatment of edema in adults. https://www.uptodate.com/contents/general-principles-of-the-treatment-of-edema-in-adults

CHAPTER 7

89. Boyer TD. Removal of ascites: what's the rush? *Gastroenterology* 1986;90(6):2022–2023.

90. Myers MG, Kearns PM, Kennedy D, Fisher R. Postural hypotension and diuretic therapy in the elderly. *Can Med Assoc J* 1978;119(6):581–585.

91. National Institute for Health and Care Excellence. *Varicose Veins: Diagnosis and Management.* Clinical Guideline CG168. London: NICE, 2013. Available at https://www.nice.org.uk/guidance/cg168 (accessed 28 May 2019).

92. Pittler MH, Ernst E. Horse chestnut seed extract for chronic venous insufficiency. *Cochrane Database Syst Rev* 2012;(11):CD003230.

93. International Society of Lymphology. The diagnosis and treatment of peripheral lymphedema: 2013 Consensus Document of the International Society of Lymphology. *Lymphology* 2013;46(1):1–11.

94. Mehrara B. Clinical staging and conservative management of peripheral oedema. https://www.uptodate.com/contents/clinical-staging-and-conservative-management-of-peripheral-lymphedema

Myocarditis

Thomas Whitehurst, Theresa McDonagh

Myocarditis (inflammation of the heart muscle) may be caused by a variety of infectious and non-infectious conditions (Table 8.1). In the general population, the most common cause of myocarditis in the northern hemisphere is viral infection. Worldwide, infection with HIV and *Trypanosoma cruzi* (Chagas disease) are responsible for most cases of myocarditis [1,2]. In the adult population, autopsy studies indicate that myocarditis is more common in males and in those aged under 40 [3,4]. The Global Burden of Diseases Study estimates the yearly prevalence as 22 per 100,000 [5].

Among patients with serious mental illness (SMI), myocarditis represents a rare but serious complication of clozapine treatment. Other considerations in this group are increased rates of risk factors for myocarditis such as substance abuse, exposure to infectious diseases, malnutrition, and exposure to toxins and unusual pathogens due to poor living conditions (see Table 8.1).

DIAGNOSTIC PRINCIPLES

International definitions of myocarditis generally specify that a diagnosis is based on immunohistochemical changes, although in clinical practice endomyocardial biopsy is rarely performed [6,32,33]. Diagnosis therefore relies on a combination of clinical presentation, biochemistry, electrocardiography (ECG), echocardiography and, potentially, cardiac magnetic resonance imaging (MRI) [6]. Myocarditis may be asymptomatic [4,34–36]. When symptoms occur, the most common is shortness of breath, followed by chest pain, flu-like symptoms, cough, and gastrointestinal disturbance [37]. Clinicians should view any presentation of acute-onset chest pain or shortness of breath as an emergency (see Chapters 67–69 for more information). The most common signs are

The Maudsley Practice Guidelines for Physical Health Conditions in Psychiatry, First Edition.
David M. Taylor, Fiona Gaughran, and Toby Pillinger.
© 2021 John Wiley & Sons Ltd. Published 2021 by John Wiley & Sons Ltd.

Table 8.1 Causes of myocarditis in the general population and special considerations in patients with serious mental illness.

	General population	Individuals with serious mental illness (SMI)
Viral	RNA viruses: enterovirsues, especially cocksackie B [3], but also coxsackie A, and polio. Also influenza, respiratory syncytial virus, mumps, rubella, dengue, yellow fever [6] DNA viruses: adenovirus, varicella, human herpes virus 6, cytomegalovirus, Epstein–Barr virus, varicella-zoster, HIV, hepatitis B and C [6]	Elevated rates of HIV and blood-borne viruses in those with schizophrenia [7,8]. Higher rates of infection with blood-borne viruses in those with substance use disorders [7,9]. Lower adherence to antiretrovirals and higher viral load in those with SMI [10,11]
Bacterial	Tuberculosis, *Streptococcus* Group A, *Staphylococcus*, *Legionella*, *Streptococcus pneumoniae*, gonorrhoea, *Chlamydia*, syphilis, *Bartonella*	Those with SMI are more likely to have any kind of bacterial infection, including a doubled risk of tuberculosis [12]. Intravenous drug use increases risk of bacterial myocardial infection. There is some evidence that clozapine may reduce immune response, thereby increasing vulnerability to infection [13]
Protozoal, fungal	*Trypanosoma cruzi* (most common cause in those living in Central and South America), *Toxoplasma*, *Aspergillus*, *Cryptococcus*, *Candida* [6]	Immunocompromise occurs in starvation, e.g. anorexia nervosa, catatonia, or depression in old age. Uncontrolled HIV more common in SMI [14]
Medication	Chemotherapy (e.g. fluorouracil, anthracyclines), Herceptin [6], antibiotics (e.g. penicillins, cephalosporins, sulfonamides, amphotericin B) [6], digoxin [15], antiepileptics [16]	Clozapine, lithium, dopamine analogues used in Parkinson's disease, barbiturates, and carbamazepine. Chlorpromazine, fluphenazine, haloperidol, and risperidone all associated with myocarditis in data-mining study of WHO adverse reactions [17]. Quetiapine [18] and olanzapine [19] in case reports only
Substances of abuse	Stimulants (e.g. cocaine [20,21], amphetamines [22], mephedrone [23], alcohol [24], cannabis [25–27], and inhalants [28])	
Systemic disorders	Diabetes mellitus, connective tissue disease, giant cell myocarditis, sarcoidosis, granulomatosis with polyangiitis, thyrotoxicosis, other autoimmune diseases	Diabetes mellitus secondary to psychotropic use. Thyroid disease in use of antipsychotics and lithium
Physiological states	Increased risk in peripartum women [29,30]	
Toxins	For example, iron, lead, arsenic Smallpox vaccine [6]	Tendency toward poorer living conditions and homeless in SMI. High prevalence of mental illness in those who have served in armed forces (who may have received smallpox vaccine) [31]

tachycardia and fever. More severe cases show evidence of heart failure, such as tachypnoea, peripheral oedema, orthopnoea (breathlessness on lying down) and raised jugular venous pressure [6].

History

History of presenting complaint

1 Most often non-specific symptoms, feeling generally unwell, flu-like illness.
2 Fever, with or without rigors.
3 Chest pain is present in about one-third of cases and has symptoms similar to those of ischaemic chest pain (heavy, central, crushing with radiation to the arm or jaw), atypical chest pain or pleuritic pain (sharp, worse on breathing deeply or leaning forward).
4 Symptoms of heart failure, starting with reduced exercise tolerance and fatigue, progressing to orthopnoea, shortness of breath at rest, and peripheral oedema.
5 Palpitations, sensation of fast heart rate and syncope.
6 Viral illness within the preceding weeks, which may have resolved prior to the onset of other symptoms. Gastroenteritis or upper respiratory tract infection are common forerunners of myocarditis.
7 Menstrual history (risk increases with pregnancy).
8 Associated symptoms may point to a systemic inflammatory/autoimmune condition: muscle aches and pains, joint pain, lymphadenopathy.
9 Recent travel history, especially to rural South America (Chagas disease).

Past medical history

1 Risk factors for myocarditis: autoimmune disease, infection screen (if HIV positive, assess concordance with treatment and last CD4 count; see Chapter 45).
2 Cardiovascular risk factors, e.g. hypertension, diabetes mellitus.

Medication history

1 See Table 8.1.
2 Check compliance, especially with potentially causative medication.

Family history

1 Similar symptoms in family members may suggest a familial cardiomyopathy.
2 Recent similar symptoms in family might suggest shared exposure to viral outbreak or environmental toxins.

Social history

1 Recreational drug use, especially cocaine, amphetamines, inhalants or barbiturates.
2 Quantify alcohol and nicotine use.

CHAPTER 8

Examination

1 Basic observations, including heart rate, blood pressure, respiratory rate, oxygen saturations, and temperature.
2 Cardiovascular and respiratory examination: signs of heart failure may include 'gallop' rhythm on auscultation, raised jugular venous pressure, peripheral oedema, bibasal crackles on auscultation of the chest (pulmonary oedema).
3 Neurological: altered consciousness indicating delirium, focal signs indicating central nervous system (CNS) infection as possible cause.
4 General: note height and weight (obesity is a poor prognostic factor) [34]. Evidence of arthritis (swelling or redness in the joints) or lymphadenopathy indicates an autoimmune cause. Evidence of liver disease (e.g. ascites, jaundice, spider naevi) might indicate alcohol/blood-borne viral cause.

Investigations

Bloods

1 C-reactive protein (CRP) and troponin are the most sensitive, if non-specific, tests for myocarditis.
2 Full blood count (FBC) may show raised white cell count and eosinophilia, the latter particularly prevalent in clozapine-induced myocarditis (CIM).
3 Urea and electrolytes.
4 Liver function tests.
5 B-type natriuretic peptide (BNP) or N-terminal pro-hormone BNP (NTproBNP) may help diagnose heart failure where there is ambiguity.
6 Where facilities allow, perform a viral screen including adenovirus, coxsackievirus A and B, cytomegalovirus, echovirus, influenza, respiratory syncytial virus, mumps, rubella, adenovirus, varicella, human herpes virus 6, Epstein–Barr virus, varicella-zoster, HIV, and hepatitis B and C.

ECG

Often normal, and not required to diagnose myocarditis. Mostly used to exclude other causes of the clinical presentation such as ischaemia. However, changes seen in myocarditis may include the following.

1 Sinus tachycardia is the most common finding in CIM [37] but is also a common benign side effect at clozapine initiation [38].
2 Of those with CIM, 24% display T-wave inversion, mostly in inferior and lateral leads (aVF, II, III, V4–V6) [37].
3 ST elevation, often in the anterior leads (V1–V3), is also common in myocarditis.
4 High-grade atrioventricular block is common in myocarditis caused by Lyme disease or sarcoidosis.

CHAPTER 8

Chest X-ray

May display cardiomegaly, pulmonary oedema, and bilateral pleural effusions if heart failure presents. Also helps to exclude other causes of raised inflammatory markers and chest pain, such as pneumonia.

Echocardiography

1 Left ventricular dysfunction.
2 Left ventricular dilation and wall motion abnormalities.

Specialist examinations

1 Cardiac MRI (examining for inflammatory hyperaemia and oedema, late gadolinium enhancement examining for scar formation).
2 Endomyocardial biopsy.

MANAGEMENT

Treat those with chest pain and ECG changes consistent with ischaemia as a medical emergency; patients should be transferred as an emergency to acute medical services (see Chapter 69). Similarly, acute rises in troponin alongside chest pain (even in the absence of ECG changes) merit immediate transfer of the patient for medical review.

The European Society of Cardiology (ESC) states that those suspected of having myocarditis who are 'haemodynamically unstable' should be managed in high dependency units [6]. For those patients awaiting transfer to such a unit, immediate supportive care is necessary and should include oxygen therapy to keep saturations above 94%, cardiac monitoring, analgesia, constant pulse oximetry, and iterative measurement of vital signs.

The ESC also recommends the hospitalisation of haemodynamically stable patients suspected as having myocarditis, because of the fast changing nature of this clinical presentation, and the potential for rapid development of arrhythmia and heart failure [6]. Those responsible for the care of psychiatric patients suspected of having myocarditis should involve cardiologists early and develop a plan of investigation and treatment together. Medical treatment includes angiotensin-converting enzyme inhibitors, diuretics, and beta-blockers [2]. Psychiatrists should review medication and consider stopping or switching treatments also known to contribute to myocarditis risk.

CLOZAPINE-INDUCED MYOCARDITIS

Myocarditis is an established complication of clozapine treatment [37]. CIM most often occurs within the first two weeks of treatment [37,39]. Some estimates of the

CHAPTER 8

prevalence of CIM are up to two orders of magnitude greater than the lowest estimates, with the highest estimates coming from studies conducted in Australia [34,40,41]. Kilian and colleagues [42] estimated that the rate of myocarditis is 2000 times higher in the first month of treatment with clozapine than it is in the general population. CIM is associated with significant mortality, although estimates vary greatly [43]. Many countries have established national monitoring protocols for CIM, and subsequent reporting of non-fatal suspected CIM to national databases in these countries has increased dramatically, without an increase in fatal cases or a comparable increase in prescription of clozapine [44,45]. Contrary to the Australian data, a 2017 retrospective study of over 800 patients commenced on clozapine at a UK institution using a similar monitoring protocol found an incidence of only 0.11% [38].

Despite the wide range of incidence estimates, most authors agree on several key points. Clozapine is an effective antipsychotic shown to reduce all-cause mortality [46]. The better the treatment of the psychiatric symptoms of those with schizophrenia, the better treated their physical health problems [38]. Clozapine is underused and discontinued too often, denying many people with schizophrenia optimum treatment [47,48]. Testing of troponin and CRP during clozapine titration is a reasonable way of monitoring for myocarditis, although there is no direct evidence that such protocols reduce mortality [38,44,45]. A recommended monitoring regimen for emergent myocarditis during the first four weeks of treatment is shown in Box 8.1.

Box 8.1 Recommended monitoring for myocarditis on starting clozapine

- Daily measurement of pulse, temperature, and respiratory rate.
- Baseline measurement of FBC, CRP, troponin, ECG, and echocardiography.
- Weekly troponin and CRP (for first four weeks).
- Stop clozapine if CRP rises above 100 mg/L *or* troponin double the upper limit of normal. Refer for echocardiography.
- Switch to daily troponin and CRP monitoring if there is fever, tachycardia plus either CRP or troponin above normal limits [49].

Clozapine re-challenge post myocarditis

There have been reports of 19 patients being re-challenged with clozapine following CIM [37]; seven developed CIM for a second time, while re-challenge was successful in the remaining 12. National Institute for Health and Care Excellence (NICE) guidelines recommend that the clinician 'discontinue permanently' clozapine in those diagnosed with CIM [37]. In patients where clozapine represents the only viable treatment option for severe psychotic symptoms, a risk–benefit decision needs to be made regarding re-challenge and must involve multidisciplinary discussion involving both psychiatry and cardiology. Considering the significant risk of myocarditis reoccurring, clozapine re-challenge after CIM should be carried out in an inpatient setting (ideally a specialist psychiatric setting) in collaboration with cardiology colleagues, with vigilant monitoring of CRP and troponin and echocardiography [39].

CHAPTER 8

References

1. Schofield CJ, Dias JCP. The Southern Cone Initiative against Chagas disease. *Adv Parasitol* 1999;42:1–27.

2. Feldman AM, McNamara D. Myocarditis. *N Engl J Med* 2000;343(19):1388–1398.

3. Friman G, Wesslen L, Fohlman J, et al. The epidemiology of infectious myocarditis, lymphocytic myocarditis and dilated cardiomyopathy. *Eur Heart J* 1995;16(Suppl O):36–41.

4. Kytö V, Saraste A, Voipio-Pulkki L-M, Saukko P. Incidence of fatal myocarditis: a population-based study in Finland. *Am J Epidemiol* 2007;165(5):570–574.

5. Vos T, Barber RM, Bell B, et al. Global, regional, and national incidence, prevalence, and years lived with disability for 301 acute and chronic diseases and injuries in 188 countries, 1990–2013: a systematic analysis for the Global Burden of Disease Study 2013. *Lancet* 2015;386(9995):743–800.

6. Caforio AL, Pankuweit S, Arbustini E, et al. Current state of knowledge on aetiology, diagnosis, management, and therapy of myocarditis: a position statement of the European Society of Cardiology Working Group on Myocardial and Pericardial Diseases. *Eur Heart J* 2013;34(33):2636–2648.

7. Bauer-Staeb C, Jörgensen L, Lewis G, et al. Prevalence and risk factors for HIV, hepatitis B, and hepatitis C in people with severe mental illness: a total population study of Sweden. *Lancet Psychiatry* 2017;4(9):685–693.

8. Hughes E, Bassi S, Gilbody S, et al. Prevalence of HIV, hepatitis B, and hepatitis C in people with severe mental illness: a systematic review and meta-analysis. *Lancet Psychiatry* 2016;3(1):40–48.

9. Degenhardt L, Charlson F, Stanaway J, et al. Estimating the burden of disease attributable to injecting drug use as a risk factor for HIV, hepatitis C, and hepatitis B: findings from the Global Burden of Disease Study 2013. *Lancet Infect Dis* 2016;16(12):1385–1398.

10. Dalseth N, Reed RS, Hennessy M, et al. Does diagnosis make a difference? Estimating the impact of an HIV medication adherence intervention for persons with serious mental illness. *AIDS Behav* 2018;22(1):265–275.

11. Rooks-Peck CR, Adegbite AH, Wichser ME, et al. Mental health and retention in HIV care: a systematic review and meta-analysis. *Health Psychol* 2018;37(6):574–585.

12. Pankiewicz-Dulacz M, Stenager E, Chen M, Stenager E. Incidence rates and risk of hospital registered infections among schizophrenia patients before and after onset of illness: a population-based nationwide register study. *J Clin Med* 2018;7(12):E485.

13. Ponsford M, Castle D, Tahir T, et al. Clozapine is associated with secondary antibody deficiency. *Br J Psychiatry* 2019;214(2):83–89.

14. Helleberg M, Pedersen MG, Pedersen CB, et al. Associations between HIV and schizophrenia and their effect on HIV treatment outcomes: a nationwide population-based cohort study in Denmark. *Lancet HIV* 2015;2(8):e344–e350.

15. Matsumori A, Igata H, Ono K, et al. High doses of digitalis increase the myocardial production of proinflammatory cytokines and worsen myocardial injury in viral myocarditis. *Jpn Circ J* 1999;63(12):934–940.

16. Zaidi AN. Anticonvulsant hypersensitivity syndrome leading to reversible myocarditis. *Can J Clin Pharmacol* 2005;12(1):e33–e40.

17. Coulter DM, Bate A, Meyboom RH, et al. Antipsychotic drugs and heart muscle disorder in international pharmacovigilance: data mining study. *BMJ* 2001;322(7296):1207–1209.

18. Roesch-Ely D, Van Einsiedel R, Kathöfer S, et al. Myocarditis with quetiapine. *Am J Psychiatry* 2002;159(9):1607–1608.

19. Vang T, Rosenzweig M, Bruhn CH, et al. Eosinophilic myocarditis during treatment with olanzapine: report of two possible cases. *BMC Psychiatry* 2016;16(1):70.

20. Peng S, French W, Pelikan P. Direct cocaine cardiotoxicity demonstrated by endomyocardial biopsy. *Arch Pathol Lab Med* 1989;113(8):842–845.

21. Karch S, Billingham M. The pathology and etiology of cocaine-induced heart disease. *Arch Pathol Lab Med* 1988;112(3):225–230.

22. Mortelmans LJ, Bogaerts PJ, Hellemans S, et al. Spontaneous pneumomediastinum and myocarditis following Ecstasy use: a case report. *Eur J Emerg Med* 2005;12(1):36–38.

23. Nicholson D, Quinn MJ, Dodd JD. Headshop heartache: acute mephedrone 'meow' myocarditis. *Heart* 2010;96(24):2051–2052.

24. Wilke A, Kaiser A, Ferency I, Maisch B. Alcohol and myocarditis. *Herz* 1996;21(4):248–257.

25. Tournebize J, Gibaja V, Puskarczyk E, et al. Myocarditis associated with cannabis use in a 15-year-old boy: a rare case report. *Int J Cardiol* 2016;203:243–244.

26. Nappe TM, Hoyte CO. Pediatric death due to myocarditis after exposure to cannabis. *Clin Pract Cases Emerg Med* 2017;1(3):166–170.

27. Tournebize J, Gibaja V, Puskarczyk E, et al. Myocarditis and cannabis: an unusual association. *Toxicologie Analytique et Clinique* 2016;28(3):236.

28. Dinsfriend W, Rao K, Matulevicius S. Inhalant-abuse myocarditis diagnosed by cardiac magnetic resonance. *Texas Heart Inst J* 2016;43(3):246–248.

29. Felker GM, Jaeger CJ, Klodas E, et al. Myocarditis and long-term survival in peripartum cardiomyopathy. *Am Heart J* 2000;140(5):785–791.

30. Midei MG, DeMent SH, Feldman AM, et al. Peripartum myocarditis and cardiomyopathy. *Circulation* 1990;81(3):922–928.

31. Hoge CW, Castro CA, Messer SC, et al. Combat duty in Iraq and Afghanistan, mental health problems, and barriers to care. *N Engl J Med* 2004;351(1):13–22.

32. Leone O, Veinot JP, Angelini A, et al. 2011 Consensus statement on endomyocardial biopsy from the Association for European Cardiovascular Pathology and the Society for Cardiovascular Pathology. *Cardiovasc Pathol* 2012;21(4):245–274.

33. Richardson P. Report of the 1995 World Health Organization/International Society and Federation of Cardiology Task Force on the definition and classification of cardiomyopathies. *Circulation* 1996;93:841–842.

34. Ronaldson KJ, Fitzgerald PB, Taylor AJ, et al. Clinical course and analysis of ten fatal cases of clozapine-induced myocarditis and comparison with 66 surviving cases. *Schizophr Res* 2011;128(1–3):161–165.

35. Burlo P, Comino A, Di Gioia V, et al. Adult myocarditis in a general hospital: observations on 605 autopsies. *Pathologica* 1995;87(6):646–649.

36. Passarino G, Burlo P, Ciccone G, Comino A. Prevalence of myocarditis at autopsy in Turin, *Italy*. *Arch Pathol Lab Med* 1997;121(6):619–622.

37. Bellissima BL, Tingle MD, Cicović A, et al. A systematic review of clozapine-induced myocarditis. *Int J Cardiol* 2018;259:122–129.

38. Joy G, Whiskey E, Bolstridge M, et al. Hearts and minds: real-life cardiotoxicity with clozapine in psychosis. *J Clin Psychopharmacol* 2017;37(6):708–712.

39. Knoph KN, Morgan RJ III, Palmer BA, et al. Clozapine-induced cardiomyopathy and myocarditis monitoring: a systematic review. *Schizophr Res* 2018;199:17–30.

40. Youssef DL, Narayanan P, Gill N. Incidence and risk factors for clozapine-induced myocarditis and cardiomyopathy at a regional mental health service in Australia. *Australas Psychiatry* 2016;24(2):176–180.

41. Reinders J, Parsonage W, Lange D, et al. Clozapine-related myocarditis and cardiomyopathy in an Australian metropolitan psychiatric service. *Aust N Z J Psychiatry* 2004;38(11–12):915–922.

42. Kilian JG, Kerr K, Lawrence C, Celermajer DS. Myocarditis and cardiomyopathy associated with clozapine. *Lancet* 1999;354(9193):1841–1845.

43. Citrome L, McEvoy JP, Saklad SR. Guide to the management of clozapine-related tolerability and safety concerns. *Clin Schizophr Relat Psychoses* 2016;10(3):163–177.

44. Ronaldson K, Fitzgerald P, McNeil J. Clozapine-induced myocarditis, a widely overlooked adverse reaction. *Acta Psychiatr Scand* 2015;132(4):231–240.

45. Neufeld NH, Remington G. Clozapine-induced myocarditis in Canada: evidence from spontaneous reports. *Schizophr Res* 2019;206:462–463.

46. Tiihonen J, Lönnqvist J, Wahlbeck K, et al. 11-year follow-up of mortality in patients with schizophrenia: a population-based cohort study (FIN11 study). *Lancet* 2009;374(9690):620–627.

47. Howes OD, Vergunst F, Gee S, et al. Adherence to treatment guidelines in clinical practice: study of antipsychotic treatment prior to clozapine initiation. *Br J Psychiatry* 2012;201(6):481–485.

48. Joy G, Bolstridge M, Whiskey E, et al. Characterisation of clozapine referrals to a tertiary cardiology unit. *Heart* 2017;103(Suppl 5):A7–A8.

49. Taylor DM, Barnes TR, Young AH. *The Maudsley Prescribing Guidelines in Psychiatry*, 13th edn. Chichester: Wiley Blackwell, 2018.

CHAPTER 8

Chapter 9

Hypercholesterolaemia
Dipen Patel, Toby Pillinger, Narbeh Melikian

Hypercholesterolaemia describes elevated total or low-density lipoprotein (LDL) cholesterol levels in the blood. Dyslipidaemia is a broader term used to describe hypercholesterolaemia accompanied by low levels of high-density lipoprotein (HDL) cholesterol and/or raised triglycerides. Dyslipidaemia plays a significant role in the development of atherosclerosis (a condition where deposition of cholesterol-rich particles in the wall of arteries results in progressive narrowing of vessels). Along with smoking, type 2 diabetes mellitus and hypertension, dyslipidaemia is a key modifiable risk factor for cardiovascular disease (CVD) [1]. It is now well recognised that reducing cholesterol levels improves cardiovascular prognosis (including reducing rates of myocardial infarction and death) in individuals with (secondary prevention) and without (primary prevention) established CVD [2,3].

Compared with the general population, people with serious mental illness (SMI) have a significantly reduced life expectancy [2]. The majority of this excess mortality is secondary to physical health conditions, in particular CVD. Mortality from CVD is approximately three times greater in people with SMI compared with the general population [3]. People with SMI have a higher prevalence of CVD risk factors, including obesity, hypertension, diabetes mellitus, and dyslipidaemia [4]. This is driven in part by physical inactivity, unhealthy dietary choices, high rates of smoking, and antipsychotic medication [5]. Common causes of hypercholesterolaemia in the general and psychiatric population are documented in Box 9.1.

The Maudsley Practice Guidelines for Physical Health Conditions in Psychiatry, First Edition.
David M. Taylor, Fiona Gaughran, and Toby Pillinger.
© 2021 John Wiley & Sons Ltd. Published 2021 by John Wiley & Sons Ltd.

Box 9.1 Causes of hypercholesterolaemia

Primary (unmodifiable) causes

- Congenital (e.g. familial hypercholesterolaemia and familial combined hyperlipidaemia)
- Increasing age
- Male gender

Secondary (modifiable) causes

- Diet[a]
- Smoking[a]
- Alcohol[a]
- Medical conditions (e.g. diabetes mellitus,[a] chronic liver or kidney disease,[a] hypothyroidism[a])
- Obesity[a]
- Medications: ciclosporin, glucocorticoids, antiretrovirals, retinoic acid derivatives, oral contraceptive pill, atypical antipsychotics,[a] some mood stabilisers[a] (e.g. sodium valproate and lithium), and antidepressants[a]

[a]Factors more common in patients with SMI compared with the general population.

DIAGNOSTIC PRINCIPLES

History

Hypercholesterolaemia is asymptomatic and usually identified during routine blood screening or when an individual presents with a clinical complication of established CVD disease (such as a myocardial infarction or stroke).

Therefore, the history should focus on (i) identifying evidence of underlying risk factors for hypercholesterolaemia (which may then be modified); (ii) identifying physical comorbidity, the presence of which may influence the management plan (e.g. presence of CVD should prompt secondary CVD prevention initiatives); and (iii) identifying symptoms suggestive of CVD which may have been hitherto undiagnosed (which will require further investigation).

As such, the following should be elucidated.

1 Symptoms indicative of CVD, for example angina (chest discomfort during exertion or stress) or intermittent arterial claudication (calf discomfort during exertion).
2 Past medical history:
   a established CVD and/or presence or classical risk factors for CVD
   b alternative risk factors for raised cholesterol, e.g. type 2 diabetes mellitus, chronic liver disease, chronic kidney disease, hypothyroidism, polycystic ovary syndrome, specific medication (such as selective immunosuppressants) that can elevate cholesterol levels (Box 9.1).
3 Social history:
   a excess alcohol
   b smoking status

 c diet (cholesterol-rich diet such as excess consumption of all dairy products, shell-fish, red meat, and fried food)

 d amount of exercise engaged in on a weekly basis.

4 Family history of premature CVD (defined as diagnosis of CVD in first-degree relative below the age of 55 years for men and 65 years for women) and hypercholesterolaemia.

Examination

Check basic observations to examine for comorbid hypertension and calculate body mass index (BMI) to guide need for weight loss. Examination may be unremarkable. However, in the case of familial hypercholesterolaemia, corneal arcus (white or grey opaque ring in margin of cornea) or tendon xanthomata (nodules attached to tendons in hands, feet, and Achilles tendon) may be observed. If history suggests presence of CVD, a cardiovascular and peripheral vascular examination is indicated (the results of which may be included in a referral to cardiology/vascular services).

Investigations

1 Blood tests:

 a fasting full lipid profile including total cholesterol, LDL cholesterol, HDL cholesterol, and triglycerides

 b urea and electrolytes

 c liver function tests

 d HbA_{1c}

 e thyroid function tests.

2 Urine dipstick: proteinuria (suggestive of kidney disease) or glucosuria (suggestive of diabetes mellitus).

3 ECG: evidence of ischaemic heart disease.

DIAGNOSTIC CRITERIA

The European Society of Cardiology (ESC) guideline considers patients in terms of different levels of risk and targets reflect the different level of risk (readers are directed to this resource for further information). However, the guidance states that in general total plasma cholesterol should be less than 5 mmol/L (<190 mg/dL) and LDL cholesterol should be less than 3 mmol/L (<115 mg/dL) (for low-risk individuals) [6]. If total cholesterol is above 7.5 mmol/L and/or there is a family history of premature heart disease, consider a diagnosis of familial hypercholesterolaemia.

MANAGEMENT

The aim of treating hypercholesterolaemia is to reduce the risk of mortality and morbidity from CVD. Management approaches should always, where possible, include non-pharmacological approaches. Of note, although raised triglyceride is a risk factor for CVD, there is currently insufficient evidence to support the practice of pharmacologically lowering triglyceride levels for CVD risk reduction.

Lifestyle modification

There is clear evidence that lifestyle modification reduces the risk of developing CVD. A recent meta-analysis found that, compared with usual care, lifestyle interventions (specifically dietary modification and exercise) achieved significant improvements in total cholesterol [7]. Patients should be advised to follow a diet that is low in fatty food, to replace saturated fats with unsaturated fats (e.g. olive oil), to limit total calorific intake (2000 kcal/day for women, 2500 kcal/day for men; see Chapter 14), and to reduce alcohol intake. Patients should also be advised to undertake at least 150 minutes of moderate-intensity aerobic activity or 75 minutes of vigorous intensity aerobic activity weekly (see Chapter 10 for further details) [8].

Rationalisation of antipsychotic medication

Clozapine, olanzapine, and quetiapine are associated with increased risk of weight gain and lipid disturbance compared with other antipsychotics [9,10]. Similarly, certain mood stabilisers and antidepressants increase risk of weight gain (see Chapter 14), and therefore by association hypercholesterolaemia. As such, where hypercholesterolaemia is identified in a patient with SMI taking a psychiatric medication that may be at least partially causative, a multidisciplinary discussion is indicated involving the psychiatrist, primary care doctor, and ideally the patient to discuss the most appropriate course of action. This will involve a risk–benefit discussion weighing up the benefits of ongoing treatment (improved mental state) versus the risks (increased CVD risk), and where appropriate consideration of alternative treatments with more benign CVD risk (see Chapter 14).

Pharmacological treatment

Lipid modification therapy should be offered to all patients with established CVD as part of secondary prevention initiatives. A high-intensity statin treatment (e.g. atorvastatin 80 mg once daily) is recommended (Box 9.2). The initial target is to achieve a 40% or greater reduction in non-HDL cholesterol after 3 months [8].

In the primary prevention of CVD, where lifestyle interventions fail to bring cholesterol levels to within optimal range, statin therapy should be considered. National Institute for Health and Care Excellence (NICE) guidelines advocate the use of the Q-RISK2 calculator to guide the need for lipid-modifying therapy. This tool estimates the risk of heart attack or stroke for a given individual over a 10-year period based on various CVD risk factors (e.g. age, ethnicity, comorbidity, and cholesterol levels). We would however advocate the use of the updated Q-RISK3 tool [11], which factors in a diagnosis of SMI and prescription of second-generation antipsychotics as part of its CVD risk calculation. Patients should be offered lipid-modification therapy (e.g. atorvastatin 20 mg daily) if they present with a 10-year CVD risk of 10% or greater. As in

Hypercholesterolaemia   83

CHAPTER 9

--

Box 9.2 Intensities of statin therapy available

All doses are once daily by mouth

High-intensity statin therapy

Atorvastatin 20–80 mg
Rosuvastatin 10–20 mg
Simvastatin 80 mg

Moderate-intensity statin therapy

Atorvastatin 10 mg
Rosuvastatin 5 mg
Simvastatin 10–40 mg
Pravastatin 40–80 mg
Lovastatin 40 mg

--

secondary prevention, the initial target is to achieve a 40% or greater reduction in non-HDL cholesterol after 3 months [8]. NICE also advises considering statin therapy for patients with type 1 diabetes who are over the age of 40, patients who have had diabetes mellitus for more than 10 years, or those with chronic kidney disease or other CVD risk factors.

In the USA, the American College of Cardiology (ACC)/American Heart Association (AHA) recommend treating those with an estimated 10-year CVD risk of 7.5% or more with 'moderate-to-high intensity' statin therapy, and those with a risk of 5–7.5% with 'moderate-intensity' therapy (see Box 9.2 for intensities of statin therapy available) [12]. Muscle/joint discomfort, indigestion, and deranged liver function tests are common side effects of treatment with statins. Serious or life-threatening side effects such as myositis, rhabdomyolysis, and liver dysfunction are rare. Discuss the risks and benefits of statin treatment so that the patient can make an informed choice about their treatment. Counsel regarding the clear cardiovascular benefits of reducing cholesterol levels using a statin. Also outline that the adverse effects of statins are generally mild, reversible, and not medically serious. Myositis and rhabdomyolysis are rare, with estimated incidences of 5 per 100,000 person-years and 1.6 per 100,000 person-years, respectively [8]. In the context of risk of myositis, if a patient has persistent generalized unexplained muscle pain (whether associated with previous lipid-lowering therapy or not) measure creatine kinase (CK) levels. If CK or liver function tests are abnormal, then stop the statin and discuss with general medical colleagues if there are concerns regarding renal or hepatic function. If tests correct after stopping the statin, then the culprit is clear, and lipid clinic advice should be sought. In the case of symptom resolution after myositis, options include switching to a moderate-intensity statin (e.g. pravastatin) if side effects occurred with a high-intensity statin, or dose reduction if the patient was on a moderate-intensity statin. Ezetimibe, which inhibits intestinal absorption of cholesterol, may be used where statin treatment is inappropriate or not tolerated (10 mg once daily by mouth). PCSK9 inhibitors (e.g. evolocumab and alirocumab), given as subcutaneous injections every two to four weeks, can also be used where statins are not tolerated [13].

When to refer

Hypercholesterolaemia can normally be managed by primary care physicians. However, a lipid clinic referral is indicated for any patient who may have a diagnosis of familial hypercholesterolaemia, if desired cholesterol level is not achieved despite appropriate intervention, or where there may be contraindications/side effects to statin therapy (e.g. persistently raised CK levels). A cardiology referral should be made in any patient where hitherto undiagnosed CVD has been identified (e.g. via a rapid-access chest pain clinic).

References

1. Helkin A, Stein JJ, Lin S, et al. Dyslipidemia Part 1. Review of lipid metabolism and vascular cell physiology. *Vasc Endovascular Surg* 2016;50(2):107–118.
2. Chesney E, Goodwin GM, Fazel S. Risks of all-cause and suicide mortality in mental disorders: a meta-review. *World Psychiatry* 2014;13(2):153–160.
3. Osborn DPJ, Levy G, Nazareth I, et al. Relative risk of cardiovascular and cancer mortality in people with severe mental illness from the United Kingdom's General Practice Research Database. *Arch Gen Psychiatry* 2007;64(2):242–249.
4. Mitchell AJ, Vancampfort D, Sweers K, et al. Prevalence of metabolic syndrome and metabolic abnormalities in schizophrenia and related disorders: a systematic review and meta-analysis. *Schizophr Bull* 2013;39(2):306–318.
5. Baller JB, McGinty EE, Azrin ST, et al. Screening for cardiovascular risk factors in adults with serious mental illness: a review of the evidence. *BMC Psychiatry* 2015;15:55.
6. Perk J, De Backer G, Gohlke H, et al. European Guidelines on cardiovascular disease prevention in clinical practice (version 2012). The Fifth Joint Task Force of the European Society of Cardiology and Other Societies on Cardiovascular Disease Prevention in Clinical Practice (constituted by representatives of nine societies and by invited experts). *Eur Heart J* 2012;33(13):1635–1701.
7. Zhang X, Devlin HM, Smith B, et al. Effect of lifestyle interventions on cardiovascular risk factors among adults without impaired glucose tolerance or diabetes: a systematic review and meta-analysis. *PLoS One* 2017;12(5):e0176436.
8. National Institute for Health and Care Excellence. Lipid modification: CVD prevention. Last revised: August 2019. https://cks.nice.org.uk/lipid-modification-cvd-prevention
9. Rummel-Kluge C, Komossa K, Schwarz S, et al. Head-to-head comparisons of metabolic side effects of second generation antipsychotics in the treatment of schizophrenia: a systematic review and meta-analysis. *Schizophr Res* 2010;123(2–3):225–233.
10. Pillinger T, McCutcheon R, Vano L, et al. Comparative effects of 18 antipsychotics on metabolic function in patients with schizophrenia, predictors of metabolic dysregulation, and association with psychopathology: a systematic review and network meta-analysis. *Lancet Psychiatry* 2020;7:64–77.
11. ClinkRisk. The QRISK3-2018 risk calculator. https://qrisk.org/three/.
12. Stone NJ, Robinson JG, Lichtenstein AH, et al. 2013 ACC/AHA guideline on the treatment of blood cholesterol to reduce atherosclerotic cardiovascular risk in adults: a report of the American College of Cardiology/American Heart Association Task Force on Practice Guidelines *Circulation* 2014;129(25 Suppl 2):S46–S48.
13. Chaudhary R, Garg J, Shah N, Sumner A. PCSK9 inhibitors: a new era of lipid lowering therapy. *World J Cardiol* 2017;9(2):76–91.

Physical Activity

Garcia Ashdown-Franks, Brendon Stubbs

Physical activity (PA) is defined as 'any bodily movement produced by skeletal muscles requiring energy expenditure' [1]. As such, PA involves a range of activities such as light workplace or leisure-time activity including housework, moving around at work, sport, leisure activities, or exercise. Exercise is a planned and structured form of PA, with the objective of improving or maintaining physical fitness [1].

In the general population, higher levels of PA are associated with healthier ageing [2], improved quality of life [3], and reduced risk of developing both psychiatric disorders [4,5] and physical health conditions such as diabetes mellitus [6] and cardiovascular disease [7]. PA has the potential to play an important role in the successful management of both the physical and mental health of patients with cancer, cardiovascular disease, chronic respiratory disease, and chronic musculoskeletal conditions [8–12]. For example, a recent network meta-analysis of 391 randomised controlled trials suggested that PA may have comparable efficacy to many common pharmacological agents in the management of hypertension [13].

PHYSICAL ACTIVITY AND SERIOUS MENTAL ILLNESS

Individuals with severe mental illness (SMI) die up to 20 years earlier than members of the general population [14], with 60% of this premature mortality attributed to physical health conditions, in particular cardiovascular disease [15,16]. Given that PA is effective in the prevention [3,6,7] and management [8–12] of various physical morbidities in the general population, there is potential for translation of PA interventions to the management of physical health conditions in people with SMI [17]. There is also potential for PA to play a role in the management of psychiatric symptoms, even those historically poorly controlled by traditional pharmacological and psychological interventions.

The Maudsley Practice Guidelines for Physical Health Conditions in Psychiatry, First Edition.
David M. Taylor, Fiona Gaughran, and Toby Pillinger.
© 2021 John Wiley & Sons Ltd. Published 2021 by John Wiley & Sons Ltd.

For example, in the general population, PA has a protective cognitive effect [18], with efficacy also observed in patients with Alzheimer's disease [19]. In major depressive disorder (MDD), 12–16 weeks of PA improves symptoms compared to control conditions, with greatest effect sizes observed when PA is delivered at moderate to vigorous intensity (e.g. cycling, running, or playing football) [17]. The beneficial effects of exercise on mood also persist over time; a recent 12-month study comparing the influence of aerobic exercise, internet-delivered cognitive-behavioural therapy (iCBT), and treatment as usual on the symptoms of MDD found that both PA and iCBT improved depressive symptoms more than usual care, with no significant difference observed between the PA and iCBT groups [20]. For schizophrenia spectrum disorder, there is evidence that aerobic PA delivered over 12–16 weeks can reduce positive, negative, and cognitive symptoms as well as improving cardiorespiratory fitness [17]. Furthermore, PA, as in the general population, has been observed to improve the quality of life of patients with schizophrenia [21].

HOW MUCH PHYSICAL ACTIVITY AND EXERCISE SHOULD PEOPLE BE DOING?

Current PA guidelines recommend a weekly combination of regular aerobic (cardiovascular training such as a brisk walk or playing a sport) and strength/resistance PA (using muscles against resistance such as using weights in a gym) [22]. Specifically, it is recommended that adults achieve at least 150 minutes per week of moderate aerobic PA (an activity that leads to the person becoming slightly short of breath, such as cycling or brisk walking), or 75 minutes per week of vigorous PA (where the person struggles to talk and breathe at the same time, such as running fast). Moreover, it is recommended that adults include strength training on two or more days each week. It is often recommended that adults participate in 30 minutes of moderate aerobic activity on five days each week, but the 150 minutes can be spread out however the individual chooses. Recent American guidelines have suggested that adults should seek to achieve 150–300 of moderate and 75–150 minutes of vigorous PA per week [23]. However, the guidelines recognise that groups with chronic physical or mental disorders may struggle to achieve such targets and emphasise that engaging in even small amounts of PA is of worth. PA can of course take the form of various activities, such as organised sport, gardening, housework, and dancing. People should be encouraged to find a PA that they enjoy, to set goals over time to increase PA levels, and to engage with PA throughout their life [24].

Individuals with SMI are significantly more sedentary and engage in lower levels of PA compared with the general population [25]; psychiatric patients are 50% less likely to meet recommended guidelines of 150 minutes of moderate to vigorous PA per week [25]. Barriers to PA in the SMI population include symptoms of psychiatric illness (e.g. low mood, negative symptoms such as amotivation, and paranoia), lack of confidence in engaging in PA, physical comorbidity, side effects of psychiatric medication (e.g. sedation or extrapyramidal side effects), and lack of support and knowledge about PA [26,27]. In a recent systematic review, up to 63% of people with SMI reported that they would exercise more if given appropriate advice by their physician [28]. Psychiatric practitioners are thus uniquely positioned to provide guidance which should increase PA levels in this population.

PRACTICAL TIPS

PA is relatively safe and inexpensive, with evidence of benefits to both mental and physical health in SMI [17]. As such, it is recommended that psychiatric practitioners discuss and encourage engagement in PA as part of routine clinical reviews with patients. One approach is to use 'physical activity vital sign' (PAVS) questions to assess the amount of activity engaged in by the patient on a weekly basis [29]. This involves asking the following questions.

1 On average, how many days per week do you engage in moderate to vigorous physical activity such as a brisk walk?
2 On those days, on average how many minutes do you engage in physical activity at this level?

The clinician can then calculate the minutes of moderate to vigorous PA completed per week and establish if the patient complies with the recommendation of 150 minutes. This provides an entry point to discuss PA and, if appropriate, how to incorporate more activity into the patient's life. PAVS scores can also act as a convenient screening tool for cardiometabolic health; low PAVS scores (i.e. fewer PA minutes per week) are associated with increased cardiometabolic risk in both schizophrenia [30] and bipolar disorder [31].

MESSAGES TO INCLUDE IN DISCUSSIONS WITH PATIENTS

- Emphasise that any activity is better than none. Advise the patient to 'start small' and to increase incidental activity in daily life. Walking has numerous recognised health benefits in SMI [32].
- Help the patient determine ways to incorporate activity into their lifestyle in simple ways. Practical examples include:
  - getting off the bus one stop early and walking the remainder of the journey
  - taking the stairs instead of elevator
  - standing up and moving around for a short walk every 30 minutes.
- Have the person find an activity that they enjoyed doing in the past [24].
- Social support is key; the patient should be encouraged to engage in PA with a friend, relative, or trainer [33,34].
- Ultimately, patients should be aiming to complete two to three sessions every week of supervised aerobic and/or aerobic and resistance training of moderate intensity for 45–60 minutes, which is associated with optimal mental and physical health benefits [20].

Psychiatric multidisciplinary teams should seek to include exercise professionals such as exercise physiologists or physiotherapists. Where access to such professionals exists, patients interested in increasing PA levels should be referred: optimal beneficial impact of PA on cardiorespiratory fitness in SMI is achieved when PA is supervised by these personnel [17]. For teams who do not have access to exercise professionals, an effort to forge links with community exercise specialists is recommended.

References

1. Caspersen CJ, Powell KE, Christenson GM. Physical activity, exercise, and physical fitness: definitions and distinctions for health-related research. *Public Health Rep* 1985;100(2):126–131.
2. Daskalopoulou C, Stubbs B, Kralj C, et al. Physical activity and healthy ageing: a systematic review and meta-analysis of longitudinal cohort studies. *Ageing Res Rev* 2017;38:6–17.
3. Gill DL, Hammond CC, Reifsteck EJ, et al. Physical activity and quality of life. *J Prev Med Public Health* 2013;46(Suppl 1):S28–S34.
4. Schuch FB, Vancampfort D, Firth J, et al. Physical activity and incident depression: a meta-analysis of prospective cohort studies. *Am J Psychiatry* 2018;175(7):631–648.
5. McDowell CP, Gordon BR, MacDonncha C, Herring MP. Physical activity correlates among older adults with probable generalized anxiety disorder: results from the Irish Longitudinal Study on Ageing. *Gen Hosp Psychiatry* 2019;59:30–36.
6. Smith AD, Crippa A, Woodcock J, Brage S. Physical activity and incident type 2 diabetes mellitus: a systematic review and dose–response meta-analysis of prospective cohort studies. *Diabetologia* 2016;59(12):2527–2545.
7. Naci H, Ioannidis JP. Comparative effectiveness of exercise and drug interventions on mortality outcomes: metaepidemiological study. *BMJ* 2013;347:f5577.
8. Wong P, Muanza T, Hijal T, et al. Effect of exercise in reducing breast and chest-wall pain in patients with breast cancer: a pilot study. *Curr Oncol* 2012;19(3):e129–e135.
9. Eisele A, Schagg D, Kramer LV, et al. Behaviour change techniques applied in interventions to enhance physical activity adherence in patients with chronic musculoskeletal conditions: a systematic review and meta-analysis. *Patient Educ Couns* 2019;102(1):25–36.
10. Billinger SA, Mattlage AE, Ashenden AL, et al. Aerobic exercise in subacute stroke improves cardiovascular health and physical performance. *J Neurol Phys Ther* 2012;36(4):159–165.
11. Lahham A, McDonald CF, Holland AE. Exercise training alone or with the addition of activity counseling improves physical activity levels in COPD: a systematic review and meta-analysis of randomized controlled trials. *Int J Chron Obstruct Pulmon Dis* 2016;11:3121–3136.
12. Welch WA, Alexander NB, Swartz AM, et al. Individualized estimation of physical activity in older adults with type 2 diabetes. *Med Sci Sports Exerc* 2017;49(11):2185–2190.
13. Naci H, Salcher-Konrad M, Dias S, et al. How does exercise treatment compare with antihypertensive medications? A network meta-analysis of 391 randomised controlled trials assessing exercise and medication effects on systolic blood pressure. *Br J Sports Med* 2019;53(14):859–869.
14. Walker ER, McGee RE, Druss BG. Mortality in mental disorders and global disease burden implications: a systematic review and meta-analysis. *JAMA Psychiatry* 2015;72(4):334–341.
15. Correll CU, Solmi M, Veronese N, et al. Prevalence, incidence and mortality from cardiovascular disease in patients with pooled and specific severe mental illness: a large-scale meta-analysis of 3,211,768 patients and 113,383,368 controls. *World Psychiatry* 2017;16(2):163–180.
16. Gardner-Sood P, Lally J, Smith S, et al. Cardiovascular risk factors and metabolic syndrome in people with established psychotic illnesses: baseline data from the IMPaCT randomized controlled trial. *Psychol Med* 2015;45(12):2619–2629.
17. Stubbs B, Vancampfort D, Hallgren M, et al. EPA guidance on physical activity as a treatment for severe mental illness: a meta-review of the evidence and Position Statement from the European Psychiatric Association (EPA), supported by the International Organization of Physical Therapists in Mental Health (IOPTMH). *Eur Psychiatry* 2018;54:124–144.
18. Blondell SJ, Hammersley-Mather R, Veerman JL. Does physical activity prevent cognitive decline and dementia? A systematic review and meta-analysis of longitudinal studies. *BMC Public Health* 2014;14:510.
19. Du Z, Li YW, Li JW, et al. Physical activity can improve cognition in patients with Alzheimer's disease: a systematic review and meta-analysis of randomized controlled trials. *Clin Interv Aging* 2018;13:1593–1603.
20. Hallgren M, Helgadottir B, Herring MP, et al. Exercise and internet-based cognitive-behavioural therapy for depression: multicentre randomised controlled trial with 12-month follow-up. *Br J Psychiatry* 2016;209(5):416–422.
21. Dauwan M, Begemann MJH, Heringa SM, Sommer IE. Exercise improves clinical symptoms, quality of life, global functioning, and depression in schizophrenia: a systematic review and meta-analysis. *Schizophr Bull* 2016;42(3):588–599.
22. Bouchard C, Blair DT, Haskell WL (eds). *Physical Activity and Health*, 2nd edn. Champaign, IL: Human Kinetics, 2012.
23. Piercy KL, Troiano RP, Ballard RM, et al. The physical activity guidelines for Americans. *JAMA* 2018;320(19):2020–2028.
24. Ekkekakis P, Parfitt G, Petruzzello SJ. The pleasure and displeasure people feel when they exercise at different intensities: decennial update and progress towards a tripartite rationale for exercise intensity prescription. *Sports Med* 2011;41(8):641–671.

25. Vancampfort D, Firth J, Schuch FB, et al. Sedentary behavior and physical activity levels in people with schizophrenia, bipolar disorder and major depressive disorder: a global systematic review and meta-analysis. *World Psychiatry* 2017;16(3):308–315.

26. Firth J, Rosenbaum S, Stubbs B, et al. Preferences and motivations for exercise in early psychosis. *Acta Psychiatr Scand* 2016;134(1):83–84.

27. Firth J, Rosenbaum S, Stubbs B, et al. Motivating factors and barriers towards exercise in severe mental illness: a systematic review and meta-analysis. *Psychol Med* 2016;46(14):2869–2881.

28. Farholm A, Sorensen M. Motivation for physical activity and exercise in severe mental illness: a systematic review of intervention studies. *Int J Ment Health Nurs* 2016;25(3):194–205.

29. Coleman KJ, Ngor E, Reynolds K, et al. Initial validation of an exercise 'vital sign' in electronic medical records. *Med Sci Sport Exerc* 2012;44(11):2071–2076.

30. Vancampfort D, Stubbs B, Probst M, et al. Physical activity as a vital sign in patients with schizophrenia: evidence and clinical recommendations. *Schizophr Res* 2016;170(2–3):336–340.

31. Vancampfort D, Probst M, Wyckaert S, et al. Physical activity as a vital sign in patients with bipolar disorder. *Psychiatry Res* 2016;246:218–222.

32. Ashdown-Franks G, Williams J, Vancampfort D, et al. Is it possible for people with severe mental illness to sit less and move more? A systematic review of interventions to increase physical activity or reduce sedentary behaviour. *Schizophr Res* 2018;202:3–16.

33. Gross J, Vancampfort D, Stubbs B, et al. A narrative synthesis investigating the use and value of social support to promote physical activity among individuals with schizophrenia. *Disabil Rehabil* 2016;38(2):123–150.

34. Cohrdes C, Bretschneider J. Can social support and physical activity buffer cognitive impairment in individuals with depressive symptoms? Results from a representative sample of young to older adults. *J Affect Disord* 2018;239:102–106.

CHAPTER 10

Part 2

Endocrinology

Diabetes Mellitus

Yuya Mizuno, Toby Pillinger, Dan Siskind, Sophie Harris

Diabetes mellitus is an umbrella term describing a group of metabolic disorders characterised by high blood glucose. It is associated with relative or total impairment in pancreatic insulin secretion, and with varying degrees of peripheral insulin resistance [1]. It is a major risk factor for both microvascular disease (retinopathy, nephropathy, and neuropathy) and macrovascular disease (coronary heart disease, peripheral arterial disease, and stroke) [2]. Type 2 diabetes mellitus (T2DM) is the most common type of diabetes in adults (>90%) and forms the focus of this chapter (see Box 11.1 for a description of type 1 diabetes mellitus and its relevance in the context of psychiatric illness). People with severe mental illness (SMI) are twice as likely to develop T2DM compared with the general population [3], with prevalence estimated at around 11% [4,5]. Furthermore, approximately three in five people with diabetes mellitus report low mood as a consequence of their condition [6]. People with SMI and T2DM receive poorer quality of diabetes management compared to people without mental illness [7,8]. Diagnosis and management of T2DM is thus important in preventing physical disability and premature mortality in this high-risk population.

DIAGNOSTIC PRINCIPLES

Although the classical symptoms of raised blood glucose are polydipsia, polyuria, blurred vision, and weight loss [9], the majority of patients with T2DM are asymptomatic and diagnosis follows routine blood screening. Emergency presentations of diabetes are discussed in Chapter 74.

The Maudsley Practice Guidelines for Physical Health Conditions in Psychiatry, First Edition.
David M. Taylor, Fiona Gaughran, and Toby Pillinger.
© 2021 John Wiley & Sons Ltd. Published 2021 by John Wiley & Sons Ltd.

> **Box 11.1** Type 1 diabetes mellitus and implications for the psychiatric population
>
> - Type 1 diabetes mellitus (T1DM) is characterised by autoimmune destruction of pancreatic beta cells, leading to total impairment of insulin secretion. As such, patients require immediate insulin therapy.
> - In the psychiatric population, T1DM can pose various therapeutic challenges. Erratic use of insulin, potentially in the context of chaotic behaviour secondary to cognitive or negative symptoms of schizophrenia, can predispose to hypoglycaemic episodes or diabetic ketoacidosis with associated acute risk to life, or chronic hyperglycaemia with associated comorbidity and premature mortality.
> - Insulin, at higher doses, is lethal and this needs to be considered in patients at risk of deliberate self-harm.
> - Diabulimia is an eating disorder in which people with T1DM deliberately give themselves less insulin than they need for the purpose of weight loss.
> - Patients with comorbid T1DM and SMI can be highly complex, and a multidisciplinary team approach to management, involving psychiatrists, psychologists, and diabetologists, is essential.

History

History of presenting complaint

Although the signs and symptoms of hyperglycaemia (polydipsia, polyuria, blurred vision, and weight loss) may be mild or absent, they should be screened for [9]. Other symptoms that may indicate complications of T2DM (generally in advanced disease) include visual symptoms of retinopathy (blurred vision, 'floaters', progressive loss of visual acuity), sensory/motor symptoms of a peripheral neuropathy (typically symmetrical and distal: numbness/reduced ability to feel pain/temperature in fingers/toes), passing of foamy urine (proteinuria of nephropathy), impotence, acanthosis nigricans (dark velvety discoloration of body folds/creases), and frequent infections (particularly candidiasis, urinary tract infection, and abscesses) [9].

Past medical history

Sociodemographic factors such as advancing age and ethnicity (particularly South Asian, Hispanic, or African-Caribbean decent) predispose to T2DM [10]. Furthermore, obesity (body mass index, BMI ≥30) [11] and increased waist circumference (>80 cm for all women; >94 cm for most men; >90 cm for South Asian men) [12,13] are important risk factors for T2DM. Screen for comorbid metabolic (i.e. hypertension, hypercholesterolaemia) and cardiovascular disease (CVD), and for medical conditions that predispose individuals to T2DM (e.g. polycystic ovary syndrome). Cushing's disease and Wilson's disease represent causes of T2DM that may also present with neuropsychiatric symptoms.

Drug history

Several psychiatric medications can predispose patients to T2DM, including antipsychotics, mood stabilisers, and antidepressants [14–16]. Non-psychiatric drugs that can increase risk of T2DM include corticosteroids, thiazide diuretics, beta-blockers, and statins.

Family history

There is a hereditary component to T2DM. Identifying family history of premature CVD may provide greater impetus to targeting other modifiable CVD risk factors alongside glucose control.

Social history

Modifiable risk factors for T2DM include levels of physical activity, dietary habits, smoking, and alcohol use [17]. Targeting these factors may form part of treatment (see Chapters 10, 14, 24, and 46).

Examination

Examination may be normal, unless the patient is presenting with a hyperglycaemic emergency (see Chapter 74) or, in patients with advanced chronic disease (which may be seen in patients with SMI presenting late to medical services), damage to multiple organ systems may be apparent. A set of basic observations may identify comorbid hypertension. General inspection should note body habitus, evidence of dehydration, and presence of skin alterations typical of T2DM (e.g. acanthosis nigricans). Consider performing cardiovascular and neurological examinations (with fundoscopy) to screen for complications of T2DM.

Investigations

The diagnostic glucose concentrations defined by the World Health Organization (WHO) are those above which it is recognised that an individual will be at high risk of developing microvascular complications [18]. Diagnosis may be made using random/ fasting plasma glucose, plasma glucose following the oral glucose tolerance test (OGTT), or HbA_{1c}. Various international and national criteria exist (Box 11.2) [18–20]. These are all broadly similar, save for the UK (NICE) guidelines [20] that provide a more narrow definition of pre-diabetes compared with the definitions of the American Diabetic Association [19] and WHO [18]. In symptomatic patients, only one glucose assessment is required to confirm diagnosis, whereas in asymptomatic patients two confirmatory glucose assessments are required. In psychiatric practice, fasting glucose assessments may be unrealistic (e.g. in patients who may not comply with fasting requirements), and the OGTT often unfeasible. As such, the HbA_{1c} represents the simplest method of glucose assessment, and two separate HbA_{1c} measurements of 6.5% or above in an asymptomatic patient will confirm diagnosis. However, clinicians should be aware that in patients with high red blood cell turnover (e.g. sickle cell anaemia, pregnancy), use of HbA_{1c} is inappropriate [21], and diagnosis will instead require assessment of plasma glucose levels.

Pre-diabetes is a condition where blood glucose levels are higher than normal but do not yet meet the criteria for diabetes mellitus. About 30% of people with pre-diabetes will progress to T2DM within 10 years. This provides opportunity to offer interventions to reduce risk of progression [22].

CHAPTER 11

Other investigations may be performed to screen for diabetes-related complications and cardiovascular risk. These should be performed at least yearly and are described in more detail in the section on annual diabetic review.

Box 11.2 Diagnostic criteria for diagnosis of type 2 diabetes mellitus

World Health Organization [18]

Diabetes mellitus

HbA_{1c} ≥48 mmol/mol (6.5%) *or*
FPG ≥7.0 mmol/L (126 mg/dL) *or*
2-hour PG after 75 g OGTT ≥11.1 mmol/L (200 mg/dL) *or*
Random PG ≥11.1 mmol/L (200 mg/dL)

Pre-diabetes

42 ≤ HbA_{1c} < 48 mmol/mol (6.0–6.4%) *or*
5.5 ≤ FPG < 7.0 mmol/L (100–125 mg/dL) *or*
7.8 ≤ 2-hour PG after 75 g OGTT < 11.1 mmol/L (140–199 mg/dL)

American Diabetic Association [19]

Diabetes mellitus

HbA_{1c} ≥48 mmol/mol (6.5%) *or*
FPG ≥7.0 mmol/L (126 mg/dL) *or*
2-hour PG after 75 g OGTT ≥11.1 mmol/L (200 mg/dL) *or*
Random PG ≥11.1 mmol/L (200 mg/dL)

Pre-diabetes

39 ≤ HbA_{1c} < 48 mmol/mol (5.7–6.4%) *or*
5.5 ≤ FPG < 7.0 mmol/L (100–125 mg/dL) *or*
7.8 ≤ 2-hour PG after 75 g OGTT <11.1 mmol/L (140–199 mg/dL)

National Institute for Health and Care Excellence [20]

Diabetes mellitus

HbA_{1c} >48 mmol/mol (6.5%) *or*
Random PG ≥11.1 mmol/L (200 mg/dL) *or*
FPG ≥7.0 mmol/L (126 mg/dL)

Pre-diabetes

42 ≤ HbA_{1c} < 48 mmol/mol (6.0–6.4%) *or*
FPG ≥7.0 mmol/L (126 mg/dL) *or*
6.1 ≤ FPG < 7.0 mmol/L (110–125 mg/dL) *or*
7.8 ≤ 2-hour PG after 75 g OGTT < 11.1 mmol/L (140–199 mg/dL)

FPG, fasting plasma glucose (defined as no caloric intake for at least eight hours); OGTT, oral glucose tolerance test; PG, plasma glucose.

MANAGEMENT

Management of T2DM is multifaceted, requiring a combination of patient education to facilitate lifestyle modification and pharmacological approaches. The overarching goals are to achieve normoglycaemia and manage/prevent vascular complications. Improving glycaemic control clearly improves outcomes in T2DM [23]. However, any approach needs to be individualised, balancing the benefits of HbA_{1c} reduction against drug side effects such as hypoglycaemia and weight gain (see Table 11.1) [24]. A recent

Table 11.1 Risks, benefits and evidence base for diabetes treatments in serious mental illness (SMI).

Drug class	Mechanism	Risk	Benefit	Evidence base in SMI
Biguanide (metformin)	Increases insulin sensitivity, reduces hepatic synthesis and release of glucose, and increases peripheral glucose uptake	Lactic acidosis B_{12} deficiency If gastrointestinal upset try modified-release formulation Contraindicated if eGFR <30 mL/min per 1.73 m³	Weight loss (3 kg) Low risk of hypoglycaemia	Good evidence for use in SMI, and should be considered first line [31] Consider in patients with pre-diabetes receiving olanzapine and clozapine [32]
Dipeptidyl peptidase-4 (DPP-4) inhibitor (e.g. sitagliptin)	Inhibits action of DPP-4 which acts to break down incretins (e.g. GLP-1). This increases incretin effect, as seen in GLP1R agonists	Possible increased hospitalisations for heart failure with alogliptin and saxagliptin Possible increased pancreatitits risk	Weight neutral Low risk of hypoglycaemia	Trial data lacking in SMI
Glucagon-like peptide-1 receptor (GLP1R)-agonists (e.g. exenatide)	Incretin mimetic: stimulates release of insulin, reduces glucagon release, delays gastric emptying, reduces appetite	Subcutaneous administration (oral now becoming available) Nausea/vomiting Possible increased pancreatitis risk	Weight loss (3–4.5 kg) Low risk of hypoglycaemia Liraglutide FDA approved for prevention of major cardiac events	Current evidence base suggests should be considered second line therapy in SMI Evidence for exenatide use in patients treated with antipsychotics, particularly olanzapine and clozapine [33, 34]
Sulphonylureas (e.g. gliclazide)	Increases endogenous production of insulin	Hypoglycaemia Weight gain		Trial data lacking in SMI
Sodium glucose transporter 2 (SGLT2) inhibitors (e.g. dapagliflozin)	Inhibits SGLT2 in the proximal renal tubule, thereby reducing glucose reabsorption of glucose promoting glucosuria	Polyuria Postural hypotension Urinary tract infection DKA can occur in stress settings Mild fracture risk	Weight loss (2–3 kg) Low risk of hypoglycaemia Empagliflozin FDA approved to reduce CV mortality Canagliflozin reduces cardiac events	Trial data lacking in SMI

(continued)

CHAPTER 11

Drug class	Mechanism	Risk	Benefit	Evidence base in SMI
Thiazolidinediones (glitazones, e.g. pioglitazone)	Improve insulin sensitivity by promoting adipogenesis and reducing circulating fatty acid and lipid availability	Weight gain Heart failure Oedema Bone fractures	May reduce stroke risk Low risk of hypoglycaemia	Rosiglitazone improves glucose homeostasis in patients treated with olanzapine [35] and clozapine [36]. However, in the UK, rosiglitazone has been withdrawn owing to risk of myocardial infarction Pioglitazone remains available as an antidiabetic medication. However, due to concerns regarding the risk of cardiovascular disease, along with their propensity to cause weight gain, they are not preferred choices in SMI
Insulin	Supplements insufficient endogenous production of insulin	Hypoglycaemia Weight gain	In poorly controlled diabetes may be only effective treatment in stabilising glucose	Trial data lacking in SMI

Table 11.1 (Continued)

DKA, diabetic ketoacidosis; eGFR, estimated glomerular filtration rate.

consensus statement by the American Diabetes Association (ADA) and the European Association for the Study of Diabetes (EASD) set out the principles by which management of hyperglycaemia in T2DM should be approached, summarised in Box 11.3 [25]. An algorithm for approaching management of T2DM in the SMI population is shown in Figure 11.1.

Non-pharmacological therapy: lifestyle modification

All patients and carers should be offered access to structured diabetes education around the time of diagnosis. In the general population, lifestyle interventions which target diet and physical activity have been effective in improving glycaemic control compared with standard treatment (see Ward et al. [26] for review). Efforts should be made to identify and improve lifestyle factors that may underlie poor glycaemic control, and address coexisting risk factors for cardiovascular disease (e.g. smoking and obesity). The reader is directed to Chapters 10, 14, and 46 for more details on weight gain, physical activity, and smoking cessation.

Pharmacological therapy

There are no diabetic treatment algorithms specific for psychiatric populations so pharmacological management should follow guidelines used in the general population. In

---

Box 11.3 Approach to glycaemic control in type 2 diabetes mellitus [25]

1 Assess key patient characteristics
  a Current lifestyle
  b Comorbidities (e.g. cardiovascular disease)
  c Clinical characteristics (e.g. BMI)
  d Comorbid psychiatric diagnoses and socioeconomic/cultural context
2 Consider specific factors that impact choice of treatment
  a HbA_{1c} target for that individual
  b Comorbid obesity or risk of hypoglycaemia
  c Side effects of medication
  d Complexity of regimen and likelihood of adherence
3 Shared decision-making
  a Educate patient and family/caregivers
  b Consider patient preference
4 Agree on management plan: 'SMART' goals
  a Specific
  b Measurable
  c Achievable
  d Realistic
  e Time limited
5 Implement management plan
  a Review patient at least every 3 months
6 Ongoing monitoring and support
  a Emotional well-being
  b Check tolerability of medication
  c Monitor glycaemic status
7 Review and agree on management plan
  a Review above decision cycle and management plan at least once/twice a year
  b Mutual agreement on any changes
  c Ensure any changes implemented in a timely manner

CHAPTER 11

---

the absence of specific guidance for SMI, the prescriber should consider an individual's risk and the side effects of their psychiatric drugs to tailor prescribing accordingly.

Where possible, rationalisation of psychiatric medications is recommended. Male sex and elevated body weight at baseline increase the risk of antipsychotic-induced glucose dysregulation [27]. Where there are concerns regarding diabetic risk in such patients, medications such as lurasidone and partial agonists (e.g. aripiprazole) are recommended [27]. However, the choice of antipsychotic treatment should be made on an individual basis, considering the clinical circumstances and preferences of patients and clinicians.

A selection of international guidelines for use in the general population are summarised in Box 11.4. The first-line pharmacological therapy for T2DM is metformin monotherapy. Second-line therapies generally involve the addition of an oral medication including dipeptidyl peptidase (DPP)-4 inhibitor, thiazolidinedione (TZD), sulphonylurea (SU), or sodium-glucose cotransporter 2 (SGLT2) inhibitor and, outside of the UK, glucagon-like peptide-1 receptor agonists (GLP1RA).

There are two considerations when selecting medications specifically for patients with SMI. As obesity is common in SMI, choosing medications which can aid in weight loss

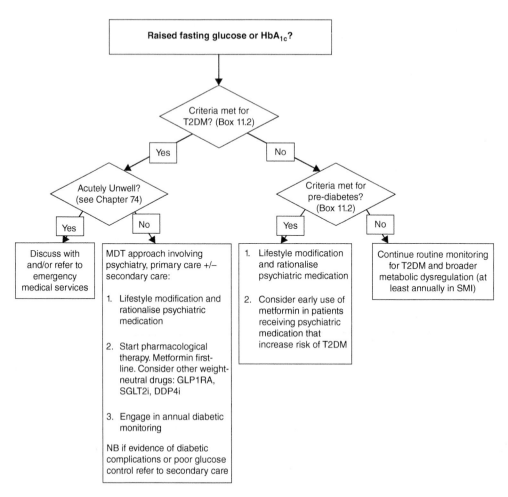

Figure 11.1 Approach to management of type 2 diabetes mellitus (T2DM) in patients with serious mental illness. DPP4i, dipeptidyl peptidase-4 inhibitor; GLP1RA, glucagon-like peptide-1 receptor agonist; SGLT2i, sodium–glucose cotransporter 2 inhibitor.

or are at least weight neutral are preferable (e.g. metformin, GLP1RAs, SGLT2 inhibitors, DPP-4 inhibitors). Furthermore, in patients with SMI characterised by disorganised behaviour or at significant risk of deliberate self-harm, medications which can result in hypoglycaemia may not be preferred (e.g. SU and insulin). Injectable agents such as insulin and GLP1RAs may require community nursing (although note that oral GLP1RAs are now emerging on the market). Multidisciplinary discussion between psychiatry and diabetology is recommended to ensure a patient receives appropriate treatment.

Pharmacological therapy should generally be initiated when the threshold is met for T2DM. A subgroup of patients whose HbA_{1c} levels are close to threshold may however choose to attempt a duration of lifestyle modification (e.g. for three to six months) to see if their diabetes can be managed without use of medication. Early prescription of metformin reduces the risk of transition from pre-diabetes to T2DM [28,29], and as

> **Box 11.4** A selection of international guidelines for use in the general population: algorithms for pharmacotherapy of type 2 diabetes mellitus
>
> ### National Institute for Health and Care Excellence [1]
>
> First line: metformin
> Second line: dual therapy with metformin plus one of DPP4i, pioglitazone, SU[a], SGLT2i
> Third line: triple therapy with one of the following combinations:
>
> Metformin + DPP4i + SU[a]
> Metformin + pioglitazone + SU[a]
> Metformin + (pioglitazone or SU[a]) + SGLT2i
>
> Fourth line: option for GLP1 mimetic alongside metformin and SU[a] if certain criteria are met:
>
> BMI >35 kg/m^2 and obesity-related medical/psychological complications
> BMI <35 kg/m^2 and insulin therapy has significant occupational implications
> If weight loss would benefit obesity-related comorbidities
>
> After exhausting the first four steps, consider insulin therapy
>
> ### Scottish Intercollegiate Guidelines Network (SIGN) [37]
>
> First line: metformin (or SU[a] if osmotic symptoms or intolerant of metformin)
> Second line: dual therapy with metformin and one of SU[a], SGLT2i, DPP4i, pioglitazone
> Third line: add either an additional oral agent from a different class (SU[a], SGLT2i, DPP4i, pioglitazone) or an injectable agent (GLP1RA or insulin)
> Fourth line: review adherence, add additional agent(s) from third line with specialist input
>
> ### American Diabetes Association [38]
>
> First line: metformin
> Second line: dual therapy with metformin plus one of DPP-4i, TZD, SU[a], GLP1 agonist, SGLT2i, insulin
> Third line: triple therapy with one of the following combinations:
>
> Metformin + SU[a] + TZD/DDP4i/SGLT2i/GLP1RA/insulin
> Metformin + TZD + SU[a]/DDP4i/SGLT2i/GLP1RA/insulin
> Metformin + DPP4i + SU[a]/TZD/SGLT2i/insulin
> Metformin + SGLT2i + SU[a]/TZD/DPP4i/GLP1RA/insulin
> Metformin + GLP1RA + SU[a]/TZD/SGLT2i/insulin
> Metformin + insulin + TZD/DDP4i/SGLT2i/GLP1RA
>
> Fourth line: combination injectable therapy[a]
>
> SU, sulphonylurea; TZD, thiazolidinedione; DPP4i, dipeptidyl peptidase-4 inhibitor; GLP1RA, glucagon-like peptide-1 receptor agonist; SGLT2i, sodium–glucose cotransporter 2 inhibitor.
>
> a Medications which can result in hypoglycaemia (e.g. SU) may not be preferred in some patients with serious mental illness where there are concerns regarding risk of overdose, or chaotic behaviour.

such recent guidelines recommend considering use of metformin in certain patients to slow progression, especially in those who are under 60 years old, have a BMI over 35 kg/m^2, or have a history of gestational diabetes [30]. We recommend considering early use of metformin in pre-diabetic patients with SMI who are receiving psychiatric treatment recognised to increase diabetic risk (e.g. second-generation antipsychotics).

Management of other comorbidities

To reduce the risk of microvascular/macrovascular complications, other cardiovascular risk factors alongside T2DM should be treated. Thus, smoking cessation, weight loss, and pharmacological treatment of hypertension and hypercholesterolaemia may be indicated (see Chapters 5, 9, 14, and 46).

Annual diabetic review

In the UK, patients with T2DM should be offered an annual diabetic review, which is generally coordinated by primary care services. This involves review of blood glucose via HbA$_{1c}$, blood pressure, cholesterol, renal function, retinal screening, neurological assessment (foot/leg), education (dietary and medication advice), smoking cessation, influenza vaccination, support if experiencing sexual side effects, psychological support, and specialist care if planning pregnancy [39].

When to refer to a specialist

T2DM can usually be managed in primary care. However, patients who have recurrent or unpredictable hypoglycaemia, suboptimal HbA$_{1c}$, or diabetic complications (e.g. neuropathy, nephropathy, or foot ulcerations) may benefit from referral to secondary care.
Information in a referral should include the following:

- brief summary of symptoms and rationale behind referral
- comorbid psychiatric diagnosis and current treatment
- any psychosocial issues that may impact on diabetic control
- summary of any potential impact of mental health on accessing/engaging with investigations/follow-up, and on concordance with recommended diabetic treatment
- contact details of the patient's mental healthcare team/support network, and if the appointment should be sent to anyone in addition to the patient
- any reasonable adjustments needed for the patient (e.g. time or duration of appointment, carer/support worker in attendance).

References

1. National Institute for Health and Care Excellence. *Type 2 Diabetes in Adults: Management*. NICE Guideline NG28. London: NICE, 2015. Available at nice.org.uk/guidance/ng28 (accessed 7 April 2019).
2. The Emerging Risk Factors Collaboration, Sarwar N, Gao P, Seshasai SR, et al. Diabetes mellitus, fasting blood glucose concentration, and risk of vascular disease: a collaborative meta-analysis of 102 prospective studies. *Lancet* 2010;375(9733):2215–2222.
3. Firth J, Siddiqi N, Koyanagi A, et al. The Lancet Psychiatry Commission: a blueprint for protecting physical health in people with mental illness. *Lancet Psychiatry* 2019;6(8):675–712.
4. Osborn DP, Wright CA, Levy G, et al. Relative risk of diabetes, dyslipidaemia, hypertension and the metabolic syndrome in people with severe mental illnesses: systematic review and metaanalysis. *BMC Psychiatry* 2008;8:84.
5. Vancampfort D, Correll CU, Galling B, et al. Diabetes mellitus in people with schizophrenia, bipolar disorder and major depressive disorder: a systematic review and large scale meta-analysis. *World Psychiatry* 2016;15(2):166–174.
6. Diabetes UK. Three in five people with diabetes experience emotional or mental health problems. https://www.diabetes.org.uk/about_us/news/three-in-five-people-with-diabetes-experience-emotional-or-mental-health-problems. 2017.
7. Frayne SM, Halanych JH, Miller DR, et al. Disparities in diabetes care: impact of mental illness. *Arch Intern Med* 2005;165(22):2631–2638.
8. Goldberg RW, Kreyenbuhl JA, Medoff DR, et al. Quality of diabetes care among adults with serious mental illness. *Psychiatr Serv* 2007;58(4):536–543.

CHAPTER 11

9. Vijan S. In the clinic. Type 2 diabetes. *Ann Intern Med* 2015;162(5):ITC1–16.

10. Public Health England. *Adult Obesity and Type 2 Diabetes*. London: PHE, 2014. Available at https://assets.publishing.service.gov.uk/government/uploads/system/uploads/attachment_data/file/338934/Adult_obesity_and_type_2_diabetes_.pdf (accessed 7 April 2019).

11. Abdullah A, Peeters A, de Courten M, Stoelwinder J. The magnitude of association between overweight and obesity and the risk of diabetes: a meta-analysis of prospective cohort studies. *Diabetes Res Clin Pract* 2010;89(3):309–319.

12. Rush E, Plank L, Chandu V, et al. Body size, body composition, and fat distribution: a comparison of young New Zealand men of European, Pacific Island, and Asian Indian ethnicities. *N Z Med J* 2004;117(1207):U1203.

13. Alberti KGMM, Zimmet P, Shaw J. Metabolic syndrome: a new world-wide definition. A consensus statement from the international diabetes federation. *Diabetic Med* 2006;23(5):469–480.

14. Smith M, Hopkins D, Peveler RC, et al. First- v. second-generation antipsychotics and risk for diabetes in schizophrenia: systematic review and meta-analysis. *Br J Psychiatry* 2008;192(6):406–411.

15. Svendal G, Fasmer OB, Engeland A, et al. Co-prescription of medication for bipolar disorder and diabetes mellitus: a nationwide population-based study with focus on gender differences. *BMC Med* 2012;10:148.

16. Barnard K, Peveler RC, Holt RIG. Antidepressant medication as a risk factor for type 2 diabetes and impaired glucose regulation: systematic review. *Diabetes Care* 2013;36(10):3337–3345.

17. Mozaffarian D, Kamineni A, Carnethon M, et al. Lifestyle risk factors and new-onset diabetes mellitus in older adults: the Cardiovascular Health Study. *Arch Intern Med* 2009;169(8):798–807.

18. Alberti KG, Zimmet PZ. *Definition, diagnosis and classification of diabetes mellitus and its complications. Report of a WHO consultation. Part 1. Diagnosis and classification of diabetes mellitus*. Geneva: WHO, 1999.

19. Cefalu WT, Berg EG, Saraco M, et al. Classification and diagnosis of diabetes: standards of medical care in diabetes 2019. *Diabetes Care* 2019;42:S13–S28.

20. National Institute for Health and Care Excellence. Diabetes – type 2. https://cks.nice.org.uk/diabetes-type-2#!diagnosisSub. Last revised: September 2019.

21. Kilpatrick ES, Atkin SL. Using haemoglobin A1c to diagnose type 2 diabetes or to identify people at high risk of diabetes. *BMJ* 2014;348:g2867.

22. NHS England. NHS Diabetes Prevention Programme (NHS DPP). https://www.england.nhs.uk/diabetes/diabetes-prevention/ (accessed 11 August 2019).

23. UK Prospective Diabetes Study (UKPDS) Group. Intensive blood-glucose control with sulphonylureas or insulin compared with conventional treatment and risk of complications in patients with type 2 diabetes (UKPDS 33). *Lancet* 1998;352(9131):837–853.

24. ADVANCE Collaborative Group, Patel A, MacMahon S, Chalmers J, et al. Intensive blood glucose control and vascular outcomes in patients with type 2 diabetes. *N Engl J Med* 2008;358(24):2560–2572.

25. Davies MJ, D'Alessio DA, Fradkin J, et al. Management of hyperglycaemia in type 2 diabetes, 2018. A consensus report by the American Diabetes Association (ADA) and the European Association for the Study of Diabetes (EASD). *Diabetologia* 2018;61(12):2461–2498.

26. Ward MC, White DT, Druss BG. A meta-review of lifestyle interventions for cardiovascular risk factors in the general medical population: lessons for individuals with serious mental illness. *J Clin Psychiatry* 2015;76(4):e477–e486.

27. Pillinger T, McCutcheon R, Vano L, et al. Comparative effects of 18 antipsychotics on metabolic function in patients with schizophrenia, predictors of metabolic dysregulation, and association with psychopathology: a systematic review and network meta-analysis. *Lancet Psychiatry* 2020;7(1):64–77.

28. Knowler WC, Barrett-Connor E, Fowler SE, et al. Reduction in the incidence of type 2 diabetes with lifestyle intervention or metformin. *N Engl J Med* 2002;346(6):393–403.

29. Diabetes Prevention Program Research Group. Long-term effects of lifestyle intervention or metformin on diabetes development and microvascular complications over 15-year follow-up: the Diabetes Prevention Program Outcomes Study. *Lancet Diabetes Endocrinol* 2015;3(11):866–875.

30. Professional Practice Committee for the Standards of Medical Care in Diabetes-2016. *Diabetes Care* 2016;39(Suppl 1):S107–S108.

31. Jarskog LF, Hamer RM, Catellier DJ, et al. Metformin for weight loss and metabolic control in overweight outpatients with schizophrenia and schizoaffective disorder. *Am J Psychiatry* 2013;170(9):1032–1040.

32. Siskind DJ, Leung J, Russell AW, et al. Metformin for clozapine associated obesity: a systematic review and meta-analysis. *PLoS One* 2016;11(6):e0156208.

33. Siskind DJ, Russell AW, Gamble C, et al. Treatment of clozapine-associated obesity and diabetes with exenatide in adults with schizophrenia: A randomized controlled trial (CODEX). *Diabetes Obes Metab* 2018;20(4):1050–1055.

34. Siskind D, Hahn M, Correll CU, et al. Glucagon-like peptide-1 receptor agonists for antipsychotic-associated cardio-metabolic risk factors: a systematic review and individual participant data meta-analysis. *Diabetes Obes Metab* 2019;21(2):293–302.

35. Baptista T, Rangel N, El Fakih Y, et al. Rosiglitazone in the assistance of metabolic control during olanzapine administration in schizophrenia: a pilot double-blind, placebo-controlled, 12-week trial. *Pharmacopsychiatry* 2009;42(1):14–19.

36. Henderson D, Fan X, Sharma B, et al. A double-blind, placebo-controlled trial of rosiglitazone for clozapine-induced glucose metabolism impairment in patients with schizophrenia. *Acta Psychiatr Scand* 2009;119(6):457–465.

37. Scottish Intercollegiate Guidelines Network (SIGN). *Pharmacological Management of Glycaemic Control in People with Type 2 Diabetes*. SIGN 154. Available at https://www.sign.ac.uk/assets/sign154.pdf (accessed 15 April 2019).

38. American Diabetes Association. Standards of medical care in diabetes-2017. *Diabetes Care* 2017;40(Suppl 1):S64–S74.

39. Diabetes UK. Annual diabetes checks. https://www.diabetes.org.uk/guide-to-diabetes/managing-your-diabetes/15-healthcare-essentials (accessed 11 August 2019).

CHAPTER 11

Chapter 12

Thyroid Disease
Harriet Quigley, Jackie Gilbert

The thyroid is a butterfly-shaped gland located at the front of the neck in front of the larynx (voice box). It produces three hormones: thyroxine (T4), triiodothyronine (T3), and calcitonin. T4 is inactive and is converted to active T3 peripherally. These hormones control the metabolic rate of the body. Calcitonin acts to reduce blood calcium.

T3 and T4 are released by the thyroid in response to thyroid stimulating hormone (TSH) which itself is produced by the pituitary gland. The pituitary gland releases TSH in response to thyrotropin releasing hormone (TRH), which is produced by the hypothalamus. Most T3/T4 in the circulation is bound to protein, and only free thyroid hormone is metabolically active. Free thyroid hormone feedbacks negatively to the hypothalamus and pituitary gland to reduce TRH and TSH production, respectively.

The three main clinical conditions arising from the thyroid gland in the general population are hypothyroidism, hyperthyroidism, and thyroid malignancy. This chapter provides an overview of the clinical presentation and management of hypothyroidism and hyperthyroidism, as well as their specific relevance to severe mental illness (SMI).

HYPOTHYROIDISM

Hypothyroidism describes the clinical state resulting from underproduction of the thyroid hormones T4 and T3. Most cases (95%) are due to an inability of the thyroid gland to produce thyroid hormones, termed primary hypothyroidism. The most common cause of primary hypothyroidism worldwide is iodine deficiency, while autoimmune thyroiditis and iatrogenic hypothyroidism (i.e. secondary to medical interventions) are common causes in regions where iodine deficiency is less prevalent. Secondary hypothyroidism accounts for the remaining 5% of cases and is due to disorders of the pituitary or hypothalamus. Other causes of hypothyroidism are described in Table 12.1.

The Maudsley Practice Guidelines for Physical Health Conditions in Psychiatry, First Edition.
David M. Taylor, Fiona Gaughran, and Toby Pillinger.
© 2021 John Wiley & Sons Ltd. Published 2021 by John Wiley & Sons Ltd.

Table 12.1 Primary and secondary causes of hypothyroidism and hyperthyroidism.

	Hypothyroidism	Hyperthyroidism
Primary	Autoimmune hypothyroidism: Hashimoto's thyroiditis and atrophic thyroiditis Iatrogenic: radioiodine treatment, surgery, radiotherapy to the neck Iodine deficiency Congenital defects (e.g. absence of thyroid gland or dyshormonogenesis) Infiltration of the thyroid (e.g. amyloidosis, sarcoidosis and haemochromatosis) Medications (see Table 12.3)	Graves' disease Toxic nodular goitre Thyroiditis Solitary thyroid nodule Follicular carcinoma of the thyroid gland Medications (see Table 12.3)
Secondary	Isolated TSH deficiency Hypopituitarism: neoplasm, infiltrative, infection, radiotherapy Hypothalamic disorders: neoplasms and trauma	TSH-secreting pituitary adenoma Gestational thyrotoxicosis Thyroid hormone resistance syndrome hCG-secreting tumour

Table 12.2 Common signs and symptoms of hypothyroidism and hyperthyroidism.

Hypothyroidism	Hyperthyroidism
Loss of outer third of eyebrows	Weight loss
Dry skin	Increased or decreased appetite
Brittle hair, hair loss	Irritability
Myxoedema	Weakness and fatigue
Tiredness, lethargy, cold intolerance	Sweating, heat intolerance
Deep hoarse voice	Tremor
Weight gain, decreased appetite	Diarrhoea
Constipation	Loss of libido
Bradycardia	Oligomenorrhoea/amenorrhoea
Delayed tendon reflex relaxation	Palmar erythema
Carpal tunnel syndrome	Tachycardia, atrial fibrillation
General slowing, physically and mentally	Hair thinning/diffuse alopecia
Myalgia	Brisk reflexes
Arthralgia	Goitre
Menorrhagia, oligomenorrhoea, amenorrhoea	Proximal myopathy
	Lid lag

Hypothyroidism often has an insidious onset but can be associated with significant morbidity. It disproportionately affects females and the elderly [1], and occurs in 2.5% of pregnant women (see Chapter 62) [2]. Clinical features are often subtle and non-specific, and may be wrongly attributed to other illnesses. Common signs and symptoms are summarised in Table 12.2. The first biochemical irregularity observed is an increase in serum TSH concentration with normal serum free T4 and free T3 (subclinical hypothyroidism). This is followed by a decrease in serum free T4, at which stage most patients have symptoms and require treatment (overt hypothyroidism). The severest form of hypothyroidism is a myxoedema or hypothyroid crisis, a severe life-threatening form of decompensated hypothyroidism associated with multiorgan failure (see Chapter 79).

DIAGNOSTIC PRINCIPLES

History

1 Symptoms of hypothyroidism: weakness, lethargy, cold sensitivity, constipation, weight gain, low mood, myalgia, menstrual irregularity, dry or coarse skin, thick tongue, eyelid/facial oedema, deep voice.
2 Past medical history:
 a iodine deficiency
 b autoimmune disorders (including type 1 diabetes and multiple sclerosis)
 c Graves' disease, and other autoimmune diseases of the thyroid
 d Turner's and Down's syndromes (both associated with increased risk of hypothyroidism)
 e primary pulmonary hypertension (associated with increased risk of hypothyroidism)
 f radiotherapy to the neck
 g infiltrative disease such as sarcoidosis (see Chapter 60) and haemochromatosis.
3 Medication history: see Table 12.3.
4 Family history: autoimmune thyroiditis.
5 Social history: history of working in the textile industry [3].

Table 12.3 Medications that cause hypothyroidism and hyperthyroidism.

	Hypothyroidism	Hyperthyroidism
General medications	Methimazole	Levothyroxine
	Carbimazole	Amiodarone
	Propylthiouracil	Interferon-alpha
	Amiodarone	
	Iodide	
	Minocycline and other tetracyclines	
	Interferon-α	
	Other cytokines (interferon-β, interleukin-2)	
	Propranolol	
	Glucocorticoids	
	Metformin	
Psychiatric medication	Lithium	Lithium
	Anticonvulsants	

CHAPTER 12

Examination

See Box 12.1.

Box 12.1 The thyroid examination

Make sure that the neck is appropriately exposed.

General inspection

- Evidence of obesity or recent rapid weight loss.
- Exophthalmos (Graves' disease).
- Dry skin (hypothyroidism).
- Hair (brittle and dry in hypothyroidism).
- Level of agitation (hyperthyroidism).

Examination of the hands

- Check pulse (bradycadia in hypothyroidism, tachycardia and atrial fibrillation in hyperthyroidism).
- Check for presence of sweating and increase in temperature (hyperthyroid).
- Onycholysis (separation of the nail from its bed).
- Thyroid acropachy: phalangeal bone overgrowth (Graves' disease).
- Ask the patient to extend his or her arms and hold hands with palms facing down; look for any tremor (hyperthyroidism).

Examination of the thyroid gland

Inspection

- Ask the patient to swallow; a thyroid mass will rise on swallowing.
- Note any asymmetry or scars from previous surgery.

Palpation

- Stand behind the patient with thumbs on the back of the neck and patient's head slightly flexed.
- Gently palpate the neck for any abnormality.
- Have the patient swallow and feel the gland move under your fingers; ask patient to protrude tongue.
- Palpation of both lobes and the isthmus: palpate again with patient swallowing. If thyroid tissue is palpable, describe size (feel for the lower border to rule out retrosternal extension), shape (uniformly enlarged or nodular), consistency (soft, rubbery or hard), tenderness (thyroiditis), and mobility (malignant neoplasm: fixed).
- Palpate lymph nodes.
- Assess tracheal position.

Percussion

- Percuss for retrosternal dullness, which may indicate retrosternal extension.

Auscultation

- Bruit is a sign of increased blood flow and can be present in thyrotoxicosis.

Examination of the eyes

- Look for lid lag and exophthalmos (Graves' disease).
- Check eye movements by asking the patient to follow your finger movements without moving their head (restricted in Graves' disease due to abnormal connective tissue deposition).
- Visual fields: bitemporal hemianopia may be suggestive of a sellar mass causing chiasmal compression (secondary hypothyroidism).

Other

- Check reflexes (slow relaxing in hypothyroidism).
- Proximal myopathy.
- Examine for pretibial myxoedema.
- Cardiovascular examination (signs of cardiac failure).

Investigations

1 Thyroid function tests (TFTs): must include measurement of serum TSH and free T4 (Table 12.4). TSH is elevated in primary hypothyroidism, and free T4 is low. In secondary hypothyroidism, free T4 is low and TSH may be low, normal, or minimally elevated. In subclinical disease, TSH is mildly elevated but free T4 normal.
2 Anti-thyroid peroxidase (anti-TPO) antibodies and anti-thyroglobulin antibodies are found in 90–95% of patients with autoimmune thyroiditis.
3 Lipid profile, creatine kinase (CK), urea and electrolytes, full blood count (FBC), and fasting blood glucose. Untreated hypothyroidism may be associated with raised cholesterol and triglycerides, a raised CK, hyponatraemia, and anaemia (normocytic or macrocytic). These abnormalities usually resolve with treatment.
4 Where secondary hypothyroidism is suspected, investigations will be guided by endocrinology, and may involve:
   a tests of pituitary function, including morning (9 a.m.) serum cortisol, prolactin, testosterone, gonadotrophins, estradiol, and insulin-like growth factor (IGF)-1
   b pituitary CT/MRI.

CHAPTER 12

Table 12.4 Biochemical findings in hypothyroidism and hyperthyroidism.

Condition	TSH	Free T4	Free T3
Primary hypothyroidism	Raised	Lowered	Lowered or normal
Secondary hypothyroidism	Lowered, normal or minimally elevated	Lowered	Lowered or normal
Subclinical hypothyroidism	Raised	Normal	Normal
Primary hyperthyroidism	Lowered	Raised	Raised or normal
Secondary hyperthyroidism	Raised	Raised	Raised or normal
Subclinical hyperthyroidism	Lowered	Normal	Normal

MANAGEMENT

Clinical primary hypothyroidism

- Guidance recommends use of thyroxine (T4) alone in the treatment of hypothyroidism, commonly prescribed as levothyroxine. For adults aged over 18 years without ischaemic heart disease, the initial dose of levothyroxine is based on the patient's body weight, i.e. 1.6 μg/kg with repeat TFT assessment after 8 weeks. The usual maintenance dose is 100–200 μg daily. There are certain patients (those with cardiac disease, the elderly) for whom the recommended initial dose of levothyroxine is 25–50 μg once daily, adjusted in steps of 25 μg every 14–21 days according to response.
- Prescribing additional T3 is currently not recommended.
- TSH should be monitored annually.

Subclinical hypothyroidism

Some patients with subclinical hypothyroidism, especially those whose TSH level is greater than 10 mU/L and who have positive anti-TPO or anti-thyroglobulin antibodies, may achieve symptomatic benefit from treatment with levothyroxine. The treatment of patients with TSH values between 4.5 and 10 mU/L is controversial, especially in older patients [4,5].

Secondary hypothyroidism

First-line treatment is levothyroxine, with adjunctive treatment for the underlying disorder.

Hypothyroidism and serious mental illness

Overt hypothyroidism can present with neuropsychiatric symptoms including cognitive deficits and depressive symptoms, and it is paramount that a diagnosis of hypothyroidism is excluded in such presentations. Moreover, there are case reports of severely hypothyroid patients presenting with frank psychotic symptoms, referred to as 'myxoedema madness' [6].

Depressive symptoms

Depression is the most common neuropsychiatric symptom in hypothyroidism, with an estimated prevalence of 60% [7]. The prevalence of overt hypothyroidism in individuals with a depressive diagnosis has been estimated to be 0.5–8% [8], and 4–10% may have subclinical hypothyroidism [9]. Most studies report an improvement in depressive symptoms in individuals with overt thyroid disease treated with thyroid hormone replacement [10–12]. However, randomised, placebo-controlled, blinded studies of thyroid hormone replacement therapy in individuals with subclinical hypothyroidism have not observed reliable improvement in depression or psychological distress scores [5,13,14].

Cognitive deficits

Overt hypothyroidism can affect a range of cognitive domains, including attention and concentration, memory, language, and executive functioning [15]. Memory is the most consistently affected; specific deficits in verbal memory are reported [16]. Thyroid hormone replacement is effective in treating these decrements, although there may not be complete reversal. Subclinical hypothyroidism is not associated with widespread or severe cognitive symptoms, though subtle deficits have been reported in memory and executive functioning. It is reasonable to initiate treatment for such patients, but realistic expectations should be set regarding symptom resolution.

Lithium

Lithium is associated with hypothyroidism. Up to 33% of patients treated with lithium have anti-thyroid antibodies; lithium also has a direct toxic effect on the thyroid gland [17]. Regular monitoring of TFTs (every 6 months) is recommended for patients on lithium therapy. When lithium-induced hypothyroidism occurs, treatment with levothyroxine is indicated as already described.

HYPERTHYROIDISM

Thyrotoxicosis describes disorders of excess thyroid hormone with or without increased synthesis of thyroid hormone (hyperthyroidism). The most common cause of primary hyperthyroidism is Graves' disease, an autoimmune disorder mediated by antibodies that stimulate the TSH receptor, accounting for approximately 75% of cases in iodine-replete areas. Toxic nodular disease accounts for 50% of cases in iodine-depleted areas. Other causes of thyrotoxicosis include thyroiditis (autoimmune, viral infection, drug induced) and excess ingestion of thyroid hormone (see Table 12.1). A hyperthyroid crisis or thyroid storm is an acute life-threatening hypermetabolic state caused by excessive release of thyroid hormone (see Chapter 79).

The prevalence of hyperthyroidism is 0.8% in Europe [18] and 1.3% in the USA [19]. Hyperthyroidism can be overt or subclinical. Overt hyperthyroidism is characterised by low serum TSH concentrations and raised serum concentrations of T4, T3, or both. Subclinical hyperthyroidism is characterised by low serum TSH, but normal serum T4 and T3 concentrations. Excess thyroid hormone affects many different organ systems (see Table 12.1). Commonly reported symptoms are palpitations, fatigue, tremor, anxiety, disturbed sleep, weight loss, heat intolerance, sweating, and polydipsia. Frequent physical findings are tachycardia, tremor of the extremities, and weight loss (see Table 12.2).

CHAPTER 12

DIAGNOSTIC PRINCIPLES

History

1 Symptoms of hyperthyroidism: heat intolerance, sweating, weight loss, palpitations, tremor, irritability, scalp hair loss.
2 Symptoms related to size of goitre: anterior pressure sensation, dyspnoea, dysphagia.
3 Past medical history:
   a radiation of the neck
   b autoimmune disease
   c trauma to thyroid gland (including surgery).
4 Medication history: see Table 12.3.
5 Drug and alcohol: tobacco use (strongly associated with Graves' hyperthyroidism, risk factor for orbitopathy) [20].
6 Family history: autoimmune thyroid disease.
7 Social history: stress may be associated with onset or relapse of Graves' disease [21].

Examination

See Box 12.1.

- Graves' disease: diffuse goitre, ophthalmopathy (proptosis, periorbital oedema, diplopia), thyroid dermopathy (pigmented thickened skin primarily involving the pretibial area), and thyroid acropachy (clubbing of the fingers and toes).
- Nodular thyroid disease: palpable thyroid nodule(s).
- Subacute thyroiditis: anterior neck pain.

Investigations

1 TFTs: TSH is the initial screening test, with reduced levels suggesting hyperthyroidism. Confirm the diagnosis with free T4 levels. If TSH is suppressed but free T4 levels are normal then, if not previously supplied, free T3 level is needed (T3 toxicosis). See Table 12.4.
2 Autoantibodies are most commonly seen in Graves' disease: TSH receptor antibodies have a sensitivity of 98% and specificity of 99% for Graves' disease [22].
3 Imaging.
   a Thyroid ultrasound scan to characterise palpable nodule(s).
   b Thyroid isotope scan (technetium-99m) to identify autonomously functioning nodule(s) (focal increased uptake); very low or absent uptake is seen in thyroiditis, factitious ingestion of thyroid hormone, or iodine-induced thyrotoxicosis.
4 Inflammatory markers: in patients with subacute thyroiditis, C-reactive protein (CRP) and erythrocyte sedimentation rate (ESR) are often raised.

MANAGEMENT

Clinical primary hyperthyroidism

1 Consider starting a beta-blocker or calcium channel blocker to control symptoms driven by the sympathetic nervous system, especially in older patients and those with cardiovascular disease.
2 Anti-thyroid medication.
   a Two methods are used (i) 'block and replace', where thionamides (e.g. carbimazole, methimazole, and propylthiouracil) are given with thyroxine replacement over a period of 6 months; and (ii) 'dose titration', where thionamides are used alone over 12–18 months and doses are titrated to achieve normalisation of thyroid hormone production. A Cochrane review suggests that both methods achieve long-term remission rates of approximately 35% [23]. Some clinicians utilise the block and replace approach when thyroid function has demonstrated marked fluctuation during treatment.
   b Propylthiouracil can cause liver failure, particularly in children [24]. As such, its use is reserved for pregnancy and thyroid storm.
   c TFTs are repeated every 4-6 weeks.
   d Thionamides can cause agranulocytosis (1–3 per 1000). It is more frequently seen early in treatment and with higher doses (>40 mg carbimazole). It is important to advise patients to stop thionamide and present for an FBC if they develop a sore throat or fever.
   e Thyrotoxicosis associated with thyroiditis is transient and resolves spontaneously; anti-thyroid drugs are not effective and should therefore be avoided.
3 Radioactive iodine.
   a Iodine-131 is the treatment of choice for toxic nodular disease and in many cases of relapsed Graves' disease. It can take three to four months to take effect.
   b Contraindicated in pregnant or breastfeeding women. Individuals are advised to avoid conception for six months.
   c Hypothyroidism is a common sequela.
4 Surgical.
   a Total thyroidectomy achieves a 98% cure rate. It is usually considered for patients who have a large goitre, compressive symptoms, significant ophthalmopathy, or who require rapid cure before pregnancy.
   b Patients should be returned to the euthyroid state with anti-thyroid drugs before surgery to avoid thyroid storm.
   c Complications are rare (<1%) but include haemorrhage, hypoparathyroidism, and vocal cord paralysis.

Subclinical hyperthyroidism

Treatment of subclinical hyperthyroidism is recommended in elderly patients due to an increased risk of atrial fibrillation, osteoporosis, bone fractures, and progression to overt disease [25].

CHAPTER 12

Hyperthyroidism and serious mental illness

Neuropsychiatric symptoms of overt hyperthyroidism include anxiety, dysphoria, emotional lability, intellectual dysfunction, and mania [9]. A subset of hyperthyroid patients, typically the elderly population, may present with depression, lethargy, pseudodementia, and apathy, with what is termed 'apathetic thyrotoxicosis' [26]. Psychotic symptoms including unusual presentations such as delusional parasitosis are rare in hyperthyroid patients, but have been reported [27,28]. Severe hyperthyroidism can result in thyroid storm, a condition that ranges in neuropsychiatric presentation from hyperirritability, anxiety, and confusion to apathy and coma.

Subclinical hyperthyroidism may be associated with agitation, irritability, and changes in mood [9]. There are no clear recommendations for treatment based on reversing neuropsychiatric symptoms associated with subclinical hyperthyroidism.

Hyperthyroidism may occur with long-term lithium treatment, though is less common than hypothyroidism. Lithium-induced hyperthyroidism is characterised by a transient and painless thyroiditis, thought to be secondary to a direct toxic effect of lithium on the thyroid gland, or through lithium-induced autoimmunity [17]. Regular monitoring of TFTs (every six months) is recommended for patients who are on lithium therapy.

Specialist input

All patients with new-onset thyrotoxicosis should be referred for assessment in secondary care to establish the aetiology and agree a management plan [29].

Consider referral for urgent admission if there is:

- atrial fibrillation or cardiac failure
- dehydration (secondary to diarrhoea).

Consider urgent referral to a thyroid surgeon if:

- symptoms of tracheal compression are present
- hyperthyroid patients present with thyroid swelling associated with voice changes, previous neck irradiation, family history of endocrine tumour, extremes of age (prepuberty, >65).

References

1. Boelaert K, Franklyn JA. Thyroid hormone in health and disease. *J Endocrinol* 2005;187(1):1–15.
2. Lazarus JH, Premawardhana LD. Screening for thyroid disease in pregnancy. *J Clin Pathol* 2005;58(5):449–452.
3. Roberts FP, Wright AL, O'Hagan SA. Hypothyroidism in textile workers. *J Soc Occup Med* 1990;40(4):153–156.
4. Franklyn JA. The thyroid: too much and too little across the ages. The consequences of subclinical thyroid dysfunction. *Clin Endocrinol* 2013;78(1):1–8.
5. Parle J, Roberts L, Wilson S, et al. A randomized controlled trial of the effect of thyroxine replacement on cognitive function in community-living elderly subjects with subclinical hypothyroidism: the Birmingham Elderly Thyroid study. *J Clin Endocrinol Metab* 2010;95(8):3623–3632.
6. Easson WM. Myxedema with psychosis. *Arch Gen Psychiatry* 1966;14(3):277–283.

7. Bathla M, Singh M, Relan P. Prevalence of anxiety and depressive symptoms among patients with hypothyroidism. *Indian J Endocrinol Metab* 2016;20(4):468–474.

8. Radhakrishnan R, Calvin S, Singh J, et al. Thyroid dysfunction in major psychiatric disorders in a hospital based sample. *Indian J Med Res* 2013;138(6):888–893.

9. Feldman AZ, Shrestha RT, Hennessey JV. Neuropsychiatric manifestations of thyroid disease. *Endocrinol Metab Clin North Am* 2013;42(3):453–476.

10. Yu J, Tian A-J, Yuan X, Cheng X-X. Subclinical hypothyroidism after ^{131}I-treatment of Graves' disease: a risk factor for depression? *PLoS One* 2016;11(5):e0154846.

11. Davis JD, Tremont G. Neuropsychiatric aspects of hypothyroidism and treatment reversibility. *Minerva Endocrinol* 2007;32(1):49–65.

12. Gulseren S, Gulseren L, Hekimsoy Z, et al. Depression, anxiety, health-related quality of life, and disability in patients with overt and subclinical thyroid dysfunction. *Arch Med Res* 2006;37(1):133–139.

13. Waterloo K, Jorde R, Nyrnes A, et al. Neuropsychological function and symptoms in subjects with subclinical hypothyroidism and the effect of thyroxine treatment. *J Clin Endocrinol Metab* 2006;91(1):145–153.

14. Kong WM, Sheikh MH, Lumb PJ, et al. A 6-month randomized trial of thyroxine treatment in women with mild subclinical hypothyroidism. *Am J Med* 2002;112(5):348–354.

15. Samuels MH. Psychiatric and cognitive manifestations of hypothyroidism. *Curr Opin Endocrinol Diabetes Obes* 2014;21(5):377–383.

16. Miller KJ, Parsons TD, Whybrow PC, et al. Verbal memory retrieval deficits associated with untreated hypothyroidism. *J Neuropsychiatry Clin Neurosci* 2007;192:132–136.

17. Kibirige D, Luzinda K, Ssekitoleko R. Spectrum of lithium induced thyroid abnormalities: a current perspective. *Thyroid Res* 2013;6(1):3.

18. Garmendia Madariaga A, Santos Palacios S, Guillen-Grima F, Galofre JC. The incidence and prevalence of thyroid dysfunction in Europe: a meta-analysis. *J Clin Endocrinol Metab* 2014;99(3):923–931.

19. Hollowell JG, Staehling NW, Flanders WD, et al. Serum TSH, T4, and thyroid antibodies in the United States population (1988 to 1994): National Health and Nutrition Examination Survey (NHANES III). *J Clin Endocrinol Metab* 2002;87(2):489–499.

20. Perros P, Krassas GE. Graves orbitopathy: a perspective. *Nat Rev Endocrinol* 2009;5(6):312–318.

21. Mizokami T, Wu Li A, El-Kaissi S, Wall JR. Stress and thyroid autoimmunity. *Thyroid* 2004;14(12):1047–1055.

22. Tozzoli R, Bagnasco M, Giavarina D, Bizzaro N. TSH receptor autoantibody immunoassay in patients with Graves' disease: improvement of diagnostic accuracy over different generations of methods. Systematic review and meta-analysis. *Autoimmun Rev* 2012;12(2):107–113.

23. Abraham P, Avenell A, McGeoch SC, et al. Antithyroid drug regimen for treating Graves' hyperthyroidism. *Cochrane Database Syst Rev* 2010;(1):CD003420.

24. British National Formulary (online). Propylthiouracil. http://www.medicinescomplete.com (accessed 23 February 2019).

25. Biondi B. Natural history, diagnosis and management of subclinical thyroid dysfunction. *Best Pract Res Clin Endocrinol Metab* 2012;26(4):431–446.

26. Arnold BM, Casal G, Higgins HP. Apathetic thyrotoxicosis. *Can Med Assoc J* 1974;111(9):957–958.

27. Özten E, Tufan AE, Cerit C, et al. Delusional parasitosis with hyperthyroidism in an elderly woman: A case report. *J Med Case Rep* 2013;7:17.

28. Lazarus A, Jaffe R. Resolution of thyroid-induced schizophreniform disorder following subtotal thyroidectomy: case report. *Gen Hosp Psychiatry* 1986;8(1):29–31.

29. Vaidya B, Pearce SHS. Diagnosis and management of thyrotoxicosis. *BMJ* 2014;349:g5128.

Hyperprolactinaemia

John Lally, Toby Pillinger, Olubanke Dzahini, Sophie Harris

Prolactin, a protein secreted from the anterior pituitary gland, is a multifunctional hormone with more than 300 direct or indirect actions reported, including effects on water and salt balance, growth and development, energy metabolism, stress adaptation, neurogenesis and neuroprotection, reproduction, and immune activity [1]. A comprehensive description of the actions of prolactin is beyond the scope of this chapter, which focuses on common causes of hyperprolactinaemia in patients with serious mental illness (SMI), the typical presentation of a patient with hyperprolactinaemia, recommended investigations, and management.

Normal prolactin levels are gender-dependent, with higher levels seen in females [2]. Normal prolactin levels are generally reported as 210–420 mIU/L for men (approximately 10–20 ng/mL), and 210–530 mIU/L for women (approximately 10–25 ng/mL) [3]. The causes of hyperprolactinaemia are listed in Box 13.1. In patients with SMI, psychiatric medication, most often antipsychotics, are implicated in most cases of hyperprolactinaemia. Prolactin secretion is tonically inhibited by dopamine released from the hypothalamus into the tuberoinfundibular system acting at D2 dopamine receptors on lactotroph cells of the anterior pituitary. Thus, antipsychotic-mediated D2 receptor blockade removes tonic inhibition of prolactin secretion. There is heterogeneity in the relative degree to which different antipsychotics affect prolactin levels (Table 13.1). As such, antipsychotics have historically been subcategorised into 'prolactin-raising' agents (so-called first-generation antipsychotics plus risperidone, paliperidone, and amisulpride) and 'prolactin-sparing' agents (so-called second-generation antipsychotics, except for risperidone, paliperidone, and amisulpride). Some antipsychotics can increase blood prolactin levels within hours of treatment initiation [4]. Prolactin levels generally fall to normal range within two to four days of stopping oral antipsychotics, although this is influenced by the half-life of the antipsychotic and the formulation in

The Maudsley Practice Guidelines for Physical Health Conditions in Psychiatry, First Edition.
David M. Taylor, Fiona Gaughran, and Toby Pillinger.
© 2021 John Wiley & Sons Ltd. Published 2021 by John Wiley & Sons Ltd.

Box 13.1 Causes of hyperprolactinaemia

Pituitary disorders

- Prolactinomas:
  Microadenomas (<10 mm): 90%
  Macroadenomas (>10 mm): 10%
- Cushing's disease
- Acromegaly
- Empty sella syndrome
- Cranial irradiation

Systemic disorders

- Hypothyroidism
- Chronic renal failure
- Liver failure
- Seizures
- Sarcoidosis
- Polycystic ovary disease
- Oestrogen-secreting tumours
- Chest wall lesions

Physiological

- Pregnancy
- Breastfeeding
- REM sleep
- Stress

Medication

- Antipsychotics (see Table 13.1)
- Tricyclic antidepressants
- Monoamine oxidase inhibitors
- Metoclopramide
- Reserpine
- Verapamil
- Methyldopa

---

which it is delivered. Some antipsychotics take up to three weeks for prolactin levels to normalise post discontinuation [4], and slower decline is seen after discontinuation of medication given in long-acting injectable form [5]. Other psychiatric medications, including tricyclic antidepressants and monoamine oxidase inhibitors, can also result in hyperprolactinaemia (see Box 13.1). Psychosocial stress can cause elevations in prolactin [6,7], a potential explanation for why hyperprolactinaemia occurs more frequently in patients with first-episode psychosis compared with healthy controls, even prior to use of antipsychotics [8].

CHAPTER 13

Table 13.1 Relative risk of hyperprolactinaemia with different antipsychotics [3,9].

Amisulpride[a]	+++
Aripiprazole	–
Asenapine	–/+
Blonanserin	+
Brexpiprazole	–
Cariprazine	–
Chlorpromazine	+++
Clozapine	–
Flupentixol	+++
Fluphenazine	+++
Haloperidol	++
Lurasidone	+
Molindone	+++
Olanzapine	+
Paliperidone[a]	+++
Perphenazine	+++
Pimozide	+++
Pipothiazine	+++
Quetiapine	–/+
Risperidone[a]	+++
Sertindole	+
Sulpiride[a]	+++
Trifluoperazine	+++
Ziprasidone	+
Zuclopenthixol	+++

[a] Amisulpride, sulpiride, risperidone, and paliperidone are generally associated with more severe prolactin changes.
+++, high risk; ++, moderate; +, low; –, very low.

CHAPTER 13

DIAGNOSTIC PRINCIPLES

Although prolactin is a multifunctional hormone, the signs and symptoms of hyperprolactinaemia generally derive from the role of prolactin in stimulating the mammary glands to produce milk, and via its influence on oestrogen levels in women and testosterone levels in men. As such, hyperprolactinaemia may be associated with hypogonadism, sexual dysfunction, acne, hirsutism, galactorrhoea (secretion of milk from nipples), and rarely gynaecomastia (the excessive growth and development of the male mammary glands) [3,10]. Sexual dysfunction due to hyperprolactinaemia in males and females may be characterised by reduced libido, and impaired arousal and orgasm [10]. Men may develop erectile dysfunction. Galactorrhoea is much more common in women than men with hyperprolactinaemia [11], and is estimated to occur in 10–20% of women treated with first-generation antipsychotics [12]. Prolonged hyperprolactinaemia, via its influence on gonadotrophin levels, can also reduce bone mineral density (therefore resulting in osteopenia/osteoporosis) in both men and women.

The degree of hyperprolactinaemia will generally influence the type and severity of clinical symptoms experienced, and the following is a guide with regard to premenopausal women [13].

- Serum prolactin levels above 2120 mIU/L (99.6 ng/mL) are associated with hypogonadism and menstrual dysfunction, including amenorrhoea and galactorrhoea.
- Serum prolactin levels between 1081 and 1590 mIU/L (50.8–74.7 ng/mL) are associated with oligomenorrhea (infrequent menstrual periods).
- Serum prolactin levels between 657 and 1060 mIU/L (30.9–49.8 ng/mL) are associated with reduced libido.

History and investigation

Many psychiatric patients with hyperprolactinaemia are asymptomatic, with raised prolactin noted on routine blood screening. However, a history should still be taken for evidence of hypogonadism, galactorrhoea, or gynaecomastia, as already detailed. Any patient presenting spontaneously to clinic with these symptoms should be investigated with a serum prolactin level.

Although the long-term consequences of raised prolactin in asymptomatic patients are yet to be clearly defined, chronically raised levels are likely to be associated with comorbidity, and as such it is recommended that prolactin levels in patients receiving antipsychotic treatment are tested routinely.

General principles regarding serum prolactin testing are as follows.

- Check serum prolactin levels in patients before starting an antipsychotic and before switching to a new antipsychotic. Consider rechecking once optimal antipsychotic dose has been reached, and annually in patients on established antipsychotic treatment.
- Since stress can elevate prolactin levels, where elevations are modest (<1000 mIU/L) repeat testing is recommended to confirm presence of hyperprolactinaemia.
- In women of childbearing age, rule out pregnancy.
- Enquire about headache or visual disturbance (pituitary adenoma) or symptoms of hypothyroidism (see Chapter 12). Physical examination may be indicated to confirm presence of a bitemporal hemianopia or evidence of hypothyroidism.
- Consider also checking thyroid, renal, and liver function (see Box 13.1).

- Where prolactin levels remain persistently elevated without an obvious cause, discussion with endocrinology and pituitary MRI is indicated (see section on management).
- Since persistent hyperprolactinaemia is associated with osteoporosis, enquire about fracture history, and family history of fractures. Also consider checking vitamin D levels and enquire about exercise levels, smoking status, and alcohol intake.

MANAGEMENT AND WHEN TO REFER TO A SPECIALIST

- Prolactin levels above 1000 mIU/L prior to antipsychotic initiation should prompt further investigations (see section History and investigation) and discussion with endocrinology.
- Hyperprolactinaemia with levels below 2500 mIU/L in asymptomatic patients where antipsychotic treatment is felt to be the most likely cause does not necessarily require further investigation or treatment. The patient should be informed and may be followed up with regular enquiry regarding emergent symptoms. Development of hypogonadism, galactorrhoea, or gynaecomastia would indicate the need for repeat serum prolactin testing and intervention. Where it is unclear whether to intervene in such patients, discussion with endocrinology is recommended.
- Where hyperprolactinaemia of less than 2500 mIU/L is likely secondary to antipsychotic treatment and the decision is made to intervene (e.g. in the case of hypogonadism), dose reduction may be considered, although whether antipsychotic-induced hyperprolactinaemia is dose dependent is unclear [14]. Alternatively, treatment can be switched to an antipsychotic with a reduced propensity to cause hyperprolactinaemia (see Table 13.1). However, this may not always be possible due to the risk of deterioration in the patient's mental state. The use of the partial dopamine agonist aripiprazole (5–10 mg daily; often 5 mg is sufficient) as an adjunctive agent is effective in reducing hyperprolactinaemia, with almost 80% of patients with antipsychotic-induced hyperprolactinaemia experiencing normalisation of prolactin levels [15]. However, aripiprazole augmentation is generally ineffective in amisulpride-induced hyperprolactinaemia [16]. Low-dose dopamine receptor agonists (e.g. bromocriptine and cabergoline) can be considered as third-line treatments, although this requires close monitoring for psychotic relapse and should only be used following endocrinology input as part of a multidisciplinary approach.
- Hypogonadism may be treated with hormone replacement. Males can be treated with testosterone administered via transdermal patches. In females, the use of a combined oral contraceptive will offset oestrogen deficiency and associated complications including bone mineral density loss [17]. However, this will not ameliorate other hyperprolactinaemia-related symptoms. Hormonal treatment should only be used following endocrinology input as part of a multidisciplinary approach.
- Prolactin levels above 2500 mIU/L should, after history and examination of the patient (see section History and investigation), prompt discussion with endocrinology regardless of whether the patient is receiving antipsychotic treatment as these levels may indicate a prolactinoma [4]. Pituitary adenomas can generally be managed

CHAPTER 13

pharmacologically using dopamine agonists, although caution should be exercised in the use of such agents in the psychiatric patient population, and a multidisciplinary approach involving both psychiatry and endocrinology is advised. Where drug treatment is not indicated, transsphenoidal surgery may be considered.

- There are currently no guidelines that stipulate which patients with hyperprolactinaemia should be assessed with dual-energy X-ray absorptiometry (DEXA). Persistent hypogonadism (e.g. amenorrhoea for over six months) is an indication to measure bone mineral density. DEXA scans are also recommended if a patient experiences a broken bone after only a minor fall, if the patient has received prolonged (more than three months) glucocorticoid treatment, if the patient has experienced early menopause, if the patient has a low body mass index (<19 kg/m^2), or if the patient has any other comorbid medical/psychiatric condition that can lead to low bone density (e.g. malabsorption syndromes, chronic renal failure, eating disorders) [18].

- The Fracture Risk Assessment Tool (FRAX) is validated for fracture risk prediction in those greater than 50 years of age [19] and can be used in people with psychotic disorders, although a diagnosis of a psychotic disorder or the use of antipsychotic medication is not currently included in the FRAX algorithm. Indeed, the FRAX calculator has been found to significantly underestimate 10-year fracture risk associated with use of psychotropic medication [20].

HYPERPROLACTINAEMIA AND OSTEOPOROSIS RISK IN SERIOUS MENTAL ILLNESS

Hyperprolactinaemia suppresses the hypothalamic–pituitary–gonadal axis which, when prolonged, reduces bone mineral density and increases risk of osteoporosis. People with schizophrenia are 2.5 times more likely to have osteoporosis and have a 72% increased risk of fracture compared to the general population [21]. The mechanisms underlying reduced bone mineral density in schizophrenia are poorly understood and multifactorial, with lifestyle factors such as increased rates of smoking, alcohol intake, low vitamin D levels, and sedentary behaviour, alongside the side effects of antipsychotic medication likely contributing [22–25]. Schizophrenia and related psychotic disorders are usually diagnosed between the ages of 16 and 30, often prior to the patient reaching peak bone mass [26]. Exposure to prolactin-raising medications at an early age, alongside the lifestyle factors, may therefore prevent development of optimum peak bone mass, thus reducing lifelong bone mineral density and predisposing patients to osteoporosis [21]. However, it is important to note that while antipsychotic-induced hyperprolactinaemia could play a role in the development of reduced bone mineral density in people with schizophrenia [27,28], there is currently insufficient evidence to be certain that antipsychotic-induced hyperprolactinaemia, in the absence of hypogonadism, constitutes an independent risk factor for the development of osteoporosis in patients with schizophrenia [29].

HYPERPROLACTINAEMIA AND CANCER RISK

Hyperprolactinaemia has been implicated in an increased risk of malignancy, particularly breast cancer [30]. Female patients with schizophrenia are at increased risk of breast cancer, although the contribution of antipsychotic-induced hyperprolactinaemia is unclear. Furthermore, studies not taking into account parity may overestimate the risk for breast cancer in schizophrenia [31]. Further work is required to determine if moderating hyperprolactinaemia in this cohort will reduce malignancy rates [32].

References

1. Bole-Feysot C, Goffin V, Edery M, et al. Prolactin (PRL) and its receptor: actions, signal transduction pathways and phenotypes observed in PRL receptor knockout mice. *Endocr Rev* 1998;19(3):225–268.
2. Melmed S, Casanueva FF, Hoffman AR, et al. Diagnosis and treatment of hyperprolactinemia: an Endocrine Society clinical practice guideline. *J Clin Endocrinol Metab* 2011;96(2):273–288.
3. Peuskens J, Pani L, Detraux J, De Hert M. The effects of novel and newly approved antipsychotics on serum prolactin levels: a comprehensive review. *CNS Drugs* 2014;28(5):421–453.
4. Haddad PM, Wieck A. Antipsychotic-induced hyperprolactinaemia: mechanisms, clinical features and management. *Drugs* 2004;64(20):2291–2314.
5. Wistedt B, Wiles D, Kolakowska T. Slow decline of plasma drug and prolactin levels after discontinuation of chronic treatment with depot neuroleptics. *Lancet* 1981;317(8230):1163.
6. Fitzgerald P, Dinan TG. Prolactin and dopamine: what is the connection? A review article. *J Psychopharmacol* 2008;22(2 Suppl):12–19.
7. Lennartsson A-K, Jonsdottir IH. Prolactin in response to acute psychosocial stress in healthy men and women. *Psychoneuroendocrinology* 2011;36(10):1530–1539.
8. Gonzalez-Blanco L, Greenhalgh AM, Garcia-Rizo C, et al. Prolactin concentrations in antipsychotic-naive patients with schizophrenia and related disorders: a meta-analysis. *Schizophr Res* 2016;174(1–3):156–160.
9. Huhn M, Nikolakopoulou A, Schneider-Thoma J, et al. Comparative efficacy and tolerability of 32 oral antipsychotics for the acute treatment of adults with multi-episode schizophrenia: a systematic review and network meta-analysis. *Lancet* 2019;394(10202):939–951.
10. Bobes J, Garc APMP, Rejas J, et al. Frequency of sexual dysfunction and other reproductive side-effects in patients with schizophrenia treated with risperidone, olanzapine, quetiapine, or haloperidol: the results of the EIRE study. *J Sex Marital Ther* 2003;29(2):125–147.
11. Wieck A, Haddad PM. Antipsychotic-induced hyperprolactinaemia in women: pathophysiology, severity and consequences. *Br J Psychiatry* 2003;182:199–204.
12. Windgassen K, Wesselmann U, Schulze Monking H. Galactorrhea and hyperprolactinemia in schizophrenic patients on neuroleptics: frequency and etiology. *Neuropsychobiology* 1996;33(3):142–146.
13. Serri O, Chik CL, Ur E, Ezzat S. Diagnosis and management of hyperprolactinemia. *Can Med Assoc J* 2003;169(6):575–581.
14. Lally J, Ajnakina O, Stubbs B, et al. Hyperprolactinaemia in first episode psychosis: a longitudinal assessment. *Schizophr Res* 2017;189:117–125.
15. Li X, Tang Y, Wang C. Adjunctive aripiprazole versus placebo for antipsychotic-induced hyperprolactinemia: meta-analysis of randomized controlled trials. *PLoS One* 2013;8(8):e70179.
16. Paulzen M, Grunder G. Amisulpride-induced hyperprolactinaemia is not reversed by addition of aripiprazole. *Int J Neuropsychopharmacol* 2007;10(1):149–151.
17. Inder WJ, Castle D. Antipsychotic-induced hyperprolactinaemia. *Aust N Z J Psychiatry* 2011;45(10):830–837.
18. Compston J, Cooper A, Cooper C, et al. UK clinical guideline for the prevention and treatment of osteoporosis. *Arch Osteoporos* 2017;12(1):43.
19. Fracture Risk Assessment Tool (FRAX). https://www.sheffield.ac.uk/FRAX/index.aspx (accessed 6 October 2019).
20. Bolton JM, Morin SN, Majumdar SR, et al. Association of mental disorders and related medication use with risk for major osteoporotic fractures. *JAMA Psychiatry* 2017;74(6):641–648.
21. Stubbs B, Gaughran F, Mitchell AJ, et al. Schizophrenia and the risk of fractures: a systematic review and comparative meta-analysis. *Gen Hosp Psychiatry* 2015;37(2):126–133.
22. De Hert M, Detraux J, Stubbs B. Relationship between antipsychotic medication, serum prolactin levels and osteoporosis/osteoporotic fractures in patients with schizophrenia: a critical literature review. *Expert Opin Drug Saf* 2016;15(6):809–823.
23. de Leon J, Diaz FJ. A meta-analysis of worldwide studies demonstrates an association between schizophrenia and tobacco smoking behaviors. *Schizophr Res* 2005;76(2–3):135–157.
24. Lally J, Ajnakina O, Singh N, et al. Vitamin D and clinical symptoms in first episode psychosis (FEP): a prospective cohort study. *Schizophr Res* 2019;204:381–388.

CHAPTER 13

25. Lally J, Gardner-Sood P, Firdosi M, et al. Clinical correlates of vitamin D deficiency in established psychosis. *BMC Psychiatry* 2016;16(1):1–9.

26. Heaney RP, Abrams S, Dawson-Hughes B, et al. Peak bone mass. *Osteoporos Int* 2000;11(12):985–1009.

27. Tseng PT, Chen YW, Yeh PY, et al. Bone mineral density in schizophrenia: an update of current meta-analysis and literature review under guideline of PRISMA. *Medicine (Baltimore)* 2015;94(47):e1967.

28. Gomez L, Stubbs B, Shirazi A, et al. Lower bone mineral density at the hip and lumbar spine in people with psychosis versus controls: a comprehensive review and skeletal site-specific meta-analysis. *Curr Osteoporos Rep* 2016;14(6):249–259.

29. Lally J, Bin Sahl A, Murphy KC, et al. Serum prolactin and bone mineral density in schizophrenia- a systematic review. *Clin Psychopharmacol Neurosci* 2019;17(3):333–342.

30. Bernichtein S, Touraine P, Goffin V. New concepts in prolactin biology. *J Endocrinol* 2010;206(1):1–11.

31. Oksbjerg Dalton S, Munk Laursen T, Mellemkjaer L, et al. Schizophrenia and the risk for breast cancer. *Schizophr Res* 2003;62(1–2):89–92.

32. Chou AIW, Wang YC, Lin CL, Kao CH. Female schizophrenia patients and risk of breast cancer: a population-based cohort study. *Schizophr Res* 2017;188:165–171.

CHAPTER 13

Chapter 14

Obesity

Yuya Mizuno, Toby Pillinger, Dan Siskind, Ian Osborne,
Kate Moffat, Donal O'Shea

The World Health Organization (WHO) defines overweight and obesity as abnormal or excessive fat accumulation that presents a risk to health [1]. A crude measure of obesity is the body mass index (BMI), with a BMI greater than or equal to 25 and 30 respectively considered overweight and obese (Box 14.1) [1]. Waist circumference and waist-to-height ratio are other indices that may be used to assess central obesity (Box 14.2). Recent global estimates indicate that 39% and 13% of adults aged 18 years and older are respectively overweight and obese [1]. In the UK, approximately 60% of adults are either overweight or obese [11]; in the USA, approximately 70% of adults meet these criteria [13]. Obesity is robustly associated with various medical conditions, including cardiometabolic disease [13,14], musculoskeletal disorders (especially osteo-arthritis), and cancer [9,11]. Accordingly, in 2014–2015 the NHS spent approximately £6 billion on overweight and obesity-related ill-health [15]. In the USA, annual medical spending attributable to obesity was approximately $150 billion in 2014 [16].

Box 14.1 Calculating body mass index and definitions of overweight and obesity [1]

Body mass index (BMI) may be calculated using the following formula:

$$BMI(kg/m^2) = \frac{mass(kg)}{(height(m))^2}$$

As a general principle, the following applies for adults.

- Ideal weight: BMI within the range 18.5–24.9.
- Overweight: BMI within the range 25.0–29.9.
- Obese: BMI greater than or equal to 30.0.

The Maudsley Practice Guidelines for Physical Health Conditions in Psychiatry, First Edition.
David M. Taylor, Fiona Gaughran, and Toby Pillinger.
© 2021 John Wiley & Sons Ltd. Published 2021 by John Wiley & Sons Ltd.

In the UK, a lower BMI cut-off value of 23 is used for black, Asian, and other minority groups due to greater risk of diabetes mellitus at lower BMI relative to white populations [2,3]. However, note that people with high muscle mass may be categorised as overweight despite having a healthy body weight. Similarly, BMI calculations will be inaccurate in patients with oedema, ascites, or who are pregnant. Furthermore, in older adults (≥65 years) being overweight is not associated with an increased risk of mortality (indeed, risk of mortality increases in those with a low-normal and low BMI) [4]. As such, an 'ideal' BMI range for older adults is 23.0–29.9 kg/m^2.

A BMI classified as overweight (except for older adults) or obese should prompt the healthcare professional to seek permission to discuss the individual's weight and its implications with them. This discussion should explore readiness and motivation for lifestyle change to manage weight. If ready, possible interventions should be discussed (see section Prevention and treatment of obesity).

Obesity is divided into three classes.

- Class 1: BMI 30–34.9.
- Class 2: BMI 35–39.9.
- Class 3: BMI 40+ ('extreme' or 'severe' obesity).

CHAPTER 14

Box 14.2 Measurement and significance of waist circumference and waist-to-height ratio

Waist circumference is an index of intra-abdominal fat mass [5]. This is important as excessive abdominal fat is associated with greater risk for cardiovascular disease, type 2 diabetes, and cancer [6]. Measure waist circumference as follows [7].

- Find the bottom of the patient's ribs and the top of the patient's hips (see Figure 14.1).
- Wrap a tape measure around the patient's waist, midway between these points.
- Have the patient breath out naturally before taking the measurement.

As a general principle, the following cut-off values apply for waist circumference, independent of height or BMI [7].

- At waist circumferences of 94 cm (37 inches) for men and 80 cm (31.5 inches) for women, losing weight should be considered.
- Waist circumferences above 102 cm (40 inches) for men and 88 cm (34.5 inches) for women are associated with a high risk of serious health conditions; these patients should be reviewed by a clinician and intervention (see section Prevention and treatment of weight gain) strongly recommended.

The waist-to-height ratio is calculated as waist circumference divided by height. A simple cut-off value of 0.5 or greater has been proposed as an indicator of increased health risk, regardless of differences in sex or ethnicity (i.e. 'keep your waist circumference to less than half your height') [8,9].

Despite the utility of waist circumference and waist-to-height ratio in assessing risk of obesity-related ill-health, it can be measured inaccurately. For example, locating anatomical landmarks may be challenging in individuals who have obesity, and tape measures can be wrapped too tightly or loosely around the waist. Furthermore, there is no universally accepted protocol for measuring waist circumference, with the World Health Organization (WHO) and National Institutes of Health having different protocols. Figure 14.1 shows the anatomical landmarks recommended by WHO for measuring waist circumference in men and women [10].

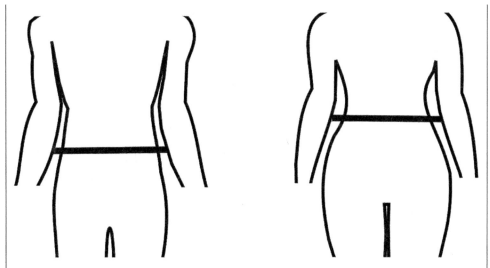

Figure 14.1 Waist circumference measurement sites for men and women based on World Health Organization recommendations. The measure is taken from midway between the highest point on the iliac crest and the bottom of the ribcage. Source: adapted from Patry-Parisien et al. [10].

Obesity is more prevalent in people with severe mental illness (SMI) compared to the general population [17,18]; for example, a 2010 North American study observed that 80% of a sample of over 10,000 people with diagnoses of schizophrenia, bipolar disorder, and depression were either overweight or obese [19]. The cause of weight gain in this population is multifactorial, including high caloric intake, genetic factors, sedentary behaviour, social isolation, and negative discrimination [20,21]. Furthermore, many antipsychotic medications [22,23], as well as some antidepressants [24] and mood stabilisers [25], are recognised to induce weight gain. In addition to the burden of physical comorbidities, obesity reduces self-worth, is associated with reduced quality of life [26] and poor concordance with psychotropic treatment [27], and is an independent predictor of psychiatric readmission [28].

Tackling obesity as a modifiable risk factor for all-cause and cardiovascular mortality represents a key component of the holistic care provided to people with SMI [29]. There is evidence that some patients with SMI (e.g. those with first-episode psychosis) present with metabolic dysregulation from illness onset and prior to psychotropic prescription [30–32]. Thus, risk of obesity and broader metabolic disturbance in this patient population should be considered from first contact with psychiatric services.

MONITORING

There are multiple guidelines focusing on the monitoring of weight gain and cardiometabolic risk in patients with schizophrenia (see De Hert et al. [33] for review). Key guidelines in the UK include the National Institute for Health and Care Excellence

CHAPTER 14

Table 14.1 Monitoring protocol for weight gain, metabolic disturbance, and cardiovascular risk in patients with serious mental illness initiating psychotropic medication (all antipsychotics, consider with some antidepressants and mood stabilisers; see text).

Parameters	Baseline[a]	When to evaluate					Comments
		+4 weeks	+8 weeks	+12 weeks	+6 months	Annually thereafter[b]	
Body weight, BMI	✓	✓	✓	✓	✓	✓	Ideally weekly for first 4–6 weeks, then every 2–4 weeks up to 12 weeks
Waist circumference	✓	✓	✓	✓	✓	✓	Not mandatory, but recommended
Waist-to-height ratio	(✓)			(✓)	(✓)	(✓)	Not mandatory
Fasting glucose, HbA$_{1c}$, and lipid profile[b]	✓			✓	✓	✓	HbA$_{1c}$ is preferable for monitoring long-term blood glucose control
Blood pressure	✓			✓	✓	✓	
Personal/family history of cardiovascular disease	✓						
History of tobacco and alcohol use	✓	✓	✓	✓	✓	✓	

[a] Before starting psychotropic, or as soon as possible after starting.
[b] Increase frequency if clinically indicated (e.g. more than 5% weight gain after a one-month period).
Source: adapted from Cooper et al. [35].

(NICE) guidelines [34] and the British Association for Psychopharmacology (BAP) guidelines [35]. The monitoring protocol recommended by the BAP forms the basis of Table 14.1. Increased monitoring frequency should be considered in certain clinical situations. For example, psychotropic-naive adults and paediatric patients are at increased risk of antipsychotic-induced weight gain [36]. Rapid weight gain following initiation of psychotropic medications (more than 5% weight gain after a one-month period) is a strong predictor of long-term weight gain and should prompt both enhanced monitoring and preventative or remedial strategies (see section Lifestyle modification) [37]. It is recommended that patients with bipolar disorder and major depressive disorder undergo the same baseline assessments as those with schizophrenia when initiating treatment [38,39]. Weight gain has been described in patients receiving antidepressants (especially mirtazapine, mianserin, tricyclics, and monoamine oxidase inhibitors) [38] and mood stabilisers (especially sodium valproate and lithium) [39]. We recommend that patients receiving those antidepressants and mood stabilisers with recognised risk of weight gain (i.e. those listed in this section) should be monitored as per the monitoring protocol shown in Table 14.1. However, this guidance is flexible, and whenever psychiatric patients appear to be gaining weight, they should be monitored closely.

As part of an assessment of a patient's weight, consider quantifying 10-year cardiovascular risk using the QRISK3 calculator [40,41]. This tool incorporates various cardiovascular risk factors detailed in Table 14.1, as well as a diagnosis of SMI and antipsychotic prescription. The QRISK3 outcome can not only be used to guide subsequent management (see Chapter 9) but also to engage with the patient on the topic of weight gain and cardiovascular risk.

PREVENTION AND TREATMENT OF WEIGHT GAIN

Figure 14.2 summarises an approach to management of weight gain in patients with SMI. As a general principle, clinicians should proactively manage weight gain before it becomes an issue.

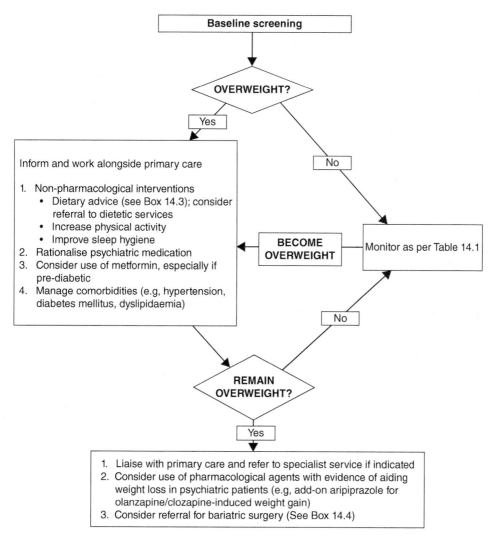

Figure 14.2 Flowchart to manage weight gain in patients with severe mental illness.

CHAPTER 14

Non-pharmacological interventions to combat weight gain

Lifestyle modification

Preventative strategies that aim to help patients achieve healthy lifestyles should be offered to everyone. These include avoiding/stopping smoking, addressing alcohol and substance misuse, improving diet, improving sleep, and increasing physical activity [29] (see Chapters 10, 24, 46, and 55). There is evidence that combined lifestyle interventions including behavioural interventions, nutrition, and exercise are effective in attenuating weight gain when introduced during early phase of antipsychotic treatment [42,43].

An individual is more likely to be successful in managing their weight if they feel ready and motivated to make the necessary lifestyle changes. Thus, if possible, explore whether weight loss is important to the individual, any motivating factors, and any potential barriers. For those who feel ready to make lifestyle changes, it is important to set realistic goals; success increases confidence and motivates further success. Make only one to three small lifestyle changes at once (selecting those that the person feels are most likely to be successful) and increase over time. In terms of weight loss targets, recommend losing 5–10% of current body weight at a rate of 0.5 kg per week, and 4 cm from around the waist.

Box 14.3 provides dietary advice/tips for weight loss. Where accessible and appropriate, consider referring to a dietician ideally with experience in treating patients with

---

Box 14.3 Dietary advice for weight loss

- Having a bowl of soup or a sugar-free drink before a main meal can help fill you up and so eat less.
- Aim to eat three regular balanced meals a day.
- A healthy weight loss plate is half vegetables/salad and the other half split equally between starch (preferably high fibre: wholemeal bread, rice, pasta, potatoes, yam, plantain chapatti) and protein (e.g. pulses, nuts, seeds, eggs, fish, poultry, or red meat).
- Increase fruit and vegetable intake, aiming for five to ten portions per day and more vegetables than fruit.
- Choose food and snacks that are low in fat, sugar, and salt.
- When reading traffic light food labels, choose those with more green and amber and fewer red.
- Choose drinks that are sugar-free/'diet' and low fat or fat-free.
- Restrict fruit juice and smoothie intake to 150 mL/day: more can cause weight gain and tooth decay.
- Take care with portion sizes: aim for a 'small' or 'medium' size when given the option.
- When having a takeaway have one main dish, one side dish, and a sugar-free drink.
- When eating aim to eat at a table rather than on the couch or in bed.
- When eating make this the only activity you are doing, i.e. no TV, no social media, no phones.
- Eat slowly, take your time, and enjoy your food.
- It takes at least 15–20 minutes for your brain to register that your stomach is full, so wait and give yourself time to feel full before considering second portions.
- A healthy dessert such as fruit and low-fat low sugar yoghurts are a better choice than second portions and can help ensure your diet is balanced.
- If you find that when taking psychiatric medication you are getting hungry very soon after having eaten a main meal, choose high-fibre, low-calorie nutritious foods such as fruits, vegetables, salad, wholegrain bread, and cereals.
- If you find that you need to eat a lot to feel full, limit eating to three main meals per day. Avoid snacking and drink water and sugar-free drinks between meals instead.

SMI. Other factors that can aid weight loss include using a food diary and regularly monitoring progress, for example weighing oneself weekly and measuring waist circumference monthly.

Rationalising psychiatric medication

When prescribing psychotropic medication, the propensity for weight gain and other metabolic adversities associated with treatments should be carefully considered. Figure 14.3 summarises the relative risk of weight gain associated with acute treatment with 18 antipsychotics relative to placebo (see Pillinger et al. [23] for ranking of antipsychotics based on other metabolic disturbance). Since all marketed antipsychotics are more effective than placebo in treating acute psychotic episodes, and drug-naive patients are particularly susceptible to weight gain, antipsychotics with high risk of weight gain should generally be avoided as first-line treatments [44]. Based on broader metabolic dysfunction associated with different antipsychotics, the following agents are thought to be safer options: aripiprazole, brexpiprazole, cariprazine, lurasidone, and ziprasidone [23]. For patients already established on an antipsychotic, there is evidence that switching treatment to aripiprazole or lurasidone is associated with weight loss (with low risk of relapse) [45,46].

For mood stabilisers, lamotrigine likely has the most benign metabolic profile [47,48]. For antidepressants, selective serotonin reuptake inhibitors (SSRIs) and serotonin/noradrenaline reuptake inhibitors (SNRIs) are reasonable options although paroxetine may be associated with a greater risk of weight gain [24]. Agomelatine is reported to

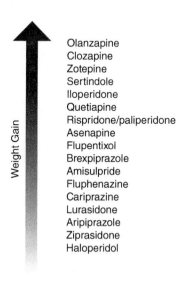

Figure 14.3 Propensity of 18 antipsychotics to induce weight gain in the acute treatment of psychosis relative to placebo [23].

have a low incidence of weight gain [49], and bupropion may have potential to induce weight loss in individuals with obesity [50].

Early use of metformin

In the general population, there is evidence that early use of metformin in patients with pre-diabetes delays progression to type 2 diabetes mellitus [51]. Metformin is also associated with weight loss in patients with schizophrenia receiving clozapine or olanzapine [52]. Therefore, in individuals who are overweight or have pre-diabetes and are receiving olanzapine or clozapine, where lifestyle interventions have not been effective, consider early prescription of metformin (aiming to reach a dose of 2 g daily in two to three divided doses, or once daily if using a modified-release preparation).

Management of comorbidities

Other components of the metabolic syndrome (hypertension, type 2 diabetes mellitus, and dyslipidaemia) should be managed to reduce cardiovascular risk. The reader is directed to the chapters on these topics (Chapters 5, 9, and 11).

Pharmacological interventions

As already described, the best evidence for pharmacological management of weight gain in patients with SMI is for the use of metformin. There are however various other agents available, which are summarised in Table 14.2. Of note, most of the evidence for these agents is based on patients with schizophrenia receiving clozapine or olanzapine. Therefore, it is unclear if the evidence is directly translatable for patients with other psychiatric diagnoses receiving other medications. When using pharmacological strategies, the risk–benefit with regard to potential side effects needs to be considered. Comorbidities may also guide prescription decisions (e.g. use of metformin or GLP1R agonists in the context of type 2 diabetes mellitus). If patients present with sedation from medications such as clozapine or olanzapine, then add-on aripiprazole or betahistine may be appropriate choices.

When to refer to a specialist

Primary care practitioners should be informed from the onset and should be involved in multidisciplinary discussions regarding the patient's weight and associated metabolic disturbance. Where available, referral to a dietician should be considered as well as supporting improved access to physical activity. Bariatric surgery may be considered for patients with morbid obesity who struggle to lose weight despite undertaking both non-pharmacological and pharmacological strategies (Box 14.4).

Table 14.2 Pharmacological interventions to counteract weight gain.

Drug	Risks/side effects	Comment
Metformin (500–2000 mg/day)	Lactic acidosis, vitamin B_{12} deficiency, GI disturbance (then try immediately after meals, if still not tolerated try modified-release formulation), contraindicated with eGFR <30 mL/min per 1.73 m²	First line for psychotropic-induced weight gain [52–56]
Glucagon-like peptide-1 receptor (GLP1R) agonists (e.g. liraglutide 3 mg/day subcutaneously)	Nausea/vomiting, possible increased pancreatitis risk.	Effective in patients treated with olanzapine or clozapine [57,58]. Weekly formulations available
Aripiprazole (5–15 mg/day)	Sleep disturbance, akathisia, GI disturbance	Evidence for use in conjunction with clozapine or olanzapine [52,59]
Amantadine (100–300 mg/day)	Theoretical risk of exacerbating psychosis	Some evidence for use in olanzapine-induced weight gain [60,61]
Bupropion (150 mg twice daily)	GI side effects reported. Potent inhibitor of cytochrome P450 isoenzyme CYP2D6 [62], so may alter other psychiatric medication levels, including clozapine	Evidence for use in the general population, including combination therapy with naltrexone [63]. Data lacking in severe mental illness and psychotropic-induced weight gain, although some evidence in depression alongside calorie restriction [64]
Betahistine (48 mg/day, although trial data suggests doses up to 144 mg/day)	Reports of headache and hypersensitivity reactions	Evidence for use in olanzapine-induced weight gain [65,66]
Methylcellulose (1500 mg before meals)	Can be difficult to swallow, bloating, laxative effect	Data lacking in severe mental illness and psychotropic-induced weight gain
Orlistat (120 mg thrice daily with meals)	A fatty diet will result in steatorrhoea and potential malabsorption of oral medication	Evidence for use in clozapine- and olanzapine-induced weight gain [67–72]. Consider referral to a dietician to support a low-fat diet
Reboxetine (4–8 mg once daily)	Difficulty sleeping, GI disturbance, dizziness, excessive sweating	Evidence for use in olanzapine-induced weight gain, and in combination with betahistine [52]
Topiramate (up to 300 mg daily)	Sedation, cognitive impairment	Evidence for use in psychotropic-induced weight gain, also for preventing weight gain [73,74]
Zonisamide (100–600 mg/day)	Sedation, diarrhea, cognitive impairment	Evidence for use in second-generation antipsychotic induced weight gain [75]

eGFR, estimated glomerular filtration rate; GI, gastrointestinal.

CHAPTER 14

> **Box 14.4** Overview of bariatric surgery [76]
>
> Bariatric surgery (also referred to as weight loss surgery) refers to a group of surgical interventions designed to reduce body weight and improve obesity-related conditions. Common types of bariatric surgery include the following.
>
> - Gastric bypass: the top part of the stomach is joined to the small intestine.
> - Sleeve gastrectomy: some of the stomach is removed.
> - Gastric banding was previously commonly performed but is no longer recommended.
>
> Bariatric surgery is available on the NHS for people who meet the following criteria.
>
> - BMI of 40 or more, or a BMI between 35 and 40 and an obesity-related condition that may improve if the person lost weight (e.g. type 2 diabetes mellitus, hypertension).
> - Attempted all other weight loss methods including lifestyle change and pharmacotherapies but have not lost significant weight.
> - Agree to long-term follow-up after surgery (e.g. making healthy lifestyle changes, attending regular check-ups).
>
> In the general population, bariatric surgery is associated with both weight loss and remission of diabetes mellitus in individuals living with obesity [77]. While there are still limited data in patients with schizophrenia, growing evidence suggests that bariatric surgery may improve short-term weight status among patients with bipolar disorder, to a comparable degree with individuals in the general population [78].

References

1. World Health Organization. Obesity and overweight. https://www.who.int/en/news-room/fact-sheets/detail/obesity-and-overweight (accessed 5 January 2020).
2. Chiu M, Austin PC, Manuel DG, et al. Deriving ethnic-specific BMI cutoff points for assessing diabetes risk. *Diabetes Care* 2011;34(8): 1741–1748.
3. WHO Expert Consultation. Appropriate body-mass index for Asian populations and its implications for policy and intervention strategies. *Lancet* 2004;363(9403):157–163.
4. Winter JE, MacInnis RJ, Wattanapenpaiboon N, Nowson CA. BMI and all-cause mortality in older adults: a meta-analysis. *Am J Clin Nutr* 2014;99(4):875–890.
5. Pouliot MC, Despres JP, Lemieux S, et al. Waist circumference and abdominal sagittal diameter: best simple anthropometric indexes of abdominal visceral adipose tissue accumulation and related cardiovascular risk in men and women. *Am J Cardiol* 1994;73(7):460–468.
6. Must A, McKeown NM. *The disease burden associated with overweight and obesity.* In: Feingold KR, Anawalt B, Boyce A, et al. (eds) *Endotext* [Internet]. South Dartmouth, MA: MDText.com Inc., 2000.
7. National Health Service. Why is my waist size important? https://www.nhs.uk/common-health-questions/lifestyle/why-is-my-waist-size-important/ (accessed 19 January 2020).
8. Ashwell M, Hsieh SD. Six reasons why the waist-to-height ratio is a rapid and effective global indicator for health risks of obesity and how its use could simplify the international public health message on obesity. *Int J Food Sci Nutr* 2005;56(5):303–307.
9. Anandacoomarasamy A, Caterson I, Sambrook P, et al. The impact of obesity on the musculoskeletal system. *Int J Obes (Lond)* 2008;32(2):211–222.
10. Patry-Parisien J, Shields M, Bryan S. Comparison of waist circumference using the World Health Organization and National Institutes of Health protocols. *Health Rep* 2012;23(3):53–60.
11. Cancer Research UK. Overweight and obesity statistics. https://www.cancerresearchuk.org/health-professional/cancer-statistics/risk/overweight-and-obesity#heading-One (accessed 5 January 2020).
12. Fryar CD, Carroll MD, Ogden CD. Prevalence of overweight, obesity, and severe obesity among adults aged 20 and over: United States, 1960–1962 through 2015–2016. https://www.cdc.gov/nchs/data/hestat/obesity_adult_15_16/obesity_adult_15_16.htm (accessed 17 January 2020).
13. Abdullah A, Peeters A, de Courten M, Stoelwinder J. The magnitude of association between overweight and obesity and the risk of diabetes: a meta-analysis of prospective cohort studies. *Diabetes Res Clin Pract* 2010;89(3):309–319.
14. Poirier P, Eckel RH. Obesity and cardiovascular disease. *Curr Atheroscler Rep* 2002;4(6):448–453.

15. Public Health England. Health matters: obesity and the food environment. https://www.gov.uk/government/publications/health-matters-obesity-and-the-food-environment/health-matters-obesity-and-the-food-environment--2 (accessed 17 January 2020).

16. Kim DD, Basu A. Estimating the medical care costs of obesity in the United States: systematic review, meta-analysis, and empirical analysis. *Value Health* 2016;19(5):602–613.

17. Dickerson FB, Brown CH, Kreyenbuhl JA, et al. Obesity among individuals with serious mental illness. *Acta Psychiatr Scand* 2006;113(4):306–313.

18. Keck PE, McElroy SL. Bipolar disorder, obesity, and pharmacotherapy-associated weight gain. *J Clin Psychiatry* 2003;64(12):1426–1435.

19. Correll CU, Druss BG, Lombardo I, et al. Findings of a U.S. national cardiometabolic screening program among 10,084 psychiatric outpatients. *Psychiatr Serv* 2010;61(9):892–898.

20. Manu P, Dima L, Shulman M, et al. Weight gain and obesity in schizophrenia: epidemiology, pathobiology, and management. *Acta Psychiatr Scand* 2015;132(2):97–108.

21. Rubino F, Puhl RM, Cummings DE, et al. Joint international consensus statement for ending stigma of obesity. *Nat Med* 2020;26(4):485–497.

22. Leucht S, Cipriani A, Spineli L, et al. Comparative efficacy and tolerability of 15 antipsychotic drugs in schizophrenia: a multiple-treatments meta-analysis. *Lancet* 2013;382(9896):951–962.

23. Pillinger T, McCutcheon R, Vano L, et al. Comparative effects of 18 antipsychotics on metabolic function in schizophrenia, predictors of metabolic dysregulation, and association with psychopathology: a systematic review and network meta-analysis. *Lancet Psychiatry* 2020;7(1):64–77.

24. Serretti A, Mandelli L. Antidepressants and body weight: a comprehensive review and meta-analysis. *J Clin Psychiatry* 2010;71(10):1259–1272.

25. Grootens KP, Meijer A, Hartong EG, et al. Weight changes associated with antiepileptic mood stabilizers in the treatment of bipolar disorder. *Eur J Clin Pharmacol* 2018;74(11):1485–1489.

26. Allison DB, Mackell JA, McDonnell DD. The impact of weight gain on quality of life among persons with schizophrenia. *Psychiatr Serv* 2003;54(4):565–567.

27. Weiden PJ, Mackell JA, McDonnell DD. Obesity as a risk factor for antipsychotic noncompliance. *Schizophr Res* 2004;66(1):51–57.

28. Manu P, Khan S, Radhakrishnan R, et al. Body mass index identified as an independent predictor of psychiatric readmission. *J Clin Psychiatry* 2014;75(6):e573–e577.

29. Firth J, Siddiqi N, Koyanagi A, et al. The Lancet Psychiatry Commission: a blueprint for protecting physical health in people with mental illness. *Lancet Psychiatry* 2019;6(8):675–712.

30. Pillinger T, Beck K, Gobjila C, et al. Impaired glucose homeostasis in first-episode schizophrenia: a systematic review and meta-analysis. *JAMA Psychiatry* 2017;74(3):261–269.

31. Pillinger T, Beck K, Stubbs B, Howes OD. Cholesterol and triglyceride levels in first-episode psychosis: systematic review and meta-analysis. *Br J Psychiatry* 2017;211(6):339–349.

32. Pillinger T, D'Ambrosio E, McCutcheon R, Howes OD. Is psychosis a multisystem disorder? A meta-review of central nervous system, immune, cardiometabolic, and endocrine alterations in first-episode psychosis and perspective on potential models. *Mol Psychiatry* 2019;24(6):776–794.

33. De Hert M, Vancampfort D, Correll CU, et al. Guidelines for screening and monitoring of cardiometabolic risk in schizophrenia: systematic evaluation. *Br J Psychiatry* 2011;199(2):99–105.

34. National Institute for Health and Care Excellence. *Psychosis and Schizophrenia in Adults: Prevention and Management*. Clical Guideline CG178. London: NICE, 2014. Available at https://www.nice.org.uk/guidance/cg178/chapter/1-Recommendations (accessed 17 November 2019).

35. Cooper SJ, Reynolds GP, Barnes T, et al. BAP guidelines on the management of weight gain, metabolic disturbances and cardiovascular risk associated with psychosis and antipsychotic drug treatment. *J Psychopharmacol* 2016;30(8):717–748.

36. Correll CU, Lencz T, Malhotra AK. Antipsychotic drugs and obesity. *Trends Mol Med* 2011;17(2):97–107.

37. Vandenberghe F, Gholam-Rezaee M, Saigi-Morgui N, et al. Importance of early weight changes to predict long-term weight gain during psychotropic drug treatment. *J Clin Psychiatry* 2015;76(11):e1417–e1423.

38. Dodd S, Malhi GS, Tiller J, et al. A consensus statement for safety monitoring guidelines of treatments for major depressive disorder. *Aust N Z J Psychiatry* 2011;45(9):712–725.

39. Ng F, Mammen OK, Wilting I, et al. The International Society for Bipolar Disorders (ISBD) consensus guidelines for the safety monitoring of bipolar disorder treatments. *Bipolar Disord* 2009;11(6):559–595.

40. Hippisley-Cox J, Coupland C, Brindle P. Development and validation of QRISK3 risk prediction algorithms to estimate future risk of cardiovascular disease: prospective cohort study. *BMJ* 2017;357:j2099.

41. ClinRisk. Welcome to the QRISK®3-2018 risk calculator. https://qrisk.org/three/ (accessed 20 January 2020).

42. Alvarez-Jimenez M, Gonzalez-Blanch C, Vazquez-Barquero JL, et al. Attenuation of antipsychotic-induced weight gain with early behavioral intervention in drug-naive first-episode psychosis patients: a randomized controlled trial. *J Clin Psychiatry* 2006;67(8):1253–1260.

43. Nyboe L, Lemcke S, Moller AV, Stubbs B. Non-pharmacological interventions for preventing weight gain in patients with first episode schizophrenia or bipolar disorder: a systematic review. *Psychiatry Res* 2019;281:112556.

44. Siskind D, Kisely S. Balancing body and mind: selecting the optimal antipsychotic. *Lancet* 2019;394(10202):900–902.

45. Barak Y, Aizenberg D. Switching to aripiprazole as a strategy for weight reduction: a meta-analysis in patients suffering from schizophrenia. *J Obes* 2011;2011:898013.

46. Stahl SM, Cucchiaro J, Simonelli D, et al. Effectiveness of lurasidone for patients with schizophrenia following 6 weeks of acute treatment with lurasidone, olanzapine, or placebo: a 6-month, open-label, extension study. *J Clin Psychiatry* 2013;74:507–515.

CHAPTER 14

47. Biton V. Effect of antiepileptic drugs on bodyweight: overview and clinical implications for the treatment of epilepsy. *CNS Drugs* 2003;17(11):781–791.
48. Bowden CL, Calabrese JR, Ketter TA, et al. Impact of lamotrigine and lithium on weight in obese and nonobese patients with bipolar I disorder. *Am J Psychiatry* 2006;163(7):1199–1201.
49. Kennedy SH, Rizvi SJ. Agomelatine in the treatment of major depressive disorder: potential for clinical effectiveness. *CNS Drugs* 2010;24(6):479–499.
50. Gadde KM, Parker CB, Maner LG, et al. Bupropion for weight loss: an investigation of efficacy and tolerability in overweight and obese women. *Obes Res* 2001;9(9):544–551.
51. Knowler WC, Barrett-Connor E, Fowler SE, et al. Reduction in the incidence of type 2 diabetes with lifestyle intervention or metformin. *N Engl J Med* 2002;346(6):393–403.
52. Mizuno Y, Suzuki T, Nakagawa A, et al. Pharmacological strategies to counteract antipsychotic-induced weight gain and metabolic adverse effects in schizophrenia: a systematic review and meta-analysis. *Schizophr Bull* 2014;40(6):1385–1403.
53. Jarskog LF, Hamer RM, Catellier DJ, et al. Metformin for weight loss and metabolic control in overweight outpatients with schizophrenia and schizoaffective disorder. *Am J Psychiatry* 2013;170(9):1032–1040.
54. Praharaj SK, Jana AK, Goyal N, Sinha VK. Metformin for olanzapine-induced weight gain: a systematic review and meta-analysis. *Br J Clin Pharmacol* 2011;71(3):377–382.
55. Siskind DJ, Leung J, Russell AW, et al. Metformin for clozapine associated obesity: a systematic review and meta-analysis. *PLoS One* 2016;11(6):e0156208.
56. Zheng W, Li XB, Tang YL, et al. Metformin for weight gain and metabolic abnormalities associated with antipsychotic treatment: meta-analysis of randomized placebo-controlled trials. *J Clin Psychopharmacol* 2015;35(5):499–509.
57. Larsen JR, Vedtofte L, Jakobsen MSL, et al. Effect of liraglutide treatment on prediabetes and overweight or obesity in clozapine- or olanzapine-treated patients with schizophrenia spectrum disorder: a randomized clinical trial. *JAMA Psychiatry* 2017;74(7):719–728.
58. Siskind DJ, Russell AW, Gamble C, et al. Treatment of clozapine-associated obesity and diabetes with exenatide in adults with schizophrenia: a randomized controlled trial (CODEX). *Diabetes Obes Metab* 2018;20(4):1050–1055.
59. Zheng W, Zheng YJ, Li XB, et al. Efficacy and safety of adjunctive aripiprazole in schizophrenia: meta-analysis of randomized controlled trials. *J Clin Psychopharmacol* 2016;36(6):628–636.
60. Praharaj SK, Sharma PS. Amantadine for olanzapine-induced weight gain: a systematic review and meta-analysis of randomized placebo-controlled trials. *Ther Adv Psychopharmacol* 2012;2(4):151–156.
61. Zheng W, Wang S, Ungvari GS, et al. Amantadine for antipsychotic-related weight gain: meta-analysis of randomized placebo-controlled trials. *J Clin Psychopharmacol* 2017;37(3):341–346.
62. Kotlyar M, Brauer LH, Tracy TS, et al. Inhibition of CYP2D6 activity by bupropion. *J Clin Psychopharmacol* 2005;25(3):226–229.
63. Greig SL, Keating GM. Naltrexone ER/Bupropion ER: a review in obesity management. *Drugs* 2015;75(11):1269–1280.
64. Jain AK, Kaplan RA, Gadde KM, et al. Bupropion SR vs. placebo for weight loss in obese patients with depressive symptoms. *Obes Res* 2002;10(10):1049–1056.
65. Barak N, Beck Y, Albeck JH. Betahistine decreases olanzapine-induced weight gain and somnolence in humans. *J Psychopharmacol* 2016;30(3):237–241.
66. Lian J, Huang XF, Pai N, Deng C. Ameliorating antipsychotic-induced weight gain by betahistine: mechanisms and clinical implications. *Pharmacol Res* 2016;106:51–63.
67. Sjostrom L, Rissanen A, Andersen T, et al. Randomised placebo-controlled trial of orlistat for weight loss and prevention of weight regain in obese patients. European Multicentre Orlistat Study Group. *Lancet* 1998;352(9123):167–172.
68. Hilger E, Quiner S, Ginzel I, et al. The effect of orlistat on plasma levels of psychotropic drugs in patients with long-term psychopharmacotherapy. *J Clin Psychopharmacol* 2002;22(1):68–70.
69. Pavlovic ZM. Orlistat in the treatment of clozapine-induced hyperglycemia and weight gain. *Eur Psychiatry* 2005;20(7):520.
70. Carpenter LL, Schecter JM, Sinischalchi J, et al. A case series describing orlistat use in patients on psychotropic medications. *Med Health R I* 2004;87(12):375–377.
71. Joffe G, Takala P, Tchoukhine E, et al. Orlistat in clozapine- or olanzapine-treated patients with overweight or obesity: a 16-week randomized, double-blind, placebo-controlled trial. *J Clin Psychiatry* 2008;69(5):706–711.
72. Tchoukhine E, Takala P, Hakko H, et al. Orlistat in clozapine- or olanzapine-treated patients with overweight or obesity: a 16-week open-label extension phase and both phases of a randomized controlled trial. *J Clin Psychiatry* 2011;72(3):326–330.
73. Correll CU, Maayan L, Kane J, et al. Efficacy for psychopathology and body weight and safety of topiramate–antipsychotic cotreatment in patients with schizophrenia spectrum disorders: results from a meta-analysis of randomized controlled trials. *J Clin Psychiatry* 2016;77(6):e746–e756.
74. Zheng W, Xiang YT, Xiang YQ, et al. Efficacy and safety of adjunctive topiramate for schizophrenia: a meta-analysis of randomized controlled trials. *Acta Psychiatr Scand* 2016;134(5):385–398.
75. Buoli M, Grassi S, Ciappolino V, et al. The use of zonisamide for the treatment of psychiatric disorders: a systematic review. *Clin Neuropharmacol* 2017;40(2):85–92.
76. National Health Service. Overview: Weight loss surgery. https://www.nhs.uk/conditions/weight-loss-surgery/ (accessed 27 January 2020).
77. Park CH, Nam SJ, Choi HS, et al. Comparative efficacy of bariatric surgery in the treatment of morbid obesity and diabetes mellitus: a systematic review and network meta-analysis. *Obes Surg* 2019;29(7):2180–2190.
78. Kouidrat Y, Amad A, Stubbs B, et al. Surgical management of obesity among people with schizophrenia and bipolar disorder: a systematic review of outcomes and recommendations for future research. *Obes Surg* 2017;27(7):1889–1895.

Part 3

Haematology

Anaemia

Sanjena Mithra, Aleksander Mijovic

The primary physiological function of haemoglobin (Hb) is to transport and deliver oxygen to body tissues. According to the World Health Organization, anaemia is defined as an Hb below 130 g/L for men and below 120 g/L for non-pregnant women, with global prevalence rates of 12.7% and 30.2%, respectively [1]. Anaemia is common in patients with serious mental illness (SMI), with observational studies estimating a prevalence of up to 35% [2], but it can also occur separately either due to an underlying condition or as a side effect of psychiatric medication [3]. It ultimately has the potential to exacerbate SMI if left untreated.

Several factors, including age, sex, nutrition, geography, ethnicity, and socioeconomic status, are known to contribute to anaemia and can therefore complicate physical or mental illness [4]. Nutritional deficiencies in eating disorders or neglect may contribute to reductions in Hb, and certain psychiatric medications are also associated with anaemia [3]. Hb levels naturally reduce with age, and differ by gender [5], ethnicity (e.g. Hb is lower in African Americans compared with Caucasians) [6], and geography (Hb increasing with altitude) [7]. Other causes of anaemia in the general population and those with SMI are documented in Table 15.1.

The Maudsley Practice Guidelines for Physical Health Conditions in Psychiatry, First Edition.
David M. Taylor, Fiona Gaughran, and Toby Pillinger.
© 2021 John Wiley & Sons Ltd. Published 2021 by John Wiley & Sons Ltd.

Table 15.1 Causes of anaemia in the general and psychiatric patient population.

	General population	Individual with serious mental illness
Medical comorbidity	Anaemia of chronic disease (e.g. chronic kidney disease, hypothyroidism, malignancy, systemic lupus erythematosus, heart failure, infection) Acute blood loss (e.g. trauma, GI bleed, deliberate self-harm) Chronic blood loss (e.g. GI bleed, urinary tract bleeding) Haematological disorders (e.g. haemoglobinopathies, myelodysplasia, haematological malignancies) Gynaecological causes (e.g. menorrhagia, fibroids)	
Nutrition	Iron/B$_{12}$/folate deficiency (e.g. old age, vegetarian diet, alcohol excess) Malabsorption (coeliac disease, Crohn's disease, following bariatric surgery)	Iron/B$_{12}$/folate deficiency (eating disorders, chronic liver disease secondary to alcohol, poor oral intake as part of spectrum of altered behaviours in serious mental illness, neglect)
Medication	Phenytoin Antibiotics (e.g. cephalosporins, trimethoprim) Chemotherapy and radiation NSAIDs Some antimalarial drugs (in glucose-6-phosphate dehydrogenase deficiency)	Mood stabilisers (e.g. carbamazepine) Antidepressants (e.g. fluoxetine, monoamine oxidase inhibitors, bupropion, duloxetine, mianserin) [8] Antipsychotics (e.g. aripiprazole, chlorpromazine, trifluoperazine) [9] Levodopa Donepezil, memantine Chlordiazepoxide Promethazine
Other	Pregnancy	

DIAGNOSTIC PRINCIPLES

The signs and symptoms associated with anaemia are dependent on its severity. Untreated progressive anaemia can cause physical symptoms such as lethargy, headaches, palpitations, and even psychiatric symptoms such as cognitive deficits and depression [10] An approach to clinical assessment of anaemia is documented in Figure 15.1, and a glossary of terms provided in Table 15.2.

Acute bleeding should be managed as a *medical emergency*, with resuscitation and emergency referral/transfer of the patient to medical services.

History

A very slowly falling Hb allows for a degree of compensation and enhancement of oxygen-carrying capacity of the blood, which means some patients may be asymptomatic. In general, elderly people tolerate anaemia less well and may present with non-specific symptoms [13,14]. Key features from a history are as follows.

1 Symptoms of anaemia: dizziness, feeling faint, fatigue, shortness of breath (either at rest or exertion), palpitations, headache, or angina (if there is pre-existing ischaemic heart disease) [5].

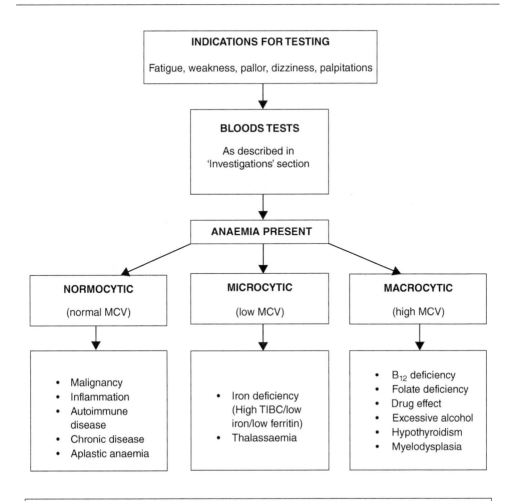

INDICATIONS FOR TESTING

Fatigue, weakness, pallor, dizziness, palpitations

BLOODS TESTS

As described in
'Investigations' section

ANAEMIA PRESENT

NORMOCYTIC

(normal MCV)

MICROCYTIC

(low MCV)

MACROCYTIC

(high MCV)

- Malignancy
- Inflammation
- Autoimmune
  disease
- Chronic disease
- Aplastic anaemia

- Iron deficiency
  (High TIBC/low
  iron/low ferritin)
- Thalassaemia

- B_{12} deficiency
- Folate deficiency
- Drug effect
- Excessive alcohol
- Hypothyroidism
- Myelodysplasia

NEXT STEPS
- Peripheral blood film evaluation
- Dietary and lifestyle modification as appropriate
- Rationalise medications (both psychiatric and non-psychiatric))
- Consider haematology opinion

Figure 15.1 An algorithmic approach to anaemia.

CHAPTER 15

2 Evidence of blood loss (per rectum bleeding, dark stool, haematemesis).
3 Symptoms that may point towards an underlying comorbidity (see Table 15.1) such as peripheral neuropathy (B_{12} deficiency), abdominal distension (hepatosplenomegaly), or any 'red flag' symptoms suggestive of malignancy, e.g. unintentional weight loss (see Chapter 25), smoking history, or change in bowel habit.
4 Past medical history including previous diagnoses of connective tissue disorders, heart disease, haematological disorders, and chronic kidney disease.

Table 15.2 Haematological tests in the work-up of anaemia.

Test	Definition
Mean corpuscular volume	The normal red cell has a volume of 80–96 femtolitres (fL) and the mean volume of red cells is called the mean corpuscular volume (MCV) [11,12]
Reticulocyte count	Reticulocytes are young red blood cells and their presence or absence can help diagnose types of anaemia [11] High count: increased red cell loss (bleeding), increased destruction (e.g. haemolytic anaemia) Low count: hypoproliferative anaemias (iron deficiency anaemia, aplastic anaemia, vitamin B_{12}/folate deficiency, kidney disease, infection)
Lactate dehydrogenase (LDH)	Enzyme that catalyses anaerobic respiratory reactions. Used as a marker for red cell breakdown in haemolysis
Direct antiglobulin test (DAT)	Also known as direct Coombs' test. Used to diagnose autoimmune haemolytic anaemias by detecting antibodies on the red cell membrane
Haptoglobin	Binds to free haemoglobin. Reduced/undetectable in hemolytic anaemias. Reduced haptoglobin alongside raised reticulocytes indicates haemolysis (of any aetiology)
Iron studies	Total iron-binding capacity (TIBC) is the total capacity of the blood to bind and transport iron. TIBC is increased in iron deficiency anaemia. Iron is transported through the blood bound to a protein called transferrin. Low transferrin saturation (expressed as a percentage) indicates reduced iron availability (e.g. in iron deficiency anaemia, or in anaemia of inflammation). Ferritin levels reflect intracellular iron stores. As such, low levels of ferritin represent low amounts of body iron. Ferritin levels below 20 µg/L are diagnostic of iron deficiency anaemia
Peripheral blood film	A way to examine the components of blood (red and white cells) under the microscope. It is also used to look for blood parasites (e.g. malaria). Red cell abnormalities may accompany anaemia, e.g. spherocytes (round cells, seen in spherocytosis and immune haemolytic anaemias), target cells (e.g. thalassaemia, post splenectomy), red cell fragments (e.g. microangiopathic haemolytic anaemia)

5 Medication history, specifically recent non-steroidal anti-inflammatory drug (NSAID) use (as prolonged treatment increases the risk of developing gastrointestinal bleeding), new medications, or antibiotic use.
6 Social and dietary history including vegan diets (iron/B_{12} deficiency), alcohol intake, socioeconomic status [10], poor diet, pregnancy. Urge to eat ice, clay, or dirt (pica) is a peculiar symptom occurring in iron deficiency anaemia.
7 Family history (hereditary anaemias: spherocytosis, sickle cell disease, thalassaemias).
8 A mental state examination should explore for evidence of symptoms of mental illness that may be contributing to poor diet, either directly (eating disorders) or indirectly (e.g. poor self-care in patients with dementia, or in those with severe depressive or psychotic symptoms).

Examination

1 General examination: is there conjunctival pallor, yellow sclerae, jaundice, or glossitis?
2 Basic observations: is there a postural drop (this can occur in the event of acute blood loss) or tachycardia?

3 Examine for lymphadenopathy (cervical, axillary, inguinal).
4 Cardiovascular examination: is there evidence of heart failure?
5 Gastrointestinal examination: is there hepatosplenomegaly?
6 Neurological examination: is there peripheral neuropathy (suggestive of B_{12} deficiency), loss of balance, or gait disorder?

Investigations

Bedside

1 Urine dip (haematuria).
2 Pregnancy test.
3 ECG (anaemia may be associated with tachycardia or induce myocardial ischaemia).

Blood tests

1 Full blood count: pay attention to Hb, mean corpuscular volume, and reticulocyte count.
2 Peripheral blood film (see Table 15.2).
3 Urea and electrolytes (upper gastrointestinal bleeding can be associated with raised urea disproportionate to the accompanying creatinine).
4 Liver function tests: for side effects of medications, evidence of chronic liver disease (e.g. secondary to alcohol abuse), and low albumin from poor nutrition.
5 C-reactive protein (infection).
6 Blood group and antibody screen in case transfusion required.
7 Lactate dehydrogenase, direct antiglobulin test, and haptoglobin (markers of haemolysis; see Table 15.2).
8 Vitamin B_{12} and folate.
9 Iron studies (see Table 15.2).
10 Hepatitis B and C, HIV serology.
11 Autoimmune screen including antinuclear antibodies, erythrocyte sedimentation rate (ESR), double-stranded DNA, and extractable nuclear antigen (if suspicion of systemic lupus erythematosus).

Imaging/special tests

1 Chest X-ray: is there any indication of pulmonary congestion or infection?
2 Cardiac echocardiogram: to evaluate myocardial function.

MANAGEMENT AND REFERRAL PATHWAYS

A blood transfusion should only be considered if there is severe acute anaemia or if the patient is particularly symptomatic (e.g. breathless or complaining of chest pain). If in doubt, discuss with general medical/haematology colleagues. Patients with acute blood loss should be assessed urgently by the on-call medical team or emergency department.

CHAPTER 15

Anaemia can usually be managed in primary care, although referral to a subspecialty may be appropriate if initial investigations reveal an underlying condition (e.g. if malignancy is suspected, if there is evidence of heart failure requiring cardiology input, or if a connective tissue disease is suspected requiring rheumatology input). If a psychiatric medication is thought to be causative, a risk–benefit decision will need to be made regarding ongoing treatment with a drug that is presumed to be responsible for the anaemia, balancing risk of continuing therapy (progressive anaemia) versus the risk of stopping treatment (deterioration in mental state). In this scenario, a multidisciplinary discussion involving psychiatry, haematology, and the patient is recommended. In the absence of a clear cause of anaemia, and where lifestyle/nutritional factors are thought to be responsible, the following approach is recommended.

Lifestyle modification

- Dietary advice (iron-rich, dark leafy green vegetables, brown rice, white and red meat). Ascorbic acid enhances iron absorption, so drinking orange juice (or indeed any food/drink high in vitamin C) may increase iron absorption. Tea impairs iron absorption, although typically this only becomes clinically significant when consumed in large volumes.
- Reduce alcohol intake.

Psychosocial interventions to improve dietary intake

- Treat symptoms of mental illness that may be contributing to poor oral intake.
- Social interventions in cases of neglect.

Pharmacological therapy

- If appropriate, rationalise psychiatric medication or, in collaboration with medical colleagues, physical health medication.
- Iron deficiency: ferrous sulfate 200 mg two to three times daily or ferrous fumarate tablets 210 mg two to three times daily. (Note that these medications can cause dark stools and abdominal cramps, and can also cause constipation; be aware when used alongside clozapine.) Hb should rise by 10 g/L per week. If oral iron replacement is not tolerated, an intravenous iron infusion can be considered, usually given every three months.
- Folate/B_{12} deficiency: folic acid 5 mg once daily *in combination with* B_{12} injections (unless normal B_{12}) as low levels of vitamin B_{12} may precipitate subacute combined degeneration of the cord. If the reason for B_{12} deficiency is purely poor dietary intake, oral supplements are appropriate. However, if compliance with oral treatment is poor or there is the risk of malabsorption, then parenteral vitamin B_{12} is preferred, as an intramuscular injection (1 mg three times per week for two weeks). If there is evidence of neuropathy, give B_{12} injections, and thereafter as a maintenance dose of 1 mg once a month. For all other cases give maintenance doses of 1 mg intramuscularly every three months (the typical maintenance dose for pernicious anaemia or post-total gastrectomy).

References

1. WHO Scientific Group on Nutritional Anaemias and World Health Organization. *Nutritional Anaemias: Report of a WHO Scientific Group.* World Health Organization Technical Report Series no. 405. Geneva: World Health Organization, 1968. https://apps.who.int/iris/handle/10665/40707

2. Korkmaz S, Yıldız S, Korucu T, et al. Frequency of anemia in chronic psychiatry patients. *Neuropsychiatr Dis Treat* 2015;11:2737–2741.

3. Stewart R, Hirani V. Relationship between depressive symptoms, anemia, and iron status in older residents from a national survey population. *Psychosom Med* 2012;74:208–213.

4. Becker M, Axelrod DJ, Oyesanmi O, et al. Hematologic problems in psychosomatic medicine. *Psychiatr Clin North Am* 2007;30:739–759.

5. Hawkins WW, Speck E, Leonard VG. Variation of the hemoglobin level with age and sex. *Blood* 1954;9:999–1007.

6. Perry GS, Byers T, Yip R, Margen S. Iron nutrition does not account for the hemoglobin differences between blacks and whites. *J Nutr* 1992;122(7):1417–1424.

7. Beall CM, Reichsman AB. Hemoglobin levels in a Himalayan high altitude population. *Am J Phys Anthropol* 1984;63(3):301–306.

8. Bosch X, Vera M. Aplastic anaemia during treatment with fluoxetine. *Lancet* 1998;351(9108):1031.

9. Stübner S, Grohmann R, Engel R, et al. Blood dyscrasia induced by psychotropic drugs. *Pharmacopsychiatry* 2004;37(Suppl 1):S70–S78.

10. Mazaira S. Haematological adverse effects caused by psychiatric drugs. *Vertex* 2008;19(82):378–386.

11. Provan D, Hickin S. Haematology. In: Longmore M, Wilkinson IB, Baldwin A, Wallin E (eds) *Oxford Handbook of Clinical Medicine,* 9th edn. Oxford: Oxford University Press, 2014:316–336.

12. Frewin R, Henson A, Provan D. ABC of Clinical haematology. Iron deficiency anaemia. *BMJ* 1997;314(7077):360–363.

13. Boksa P. Smoking, psychiatric illness and the brain. *J Psychiatry Neurosci* 2017;42(3):147–149.

14. Smith JR, Landaw SA. Smokers' polycythemia. *N Engl J Med* 1978;298:6–10.

Chapter 16

Neutropenia

John Lally, Toby Pillinger, Aleksander Mijovic

The neutrophil is the most abundant type of white blood cell in the body. Neutrophils are the first line of defence against invading microbes by employing phagocytosis of pathogens and/or release of antimicrobial factors contained within specialised granules. They also represent a key role in the interface between innate and adaptive immunity. Neutropenia is defined as an absolute neutrophil count (ANC) below 1.5×10^9/L. Based on ANC, neutropenia can be categorised as mild ($1.0–1.5 \times 10^9$/L), moderate ($0.5–1.0 \times 10^9$/L), and severe ($<0.5 \times 10^9$/L). Agranulocytosis is commonly defined as an ANC less than 0.5×10^9/L.

Neutropenia is generally caused by decreased granulocyte production or increased peripheral destruction of neutrophils. Neutrophil pooling leading to neutropenia occurs in specific settings, e.g. splenomegaly and haemodialysis. Common causes of neutropenia are listed in Box 16.1.

Box 16.1 Causes of neutropenia in the general population

Nutritional

- Vitamin and mineral deficiencies (e.g. B_{12}, folate, copper): in the SMI population, consider this differential in those with eating disorders or alcohol dependency.

Infection

- Viral (e.g. HIV, infectious mononucleosis), bacterial (e.g. brucellosis, tuberculosis), parasitic (e.g. malaria, kala-azar), and rickettsial infections.

Rheumatological/autoimmune

- Primary autoimmune neutropenia.
- Secondary, e.g. in rheumatoid arthritis, systemic lupus erythematosus, common variable immunodeficiency.

The Maudsley Practice Guidelines for Physical Health Conditions in Psychiatry, First Edition.
David M. Taylor, Fiona Gaughran, and Toby Pillinger.
© 2021 John Wiley & Sons Ltd. Published 2021 by John Wiley & Sons Ltd.

Chronic idiopathic neutropenia

- Long-standing neutropenia of unknown cause. Usually runs a benign course, but patients may be prone to bacterial/fungal infections. Exact mechanism is unknown, but there is a high degree of overlap with autoimmune neutropenia.

Congenital neutropenias

- Benign ethnic neutropenia (BEN) describes an inherited neutropenia in people of African ethnicity, but also in some Middle Eastern populations. It is not associated with increased risk of infection. Although its pathophysiology is unclear, BEN has a genetic basis, being associated with a polymorphism of the Duffy antigen receptor for chemokines (*DARC*) gene [11]. Unexplained mild familial neutropenia in ethnic groups not associated with BEN can also occur.
- Cyclic neutropenia (CyN) is a rare autosomal dominant disorder with an incidence of 1–2 per million. Heterozygous mutation of the *ELANE* (formerly *ELA2*) gene occurs in almost all cases of CyN [12]. Severe neutropenia typically recurs every two to four weeks, with fever, pharyngitis, and mouth sores. Prognosis is typically benign, but there are reports of overwhelming infection and death in association with CyN.
- Severe congenital neutropenia (SCN) is a genetically heterogeneous disorder, characterised by early-onset severe neutropenia and bacterial infections, often requiring prolonged treatment with G-CSF. SCN is a preleukaemic condition, regardless of treatment with G-CSF.
- Other congenital neutropenias include rare entities such as Shwachman–Diamond syndrome and WHIM (warts, hypogammaglobulinaemia, immunodeficiency, and myelokathexis) syndrome, among others.

Haematological malignancies

- Myelodysplastic syndromes and acute myeloid leukaemia (although rarely present with isolated neutropenia).
- Neutropenia with large granular lymphocyte (LGL) proliferation, with its two subtypes: T lymphocyte, and natural killer lymphocytes. Often associated with rheumatoid arthritis and sometimes indistinguishable from Felty's syndrome.

Hypersplenism

- Hypersplenism is due to an increase in the marginated granulocyte pool, a portion of which is located in the spleen. Non-haematological causes of hypersplenism include liver cirrhosis, heart failure, infection, rheumatological disease (e.g. rheumatoid arthritis, systemic lupus erythematosus, and sarcoid), and infiltrative disease (e.g. amyloid). It can occur in haematological cancers with a bulky spleen, e.g. primary myelofibrosis.

Drugs

See Box 16.2.

CHAPTER 16

A significant proportion of people of African heritage have neutrophil counts lower than the laboratory standard ranges [1]. This is often not pathological and a diagnosis of benign ethnic neutropenia (BEN) is made where a reduced ANC exists in the absence of secondary causes.

DRUG-INDUCED NEUTROPENIA AND AGRANULOCYTOSIS

A wide range of medications, and in particular psychotropic agents, are associated with neutropenia (Box 16.2), with various pathoaetiological mechanisms proposed. All antipsychotics have been associated with neutropenia, although the highest risk is traditionally considered to be with clozapine (approximate frequency 3%). Mood stabilisers are also associated with disturbances of white cell count: the risk of neutropenia with carbamazepine is 0.5–2% [2,3] while sodium valproate is associated with leucopenia in approximately 1 in 400 patients [3]. A hospital-based cohort study identified leucopenia in 0.3% of patients treated with tricyclic antidepressants [3].

Box 16.2 Medications associated with neutropenia/leucopenia/agranulocytosis

- Anti-inflammatory agents (e.g. NSAIDs, sulfasalazine): time course unclear, occurs in <1% of users.
- Antibiotics (e.g. β-lactams): typically occurs in patients receiving treatment for two weeks or more.
- Antimalarials (e.g. chloroquine, quinine): time course unclear, rare.
- Diuretics (e.g. thiazides, furosemide, spironolactone): time course unclear.
- Cardiovascular agents (e.g. ACE inhibitors): risk of ACE inhibitor-related neutropenia may be higher risk in patients with renal failure, typically occurs in first 90 days.
- Antithyroid agents (e.g. carbimazole, propylthiouracil): with carbimazole, usually in first two months of treatment.
- Chemotherapy (virtually all chemotherapy drugs): at any time, but usually within first few weeks of treatment.
- Gastrointestinal agents (e.g. histamine H_2 receptor antagonists): time course unclear, rare.
- Antipsychotics (e.g. clozapine, olanzapine, haloperidol, risperidone, paliperidone, chlorpromazine, lurasidone, ziprasidone, fluphenazine, cariprazine, asenapine): with clozapine, usually in first three months but may occur at any time.
- Anticonvulsants/mood stabilisers (e.g. sodium valproate, carbamazepine, lamotrigine): neutropenia typically occurs in first few weeks to months of treatment.
- Antidepressants (e.g. mirtazapine, mianserin, sertraline, trazodone): usually within first few weeks of treatment.

Drug-induced agranulocytosis from any cause is rare, with an annual incidence of 3–12 per million population [4]. Agranulocytosis occurs in 0.2–0.9% of clozapine-treated patients [5–7], although incidence is reduced with more regular monitoring of neutrophil counts. The one-year prevalence of clozapine-induced neutropenia is 2.7% in the first year, with the peak incidence occurring at 6–18 weeks [8].

There are case reports of agranulocytosis with lamotrigine [9], and during clinical trials of mirtazapine, agranulocytosis was reported in three of 2796 patients (occurring in the first three months of treatment), with neutrophil counts recovering on discontinuation of mirtazapine in all cases [10]. Risk of mirtazapine-induced agranulocytosis increases with age (>65 years) [10].

DIAGNOSTIC PRINCIPLES

Neutropenia may be an incidental finding in an asymptomatic patient on routine blood testing, or instead may present as a clinical emergency with neutropenic sepsis. The urgency with which a patient is examined and investigated will therefore be defined by the patient's presenting complaint, and the severity of neutropenia.

Neutropenic patients with evidence of sepsis (e.g. fever, rigors, shortness of breath, confusion, hypotension, tachycardia, or low urine output) should be managed as a *medical emergency*. Resuscitation and referral to emergency services is indicated (see Chapter 72).

History

A history should screen for the common causes of neutropenia described in Boxes 16.1 and 16.2. This will include clarifying the patient's ethnicity, enquiring about recent/ongoing infection, recurrent infections, episodic aphthous ulcers (may suggest cyclic neutropenia), previous haematological malignancy, recent weight loss/other 'red flag' signs for malignancy, history of malabsorption or conditions that predispose to malabsorption (e.g. inflammatory bowel disease), liver disease, rheumatological/autoimmune disease, family history of neutropenia, alcohol intake, diet, travel history, and medication history.

Examination

1 Check temperature, blood pressure, pulse, respiratory rate, and oxygen saturation.
2 Examine for evidence of infection, including the oral cavity (gingivitis, mouth ulcers), skin (cellulitis), nails (paronychia), lungs, and perirectal area.
3 Examine for evidence of conditions that might underlie neutropenia: joint swelling of rheumatological disease, hepatomegaly/jaundice, lymphadenopathy suggestive of haematological malignancy, splenomegaly suggestive of haematological/liver disease, or parasitic infection (e.g. leishmaniasis).

Investigations

The following blood tests are recommended in the neutropenic patient.

1 Full blood count (FBC) for comparison with previous FBCs if available; blood film for examination of neutrophil morphology and for other haematological diagnoses.
2 If concerns regarding infection, consider collecting blood, urine, stool, or sputum samples (as appropriate) for microscopy, culture, and sensitivity. Nose, mouth, and skin swabs are also required.
3 Urea and electrolytes (renal function).
4 Liver function tests.
5 C-reactive protein (CRP).
6 HIV serology, hepatitis B and C serology, hepatitis C RNA.
7 Rheumatoid factor, antinuclear antibodies, autoimmune screen.

8 Serum vitamin B_{12}/folate.
9 Thyroid function tests.
10 Serum protein electrophoresis and immunoglobulins.

MANAGEMENT

Management of neutropenic sepsis will involve urgent admission under acute medical services for appropriate supportive care and antimicrobial treatment. Any presumed causative agent(s) should also be discontinued.

Patients with an ANC below 0.5×10^9/L, even if systemically well, should be reviewed medically. The urgency of this medical referral will be guided by the patient's clinical presentation, the severity of neutropenia, and the results of screening blood tests described in the preceding section.

Asymptomatic incidental neutropenia with an ANC above 1.0×10^9/L can be monitored on an outpatient basis. If there is resolution over the following weeks, the most likely diagnosis is a transient neutropenia secondary to viral infection or medication. No further investigations will likely be required.

Stable mild neutropenia is usually secondary to BEN, familial neutropenia, diet, rheumatological conditions, or an indolent haematological malignancy. In cases of systemic conditions resulting in neutropenia, appropriate targeted therapy may improve blood counts.

In systemically well patients, and where a psychiatric drug is felt to be causative, a risk–benefit decision will need to be made regarding ongoing treatment with a drug that is presumed to be responsible for the neutropenia, balancing risk of continuing therapy (worsened neutropenia and infection liability) versus the risk of stopping treatment (e.g. deterioration in mental state). In this scenario, a multidisciplinary discussion involving psychiatry, haematology, and the patient is recommended.

Neutropenia and clozapine

During clozapine treatment, transient fluctuations in neutrophil counts can occur that may not necessarily progress to agranulocytosis; however, even if clozapine is continued, current UK licensing requires discontinuation [13] at a neutrophil count of less than 1.5×10^9/L (or $<1.0 \times 10^9$/L in patients with BEN). In the USA, a lower neutrophil count ($<1.0 \times 10^9$/L) is allowed (or $<0.5 \times 10^9$/L in patients with BEN).

Differentiating between a clozapine-induced neutropenia and a transient natural dip in neutrophils can be difficult. Where possible, all cases of neutropenia with clozapine should be assessed as described in the Diagnostic principles section, which will serve to identify any intercurrent conditions (e.g. infections) or co-administered drugs (e.g. valproate) [14] that may be causative. Specific considerations that suggest a neutropenic episode was related to clozapine are as follows:

■ if the decrease in neutrophil count was inconsistent with previous counts (i.e. not in a patient who presents with labile ANCs which often 'naturally' dip in to neutropenia territory)

- if ANC dropped below 0.5×10^9/L
- if neutropenia was prolonged for longer than 10 days
- if neutropenia occurred within 18 weeks of clozapine initiation
- if no alternative causes for the neutropenia/agranulocytosis, such as concurrent medication or infection, were identified [15,16].

Re-challenge with clozapine after neutropenia is 'off licence' but has been observed to be successful in approximately 70% of cases, although this figure includes re-challenge in some cases where clozapine was not the likely cause [17]. There are some non-pharmacological and pharmacological strategies that can be employed to avoid recurrent modest dips in neutrophil counts that may result in extra blood tests or temporary interruption in clozapine administration. For example, some people have a marked circadian rhythm in their neutrophil count, with higher levels in the afternoon compared to the morning, and thus venepuncture later in the day may be associated with higher ANCs. Moderate to heavy exercise can also increase ANCs. Lithium can be used to promote granulopoiesis, with evidence of serum levels above 0.4 mmol/L promoting neutrophil proliferation in the absence of left shift (i.e. the increased ANC is not a consequence of excessive numbers of immature neutrophils; the neutrophils are mature and function normally) [18]. However, caution with these approaches is required, as neither will prevent drug-induced agranulocytosis from occurring.

In some cases, granulocyte colony-stimulating factor (G-CSF) may be used to support clozapine re-challenge and maintenance following neutropenia. These agents are more typically administered during chemotherapy to reduce the incidence or duration of neutropenia [19,20]. They stimulate proliferation and differentiation of committed myeloid progenitor cells in the bone marrow [21]. Filgrastim and lenograstim are the most commonly used G-CSFs, and are administered by subcutaneous injection. A systematic review providing the largest synthesis of clozapine re-challenge following neutropenia to date reported relatively high success but highlighted the likelihood of publication bias [16]. Consultation with a haematologist is recommended before considering the use of lithium and certainly before use of G-CSF in the context of clozapine-associated neutropenia. It is important to note that while G-CSF will help maintain an adequate baseline ANC to allow administration within licensing guidelines, it is unlikely to prevent progression from neutropenia to a true clozapine-related agranulocytosis.

Management of clozapine-induced agranulocytosis

As with any drug, if clozapine is considered the causative agent in the context of agranulocytosis, it should be stopped and clinical review conducted as described. Following cessation, G-CSF shortens time to neutrophil recovery from a median of 12 days to 7 days, and may therefore be considered [22]. Because of the high risk of recurrence, re-challenge following clozapine-induced agranulocytosis, with or without lithium or G-CSF, and certainly outside of specialist care settings, is not recommended.

References

1. Shoenfeld Y, Alkan ML, Asaly A, et al. Benign familial leukopenia and neutropenia in different ethnic groups. *Eur J Haematol* 1988;41(3):273–277.
2. Duggal HS, Singh I. Psychotropic drug-induced neutropenia. *Drugs Today (Barc)* 2005;41(8):517–526.
3. Tohen M, Castillo J, Baldessarini RJ, et al. Blood dyscrasias with carbamazepine and valproate: a pharmacoepidemiological study of 2,228 patients at risk. *Am J Psychiatry* 1995;152(3):413–418.
4. Andres E, Noel E, Kurtz JE, et al. Life-threatening idiosyncratic drug-induced agranulocytosis in elderly patients. *Drugs Aging* 2004;21(7):427–435.
5. Myles N, Myles H, Xia S, et al. Meta-analysis examining the epidemiology of clozapine-associated neutropenia. *Acta Psychiatr Scand* 2018;138(2):101–109.
6. Honigfeld G, Arellano F, Sethi J, et al. Reducing clozapine-related morbidity and mortality: 5 years of experience with the Clozaril National Registry. *J Clin Psychiatry* 1998;59:3–7.
7. Tang YI, Mao PX, Jiang F, et al. Clozapine in China. *Pharmacopsychiatry.* 2008;41(1):1–9.
8. Munro J, O'Sullivan D, Andrews C, et al. Active monitoring of 12,760 clozapine recipients in the UK and Ireland. Beyond pharmacovigilance. *Br J Psychiatry* 1999;175:576–580.
9. Ahn YM, Kim K, Kim YS. Three cases of reversible agranulocytosis after treatment with lamotrigine. *Psychiatry Investig* 2008;5(2):121–123.
10. Remeron (mirtazapine). *Physicians' Desk Reference.* Montvale, NJ: Medical Economics, 1996:1878–1881.
11. Reich D, Nalls MA, Kao WHL, et al. Reduced neutrophil count in people of African descent is due to a regulatory variant in the Duffy antigen receptor for chemokines gene. *PLoS Genet* 2009;5(1):e1000360.
12. Horwitz MS, Corey SJ, Grimes HL, Tidwell T. ELANE mutations in cyclic and severe congenital neutropenia:genetics and pathophysiology. *Hematol Oncol Clin North Am* 2013;27(1):19–41, vii.
13. Ingimarsson O, MacCabe JH, Haraldsson M, et al. Neutropenia and agranulocytosis during treatment of schizophrenia with clozapine versus other antipsychotics: an observational study in Iceland. *BMC Psychiatry* 2016;16(1):441.
14. Malik S, Lally J, Ajnakina O, et al. Sodium valproate and clozapine induced neutropenia: a case control study using register data. *Schizophr Res* 2018;195:267–273.
15. Taylor DM, Barnes TRE, Young AH. *The Maudsley Prescribing Guidelines in Psychiatry*, 13th edn. Chichester: Wiley Blackwell, 2018.
16. Lally J, Malik S, Krivoy A, et al. The use of granulocyte colony-stimulating factor in clozapine rechallenge: a systematic review. *J Clin Psychopharmacol* 2017;37(5):600–604.
17. Manu P, Sarpal D, Muir O, et al. When can patients with potentially life-threatening adverse effects be rechallenged with clozapine? A systematic review of the published literature. *Schizophr Res* 2012;134(2–3):180–186.
18. Meyer N, Gee S, Whiskey E, et al. Optimizing outcomes in clozapine rechallenge following neutropenia: a cohort analysis. *J Clin Psychiatry* 2015;76(11):e1410–e1416.
19. Renner P, Milazzo S, Liu JP, et al. Primary prophylactic colony-stimulating factors for the prevention of chemotherapy-induced febrile neutropenia in breast cancer patients. *Cochrane Database Syst Rev* 2012;10:CD007913.
20. Kuderer NM, Dale DC, Crawford J, Lyman GH. Impact of primary prophylaxis with granulocyte colony-stimulating factor on febrile neutropenia and mortality in adult cancer patients receiving chemotherapy: a systematic review. *J Clin Oncol* 2007;25(21):3158–3167.
21. Lieschke GJ, Burgess AW. Granulocyte colony-stimulating factor and granulocyte-macrophage colony-stimulating factor. *N Engl J Med* 1992;327(1):28–35.
22. Lally J, Malik S, Whiskey E, et al. Clozapine-associated agranulocytosis treatment with granulocyte colony-stimulating factor/granulocyte-macrophage colony-stimulating factor: a systematic review. *J Clin Psychopharmacol* 2017;37(4):441–446.

Thrombocytopenia

Sanjena Mithra, Aleksander Mijovic

Platelets are tiny cell fragments within the blood that, along with coagulation factors, allow blood to clot. They are shed from the cytoplasm of megakaryocytes and circulate for a lifespan of 7–10 days or until they are activated by a specific trigger [1]. A normal platelet count is $150–400 \times 10^9$/L, but levels can vary depending on several factors including menstrual cycle, pregnancy (gestational thrombocytopenia), and in response to inflammation [2]. Thrombocytopenia can be subdivided into mild (platelet count $100–150 \times 10^9$/L), moderate ($50–100 \times 10^9$/L), and severe ($<50 \times 10^9$/L) [3]. Risk of bleeding is highest in patients with severe thrombocytopenia.

Thrombocytopenia may occur due to accelerated destruction, ineffective production, or splenic sequestration of platelets (Table 17.1) [4]. Patients with serious mental illness (SMI) are at increased risk of various conditions that may in turn result in thrombocytopenia, such as vitamin B_{12}/folate deficiency [5,6] and splenomegaly secondary to cirrhosis of the liver and portal hypertension [7]. Certain medications, including psychiatric medication, are associated with development of thrombocytopenia (Box 17.1). Indeed, alongside immune thrombocytopenic purpura (ITP), medication is the most common cause of thrombocytopenia [4]. Drug-induced thrombocytopenia is thought to be due to the actions of drug-dependent antibodies [8], and generally occurs within one to two weeks of starting a new drug. If the drug is stopped, there is usually resolution within 5–10 days. In addition, some foods and drink have been implicated in causing thrombocytopenia, such as tonic water (which contains quinine) [9], herbal remedies [10], walnuts [11], and even cows' milk [12].

The Maudsley Practice Guidelines for Physical Health Conditions in Psychiatry, First Edition.
David M. Taylor, Fiona Gaughran, and Toby Pillinger.
© 2021 John Wiley & Sons Ltd. Published 2021 by John Wiley & Sons Ltd.

Table 17.1 Causes of isolated thrombocytopenia.

Mechanism	Pathology
Accelerated destruction	Immune thrombocytopenic purpura (ITP) Thrombotic thrombocytopenic purpura (TTP) and related disorders Disseminated intravascular coagulation (DIC) Systemic lupus erythematosus, antiphospholipid syndrome Medication (see Box 17.1)
Decreased production	Congenital thrombocytopenias Vitamin B_{12}/folate deficiency Haematological disorders (e.g. leukaemia, aplastic anaemia, myelodysplastic syndrome) Sepsis Medication (see Box 17.1)
Splenic sequestration	Portal hypertension with splenomegaly: cirrhosis due to viral disease or alcohol, hepatic vein thrombosis (Budd–Chiari syndrome), splanchnic vein thrombosis, cardiac failure Viral infections with splenomegaly (e.g. Epstein–Barr virus, cytomegalovirus) Myelofibrosis Gaucher's disease (inherited lysosomal storage disease characterised by hepatosplenomegaly, pancytopenia, bone pain, and neurological symptoms)

Box 17.1 Medications associated with thrombocytopenia

- Methotrexate (and other cytotoxic drugs, including chemotherapy)
- Histamine H_2 receptor antagonists (ranitidine, cimetidine)
- Heparin (occurs within five days)
- Antibiotics (e.g. penicillin, quinine, trimethoprim, ciprofloxacin) [8,13]
- Antifungals (e.g. fluconazole) [8,13]
- Antiplatelet drugs: can occur after first administration (e.g. tirofiban and abciximab) [8]
- Mood stabilisers (carbamazepine, phenytoin, valproic acid, lamotrigine) [13,14]
- Antidepressants (tricyclic antidepressants, escitalopram, venlafaxine, buproprion, duloxetine, fluoxetine, mirtazapine, sertraline) [13,14]
- Antipsychotics (haloperidol, chlorpromazine, clozapine, fluphenazine, olanzapine, quetiapine, risperidone/paliperidone, trifluoperazine, ziprasidone)
- Benzodiazepines
- Donepezil
- Recreational drugs (e.g. alcohol, cocaine)
- Miscellaneous (gold, furosemide) [8]

DIAGNOSTIC PRINCIPLES

Mild to moderate thrombocytopenia is generally asymptomatic. Clinical signs and symptoms of thrombocytopenia generally start to manifest at platelet levels of approximately 30×10^9/L [15]. Determining the aetiology of thrombocytopenia can be challenging. Often, if a drug is suspected then the diagnosis is empirical and based on confirmation of platelet count recovery after discontinuation of the offending drug, or even following recurrence of thrombocytopenia following re-exposure to the drug in question. To make a laboratory diagnosis of a drug-induced thrombocytopenia would be time-consuming and costly, involving the demonstration of drug-dependent anti-platelet antibodies by methods such as flow cytometry, platelet immunofluorescence test, and ELISA [8].

History

Eliciting a full medical history is vital for determining the aetiology of thrombocytopenia and whether this is accompanied by suppression of other cell lines (red and white blood cells).

1 Duration of symptoms (drug-induced thrombocytopenia is associated with a shorter duration of symptoms, usually days to weeks).
2 Ask about any concurrent symptoms suggestive of infection.
3 Clinical signs: petechial rash, bruises or superficial bleeding after minor trauma (such as shaving or brushing teeth), or prolonged menstrual bleeding.
4 Presentations suggestive of more severe bleeding: fatigue (due to blood loss and anae-mia), headache or fluctuating conscious level (which may suggest cerebral haemor-rhage), haematemesis, or melaena (indicative of gastrointestinal bleeding).
5 Past medical history: red flag screening for haematological malignancy (uninten-tional weight loss, lymphadenopathy, night sweats), venous thromboembolism or atrial fibrillation and stroke requiring anticoagulation.
6 Family history: bleeding disorders.
7 Medication history: new medications and antibiotics, as well as non-steroidal anti-inflammatory drugs (NSAIDs), aspirin, or anticoagulants that could further increase likelihood of bleeding.

Examination

This should predominantly focus on determining the location and severity of any bleed-ing, although evidence of infection or hepatosplenomegaly may point towards an underlying pathology.

1 Observations including temperature (fever may signal underlying infection).
2 General: skin examination (looking for petechiae).
3 Abdominal examination for hepatosplenomegaly.
4 Neurological examination to assess conscious level and any focal neurology.

Investigations

1 Bedside: urine dip.
2 Blood tests:
  a full blood count to determine if thrombocytopenia is isolated or associated with low haemoglobin and white cells
  b blood film to confirm if the low count represents true thrombocytopenia or if there is any 'clumping', and also to assess platelet size (larger may suggest a hereditary cause)

    c coagulation screen (international normalised ratio, activated partial thromboplastin time)

    d urea and electrolytes, liver function tests, C-reactive protein.

3 Imaging/special tests:

    a chest X-ray if any suspicion of infection

    b consider CT head if fluctuating conscious level or suspicion of intracranial bleed

    c mixing clotting studies are used to distinguish between clotting factor deficiency and clotting factor inhibitors (e.g. antibodies such as 'lupus anticoagulant').

MANAGEMENT AND WHEN TO REFER

Acute bleeding should be managed as a *medical emergency*, with emergency transfer of the patient to medical services.

Finding the causative agent of thrombocytopenia is difficult and is made more so by polypharmacy and lack of specific laboratory tests. The mainstay of treatment is to stop the agent thought to have caused the thrombocytopenia. Drug-induced thrombocytopenia usually occurs within weeks of starting a new drug (within days in the case of heparin), and the causative drug is usually the most recent drug to have been prescribed.

If a psychiatric medication is thought to be responsible, multidisciplinary discussion involving psychiatry, haematology, and the patient should be sought. If there is evidence of associated acute pathology or bleeding, the patient should be referred urgently to the emergency department or acute medical team for assessment. A platelet transfusion is considered if levels drop below 10×10^9/L, or below 20×10^9/L with evidence of bleeding [15]. Other interventions that may be considered following haematology input include intravenous immunoglobulin (e.g. for ITP), steroids (e.g. for immune-mediated thrombocytopenia), or plasmapheresis (e.g. for TTP) [15]

References

1. Stasi R. How to approach thrombocytopenia. *Hematology Am Soc Hematol Educ Program* 2012;2012:191–197.
2. Neunert C, Lim W, Crowther M, et al. The American Society of Hematology 2011 evidence-based practice guideline for immune thrombocytopenia. *Blood* 2011;117(16):4190–4207.
3. Williamson DR, Albert M, Heels-Ansdell D, et al. Thrombocytopenia in critically ill patients receiving thromboprophylaxis: frequency, risk factors, and outcomes. *Chest* 2013;144(4):1207–1215.
4. Izak M, Bussel JB. Management of thrombocytopenia. *F1000Prime Rep* 2014;6:45.
5. Carmel R, Gott PS, Waters CH, et al. The frequently low cobalamin levels in dementia usually signify treatable metabolic, neurologic and electrophysiologic abnormalities. *Eur J Haematol* 1995;54(4):245–253.
6. Silver H. Vitamin B12 levels are low in hospitalized psychiatric patients. *Israel J Psychiatry* 2000;37(1):41–45.
7. Hsu JH, Chien IC, Lin CH, et al. Increased risk of chronic liver disease in patients with schizophrenia: a population-based cohort study. *Psychosomatics* 2014;55(2):163–171.
8. George JN, Aster RH. Drug-induced thrombocytopenia: pathogenesis, evaluation, and management. *Hematology Am Soc Hematol Educ Program* 2009;2009:153–158.
9. Davies JK, Ahktar N, Ranasinge E. A juicy problem. *Lancet* 2001;358(9299):2126.
10. Royer DJ, George JN, Terrell DR. Thrombocytopenia as an adverse effect of complementary and alternative medicines, herbal remedies, nutritional supplements, foods, and beverages. *Eur J Haematol* 2010;84(5):421–429.
11. Achterbergh R, Vermeer HJ, Curtis BR, et al. Thrombocytopenia in a nutshell. *Lancet* 2012;379(9817):776.
12. Caffrey EA, Sladen GE, Isaacs PE, Clark KG. Thrombocytopenia caused by cows milk. *Lancet* 1981;318(8241):316.
13. Aster RH, Curtis BR, McFarland JG, Bougie DW. Drug-induced immune thrombocytopenia: pathogenesis, diagnosis, and management. *J Thromb Haemost* 2009;7(6):911–918.
14. Song HR, Jung YE, Wang HR, et al. Platelet count alterations associated with escitalopram, venlafaxine and bupropion in depressive patients. *Psychiatry Clin Neurosci* 2012;66(5):457–459.
15. Provan D, Hickin S. Haematology. In: Longmore M, Wilkinson IB, Baldwin A, Wallin E (eds) *Oxford Handbook of Clinical Medicine*, 9th edn. Oxford: Oxford University Press, 2014:316–336.

Venous Thromboembolism and Anticoagulation

Helen Doolittle, Lara Roberts, Roopen Arya

The term 'venous thromboembolism' (VTE) comprises deep vein thrombosis (DVT), most commonly in the pelvic or deep leg veins, and the movement of the clot through the vasculature to the lungs, i.e. pulmonary embolism (PE). VTE is associated with significant morbidity and mortality. Venous thrombosis may occur in other sites, such as the intra-abdominal veins, cavernous sinus, deep veins of the upper limbs, and superficial veins. There is some overlap between the provoking factors and management of these atypical thromboses, but these are beyond the scope of the guidance given here.

RISK FACTORS

There are many recognised risk factors for VTE. In psychiatric patients it is important to consider underlying medical conditions, features of the psychiatric illness (e.g. immobility), and psychiatric treatments (antipsychotics) which may all increase risk of developing VTE (Box 18.1).

Box 18.1 Risk factors for venous thromboembolism (VTE)

Inherited

- Inherited thrombophilia (including protein C deficiency, protein S deficiency, antithrombin deficiency, prothrombin gene polymorphism, factor V Leiden)
- History of VTE in first-degree relative

Acquired: persistent

General physical/lifestyle factors

- Increasing age
- Body mass index (BMI) >30 kg/m²
- Previous/current intravenous drug use

Medical conditions

- Cancer (active disease/receiving anticancer therapy)
- Chronic inflammatory/metabolic conditions
- Myeloproliferative disorders
- Paroxysmal nocturnal haemoglobinuria
- Antiphospholipid syndrome
- Previous personal history of VTE

Acquired: transient/reversible

General physical/lifestyle factors

- Pregnancy/postpartum
- Prolonged periods of immobility, including paresis, long-distance travel (>4 hours), catatonia, stupor

Medical conditions

- Post surgery
- Acute medical illness
- Hospitalisation
- Trauma/fracture especially to lower limbs

Medications

- Oestrogen-containing/oestrogen receptor-targeting medications (including combined hormonal contraception, oral hormone replacement therapy, tamoxifen)
- Antipsychotics (see text)

Antipsychotics and venous thromboembolism

Studies have demonstrated an increased risk of VTE in patients treated with antipsychotic medications of 1.3 to 7-fold [1]. The mechanism by which antipsychotics increase VTE risk is not clear but the risk appears to be highest in the first three months of treatment, in younger patients, and is probably dose related [1]. While clozapine was the first antipsychotic widely acknowledged to carry an increased VTE risk, a broad variety of antipsychotic medications have now been implicated [1,2]. Evidence is still lacking as to whether there are significant differences in the risk associated with different drugs or classes of antipsychotics [3,4].

PROPHYLAXIS

Prophylaxis has been shown to reduce the risk of VTE in selected patient groups, such as acutely unwell medical and postoperative patients. Prophylaxis includes mechanical and pharmacological measures. The decision regarding whether VTE prophylaxis is warranted during an acute hospital admission and the selection of the most appropriate prophylactic measure are based on assessing the patient's risk of developing VTE alongside their bleeding risk.

Several international guidelines have been developed for the appropriate assessment of hospitalised patients and provision of VTE prophylaxis [5–7], although most do not specifically discuss assessment and management of psychiatric patients. However, the UK-based National Institute for Health and Care Excellence (NICE) guidance (2018) recommends that acute psychiatric inpatients are assessed similarly to acutely unwell medical inpatients using the Department of Health VTE risk assessment tool (http://www.nice.org.uk/guidance/ng89/resources) or an equivalent published tool [5]. The initial assessment should take place as soon as possible after admission to hospital, with reassessment at the time of the patient's consultant review and when the patient's condition changes. Further work is required to determine if existing risk assessment tools need adaptation for psychiatric patients.

Before employing pharmacological VTE prophylaxis, the risk of bleeding should be also assessed; the IMPROVE bleeding assessment model is sometimes used to assess bleeding risk in medical patients [8]. Again, further work is required to see if such tools are valid for use in psychiatric patients. Where pharmacological VTE prophylaxis is indicated, the use of low-molecular-weight heparin (LMWH) is usually recommended. Fondaparinux can be considered if LMWH is contraindicated, such as inpatients wishing to avoid animal products or with hypersensitivity reactions to LMWH (especially thrombocytopenia). Dose adjustment, additional monitoring, or alternative drugs may be required in patients with renal impairment.

The use of mechanical thromboprophylaxis with graduated compression stockings has only been evaluated and demonstrated to benefit patients in the surgical setting. There is no evidence to support their use in medical or obstetric patients, or indeed psychiatric patients. The UK-based NICE and Asian VTE guidelines therefore no longer recommend the use of graduated compression stockings for acute medical patients, although the American Society of Hematology suggests they can be considered for medical patients where pharmacological prophylaxis is contraindicated [5–7]. If graduated compression stockings are used they should be fitted by staff trained in their use. They are not recommended for patients with peripheral arterial disease (suspected or known), peripheral arterial bypass grafting, peripheral sensory impairment, and local skin or soft tissue conditions (where stockings can cause further damage and severe leg oedema) [5]. In selected situations, intermittent pneumatic compression is recommended as an alternative form of mechanical VTE prophylaxis [5–7].

Early mobilisation and maintaining hydration are also proposed to reduce the risk of VTE.

DIAGNOSIS

Deep vein thrombosis

A diagnosis of DVT should be considered in a patient with unilateral calf swelling and/ or pain. The clinical assessment should be based around calculating the Revised Wells Score for suspected DVT [9] (Table 18.1) and considering other causes for the patient's presentation such as cellulitis, trauma, or ruptured Baker's cyst. This is usually done by a DVT clinic or following referral of the patient to the nearest emergency or medical team. An algorithm outlining the investigation and management of a suspected DVT is presented in Figure 18.1.

Table 18.1 Revised Wells Score for suspected deep vein thrombosis (DVT) [9].

Clinical characteristic	Score
Active cancer (treatment for cancer within previous 6 months/ongoing palliative treatment)	1
Paralysis, paresis, or plaster immobilisation of lower limbs	1
Recently bedridden for ≥3 days, or major surgery within 12 weeks requiring general or regional anaesthesia	1
Localised tenderness along the distribution of the deep venous system	1
Entire leg swollen	1
Calf swelling ≥3 cm than asymptomatic side (measured at 10 cm below tibial tuberosity)	1
Pitting oedema in the symptomatic leg only	1
Collateral superficial veins (non-varicose)	1
Previous DVT	1
Alternative diagnosis at least as likely as DVT	−2

Score ≥2 indicates DVT likely; score <2 indicates DVT unlikely.

Pulmonary embolism

A diagnosis of PE should be considered in a patient with new or progressive hypoxia, pleuritic chest pain, unexplained tachycardia, or collapse (see Chapters 67 and 68). If such symptoms or signs are present, urgent assessment should be sought at the nearest acute medical or emergency unit. Direct admission to an acute hospital will be required if the patient has significant hypoxia or is haemodynamically unstable. Initial assessment of a patient with a suspected PE should include calculation of the Revised PE Wells Score [11] (Table 18.2) and consideration of other causes for the presentation such as pneumonia, chest wall pain (secondary to trauma or malignant disease), gastro-oesophageal reflux, cardiac chest pain (secondary to ischaemia, pericarditis, or aortic dissection/aneurysm rupture), as well as any neurological or other cardiovascular causes of collapse. An algorithm for the investigation and management of suspected PE is presented in Figure 18.2.

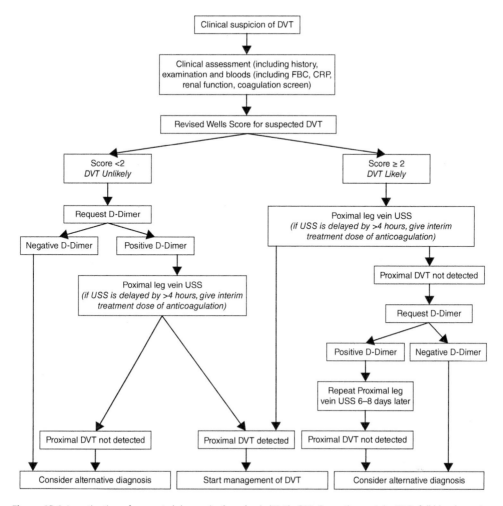

Figure 18.1 Investigation of suspected deep vein thrombosis (DVT). CRP, C-reactive protein; FBC, full blood count; USS, ultrasound scan. Source: adapted from National Institute for Health and Care Excellence [10].

Table 18.2 Wells Score for suspected pulmonary embolus (PE) [11].

Clinical characteristic	Score
Clinical signs and symptoms of DVT (including leg swelling and pain over deep veins)	3
Alternative diagnosis less likely than PE	3
Heart rate >100 beats per minute	1.5
Immobilisation or surgery within previous 4 weeks	1.5
Previous DVT/PE	1.5
Haemoptysis	1
Active cancer (treatment for cancer within previous 6 months/ongoing palliative treatment)	1

Score >4 indicates PE likely; score ≤4 indicates PE unlikely.

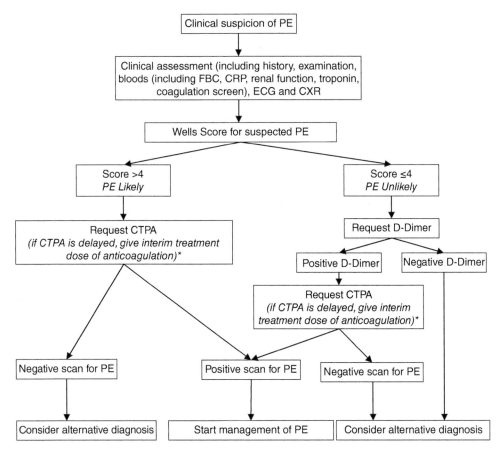

Figure 18.2 Investigation of suspected pulmonary embolus (PE). ECG, electrocardiogram; CXR, chest X-ray; CTPA, computed tomography pulmonary angiogram. *If patient has renal impairment, allergy to contrast media or with high irradiation risk, ventilation–perfusion single photon emission computed tomography scan can be considered as an alternative to CTPA. Source: adapted from National Institute for Health and Care Excellence [10].

MANAGEMENT

Anticoagulation

Anticoagulation is the recommended treatment of DVT or PE. The majority of patients with DVT and a significant proportion of patients with PE are now managed without hospital admission. The minimum duration of therapy is usually three months, with a minimum of six months recommended for those with active cancer. This allows resolution of the VTE and prevention of early recurrent VTE. Anticoagulation may be extended beyond this, based on individual characteristics and particularly in the absence of provoking factors for VTE. The risk of bleeding will also need to be considered in this decision-making process, along with the patient's preferences.

Initial management of VTE can be with LMWH, fondaparinux, or a direct oral anticoagulant (apixaban or rivaroxaban). Long-term anticoagulants include direct oral anticoagulants, warfarin, LMWH, or fondaparinux. The characteristics of the different agents are summarised in Table 18.3. These can all be used to manage VTE, and the choice should be made based on the patient's medical comorbidities and concomitant medications. LMWH is generally recommended for use in patients with active cancer, at least in the initiation phase [12]. Selection of appropriate anticoagulation will usually be made by the DVT clinic or acute medical unit managing the patient. Patients with absolute or relative contraindications to anticoagulation should be discussed with haematology for specialist guidance.

If VTE occurs in the context of prior therapeutic anticoagulation, a discussion regarding adherence to medication is needed. If compliance to prior anticoagulation therapy is established, the patient should be discussed with the haematology team. Increased intensity of anticoagulation may be indicated. Temporary inferior vena cava filters may also be considered.

Use of anticoagulants alongside antipsychotic drugs

If a patient requires treatment for VTE and is taking an antipsychotic drug, the role of that drug in causing the event requires consideration by the psychiatric and haematology teams involved in the patient's care. This might have implications as to the choice of antipsychotic agent. This decision may also affect the duration of anticoagulation. If extended anticoagulation is required, low-dose direct oral anticoagulants are a convenient option.

Since the co-prescription of selective serotonin reuptake inhibitors (SSRIs) may increase risk of bleeding, SSRIs should generally be avoided alongside anticoagulation [13]. For patients taking SSRIs in whom anticoagulation is indicated, a multidisciplinary discussion involving both psychiatry and haematology should take place. If SSRI use cannot be avoided, monitor closely, avoid concomitant use of non-steroidal anti-inflammatories or antiplatelet medications, and consider prescribing gastroprotection (e.g. a proton pump inhibitor). Given the bleeding risk associated with SSRIs is thought to be due to reduced serotonin uptake by platelets, reducing platelet function, caution is also recommended with the use of serotonin/noradrenaline reuptake inhibitors (SNRIs) [14]. Whether a true increased bleeding risk exists with SNRIs remains a point of debate and a selected population-based study did not observe excess bleeding in SNRI users [15].

Follow-up and referral to anticoagulation clinic

All patients started on anticoagulation should be given information about the treatment, its duration and side effects, and when to seek medical attention in the event of bleeding. It is best practice to provide written patient information and an anticoagulant alert card. Appropriate follow-up in primary or secondary care should be arranged, with NICE recommending treatment-duration review within three months for all

Table 18.3 Anticoagulants for use in long-term treatment of DVT/PE and prevention of recurrent DVT/PE in adults.

Drug group	Drug	Delivery	Monitoring	Reversal agent	Use in renal impairment	Drug interactions/cautions[a]	Initiation of treatment in acute VTE
Direct thrombin inhibitor	Dabigatran	Oral	Not routinely required	Idarucizumab	CrCl 30–50 mL/min: dose reduction to 110 mg b.d. CrCl <30 mL/min: contraindicated	Amiodarone Antifungals Carbamazepine Ciclosporin Clarithromycin Phenytoin Protease inhibitors Rifampicin St John's Wort Drugs associated with bleeding risk[b]	Start after >5 days of parenteral anticoagulation with LMWH/UFH
Direct factor Xa inhibitors	Apixaban Edoxaban Rivaroxaban	Oral Note: rivaroxaban doses of 15 mg or more should be taken *with* food	Not routinely required	Protocols using prothrombin complex concentrate often used in emergency situations Andexanet (reversal of apixaban/rivaroxaban) is not currently available in UK	*Apixaban* CrCl 15–30 mL/min: use with caution CrCl <15 mL/min: contraindicated *Edoxaban* CrCl 15–50 mL/min: dose reduction to 30 mg CrCl <15 mL/min: contraindicated *Rivaroxaban* CrCl 15–30 mL/min: use with caution and consider dose reduction CrCl <15 mL/min: contraindicated	Antifungals Carbamazepine Ciclosporin Erythromycin Phenytoin Protease inhibitors Rifampicin St John's Wort Drugs associated with bleeding risk[b]	Apixaban/rivaroxaban: no prior parenteral anticoagulation required Edoxaban: start after >5 days of parenteral anticoagulation with LMWH/UFH

	Drugs	Route	Monitoring	Reversal	Renal considerations	Interactions	Comments
LMWH	Dalteparin Enoxaparin	Subcutaneous	Only required in selected patient groups as per haematology guidance (anti-Xa level)	Protamine partially effective	*Dalteparin* CrCl 15–30 mL/min: use with caution and adjust dose according to anti-Xa monitoring CrCl <15 mL/min: not recommended *Enoxaparin* CrCl 15–30 mL/min: dose reduction ± anti-Xa monitoring CrCl <15 mL/min: not recommended	Antihistamines Cardiac glycosides Tetracyclines Ascorbic acid Drugs associated with bleeding risk[b]	Suitable for use in the initial management of acute VTE
Fondaparinux	Fondaparinux	Subcutaneous	Not required	Not available	CrCl 30–50 mL/min: use with caution CrCl <30 mL/min: contraindicated	Drugs associated with bleeding risk[b]	Suitable for use in the initial management of acute VTE
Vitamin K antagonists	Warfarin	Oral	Required (INR)	Vitamin K and prothrombin complex concentrate	No renal excretion	Many drugs and foods interact with warfarin, so care is required with all concomitant therapy. Clinicians should refer to drug SPC or BNF for individual details	Parenteral anticoagulation required for >5 days and until INR ≥2 for 24 hours (whichever is longer)

[a] Underlined drugs are those which reduce the drug plasma concentrations.

[b] Drugs associated with bleeding risk include anticoagulants, antiplatelet agents, non-steroidal anti-inflammatory drugs, selective serotonin reuptake inhibitors, and serotonin/noradrenaline reuptake inhibitors.

BNF, British National Formulary; CrCl, creatinine clearance; INR, international normalised ratio; LMWH, low-molecular-weight heparin; SPC, summary of product characteristics; UFH, unfractionated heparin; VTE, venous thromboembolism.

patients with a new VTE diagnosis [10]. Other indications for referral to anticoagulation clinic include:

1 blood monitoring of warfarin (if this is not available with the patient's general practitioner)
2 unprovoked proximal DVT/PE or recurrent VTE on anticoagulation for further investigation and counselling regarding anticoagulation dose and duration.

References

1. Jonsson AK, Schill J, Olsson H, et al. Venous thromboembolism during treatment with antipsychotics: a review of current evidence. *CNS Drugs* 2018;32(1):47–64.
2. Hagg S, Spigset O, Soderstrom TG. Association of venous thromboembolism and clozapine. *Lancet* 2000;355(9210):1155–1156.
3. Zhang R, Dong L, Shao F, et al. Antipsychotics and venous thromboembolism risk: a meta-analysis. *Pharmacopsychiatry* 2011;44(5):183–188.
4. Barbui C, Conti V, Cipriani A. Antipsychotic drug exposure and risk of venous thromboembolism: a systematic review and meta-analysis of observational studies. *Drug Saf* 2014;37(2):79–90.
5. National Institute for Health and Care Excellence. *Venous Thromboembolism in Over 16s: Reducing the Risk of Hospital-acquired Deep Vein Thrombosis or Pulmonary Embolism*. NICE Guideline NG89. London: NICE, 2018. Available at https://www.nice.org.uk/guidance/ng89/resources
6. Liew NC, Alemany GV, Angchaisuksiri P, et al. Asian venous thromboembolism guidelines: updated recommendations for the prevention of venous thromboembolism. *Int Angiol* 2017;36(1):1–20.
7. Schunemann HJ, Cushman M, Burnett AE, et al. American Society of Hematology 2018 guidelines for management of venous thromboembolism: prophylaxis for hospitalized and nonhospitalized medical patients. *Blood Adv* 2018;2(22):3198–3225.
8. Rosenberg DJ, Press A, Fishbein J, et al. External validation of the IMPROVE Bleeding Risk Assessment Model in medical patients. *Thromb Haemost* 2016;116(3):530–536.
9. Wells PS, Anderson DR, Rodger M, et al. Evaluation of D-dimer in the diagnosis of suspected deep-vein thrombosis. *N Engl J Med* 2003;349(13):1227–1235.
10. National Institute for Health and Care Excellence. *Venous Thromboembolic Diseases: Diagnosis, Management and Thrombophilia Testing*. Clinical Guideline CG144. London: NICE, 2012.
11. Wells PS, Anderson DR, Rodger M, et al. Derivation of a simple clinical model to categorize patients probability of pulmonary embolism: increasing the models utility with the SimpliRED D-dimer. *Thromb Haemost* 2000;83(3):416–420.
12. Watson HG, Keeling DM, Laffan M, et al. Guideline on aspects of cancer-related venous thrombosis. *Br J Haematol* 2015;170(5):640–648.
13. Schalekamp T, Klungel OH, Souverein PC, de Boer A. Increased bleeding risk with concurrent use of selective serotonin reuptake inhibitors and coumarins. *Arch Intern Med* 2008;168(2):180–185.
14. Maurer-Spurej E, Pittendreigh C, Solomons K. The influence of selective serotonin reuptake inhibitors on human platelet serotonin. *Thromb Haemost* 2004;91(1):119–128.
15. Cheng YL, Hu HY, Lin XH, et al. Use of SSRI, but not SNRI, increased upper and lower gastrointestinal bleeding: a nationwide population-based cohort study in Taiwan. *Medicine (Baltimore)* 2015;94(46):e2022.

Part 4

Gastroenterology

Gastro-oesophageal Reflux and Peptic Ulcer Disease

Luke Vano, Seema Varma, John O'Donohue

GASTRO-OESOPHAGEAL REFLUX DISEASE

As part of normal digestion, food is passed from the mouth to the stomach via the oesophagus. The lower oesophageal sphincter (LOS) is a ring of muscle that encircles the bottom end of the oesophagus where it meets the stomach. This sphincter helps to prevent stomach contents from refluxing back into the oesophagus.

In gastro-oesophageal reflux disease (GORD), acidic stomach contents are refluxed back into the oesophagus, which is lined by squamous epithelium and, unlike the specialised gastric mucosa, can be inflamed by acid. Exposure of the oesophagus to acid may lead to retrosternal discomfort and burning ('heartburn'). Reflux may also cause other symptoms, including cough, wheeze, and hoarseness. GORD is a common condition that affects up to 20% of the Western world [1]. Complications that may arise from GORD include erosive oesophagitis, oesophageal strictures, Barrett's oesophagus (pre-cancerous cell changes), and oesophageal cancer [2].

Table 19.1 documents common causes of GORD in the general and psychiatric population. If the LOS is weakened from previous surgery (e.g. for achalasia), anatomical abnormalities (e.g. hiatus hernia), or by use of medications that relax smooth muscle (e.g. calcium channel blockers or nitrates), the likelihood of GORD increases. Conditions that increase pressure on the stomach (e.g. obesity or pregnancy) can also lead to GORD as stomach contents are more readily refluxed. Diets high in fat have been observed to increase the risk of developing GORD, while diets high in fibre are protective [3].

In the psychiatric population, bulimia nervosa and binge eating disorder increase the risk of GORD [4]. Medications with anticholinergic effects (e.g. tricyclic antidepressants, anticholinergics, and antipsychotics) decrease LOS tone, which can lead to reflux. Depression, even in the absence of antidepressant use, is a risk factor for GORD [5–7]. It has been observed that people who score highly on psychosomatic symptom checklists are at higher risk of GORD. Mechanistically, it has been postulated that people

Table 19.1 Common causes of GORD in the general and psychiatric patient population [1–9].

	General population	Psychiatric population
Medication	NSAIDs (e.g. ibuprofen) Nitrates (e.g. isosorbide mononitrate) Calcium channel blockers (e.g. amlodipine) Bisphosphonates Corticosteroids Theophylline	As for general population Tricyclic antidepressants Anticholinergics Antipsychotics Benzodiazepines
Past medical history	Asthma Previous oesophageal surgery Hiatus hernia Lower oesophageal sphincter dysfunction	As for general population
Lifestyle factors	Obesity Alcohol consumption Overeating Diet (high fat, low fibre) Smoking	As for general population
Non-modifiable factors	Older age Family history of GORD Male gender Pregnancy	As for general population
Psychiatric conditions	N/A	Bulimia nervosa Binge eating disorder Depression Presence of psychosomatic symptoms

with psychosomatic symptoms are more likely to take non-steroidal anti-inflammatory drugs (NSAIDs), a risk factor for GORD [8].

Diagnostic principles

An algorithm for approaching diagnosis and management of GORD is shown in Box 19.1.

History

1 Symptoms:
   a Typical: heartburn (burning feeling in the chest occurring after meals that is often worse on lying or bending down), acid regurgitation (sour or bitter taste at the back of mouth).
   b Atypical: belching, bloating, nausea, dyspepsia (indigestion), epigastric (upper abdominal) pressure/pain, odynophagia (painful swallowing).
   c Extra-oesophageal: nocturnal asthma (breathlessness and wheeze), laryngitis (hoarse voice), sinusitis, chronic cough, dental erosions [1].

Box 19.1 Approach to diagnosis and management of gastrointestinal oesophageal reflux disease

History

- Screen for typical, atypical, extra-oesophageal, and red flag symptoms
- Gastrointestinal history
- Past medical and surgical histories
- Medication history
- Social history
- Family history

Examination

- Gastrointestinal examination
- Height and weight measurements

Management

Where possible, rationalise psychiatric medication and offer non-pharmacological interventions

Typical symptoms

- Start once-daily PPI for four weeks then review
- If symptoms persist, increase PPI to twice daily and refer to gastroenterology
- If symptoms improve with four-week trial PPI, continue for a further four weeks before discontinuing
- Re-prescribe PPI if symptoms return and refer to gastroenterology

Atypical symptoms present

- Start once-daily PPI for four weeks, to be reviewed, and refer to gastroenterology
- If symptoms persist, then increase dose to twice daily and await gastroenterology review

Red flag symptoms present

- Do not start a PPI
- Discuss with a medical doctor if any acute concerns
- Refer for urgent 'two-week wait' upper gastrointestinal endoscopy and gastroenterology review

---

2 Ask about 'red flag' symptoms which may indicate a more serious condition: bleeding (haematemesis or melaena; see Chapter 20), symptoms of anaemia or unexplained anaemia on full blood count (see Chapter 15), persistent vomiting (see Chapter 21), weight loss (see Chapter 25), dysphagia (difficulty swallowing; see Chapter 22), and cardiac sounding chest pain (see Chapter 67).

3 Medication history (see Table 19.1).

4 Any recent changes in diet or weight.

5 Family history of any gastrointestinal disease, especially GORD or gastrointestinal cancer.
6 Past medical history (see Table 19.1).
7 Social history, including smoking and alcohol history.

Examination

1 Abdominal examination is often unremarkable in GORD. Halitosis (bad breath) is more likely in patients with GORD. There may be evidence of pallor (unusually pale skin) if anaemia is present.
2 Possible Russell's sign (calluses on the back of hands) if patient has bulimia nervosa.
3 Height and weight measures.

Diagnosis

GORD is a clinical diagnosis. Typical symptoms of either heartburn or acid regurgitation are both highly specific, though low in sensitivity for GORD [1]. Treatment should therefore be started empirically if either of these symptoms are present and GORD is suspected (see section Management).

Differential diagnoses include coronary artery disease, peptic ulcer disease, achalasia, gastritis, dyspepsia, gastroparesis, and 'functional' heartburn. Red flag symptoms may indicate oesophagitis, peptic stricture, or malignancy.

Management

In patients with suspected GORD, rationalisation of medication, non-pharmacological therapy, and pharmacological therapy should be considered. In the absence of atypical or red flag symptoms and where GORD is successfully treated with an eight-week trial of a proton-pump inhibitor, no further investigations are required. Where atypical or red flag symptoms are present, referral to specialist services are indicated.

Rationalising psychiatric medication

Tricyclic antidepressants have been shown to increase the risk of GORD, with clomipramine possibly having the greatest effect [6]. Selective serotonin reuptake inhibitors have little, if any, impact on risk of GORD [6,7]. If a patient with GORD is on a tricyclic antidepressant, the prescriber may consider offering a switch to an alternative antidepressant, having considered the risks and benefits of such a decision, and after discussion with the patient.

Anticholinergics have been shown to increase the number of reflux episodes in patients with pre-existing GORD [10–12]. In patients with GORD who are experiencing acute extrapyramidal side effects, appropriate treatment with anticholinergics should not be withheld (see Chapter 56), but GORD treatment regimens may need to be intensified. If a patient receiving long-term anticholinergic treatment develops

GORD, then a risk–benefit conversation should be engaged in with the patient to determine whether continued anticholinergic treatment is necessary.

Antipsychotics may increase the risk of developing GORD [13,14], with clozapine associated with higher rates of GORD (up to five times the prevalence) compared with other antipsychotics [15,16]. However, it is considered safe to continue prescribing antipsychotics in patients with GORD.

Hypnotics and benzodiazepines may increase the risk of developing GORD, but the quality of this evidence is not strong enough to advise any changes to practice of prescribing these medications [17,18].

Non-pharmacological: lifestyle modification [1,3,5,19]

- Avoid eating meals within three hours of bedtime.
- Raise the head of the bed.
- Weight loss.
- Smoking cessation.
- Reduce alcohol intake or, if safe, stop drinking alcohol entirely (see Chapter 24).
- Encourage a low-fat, high-fibre diet.
- If patient notices any relationship between certain foods (e.g. chocolate or caffeine) and their symptoms, then a trial elimination of these foods from their diet may be considered.

Pharmacological

GORD is treated by suppressing stomach acid production. Proton-pump inhibitors (PPIs), histamine H_2-receptor antagonists, and antacids can all be used; however, note that ranitidine was recently withdrawn from international markets owing to concerns regarding carcinogenicity. PPIs have been shown to be more effective at treating GORD than histamine H_2-receptor antagonists, but are also costlier [1,5,19,20].

Patients with no red flag or atypical symptoms but who are suspected of suffering with GORD should be given an eight-week trial of a PPI. This provides rapid symptomatic relief in 70–80% of patients [20]. All PPIs have been shown to be of roughly equal efficacy. They should be taken around 30–60 minutes prior to food for maximum benefit [1,5,19,20]. Doses of commonly prescribed PPIs are omeprazole 20 mg, lansoprazole 30 mg, esomeprazole 20 mg, and pantoprazole 40 mg, all given orally once daily. If the patient does not fully respond to PPI treatment within four weeks, then the dose of PPI should be increased to twice daily, with doses being taken before breakfast and before dinner, and a referral to gastroenterology should be completed [20].

Long-term PPI use has been associated with increased risk of various comorbid complaints, including pneumonia [21], osteoporosis and fractures [22], *Clostridium difficile* infection [23], and increased all-cause mortality [24]. Although association does not imply causality, and confounding has been implicated in some of these population-based analyses [25], the judicious prescriber may consider limiting long-term PPI use where possible. Moreover, PPIs may influence plasma levels of other medications (including psychiatric drugs), either through alterations in absorption secondary to changes in gut pH, or via cytochrome P450 interactions [26].

When to refer to a specialist

Where atypical symptoms are present then treatment should be started as described, and the patient referred to gastroenterology. If any red flag symptoms are detected, then a 'two-week wait' urgent referral for endoscopy should be made, alongside a referral to gastroenterology. Avoid PPIs and histamine H_2-receptor antagonists for two weeks prior to endoscopy.

In patients who experience a relapse of symptoms when the PPI is discontinued, the PPI should be reinstated and a referral to gastroenterology made [20]. Gastrointestinal endoscopy should be considered in those whose symptoms repeatedly recur after PPIs are stopped, or in those who require maintenance PPIs. This enables risk stratification of GORD (non-erosive, erosive) and to exclude Barrett's oesophagus.

Information to include in a referral letter

When writing a referral letter to either the two-week wait service or the gastroenterology team, it is important to include the following information: gastrointestinal history, past medical and surgical histories, current medication along with allergy status, a brief social history, and any findings from clinical examination. Ensure that the patient's psychiatric history is included in the letter.

PEPTIC ULCER DISEASE

The typical presentation of peptic ulcer disease (PUD) is of chronic epigastric pain associated with eating. There may also be pain on palpation of the epigastrium. It is most often caused by *Helicobacter pylori* infection or use of NSAIDs. PUD may coexist with GORD or may be difficult to distinguish from it, but should be suspected when epigastric pain is the primary presenting complaint, or if treatment for GORD has been ineffective. If there are any red flag symptoms (as described for GORD), or the patient does not respond to treatment, then specialist advice from gastroenterology should be sought. An algorithm for approaching diagnosis and management of PUD is shown in Box 19.2.

Investigation of new symptoms of PUD

1 Full blood count: anaemia may indicate gastrointestinal bleeding.
2 If aged under 55 years, *H. pylori* breath or stool testing is the first-line investigation. Testing should not be performed if PPIs, bismuth or antibiotics have been used in the two weeks prior to testing in order to reduce the chance of a false-negative result.
3 In those aged 55 years or older, and also in those (at any age) who have associated weight loss, vomiting, anaemia or dysphagia, upper gastrointestinal endoscopy should be requested. If an ulcer is found, then *H. pylori* testing is indicated. In patients with no weight loss, *H. pylori* testing should be organised as the first-line investigation.

> **Box 19.2** Approach to diagnosis and management of peptic ulcer disease
>
> **History**
>
> - Gastrointestinal history including screen for red flag symptoms
> - Past medical and surgical histories
> - Medication history
> - Social history
> - Family history
>
> **Examination and investigations**
>
> - Gastrointestinal examination
> - Full blood count
> - Age <55: *H. pylori* testing
> - Age ≥55 or with weight loss, anaemia, vomiting or dysphagia: endoscopy and *H. pylori* testing if ulcer present
>
> **Management**
>
> - Stop NSAIDs if possible
> - If NSAIDs to continue, offer long-term PPI therapy
> - Refer to specialists if red flag symptoms present or not responding to treatment
>
> *Active bleeding*
>
> - Resuscitation and transfer to emergency services
>
> *H. pylori test negative*
>
> - Once-daily PPI for four to eight weeks
>
> *H. pylori test positive*
>
> - One- to two-week course of triple therapy (PPI and antibiotics), as defined by local guidelines
> - See local guidelines for alternative regimen if symptoms persist
> - *H. pylori* testing four weeks after successful therapy to confirm eradication

Management

NSAIDs should be stopped unless the patient is using aspirin as an antiplatelet agent for primary/secondary prevention of cardiovascular disease [27]. In this instance, aspirin should be continued, and the patient started on long-term acid suppression therapy (PPI) [27]. NSAIDs for pain management should be used at the lowest dose for the shortest period of time.

Active bleeding

Start resuscitation and call for ambulance/emergency assistance. Active bleeding will require endoscopy/surgery, PPI, and possible blood transfusion. PPI will be continued for around four to eight weeks post intervention but be guided by specialist advice.

H. pylori test negative

Once daily PPI for four to eight weeks (see section on pharmacological management of GORD for medication and doses).

H. pylori test positive

A one- to two-week period of triple therapy is needed, for example PPI twice daily (see section on pharmacological management of GORD for medication and doses), clarithromycin 500 mg twice daily, and amoxicillin 1 g twice daily (use metronidazole if allergic to penicillin). Most patients will not need continued PPI prescribing thereafter. If symptoms persist, then an alternative treatment regimen may be trialled (refer to local guidelines). Testing for *H. pylori* should be repeated four weeks after the end of therapy to confirm eradication. This should ideally by performed using carbon-14 urea breath testing which, unlike stool testing, is validated in the post-eradication setting.

References

1. Badillo R, Francis D. Diagnosis and treatment of gastroesophageal reflux disease. *World J Gastrointest Pharmacol Ther* 2014;5(3):105–112.
2. Chait MM. Gastroesophageal reflux disease: important considerations for the older patients. *World J Gastrointest Endosc* 2010;2(12):388–396.
3. El-Serag HB, Satia JA, Rabeneck L. Dietary intake and the risk of gastro-oesophageal reflux disease: a cross sectional study in volunteers. *Gut* 2005;54(1):11–17.
4. Denholm M, Jankowski J. Gastroesophageal reflux disease and bulimia nervosa: a review of the literature. *Dis Esophagus* 2011;24(2):79–85.
5. Keung C, Hebbard G. The management of gastro-oesophageal reflux disease. *Aust Prescr* 2016;39(1):6–10.
6. van Soest EM, Dieleman JP, Siersema PD, et al. Tricyclic antidepressants and the risk of reflux esophagitis. *Am J Gastroenterol* 2007;102(9):1870–1877.
7. Martin-Merino E, Ruigomez A, Garcia Rodriguez LA, et al. Depression and treatment with antidepressants are associated with the development of gastro-oesophageal reflux disease. *Aliment Pharmacol Ther* 2010;31(10):1132–1140.
8. Locke GR III, Talley NJ, Fett SL, et al. Risk factors associated with symptoms of gastroesophageal reflux. *Am J Med* 1999;106(6):642–649.
9. Theodoropoulos DS, Lockey RF, Boyce HW Jr, Bukantz SC. Gastroesophageal reflux and asthma: a review of pathogenesis, diagnosis, and therapy. *Allergy* 1999;54(7):651–661.
10. Ciccaglione AF, Grossi L, Cappello G, et al. Effect of hyoscine N-butylbromide on gastroesophageal reflux in normal subjects and patients with gastroesophageal reflux disease. *Am J Gastroenterol* 2001;96:2306–2311.
11. Koerselman J, Pursnani KG, Peghini P, et al. Different effects of an oral anticholinergic drug on gastroesophageal reflux in upright and supine position in normal, ambulant subjects: a pilot study. *Am J Gastroenterol* 1999;94(4):925–930.
12. Lidums I, Checklin H, Mittal RK, Holloway RH. Effect of atropine on gastro-oesophageal reflux and transient lower oesophageal sphincter relaxations in patients with gastro-oesophageal reflux disease. *Gut* 1998;43:12–16.
13. Dziewas R, Warnecke T, Schnabel M, et al. Neuroleptic-induced dysphagia: case report and literature review. *Dysphagia* 2007;22(1):63–67.
14. Crouse EL, Alastanos JN, Bozymski KM, Toscano RA. Dysphagia with second-generation antipsychotics: a case report and review of the literature. *Ment Health Clin* 2017;7(2):56–64.
15. Taylor D, Olofinjana O, Rahimi T. Use of antacid medication in patients receiving clozapine: a comparison with other second-generation antipsychotics. *J Clin Psychopharmacol* 2010;30(4):460–461.
16. van Veggel M, Olofinjana O, Davies O, Taylor D. Clozapine and gastro-oesophageal reflux disease (GORD): an investigation of temporal association. *Acta Psychiatr Scand* 2013;127(1):69–77.
17. Rushnak MJ, Leevy CM. Effect of diazepam on the lower esophageal sphincter. A double-blind controlled study. *Am J Gastroenterol* 1980;73:127–130.
18. Singh S, Bailey RT, Stein HJ, et al. Effect of alprazolam (Xanax) on esophageal motility and acid reflux. *Am J Gastroenterol* 1992;87:483–488.
19. Sandhu DS, Fass R. Current trends in the management of gastroesophageal reflux disease. *Gut Liver* 2018;12(1):7–16.
20. Katz PO, Gerson LB, Vela MF. Guidelines for the diagnosis and management of gastroesophageal reflux disease. *Am J Gastroenterol* 2013;108(3):308–328.

21. Zirk-Sadowski J, Masoli JA, Delgado J, et al. Proton-pump inhibitors and long-term risk of community-acquired pneumonia in older adults. *J Am Geriatr Soc* 2018;66(7):1332–1338.

22. Andersen BN, Johansen PB, Abrahamsen B. Proton pump inhibitors and osteoporosis. *Curr Opin Rheumatol* 2016;28(4):420–425.

23. McDonald EG, Milligan J, Frenette C, Lee TC. Continuous proton pump inhibitor therapy and the associated risk of recurrent *Clostridium difficile* infection. *JAMA Intern Med* 2015;175(5):784–791.

24. Xie Y, Bowe B, Li T, et al. Risk of death among users of proton pump inhibitors: a longitudinal observational cohort study of United States veterans. *BMJ Open* 2017;7(6):e015735.

25. Othman F, Crooks CJ, Card TR. Community acquired pneumonia incidence before and after proton pump inhibitor prescription: population based study. *BMJ* 2016;355:i5813.

26. Frick A, Kopitz J, Bergemann N. Omeprazole reduces clozapine plasma concentrations. A case report. *Pharmacopsychiatry* 2003;36(3):121–123.

27. Cryer B, Mahaffey KW. Gastrointestinal ulcers, role of aspirin, and clinical outcomes: pathobiology, diagnosis, and treatment. *J Multidiscip Healthc* 2014;7:137–146.

28. Nissen SE, Yeomans ND, Solomon DH, et al. Cardiovascular safety of celecoxib, naproxen, or ibuprofen for arthritis. *N Engl J Med* 2016;375(26):2519–2529.

29. Whittle BJ. COX-1 and COX-2 products in the gut: therapeutic impact of COX-2 inhibitors. *Gut* 2000;47:320–325.

CHAPTER 19

Chapter 20

Gastrointestinal Bleeding

Douglas Corrigall, David Dewar

Gastrointestinal (GI) bleeding refers to blood loss from within the gastrointestinal tract. Upper GI bleeding is defined as bleeding occurring proximal to the ligament of Treitz; that is to say from the oesophagus, stomach, or duodenum. Lower GI bleeding is that originating from the small bowel or colon. Acute small bowel bleeding is rare, so we focus here on investigation and management of upper GI bleeds and colonic bleeding.

Acute upper GI bleeding can be life-threatening, with mortality rates ranging between 10 and 50% in general medical inpatient settings [1,2], depending on severity and aetiology. This therefore is the focus of the chapter. Assessment of GI bleeding in a psychiatric inpatient setting must focus on the rapid identification of patients who will require urgent medical interventions that necessitate transfer. We would advise timely discussion with medical/gastroenterological colleagues in the case of all suspected acute GI bleeds. As 70% of blood loss from the GI tract is due to upper GI causes, the usual approach is to rule these out before considering lower GI investigations [3].

Common causes in the general population and specific considerations in individuals with serious mental illness (SMI) are summarised in Box 20.1. Specific considerations for psychiatric patients include the fact that some selective serotonin reuptake inhibitors (SSRIs) have been shown in observational studies to increase the risk of both upper and lower GI bleeding (potentially via inhibition of platelet function; see Chapter 17) [4]. Variceal bleeding as a result of chronic liver disease is usually secondary to alcohol-related liver disease (see Chapter 24) or chronic viral hepatitis (consider this in patients with risk factors such as a history of intravenous drug misuse; see Chapter 43). Variceal bleeding is a medical emergency, with mortality rates approaching 50% [3]. Any signs of upper GI bleeding in patients with known liver disease should be treated as a variceal bleed until proven otherwise [5]. Patients with eating disorders such as bulimia with frequent vomiting/purging may develop Mallory–Weiss tears at the gastro-oesophageal junction [6].

The Maudsley Practice Guidelines for Physical Health Conditions in Psychiatry, First Edition.
David M. Taylor, Fiona Gaughran, and Toby Pillinger.
© 2021 John Wiley & Sons Ltd. Published 2021 by John Wiley & Sons Ltd.

Box 20.1 Common causes/risk factors for GI bleeds in the general and psychiatric patient population

Upper GI tract

- Gastric/duodenal ulcer
- Varices (gastric or oesophageal)
- Mallory–Weiss tear
- Oesophagitis
- Arteriovenous malformations
- Gastrointestinal stromal tumours

Lower GI tract

- Anal fissures
- Angiodysplasia
- Colitis (radiation, ischaemic, infectious)
- Colonic polyps
- Colonic carcinoma
- Diverticular disease
- Inflammatory bowel disease
- Haemorrhoids

Small bowel (rare)

- Arteriovenous malformations
- Meckel's diverticulum
- Tumours

Medication

- NSAID use can cause ulcers
- Bisphosphonates can cause oesophagitis

Infection

- *Helicobacter pylori* can cause ulcers/gastritis

Liver disease

- Variceal bleed
- Portal hypertensive gastropathy

Kidney disease

- Angiodysplasia

Malignancy

- Blood loss from friable tumours or vessel invasion

Alcohol

- Can cause oesophagitis, gastritis, ulcers
- Association with liver disease

Patients with SMI

- SSRI prescription
- Liver disease, portal hypertension and resultant varices
- Mallory–Weiss tear secondary to purging behaviours

A further consideration for SMI patients, especially those who may be survivors of abuse, is that endoscopy is an invasive and for some unpleasant test which can provoke a great deal of anxiety [7]. The sedation typically given during endoscopy consists of an anxiolytic, usually 2–5 mg of midazolam, which can be given with a short-acting opiate such as pethidine or fentanyl, so any interactions with other medications should also be considered and advice regarding interactions with psychiatric medications will be gratefully received. Furthermore, tolerance to benzodiazepines in those on long-term benzodiazepine treatment may occur, potentially necessitating higher doses of sedation.

DIAGNOSTIC PRINCIPLES

Mortality from acute upper GI bleeds, even those occurring in hospital, remains high and this has not changed significantly for decades [8]. Therefore, when faced with a possible GI bleed in an inpatient setting it is important first to exclude this and patients must be assessed and triaged for early resuscitation and endoscopy [8]. The signs and symptoms of lower GI bleeding, including fresh blood per rectum, can be due to an acute upper GI source and this will need to be excluded (by upper GI endoscopy) in most cases before proceeding to further investigations [3]. As always, careful history and examination is vital in guiding appropriate investigations and avoiding unnecessary tests. The aim is to identify those with acute bleeds who need urgent management, and those with chronic blood loss who can be managed on an outpatient basis. Most if not all patients with suspected GI blood loss will require an endoscopy; the question is how soon it should occur.

History

1 Ask about the timing of bleeding, estimated volume, the colour of any vomit (resist the temptation to mention coffee grounds; the patient will often describe the vomitus as this unprompted, which is useful in arriving at the diagnosis), and the frequency of haematemesis/melaena.
2 For lower GI blood loss ask about stool frequency, volumes of blood, and whether it is mixed in with the stool or fresh on the tissue (suggesting haemorrhoids).
3 Systemic symptoms such as weight loss, loss of appetite, dysphagia, or dypsepsia which may suggest malignancy.
4 Medication history, specifically non-steroidal anti-inflammatory drugs (NSAIDs) or bisphosphonates.
5 Any symptoms suggestive of volume loss, including dizziness or syncope.
6 Symptoms of anaemia: tiredness, fatigue, and shortness of breath.
7 Family history of gastrointestinal disease, liver disease, or malignancy.
8 Past medical history: previous ulcers/bleeding, liver disease.
9 Social history, including alcohol and smoking and any other non-prescribed medications.

CHAPTER 20

Signs of upper GI bleeding

1 Haematemesis (vomiting fresh blood; however, note that occasionally regurgitation of bright red food or drink can be mistaken for haemetemesis). Frank haematemesis suggests moderate to severe bleed usually from stomach or oesophagus, which may be ongoing.
2 Coffee ground vomitus (altered blood from an upper GI source that has been in the stomach for a period of time): bleeding may still be ongoing.
  Melaena (blood altered by passage through the GI tract):
  a characteristic sickly sweet smell
  b present in 70% of upper GI bleeds
  c black tarry stool indicates at least 50 mL of blood loss
  d generally means blood has been in GI tract for eight hours or more [9]
  e oral iron supplementation causes tarry black stool so beware.
3 Haematochezia (frank blood per rectum): can represent upper GI bleed [10].

Signs of lower GI bleeding

1 Blood per rectum can occur with any GI source of blood loss.
2 Haematochezia:
  a can be frank blood or dark red stool
  b can be due to large upper GI bleeds [11].
3 Blood in toilet/on tissue (suggests haemorrhoid source): toilet water can appear bright red from only 5 mL of blood.

Examination

1 Basic observations: haemodynamic instability suggests a possible large upper GI bleed and should prompt rapid transfer to a resuscitation area.
2 Cardiovascular examination:
  a Look for signs of hypoperfusion such as increased capillary return time.
  b Flow murmur on auscultation can occur in high-output states.
  c Young fit patients: resting tachycardia or postural tachycardia should be treated with caution, since this can represent significant blood loss (with associated physiological compensation).
3 Respiratory examination: listen for any crepitations which may suggest that aspiration of vomit has occurred. Aspiration of blood can cause a severe pneumonitis.
4 Abdominal examination:
  a Look for signs of chronic liver disease and in particular signs of hepatic decompensation such as ascites or jaundice.
  b Per rectum examination to check for fresh blood or melaena. Ensure visual inspection for haemorrhoids.

5 Neurological examination:
   a Any signs of altered consciousness could be due to hypoperfusion or hepatic encephalopathy in decompensated chronic liver disease.
   b Check for asterixis ('liver flap'), which is suggestive of hepatic encephalopathy.

Investigations

These will obviously be dependent on the facilities available. If results of tests are not immediately available, this may necessitate transfer to a medical environment.

1 ECG to check for any signs of cardiac ischaemia secondary to blood loss.
2 Bloods:
   a Full blood count: this may be misleadingly normal in the hyperacute situation before haemodilution has occurred.
   b Urea and electrolytes.
   c Clotting screen.
   d Liver function tests.
   e Iron studies: iron deficiency anaemia can represent chronic GI blood loss.
   f Blood cultures if signs of liver disease (infection is a frequent cause of decompensating events).
   g Group and save if an inpatient. If there is a suggestion of a large bleed, cross-match at least 4 units immediately. If in the psychiatric setting and group and save is being considered, urgent referral and transfer to medical services should have been requested.

MANAGEMENT

If an inpatient, ensure the patient is kept nil by mouth until decisions about endoscopy have been made [4]. If there is frank active bleeding and haemodynamic instability, do not delay transfer by requesting investigations. This is a medical emergency which requires rapid transfer to a medical unit where resuscitation can continue. If possible and appropriate, ensure the following.

1 Airway patent and secure.
2 If facilities allow, gain intravenous access with two large-bore cannulae.
3 If blood pressure is low, and if facilities allow, commence fluid resuscitation (e.g. normal saline 0.9%) while rapid transfer is arranged.
4 If haemodynamically stable, there is no sign of ongoing bleeding, and blood results can be obtained in a timely manner, it may after discussion with the medical/gastroenterology teams be appropriate to await these and calculate the Blatchford score [12] (Table 20.1) before transfer.

The Blatchford score is a validated scoring system that can be used to predict clinical outcomes [12]. Low-risk patients with a Blatchford score of zero can be considered for non-urgent or outpatient endoscopy [4]. Those patients with higher risk scores can be prioritised for urgent (within 24 hours) or emergent inpatient endoscopy.

CHAPTER 20

Table 20.1 Blatchford score for GI bleeds.

Risk marker		Score
Haemoglobin (g/L)		
Male	*Female*	
120–130	100–120	1
100–120		3
<100	<100	6
Urea (mmol/L)		
6.5–8		2
8–10		3
10–25		4
>25		6
Systolic blood pressure (mmHg)		
100–109		1
90–99		2
<90		3
Other markers		
Pulse >100		1
Melaena		1
Syncope		2
Hepatic disease		2
Cardiac failure		2

Non-pharmacological therapy

Endoscopy is the definitive investigation and usually the definitive therapeutic modality in GI bleeds. Depending on what is seen at endoscopy, the risk of rebleeding can be estimated.

In cases of intractable bleeding, depending on the site, embolisation via interventional radiology to occlude the bleeding vessel can be attempted, or surgery such as partial gastrectomy can be attempted [13].

Pharmacological therapy

In an outpatient setting where the patient is stable, consider oral PPI therapy while waiting for gastroenterology review if you suspect reflux disease, gastritis, or peptic ulcer disease.

In inpatients, practice continues to vary widely around the use of intravenous PPI therapy prior to endoscopy [4,14]. You may be advised to commence intravenous PPIs in patients awaiting endoscopy, although some authorities feel there is little evidence for their benefit [4]. Similarly, while there is a paucity of high-quality evidence for the use of tranexamic acid, this is sometimes given in an attempt to slow bleeding [15].

In the case of variceal bleeds, antibiotics are given along with terlipressin [4] or octreotide [16] infusions to attempt to reduce portal pressure. Terlipressin and octreotide require close monitoring so should not be given in the psychiatric setting.

When to refer to a specialist

In view of the high in-hospital mortality and potential for deterioration it is important that all suspected inpatient acute GI bleeds are discussed immediately with the local medical or gastroenterological team and most should receive timely endoscopy within 24 hours [4] or on an emergent basis in the case of suspected variceal bleeds or if there is ongoing haemodynamic instability.

In stable patients in the community with a Blatchford score of zero, urgent outpatient management can be appropriate as outlined in Box 20.2 [8]. If there is any uncertainty at all, discuss with your local medical or gastroenterology on-call team.

Box 20.2 When to consider outpatient management for suspected acute GI bleeds

Consider for urgent outpatient management

- Age <60 years *and*
- Haemodynamically stable *and*
- No significant cardiac disease, liver disease, malignancy or other major comorbidity *and*
- Not currently an inpatient *and*
- No witnessed haematemesis/haematochezia

Consider admission/early endoscopy

- Age >60 years *or*
- Witnessed haematemesis/haematochezia or suspected continued bleeding *or*
- Haemodynamic instability *or*
- Liver disease/known varices *or*
- Current inpatient (medical or psychiatric)

Chronic GI bleeding generally presents with iron deficiency anaemia or a positive faecal test for occult blood (in the UK, a faecal immunochemical test). It can be managed on an outpatient basis and in the first instance urgent referral to gastroenterology outpatients or a medical consultation should be sought [17] and upper and lower GI endoscopy arranged. Anaemia is not a diagnosis and the cause must be established. Box 20.3 provides a diagnostic summary to guide investigation and management.

Box 20.3 Diagnostic summary

History

- Define symptoms: suggestive of acute or chronic blood loss?
- Explore risk factors/symptoms suggesting malignancy
- Past medical history, including previous GI bleeds and liver disease
- Medication history
- Alcohol/smoking
- Family history of malignancy

Examination

- Establish if any ongoing bleeding/haemodynamic instability
- Examine for signs of liver disease

Investigations

- Bloods
- Endoscopy

Management

- Stratify risk: does this patient need urgent/emergent endoscopy?
- Decide on urgent inpatient investigations or outpatient follow-up

References

1. Rockall TA, Logan RF, Devlin HB, Northfield TC. Incidence of and mortality from acute upper gastrointestinal haemorrhage in the United Kingdom. *BMJ* 1995;311(6999):222–226.
2. Hearnshaw SA, Logan RFA, Lowe D, et al. Acute upper gastrointestinal bleeding in the UK: patient characteristics, diagnoses and outcomes in the 2007 UK audit. *Gut* 2011;60(10):1327–1335.
3. Oakland K, Chadwick G, East JE, et al. Diagnosis and management of acute lower gastrointestinal bleeding: guidelines from the British Society of Gastroenterology. *Gut* 2019;68(5):776–789.
4. National Institute for Health and Care Excellence. *Acute Upper Gastrointestinal Bleeding in Over 16s: Management.* Clinical Guideline CG141. London: NICE, 2012. Available at https://www.nice.org.uk/guidance/cg141
5. Tripathi D, Stanley AJ, Hayes PC, et al. UK guidelines on the management of variceal haemorrhage in cirrhotic patients. *Gut* 2015;64(11):1680–1704.
6. Forney KJ, Buchman-Schmitt JM, Keel PK, Frank GKW. The medical complications associated with purging. *Int J Eat Disord* 2016;49(3):249–259.
7. Davy E. The endoscopy patient with a history of sexual abuse: strategies for compassionate care. *Gastroenterol Nurs* 2006; 29(3):221–225.
8. Scottish Intercollegiate Guidelines Network. *Management of Acute Upper and Lower Gastrointestinal Bleeding: A National Clinical Guideline.* SIGN Guideline 105, 2008.
9. Schiff L, Shapiro N, Stevens RJ. Observations on the oral administration of citrated blood in man. *Am J Med Sci* 1939;207(4):465–467.
10. Srygley FD, Gerardo CJ, Tran T, Fisher DA. Does this patient have a severe upper gastrointestinal bleed? *JAMA* 2012;307(10):1072.
11. Sittichanbuncha Y, Senasu S, Thongkrau T, et al. How to differentiate sites of gastrointestinal bleeding in patients with hematochezia by using clinical factors? *Gastroenterol Res Pract* 2013;2013:265076.
12. Blatchford O, Murray WR, Blatchford M. A risk score to predict need for treatment for upper gastrointestinal haemorrhage. *Lancet* 2000;356(9238):1318–1321.

13. Siau K, Chapman W, Sharma N, et al. Management of acute upper gastrointestinal bleeding: an update for the general physician. *J R Coll Physicians Edinb* 2017;47(3):218–230.

14. Laine L, Jensen DM. Management of patients with ulcer bleeding. *Am J Gastroenterol* 2012;107(3):345–360.

15. Bennett C, Klingenberg SL, Langholz E, Gluud LL. Tranexamic acid for upper gastrointestinal bleeding. *Cochrane Database Syst Rev* 2014;(11):CD006640.

16. LaBrecque D, Khan AG, Sarin SK, Le Mair AW. Esophageal varices. World Gastroenterology Organisation Global Guidelines, 2014. http://www.worldgastroenterology.org/UserFiles/file/guidelines/esophageal-varices-english-2014.pdf (accessed 21 May 2019).

17. Goddard AF, James MW, McIntyre AS, Scott BB. Guidelines for the management of iron deficiency anaemia. *Gut* 2011;60(10):1309–1316.

CHAPTER 20

Nausea and Vomiting

Mary Denholm, Matthew Cheetham

Nausea is the unpleasant feeling of the need to vomit, which may be accompanied by additional autonomic symptoms (e.g. tachycardia and sweating). Vomiting, as distinct from expectoration or regurgitation, is expulsion of gastric contents through the mouth. Regurgitation is the return of substances from the oesophagus to the hypopharynx with minimal effort [1]. Clinically it is important to distinguish acute presentations from those of a more chronic nature. Both can indicate significant pathology, but some acute causes, such as bowel obstruction or acute pancreatitis, require immediate medical attention.

Nausea and vomiting are prompted by activation of specific 'trigger areas' within the body, some of which are located in the gastrointestinal tract and some in the central nervous system (CNS), in the latter mainly the floor of the fourth ventricle (the chemoreceptor trigger zone) and the medulla (the nucleus tractus solitarius) [2]. Afferent signals can come from different locations, hence the association of nausea and vomiting with a wide range of conditions. Common causes are listed in Box 21.1 [1,3–8].

Nausea and/or vomiting in patients with serious mental illness (SMI) may be the feature of a primary psychiatric diagnosis (e.g. bulimia nervosa), a consequence of autonomic activation in the context of psychological symptoms (e.g. anxiety/panic), or secondary to psychiatric treatment. For example, nausea and vomiting is a recognised side effect of selective serotonin reuptake inhibitors (SSRIs), likely secondary to stimulation of 5-HT$_3$ receptors [9], and may also accompany SSRI discontinuation [10]. Although several antipsychotics have anti-emetic activity, D2 dopamine receptor partial agonists such as aripiprazole may be associated with nausea, especially early during treatment [11]. Psychostimulants (e.g. methylphenidate) and mood stabilisers (e.g. sodium valproate and lithium) can also be associated with nausea. Indeed, nausea and vomiting in a patient receiving lithium treatment may herald toxicity. Functional disorders associated with nausea and vomiting (e.g. cyclic vomiting disorder) are diagnoses of exclusion.

The Maudsley Practice Guidelines for Physical Health Conditions in Psychiatry, First Edition.
David M. Taylor, Fiona Gaughran, and Toby Pillinger.
© 2021 John Wiley & Sons Ltd. Published 2021 by John Wiley & Sons Ltd.

Box 21.1 Common causes of nausea and vomiting

Gastrointestinal

Gastric stasis, intestinal obstruction or pseudo-obstruction/ileus, constipation, presence of ascites, gastritis, peptic ulceration, gastroenteritis, pyloric stenosis, acute pancreatitis, cholecystitis, gastric cancer, oesophageal reflux, appendicitis

Metabolic

Hypercalcaemia, renal failure/uraemia, hyponatraemia, Addisonian crisis, diabetic ketoacidosis

Neurological

Raised intracranial pressure, meningitis, encephalitis, migraine, Ménière's disease, labyrinthitis, autonomic neuropathy, head injury, benign paroxysmal positional vertigo

Infection

Viral or bacterial gastrointestinal infections, mucocutaneous candidiasis, urinary tract infection, sepsis syndromes

Pain

Usually acute and severe pain

Pregnancy

First trimester but may persist

Alcohol and recreational drugs

For example, cannabis (cannabinoid hyperemesis syndrome)

Drugs

Opiates (e.g. codeine phosphate), chemotherapy, iron, antibiotics, NSAIDs, digoxin

Psychiatric drugs

Selective serotonin reuptake inhibitors
Dopamine D2 receptor partial agonists (e.g. aripiprazole)
Mood stabilisers (e.g. lithium, sodium valproate, and lamotrigine)
Psychostimulants (e.g. methylphenidate)

Psychiatric

Anxiety, panic disorder, bulimia nervosa

Functional disorders

For example, cyclic vomiting disorder, chronic nausea and vomiting syndrome (diagnoses of exclusion)

Miscellaneous

Normal physiological response to stress, travel sickness, radiation therapy, hepatic and biliary disease (e.g. cirrhosis), testicular torsion, twisted ovarian cyst

Rumination syndrome

A chronic motility disorder commonly misdiagnosed as vomiting

DIAGNOSTIC PRINCIPLES

History, examination, and investigations are primarily performed to screen for acute underlying conditions that may require urgent medical attention (e.g. appendicitis), chronic but severe underlying conditions that may require expedited medical/surgical referral (e.g. malignancy), or complications secondary to vomiting/poor oral intake that may require urgent medical attention (e.g. electrolyte disturbance).

History [3,12]

- Duration (acute or chronic).
- Amount and frequency.
- Colour/contents (e.g. liquid, bile, feculent).
- Ask about any contacts or family members unwell with similar symptoms (gastroenteritis).
- Presence or absence of blood: fresh red, dark 'coffee ground' (GI bleeding).
- Timing:
  - Time of day: early morning (pregnancy) and with headaches (raised intracranial pressure, ICP).
  - Relation to eating: few hours after food suggests gastric outlet obstruction.
- Systemic symptoms, e.g. fevers, unintentional weight loss (malignancy).
- Headaches: nausea/vomiting may be associated with migraine or raised ICP.
- Vertigo (possible acute viral labyrinthitis).
- Abdominal pain: right upper quadrant pain may suggest biliary colic or cholecystitis, right iliac fossa pain may suggest appendicitis (see Chapter 88).
- 'Red flag' gastrointestinal symptoms that may point towards malignancy, e.g. dysphagia (see Chapter 22), weight loss, and melaena (see Chapter 20).
- Reflux symptoms and nausea might suggest gastro-oesophageal reflux disease (see Chapter 19).
- Abdominal bloating/distension.
- Bowel habit (diarrhoea suggestive of gastroenteritis).
- Past medical history: previous malignancy (intracranial metastases), diabetes mellitus (autonomic neuropathy), active cancer treatment (chemotherapy-induced nausea and vomiting, immunosuppression and risk of CNS infection).

- Medication history (see Box 21.1).
- Dietary history.
- Social history: alcohol use, recreational drug use.

Examination

- Basic observations including temperature, heart rate, and blood pressure to assess for hypovolaemia.
- Clinical hydration status: check mucous membranes, skin turgor, and jugular venous pressure; assess for pedal oedema.
- Abdominal examination: tenderness, distension, masses, bowel sounds for evidence of obstruction.
- Rectal/genital/pelvic examination if indicated to exclude faecal impaction, testicular/ovarian cyst, torsion.
- Physical signs of self-induced vomiting/bulimia: dental enamel erosion, calluses on the dorsal surface of the hands, enlargement of the parotid glands [13,14].
- Neurological: check fundi for papilloedema if concerned about raised ICP, although absence does not exclude raised ICP.
- In a patient receiving lithium therapy, examine for other clinical features that may suggest toxicity, e.g. coarse tremor, nystagmus, ataxia, and altered consciousness.

Investigations

For short-lived causes of nausea and vomiting such as gastroenteritis, where the patient is clinically stable and able to tolerate oral fluids, generally symptoms will be self-limiting, and no further investigations are required.

In cases of persistent vomiting, if signs/symptoms suggest severe systemic pathology (see Box 21.1), or where oral fluids are not tolerated, investigations that may be considered are as follows.

- Bloods:
  - urea and creatinine
  - electrolytes including potassium and magnesium
  - full blood count
  - liver function tests
  - C-reactive protein
  - serum amylase
  - bone profile (to include corrected calcium)
  - blood cultures if pyrexial
  - glucose levels if patient is diabetic
  - lithium levels if receiving lithium (possible toxicity).
- ECG: particularly in context of electrolyte disturbance, or to calculate QTc interval before initiation of an anti-emetic which may interact with other prescribed medications to cause prolongation.
- Urinalysis including pregnancy test.
- Stool cultures if associated prolonged diarrhoea.

If the patient requires transfer from psychiatric to medical care (e.g. in the setting of acute infection/volume depletion), then the following investigations may be considered.

- Venous blood gas to check lactate (hydration status, indicators of ischaemia, e.g. some cases of bowel obstruction) and for acidosis (renal failure) or metabolic alkalosis (pyloric stenosis or gastric outlet obstruction).
- Abdominal X-ray: look for signs of bowel obstruction or toxic megacolon.
- Ultrasound abdomen/pelvis.
- CT head if concerns over raised ICP.
- Lumbar puncture (bacterial meningitis/viral encephalitis).

MANAGEMENT [15]

Acute management of nausea and vomiting

- For acute cases where the patient can still tolerate oral fluids or diet, only supportive management is required: oral fluids (ideally oral rehydration therapy), simple analgesia such as paracetamol for headache or abdominal pain, and anti-emetics (Table 21.1).
- Referral to acute medical services may be necessary for the following.
  - Severe gastroenteritis, hyperemesis gravidarum, or any cause where the patient is no longer able to tolerate oral fluids and requires intravenous fluids and electrolyte replacement.
  - Targeted management of the underlying cause, e.g. bowel obstruction, management of underlying infections (e.g. meningitis, cholecystitis), steroids if raised ICP due to intracranial lesion.

Management of chronic nausea and vomiting

Rationalise medication

- Nausea in the context of psychiatric medication may be dose-related. For example, SSRI-related nausea may resolve with dose reduction [9]. Nausea can also be associated with SSRI discontinuation, generally emerging within a week of discontinuing the drug and resolving within three weeks [10]. In this situation, consider slowing the rate of SSRI tapering.
- Nausea has also been reported as a side effect of dopamine D2 receptor partial agonists such as aripiprazole [11], brexpiprazole [16], and cariprazine [17]. This may be dose-related (consider slowing dose titration rate) and usually occurs early in treatment, with most patients developing tolerance [11].
- Nausea has been reported in association with prescription of psychostimulants (e.g. methylphenidate) for attention deficit hyperactivity disorder, although a recent meta-analysis observed that the risk of nausea was not significantly increased in patients receiving methylphenidate compared with placebo [18].

CHAPTER 21

- Nausea and vomiting can be associated with prescription of mood stabilisers, such as sodium valproate [19], lamotrigine [20], and lithium. Indeed, nausea has been documented in up to 20% of lithium-treated patients, although it tends to be more likely early in treatment, with most patients developing tolerance [21]. Plasma lithium levels should be checked in a nauseated patient receiving lithium to rule out lithium toxicity. In the absence of toxicity, taking lithium after meals or using a sustained-release preparation may diminish associated nausea.

Table 21.1 Commonly prescribed anti-emetics.

Drug	Mechanism	Particular indications	Dose	Side effects/cautions
Cyclizine	Antihistamine	Good general anti-emetic	50 mg t.d.s. (IV/IM/SC/PO)[a]	Can cause acute reaction when given intravenously Dry mouth, drowsiness
Ondansetron	5-HT$_3$ antagonist	Opiate-induced nausea and vomiting	4–8 mg t.d.s. (PO/IV)	Constipation: avoid in bowel obstruction Headache
Haloperidol	Dopamine (D2) receptor antagonist	Metabolic causes (see Box 21.1) Drug-induced nausea and vomiting	0.5–1.5 mg b.d. (PO/SC/IM)	Sedation EPSE Caution using alongside ondansetron due to risk of QTc prolongation
Prochlorperazine	Dopamine (D2) receptor antagonist	Metabolic causes (see Box 21.1)	Oral: 5–10 mg t.d.s. Buccal: 3–6 mg b.d.	Sedation EPSE (although rare at this dose, risk increased in the elderly)
Metoclopramide	Prokinetic Dopamine (D2) antagonist and 5-HT$_4$ agonist	Delayed gastric emptying/gastroparesis (prokinetic)	10 mg t.d.s. (PO/IV)	Do not give in bowel obstruction: can cause severe colic EPSE (although rare at this dose)
Domperidone	Dopamine (D2) antagonist	Delayed gastric emptying/gastroparesis (prokinetic)	10 mg t.d.s. (PO)	EPSE rarer than with metoclopramide (reduced BBB permeability) Increased risk of serious cardiac side effects, particularly if aged >60, with higher doses, and if taking other medication that prolong the QTc or inhibit CYP3A4 [24]
Levomepromazine	Antagonist at muscarinic, histamine, 5HT$_2$ and dopamine (D2) receptors	Metabolic causes (see Box 21.1) Useful in palliative care: also has anxiolytic properties	6.25 mg b.d. initially (should not be used outside oncology and palliative care without specialist advice)	Sedation

Table 21.1 (Continued)

Drug	Mechanism	Particular indications	Dose	Side effects/cautions
Hyoscine hydrobromide	Antimuscarinic	Licensed for motion sickness, but also used (unlicensed) in treatment of clozapine-associated hypersalivation	300 μg up to t.d.s. (PO) or as transdermal patch (1.5 mg every 72 hours)	
Cinnarizine	Antihistamine	Motion sickness, vestibular disorders (e.g. Ménière's disease)	30 mg t.d.s. (PO) for vestibular disorders, 30 mg 2 hours prior to travel if motion sickness, followed by 15 mg every 8 hours as required during journey	Sedation

[a] IV, intravenous; IM, intramuscular; SC, subcutaneous; PO, by mouth.
EPSE, extrapyramidal side effects; BBB, blood–brain barrier.

Other management options

- Non-pharmacological management:
  - acupressure wrist bands
  - small snacks instead of larger meals.
- Anti-emetic therapy (see Table 21.1).
- Investigation and management of underlying causes: if malignancy is suspected (weight loss, dysphagia, anaemia), consider an urgent referral for endoscopy and gastroenterology. In absence of red flag signs/symptoms, a routine referral can be made to gastroenterology.

Anti-emetic therapy

The properties of commonly used anti-emetics are listed in Table 21.1. Anti-emetics should be given regularly for the duration of symptoms rather than on an as-required basis for best efficacy. Haloperidol and levomepromazine are used most commonly in palliative care settings but are not first-choice options for acute settings and should not be used without specialist advice. Of course, some patients with SMI may already be prescribed these drugs. Care must be taken over the risk of QTc prolongation and risk of arrhythmia, particularly if patients are taking antipsychotics, antiarrhythmics (e.g. amiodarone, flecainide), antibiotics (macrolides such as clarithromycin, erythromycin and azithromycin, or fluoroquinolones such as ciprofloxacin), antifungal medication (e.g. fluconazole), or antimalarial medication (e.g. chloroquine) [4,22].

In the SMI population, dopamine antagonists such as metoclopramide are more likely to cause acute movement disorders when used in patients already receiving antipsychotic treatment. This risk increases in the elderly. Alternatives such as cyclizine and 5-HT$_3$ antagonists (e.g. ondansetron) may be preferred, although care should be taken over avoiding constipation with ondansetron [23].

References

1. American Gastroenterological Association. American Gastroenterological Association medical position statement: nausea and vomiting. *Gastroenterology* 2001;120(1):261–263.
2. Hornby PJ. Central neurocircuitry associated with emesis. *Am J Med* 2001;111(Suppl 8A):106S–112S.
3. Metz A, Hebbard G. Nausea and vomiting in adults: a diagnostic approach. *Aust Fam Physician* 2007;36:688–692.
4. Watson M, Lucas C, Hoy A, Wells J. Gastrointestinal symptoms: nausea and vomiting. In: *Oxford Handbook of Palliative Care*, 2nd edn. Oxford: Oxford University Press, 2010:308–315.
5. Herrell HE. Nausea and vomiting of pregnancy. *Am Fam Physician* 2014;89:965–970.
6. Bollom A, Austrie J, Hirsch W, et al. Emergency department burden of nausea and vomiting associated with cannabis use disorder: US trends from 2006 to 2013. *J Clin Gastroenterol* 2018;52(9):778–783.
7. Stanghellini V, Chan FK, Hasler WL, et al. Gastroduodenal disorders. *Gastroenterology* 2016;150:1380–1392.
8. Brzana RJ, Koch KL. Gastroesophageal reflux disease presenting with intractable nausea. *Ann Intern Med* 1997;126:704–707.
9. Goldstein BJ, Goodnick PJ. Selective serotonin reuptake inhibitors in the treatment of affective disorders: III. Tolerability, safety and pharmacoeconomics. *J Psychopharmacol* 1998;12(3 Suppl B):S55–S87.
10. Haddad P. The SSRI discontinuation syndrome. *J Psychopharmacol* 1998;12:305–313.
11. Fleischhacker WW. Aripiprazole. *Expert Opin Pharmacother* 2005;6:2091–2101.
12. Scorza K, Williams A, Phillips JD, Shaw J. Evaluation of nausea and vomiting. *Am Fam Physician* 2007;76:76–84.
13. Harrington BC, Jimerson M, Haxton C, Jimerson DC. Initial evaluation, diagnosis, and treatment of anorexia nervosa and bulimia nervosa. *Am Fam Physician* 2015;91:46–52.
14. Carney CP, Andersen AE. Eating disorders. Guide to medical evaluation and complications. *Psychiatr Clin North Am* 1996;19:657–679.
15. Singh P, Yoon SS, Kuo B. Nausea: a review of pathophysiology and therapeutics. *Therap Adv Gastroenterol* 2016;9:98–112.
16. Ishigooka J, Iwashita S, Tadori Y. Efficacy and safety of brexpiprazole for the treatment of acute schizophrenia in Japan: a 6-week, randomized, double-blind, placebo-controlled study. *Psychiatry Clin Neurosci* 2018;72:692–700.
17. Campbell RH, Diduch M, Gardner KN, Thomas C. Review of cariprazine in management of psychiatric illness. *Ment Health Clin* 2017;7:221–229.
18. Holmskov M, Storebø OJ, Moreira-Maia CR, et al. Gastrointestinal adverse events during methylphenidate treatment of children and adolescents with attention deficit hyperactivity disorder: a systematic review with meta-analysis and Trial Sequential Analysis of randomised clinical trials. *PLoS One* 2017;12(6):e0178187.
19. Carpay JA, Aldenkamp AP, van Donselaar CA. Complaints associated with the use of antiepileptic drugs: results from a community-based study. *Seizure* 2005;14:198–206.
20. Mackay FJ, Wilton LV, Pearce GL, et al. Safety of long-term lamotrigine in epilepsy. *Epilepsia* 1997;38:881–886.
21. Schou M, Baastrup PC, Grof P, et al. Pharmacological and clinical problems of lithium prophylaxis. *Br J Psychiatry J Ment Sci* 1970;116:615–619.
22. Goldstein EJC, Owens RC, Nolin TD. Antimicrobial-associated QT interval prolongation: pointes of interest. *Clin Infect Dis* 2006;43:1603–1611.
23. Howard LM, Barley EA, Davies E, et al. Cancer diagnosis in people with severe mental illness: practical and ethical issues. *Lancet Oncol* 2010;11(8):797–804.
24. Medicines and Healthcare Products Regulatory Agency. Domperidone: risks of cardiac side effects. https://www.gov.uk/drug-safety-update/domperidone-risks-of-cardiac-side-effects (accessed 30 March 2019).

Chapter 22

Dysphagia
Mary Denholm, Jason Dunn

Dysphagia is defined as the subjective sensation of difficulty or abnormality in swallowing. Odynophagia is defined as pain or discomfort on swallowing. Dysphagia is commonly subdivided into oropharyngeal dysphagia and oesophageal dysphagia [1]. Oropharyngeal dysphagia is characterised by difficulty initiating a swallowing action and with passage of food through the mouth or throat. Oesophageal dysphagia describes difficulty in movement of food or liquid down the oesophagus. Oesophageal dysphagia is the more common of the two, and accounts for most cases in the adult population. A comprehensive history has been shown to be able to differentiate between the two types in 80–85% of cases [2]. Dysphagia is common, with an estimated prevalence in adult populations of approximately 3% [3]. Dysphagia can be a 'red flag' for malignancy, and persistent dysphagia in almost all cases will require prompt assessment and referral for further investigation.

CAUSES OF DYSPHAGIA IN THE GENERAL POPULATION

Box 22.1 provides a list of non-acute causes of oropharyngeal and oesophageal dysphagia. Both types of dysphagia can coexist in some neurological conditions including Parkinson's disease and myotonic dystrophy, and in acute conditions including *Candida* infection. An acute presentation with sudden dysphagia and inability to swallow solids, liquids or, in some cases, even saliva suggests the presence of a foreign body in the oesophagus, usually a food bolus [4]. This requires immediate attention and referral to an acute hospital.

The Maudsley Practice Guidelines for Physical Health Conditions in Psychiatry, First Edition.
David M. Taylor, Fiona Gaughran, and Toby Pillinger.
© 2021 John Wiley & Sons Ltd. Published 2021 by John Wiley & Sons Ltd.

Box 22.1 Common causes of oropharyngeal and oesophageal dysphagia [5,6]

Oropharyngeal dysphagia

Neuromuscular disturbance
   Central nervous system, e.g. stroke, motor neurone disease or multiple sclerosis (bulbar palsy),
      cranial nerve deficits
   Myasthenia gravis, oculopharyngeal muscular dystrophy
   Drug induced (see Box 22.2)
Thyromegaly/goitre
Lymphadenopathy
Infection
Cancer of the head and neck
Strictures post surgery or radiotherapy
Eosinophilic oesophagitis
Cervical osteophytes

Oesophageal dysphagia

Peptic stricture (benign)
Oesophageal cancer
Oesophageal webs and rings
Eosinophilic oesophagitis
Achalasia
Spastic motility disorders
Iatrogenic strictures, e.g. post surgery or radiotherapy
Scleroderma
Functional dysphagia, e.g. globus (diagnosis of exclusion)

Rarer causes

Lymphocytic oesophagitis
Oesophageal involvement from Crohn's disease
Caustic injury from artificial substances

Additional causes of dysphagia in patients with serious mental illness

Adults with serious mental illness (SMI) have higher rates of dysphagia and are considered especially vulnerable to its complications, including asphyxiation and aspiration. This relates particularly to oropharyngeal dysphagia, with one study showing rates of up to 35% in an SMI cohort compared with 6% in the general population [7]. Box 22.2 summarises factors predisposing patients with SMI to dysphagia.

DIAGNOSTIC PRINCIPLES

History [5]

- Is the onset of symptoms sudden or progressive?
- Is there difficulty swallowing solids, liquids or both? Did the symptoms start with solids then progress to liquids?

> **Box 22.2** Additional causes of dysphagia in patients with serious mental illness [7,8]
>
> **Medication**
>
> - Antipsychotics
>   - May affect the oral and pharyngeal phases of swallowing
>   - Acute dystonia
>   - Anticholinergic side effects, e.g. dry mouth (see Chapter 26)
> - Benzodiazepines
> - Anti-seizure medication
>
> **Extrapyramidal symptoms**
>
> - Drug-induced
> - Disease-related, e.g. Parkinson's disease
>
> **Poor chewing skills and concentration in dementia patients**

- Is there pain on swallowing?
- Are the symptoms constant or intermittent?
- Can the patient initiate and complete the swallowing action? Do they repeat the swallowing action numerous times trying to initiate it?
- Is there a previous history of acid reflux, dyspepsia, or Barrett's oesophagus?
- Is there a history of atopy (associated with eosinophilic oesophagitis)?
- Has there been associated weight loss?
- Has there been any recent change in bowel habit or melaena?
- Has there been any previous oesophageal treatment/intervention?
- Have there been episodes of coughing/choking, or nasal regurgitation?
- Has the patient had recurrent lower respiratory tract infections or pneumonia?

Key features in the history to suggest a particular cause

- Dysphagia starting with solids and progressively worsening to include softer foods and liquids is suspicious of a stricture/tumour.
- Dysphagia to both solids and liquids from the outset and which is not worsening may be more suggestive of a motility disorder.
- Accompanying chest pain/oesophageal spasm can be more suggestive of a motility disorder (but oesophageal spasm as a cause for acute chest pain must be a diagnosis of exclusion to avoid missing acute cardiac events and other serious causes).
- Patients with peptic (benign) strictures frequently have a long pre-existing history of acid reflux symptoms, and usually do not exhibit weight loss.
- History of acid reflux or Barrett's oesophagus is a risk factor for development of oesophageal cancer.
- History of smoking and excess alcohol use are risk factors for oesophageal cancer.
- Dysphagia that is intermittent and associated with instances of food impaction may indicate eosinophilic oesophagitis.

CHAPTER 22

Examination

- Halitosis: may suggest long-standing obstruction.
- Evidence of recent weight loss.
- Oral *Candida* infection.
- Lymphadenopathy: cervical and supraclavicular nodes in particular.
- Umbilical nodule (Sister Mary Joseph nodule): underlying gastrointestinal malignancy.
- Neurological examination including cranial nerves: look for diplopia, ptosis, dysarthria.
- Features of Parkinson's disease: rigidity, tremors, shuffling gait, autonomic dysfunction (e.g. postural hypotension).
- Features of systemic scleroderma: calcinosis, Raynaud's phenomenon, sclerodactyly, telangiectasia.

Investigations

- Bloods:
  - full blood count
  - haematinics, e.g. B_{12}, folate, iron studies if anaemic
  - creatinine, urea and electrolytes (including phosphate and magnesium)
  - bone profile including calcium
  - liver function tests including albumin.
- A bedside swallow test may be performed as an initial screening test [9].
- Chest X-ray may be indicated if there are concerns regarding aspiration.

Further investigations that may be undertaken in hospital

Oropharyngeal dysphagia may be investigated using video fluoroscopy. Oesophageal dysphagia may be investigated using endoscopy, barium swallow, or oesophageal manometry. CT imaging may be indicated if malignancy is suspected.

Onward referral

- Patients with acute dysphagia should be referred as an emergency to hospital for urgent assessment.
- Patients with subacute symptoms that have progressed to complete dysphagia will also require admission for alternative nutrition and hydration while diagnostic investigations are undertaken.
- New presentations of oesophageal dysphagia may warrant an urgent 'two-week wait' referral to gastroenterology to rule out malignancy, and referral should certainly be made if dysphagia is accompanied by other red flag symptoms (Box 22.3).
- If in doubt regarding the correct referral route, liaise with your local gastroenterology service.

CHAPTER 22

> **Box 22.3** Red flag features indicating urgent referral to gastroenterology
>
> - Symptom duration <4 months
> - Unexplained weight loss
> - Progression of symptoms from solids to liquids
> - Anaemia
> - Vomiting
> - Evidence of gastrointestinal bleeding: haematemesis, melaena
> - Age >50 years

Key information required for referral

- Full clinical details including comorbidities, current medication, nutritional status, degree of weight loss.
- Any recent blood results.
- Any imaging done to date.
- Functional status and ability to live independently/support required.
  - Facilitates prompt organisation of support required to attend appointments.
  - Allows specialty teams to consider further appropriate onward referrals and treatment decisions
  - All patients with a diagnosis of cancer will be discussed at a multidisciplinary team meeting and functional status is key in deciding on appropriate treatments, e.g. radical surgery/chemoradiotherapy or palliative chemotherapy in the case of metastatic disease.

MANAGEMENT

Management will depend on the cause of the dysphagia (some examples are summarised in Box 22.4) [5,10]. Where nutritional intake is compromised, dietetic review is essential as well as consideration of alternative routes of feeding if indicated and appropriate for the patient. Speech and language therapy review is a cornerstone of diagnosis and management, particularly for oropharyngeal dysphagia. In the SMI population, if psychiatric medication is felt to be contributing, consider rationalisation of treatment (reduce dose of causative agent or switch to alternative therapy). A multidisciplinary approach is recommended, involving as appropriate the psychiatrist, gastroenterology, and speech and language therapists.

OESOPHAGEAL CANCER IN PSYCHIATRIC POPULATIONS

The prognosis of oesophageal cancer remains poor for the general population, and this is potentially further exacerbated by delays to diagnosis in the SMI population. Patients with psychiatric illnesses have been shown to have delayed diagnosis of oesophageal

> **Box 22.4** Management of dysphagia
>
> **Management of oropharyngeal dysphagia**
>
> Neurological causes (e.g. Parkinson's disease): pharmacological management of underlying condition
> Neoplastic causes
>   Surgical resection
>   Chemotherapy/radiotherapy
> Aftercare of stroke, post trauma, or post treatment complications
>   Rehabilitation
>   Techniques to increase safe oral intake or alternative feeding routes if not possible
>
> **Management of oesophageal dysphagia**
>
> Oesophageal cancer
>   Surgery/radical chemoradiotherapy for localised disease amenable to resection
>   Palliative chemotherapy for metastatic disease
>   Stenting or palliative radiotherapy for local control if unsuitable for radical resection
> Peptic stricture: antacid therapy (e.g. proton pump inhibitor), soft food, dilatation of stricture
> Eosinophilic oesophagitis: oral topical steroids (budesonide oro-dispersible tablets), elimination diets (removing food from diet that may be responsible), proton pump inhibitors
> Achalasia: surgery (Heller's myotomy), per oral endoscopic myotomy (POEM), pneumatic balloon dilatation, botulinum toxin injections
> Oesophageal spasm: nitrates, calcium-channel blockers
> Infection: treatment of underlying infection, e.g. *Candida*

cancer, and more advanced presentations at diagnosis, thereby limiting therapeutic options. Even in those patients presenting earlier, psychiatric illness is associated with lower rates of curative surgery [11,12].

DYSPHAGIA IN THE ELDERLY

Dysphagia in the older patient population is increasingly recognised as complex and multi-factorial, as well as producing difficult ethical situations. It is common in those with dementia, as well as other acute illnesses and conditions such as cerebrovascular disease/stroke. It is estimated that the normal ageing process can cause mild abnormalities in oesophageal motility, but these are usually insufficient to cause symptoms, and dysphagia in older patients should not be attributed to ageing alone without appropriate investigation [13]. The British Geriatrics Society recommends a multidisciplinary approach to dysphagia, and emphasises need to assess capacity [14]: decisions to commence artificial enteral feeding in this population are highly complex and should not be taken in isolation.

References

1. Liu LWC, Andrews CN, Armstrong D, et al. Clinical practice guidelines for the assessment of uninvestigated esophageal dysphagia. *J Can Assoc Gastroenterol* 2018;1:5–19.
2. Hila A, Castell DO. Upper gastrointestinal disorders. In: Hazzard WR, Blass JP, Halter JB, et al. (eds) *Principles of Geriatric Medicine and Gerontology*. New York: McGraw-Hill Professional, 2003:613–640.

3. Cho SY, Choung RS, Saito YA, et al. Prevalence and risk factors for dysphagia: a USA community study. *Neurogastroenterol Motil* 2015;27:212–219.

4. Ginsberg GG. Food bolus impaction. *Gastroenterol Hepatol* 2007;3:85–86.

5. Malagelada J-R, Bazzoli F, Boeckxstaens G, et al. World Gastroenterology Organisation Global Guidelines: dysphagia. Global guidelines and cascades update September 2014. *J Clin Gastroenterol* 2015;49:370–378.

6. Aziz Q, Fass R, Gyawali CP, et al. Functional esophageal disorders. *Gastroenterology* 2016;150(6):1368–1379.

7. Regan J, Sowman R, Walsh I. Prevalence of dysphagia in acute and community mental health settings. *Dysphagia* 2006;21:95–101.

8. Cicala G, Barbieri MA, Spina E, de Leon J. A comprehensive review of swallowing difficulties and dysphagia associated with antipsychotics in adults. *Expert Rev Clin Pharmacol* 2019;12:219–234.

9. Martino R, Silver F, Teasell R, et al. The Toronto Bedside Swallowing Screening Test (TOR-BSST): development and validation of a dysphagia screening tool for patients with stroke. *Stroke* 2009;40:555–561.

10. Sami SS, Haboubi HN, Ang Y, et al. UK guidelines on oesophageal dilatation in clinical practice. *Gut* 2018;67:1000–1023.

11. Howard LM, Barley EA, Davies E, et al. Cancer diagnosis in people with severe mental illness: practical and ethical issues. *Lancet Oncol* 2010;11:797–804.

12. O'Rourke RW, Diggs BS, Spight DH, et al. Psychiatric illness delays diagnosis of esophageal cancer. *Dis Esophagus* 2008;21:416–421.

13. Shamburek RD, Farrar JT. Disorders of the digestive system in the elderly. *N Engl J Med* 1990;322:438–443.

14. British Geriatrics Society. Dysphagia management for older people towards the end of life. Good Practice Guide, 2012. https://www.bgs.org.uk/resources/dysphagia-management-for-older-people.

CHAPTER 22

Deranged Liver Function Tests

John Lally, Aisling Considine, Kosh Agarwal

Serum parameters traditionally termed as 'liver function tests' (LFTs) include the liver enzymes alanine aminotransferase (ALT), aspartate aminotransferase (AST), alkaline phosphatase (ALP), and gamma-glutamyltransferase (GGT) alongside bilirubin and albumin. Specifically, liver enzymes with bilirubin are markers of liver injury (with ALT and AST released from damaged hepatocytes), while albumin, bilirubin, and clotting (prothrombin time, international normalised ratio) are markers of liver function. There are many causes of deranged LFTs (Box 23.1), and partly owing to the frequency with which LFTs are routinely requested, deranged LFTs are a common observation in day-to-day clinical practice [1]. Patients with serious mental illness present with a number of risk factors for liver injury, including increased rates of obesity (and therefore non-alcoholic fatty liver disease, NAFLD), alcohol abuse, viral hepatitis [2], use of potentially hepatotoxic psychiatric drugs (Box 23.2), and deliberate self-harm (e.g. paracetamol overdose) [3]. Thus, deranged LFTs will be a relatively frequent observation in psychiatric practice. This chapter provides an approach to the assessment, investigation, and management of a patient presenting with deranged LFTs. The reader is also directed to Chapters 24 and 43 for relevant information on alcohol and liver disease and on viral hepatitis, respectively.

DIAGNOSTIC PRINCIPLES

The clinical presentation of a patient with deranged LFTs will depend on the degree of liver injury and patient comorbidity. In mild cases, patients may be asymptomatic with normal clinical examination, while in severe cases patients may present with signs and symptoms of hepatic decompensation and haemodynamic instability. Severe cases should be managed as medical emergencies, potentially with early referral to a specialist hepatology provider (e.g. in cases where transplantation may be indicated). In the

The Maudsley Practice Guidelines for Physical Health Conditions in Psychiatry, First Edition.
David M. Taylor, Fiona Gaughran, and Toby Pillinger.
© 2021 John Wiley & Sons Ltd. Published 2021 by John Wiley & Sons Ltd.

Box 23.1 Causes of deranged liver function tests

Non-alcoholic fatty liver disease

Alcohol-related liver disease

Cirrhosis of any aetiology

Viral hepatitis

- Hepatitis A, B, C, D, and E
- Cytomegalovirus (CMV), Epstein–Barr virus (EBV), herpesvirus, parvoviruses, varicella zoster virus

Ischaemic hepatitis

- Systemic hypotension
- Sepsis
- Primary cardiac, circulatory, respiratory failure
- Budd–Chiari syndrome

Reversible causes

- Autoimmune hepatitis
- Haemochromatosis
- Leptospirosis, hepatic amoebiasis, malaria, rickettsial diseases

Pregnancy-specific liver diseases

- Acute fatty liver of pregnancy
- HELLP syndrome (haemolysis, elevated liver enzymes, and a low platelet count)
- Pre-eclampsia-associated liver diseases

Miscellaneous

- Primary biliary cirrhosis
- Primary sclerosing cholangitis
- Wilson's disease
- α_1-Antitrypsin deficiency
- Hypothyroidism
- Addison's disease
- Coeliac disease
- Glycogen storage diseases
- Strenuous exercise
- Skeletal muscle damage/rhabdomyolysis
- Malignancy including hepatocellular carcinoma
- Toxin related
    - Paracetamol overdose
    - Recreational drugs including methamphetamine, cocaine
    - Use of unregulated supplements/herbal remedies
    - Associated with psychiatric/physical health prescription
    - Medications associated with hepatoxicity, e.g. rifampicin, isoniazid, statins, efavirenz (see Box 23.2)
    - Alcohol

Box 23.2 Medications associated with liver injury and abnormal liver function tests [4,5]

Psychiatric medication

Antipsychotics

Clozapine, olanzapine, risperidone, quetiapine, aripiprazole, haloperidol, chlorpromazine

Antidepressants

Sertraline, paroxetine, fluoxetine, citalopram/escitalopram, fluvoxamine, venlafaxine, duloxetine, mirtazapine, agomelatine, bupropion, trazodone, imipramine, amitriptyline, iproniazid, phenelzine, moclobemide

Mood stabilisers

Carbamazepine, sodium valproate, lamotrigine, topiramate, pregabalin, lithium, benzodiazepines

Physical health medication

Antibiotics

Amoxicillin/clavulanic acid, flucloxacillin, erythromycin, ciprofloxacin, nitrofurantoin, minocycline, dapsone, doxycycline, trimethoprim

Antifungals

Ketoconazole

Antiretrovirals

Efavirenz, didanosine, abacavir

Anticonvulsants

Sodium valproate, phenytoin, carbamazepine

Analgesics

Paracetamol in doses in excess of maximum licenced daily dose for weight/age
  Non-steroidal anti-inflammatories

Anti-tuberculosis drugs

Isoniazid, rifampicin, pyrazinamide

Miscellaneous

Propylthiouracil, statins, amiodarone, baclofen, methotrexate, methyldopa, lisinopril
  Herbal medicines, in particular Chinese herbal medicines
  Khat

CHAPTER 23

non-acute setting, there may be an opportunity for the psychiatric practitioner, in combination with input from pharmacy and/or dialogue with gastroenterology, to explore the aetiology of liver dysfunction. Such an approach is described in this chapter. Where medication-induced liver injury is the most likely cause, removal of said treatment and subsequent normalisation of LFTs might avoid a referral to medical services. Even if a gastroenterology review is ultimately required, the referral will be strengthened by the history, examination, and investigations described here.

History

A history should screen for the common causes of abnormal LFTs described in Boxes 23.1 and 23.2. This will include the following.

1 History of presenting complaint:
   a Patients may present with malaise, fatigue, nausea, jaundice, abdominal pain, and pruritus.
   b Red flag symptoms of malignancy (e.g. weight loss).
   c Associated symptoms that may suggest a causative comorbidity include:
      i shortness of breath, peripheral oedema (heart failure)
      ii skin pigmentation, diabetes mellitus, arthritis (haemochromatosis)
      iii right upper quadrant pain (gallstones); cholestasis may be associated with dark urine and pale stool.
2 Past medical history:
   a pre-existing liver disease or autoimmune disorders
   b metabolic syndrome
   c inflammatory bowel disease (primary sclerosing cholangitis)
   d previous cholecystectomy.
3 Drug history:
   a recent medication changes
   b over-the-counter and herbal remedies.
4 Family history of liver or autoimmune disease.
5 Social history:
   a alcohol (see Chapter 24 for screening questions)
   b recreational drug use
   c other risk factors for viral hepatitis, e.g. tattoos or intravenous drug use (see Chapter 43)
   d exposure to potential hepatotoxins.
6 As part of a mental state examination, enquire regarding deliberate self-harm. Overdose should be managed as a medical emergency (see Chapter 83).

Examination

1 Basic observations: temperature, blood pressure, pulse, respiratory rate, and oxygen saturations.
2 Calculate body mass index (BMI).

3 On general inspection there may be evidence of chronic liver disease: finger clubbing, palmar erythema, spider naevi, telangectasia, ascites, and jaundice. If there is decompensated liver function, there may be signs of easy bruising. There may be evidence of routes of transmission such as tattoos or needle marks.
4 Hepatic encephalopathy may be accompanied by changes in mental state, e.g. fluctuating levels of consciousness, inattention, mood changes, irritability, drowsiness, lethargy, and confusion.
5 A focused abdominal examination should look for asterixis, hepatosplenomegaly, ascites, and peripheral oedema.

Investigations

A key step in the interpretation of abnormal LFTs is to consider them in the context of historical blood test results in order to determine if this is an acute or chronic presentation. The pattern of LFT derangement may provide insight into the underlying pathoaetiology. For example, a predominant increase in ALT and AST points towards hepatocellular pathology, such as a viral or toxic (drugs/alcohol) hepatitis or a cirrhosis, while a predominant increase in ALP points towards cholestatic pathology (gallstones, stricture, or malignancy). Raised bilirubin may be seen in either hepatocellular or cholestatic disease. An AST/ALT ratio above 2 is suggestive of alcoholic hepatitis, rather than other causes of hepatitis (e.g. viral). Raised GGT is a marker of recent alcohol use (24 hours to two weeks). Where LFTs are deranged, clotting should be requested to assess synthetic function. Other tests that may be requested, depending on history or examination, are as follows.

Bloods

1 Routine bloods: full blood count, renal function, C-reactive protein, HbA$_{1c}$, lipid profile.
2 Viral hepatitis screen: hepatitis B surface antigen (HBsAg), IgM anti-hepatitis B core antigen (anti-HBc), antibody to HBsAg (anti-HBs), anti-hepatitis C virus antibody (HCV), hepatitis C viral RNA.
3 Autoantibody screen:
   a antinuclear antibody/anti-smooth muscle antibody (autoimmune hepatitis)
   b anti-liver/kidney microsomal antibody (autoimmune hepatitis)
   c anti-mitochondrial antibody (primary biliary cirrhosis)
   d anti-neutrophil cytoplasmic antibodies (consider if cholestatic picture: primary sclerosing cholangitis).
4 Pregnancy test if a female of childbearing age.
5 Creatine kinase if considering a muscle disorder.
6 Toxicology screen including paracetamol (acetaminophen) level.
7 If Wilson's disease is suspected: plasma ceruloplasmin level and urinary copper quantitation.
8 If haemochromatosis is suspected: iron studies.
9 If hepatocellular carcinoma suspected: alpha-fetoprotein.

CHAPTER 23

Imaging

Abdominal ultrasound should be used to image the liver (masses, cirrhosis, or fatty liver) and biliary tract (obstruction), with Doppler imaging for vascular occlusion (Budd–Chiari syndrome). Liver biopsy may be considered if the diagnosis remains unclear after these tests, or to assess the degree of liver damage.

MANAGEMENT

Abnormal LFTs do not always indicate hepatitis or liver disease, and therefore may not require specific management. In members of the general population with abnormal LFTs, defined as ALT twice the upper limit of normal (ULN), one-third of males and one-quarter of females had no identifiable cause [6]. Furthermore, 20% of healthy volunteers treated with placebo in clinical trials have ALT increases of between one and three times ULN [7], and 12% of the general population have one abnormal LFT measure [8]. When assessing abnormal LFTs it is important to consider the clinical context in which they have occurred and the pattern and degree of increase. If the increase in ALT/AST is less than three times ULN, and if the patient has evidence of obesity and/or the metabolic syndrome and no other clear risk factors for liver disease, then a diagnosis of NAFLD is likely [9]. Lifestyle advice should be offered, with recommendations to reduce or discontinue alcohol use. Increased exercise and dietary changes to aid weight loss are recommended (see Chapter 14). LFTs should then be rechecked two to three months later. Increases in ALT/AST of more than three times ULN or raised ALP should prompt assessment for other causes, including a blood and imaging liver screen as described. When in doubt, discuss the case with general medical/gastroenterology colleagues. Management will then depend on the underlying cause.

Drug-induced liver injury

A number of drugs can cause LFT derangements. In the psychiatric patient population, psychotropic medications are potentially responsible, and rationalising pharmacotherapy may be required. Up to one-third of people treated with antipsychotic medications have one or more abnormal LFTs recorded, and 4% have at least one LFT of more than three times ULN [4]. The time to onset of LFT changes after starting antipsychotic medications is generally short, with the majority occurring within one to six weeks [4,10]. However, antipsychotic-induced liver injury is generally mild and transient [4], so stopping treatment is not always necessary. Clozapine is one of the psychotropic agents more frequently associated with abnormal LFTs. The median rate of clozapine-associated hepatitis (defined as ALT more than twice ULN) is 17%, although for most patients this does not result in progression to severe liver injury [4], and LFTs will normalise in up to 60% of cases with continued treatment [11]. Hepatotoxicity is associated with all antidepressants and is more common in the elderly and with polypharmacy. Antidepressants are associated with mild transient increases in transaminases in 0.5–3% of patients treated [5]. Clinically significant liver impairment or damage is however rare.

Most episodes of drug-induced hepatitis are benign and improve following discontinuation of the offending agent. Medications such as paracetamol cause a predictable dose-dependent liver toxicity. However, antipsychotic and other psychotropic medication-induced hepatitis are idiosyncratic reactions, being unpredictable and not dose dependent. Risk factors for drug-induced hepatitis include older age, female gender, alcohol use, NAFLD, obesity, and pre-existing liver disease. Although a transient and mild transaminitis may be seen with many antipsychotics and antidepressants, it is important to recognise progressive drug-induced hepatitis to allow for the withdrawal of the medication and prevent progression to liver failure. As a guide, if serum ALT or AST is more than three times ULN, and serum total bilirubin is elevated to more than twice ULN [12] and there is a likely drug cause, then consider discontinuing the treatment. If ALT is increased more than five times ULN, then immediate discontinuation is indicated [13]. If ALT was already raised at baseline, then increases in ALT more than three times the baseline level should prompt consideration of discontinuing treatment. However, this is only a guide, and any decision should balance the risk of continuing treatment (progressive and potentially irreversible liver damage) against the risk of stopping treatment (deterioration in mental state). A multidisciplinary team (MDT) approach involving the patient is recommended. A similar MDT approach is recommended if re-challenge of a potentially causative agent is being considered.

Some patients with drug-induced liver injury may present with a more severe clinical picture, with features of systemic hypersensitivity, fever, raised inflammatory markers, eosinophilia, and cutaneous or multiorgan involvement. The patient should be transferred to the care of medical colleagues. Management involves discontinuation of the medication and supportive management (i.e. there are no specific treatments for psychotropic-induced hepatitis/liver failure). Monitoring of transaminases, bilirubin, and clotting should be initiated and continued until markers stabilise. Patients should be monitored for emerging clinical features of liver dysfunction, haemodynamic instability, or encephalopathy.

References

1. Pratt DS, Kaplan MM. Evaluation of abnormal liver-enzyme results in asymptomatic patients. *N Engl J Med* 2000;342(17):1266–1271.

2. Hughes E, Bassi S, Gilbody S, et al. Prevalence of HIV, hepatitis B, and hepatitis C in people with severe mental illness: a systematic review and meta-analysis. *Lancet Psychiatry* 2016;3(1):40–48.

3. David S, Hamilton JP. Drug-induced liver injury. *US Gastroenterol Hepatol Rev* 2010;6:73–80.

4. Marwick KF, Taylor M, Walker SW. Antipsychotics and abnormal liver function tests: systematic review. *Clin Neuropharmacol* 2012;35(5):244–253.

5. Voican CS, Corruble E, Naveau S, Perlemuter G. Antidepressant-induced liver injury: a review for clinicians. *Am J Psychiatry* 2014;171(4):404–415.

6. Ruhl CE, Everhart JE. Upper limits of normal for alanine aminotransferase activity in the United States population. *Hepatology* 2012;55(2):447–454.

7. Rosenzweig P, Miget N, Brohier S. Transaminase elevation on placebo during phase I trials: prevalence and significance. *Br J Clin Pharmacol* 1999;48(1):19–23.

8. Rosalki SB, Dooley JS. Liver function profiles and their interpretation. *Br J Hosp Med* 1994;51(4):181–186.

9. Chalasani N, Younossi Z, Lavine JE, et al. The diagnosis and management of nonalcoholic fatty liver disease: practice guidance from the American Association for the Study of Liver Diseases. *Hepatology* 2018;67(1):328–357.

10. Lally J, Al Kalbani H, Krivoy A, et al. Hepatitis, interstitial nephritis, and pancreatitis in association with clozapine treatment: a systematic review of case series and reports. *J Clin Psychopharmacol* 2018;38(5):520–527.

11. Hummer M, Kurz M, Kurzthaler I, et al. Hepatotoxicity of clozapine. *J Clin Psychopharmacol* 1997;17(4):314–317.

12. Chalasani NP, Hayashi PH, Bonkovsky HL, et al. ACG Clinical Guideline: the diagnosis and management of idiosyncratic drug-induced liver injury. *Am J Gastroenterol* 2014;109(7):950–966; quiz 967.

13. Aithal GP, Watkins PB, Andrade RJ, et al. Case definition and phenotype standardization in drug-induced liver injury. *Clin Pharmacol Ther* 2011;89(6):806–815.

CHAPTER 23

Alcohol and Physical Health

Musa Sami, Joseph Cooney, Michael Heneghan

Alcohol (ethanol) is the most commonly used drug in the world [1]. For most people who consume it, alcohol causes little or no harm. However, alcohol is a toxin with the potential to damage multiple organ systems.

WHAT IS HARMFUL USE?

There is no global consensus on recommended maximum intake (or safe limits) of alcohol. In the UK, alcohol units can be quantified by multiplying volume (litres) by percentage alcohol concentration. A glass of red wine (175 mL, 12% alcohol) constitutes $0.175 \times 12 = 2.1$ units and a bottle of vodka (700 mL, 37.5%) $0.7 \times 37.5 = 26.25$ units. In the UK, current safe recommended intakes are less than 14 units of alcohol per week for both men and women [2].

Harmful use is that which causes damage to physical or mental health. Alcohol dependence is characterised by inability to control use (*compulsion*), priority given to drinking over other substances (*salience*), and *persistence* of use despite negative consequences. *Craving* and physical *tolerance* (needing increasing amounts to get the same effect) and *withdrawal* symptoms (tremor, tachycardia, sweats, anxiety, and nausea on cessation or reduction of use) may also be present. Alcohol use disorder refers to both harmful use and dependence. The terms 'alcoholic' and 'alcoholism' are used colloquially, but they do not adequately distinguish between harmful use and dependence, can be stigmatising, and are best avoided by health professionals.

In pregnancy, alcohol crosses the placenta and there is a risk of fetal alcohol spectrum disorders (an umbrella term encompassing a spectrum of disorders that includes decreased IQ, distinctive facies, and attentional and behavioural difficulties). Pregnant women and those planning pregnancies should be advised there is no safe minimum level of alcohol intake and to minimise consumption (see Chapter 62) [2].

The Maudsley Practice Guidelines for Physical Health Conditions in Psychiatry, First Edition.
David M. Taylor, Fiona Gaughran, and Toby Pillinger.
© 2021 John Wiley & Sons Ltd. Published 2021 by John Wiley & Sons Ltd.

PHYSICAL COMPLICATIONS OF ALCOHOL USE

Acute presentations

These will require immediate referral to emergency services.

- *Delirium tremens*: a severe form of alcohol withdrawal that usually occurs two to three days after alcohol cessation, characterised by severe tremor, perspiration, fever, and tachycardia. Can be associated with dramatic florid or bizarre visual/tactile hallucinations. Occasionally, hallucinations are predominant and physical signs less apparent, so the patient may present on a psychiatric ward before diagnosis is made. Main risks are of dehydration from increased perspiration or alcohol withdrawal seizures. Manage in a medical unit with a benzodiazepine detoxification regimen, fluids, and vitamin replacement (thiamine).
- *Alcohol withdrawal seizures.*
- *Gastrointestinal bleeding*: cirrhosis leads to portal venous hypertension and oesophageal/gastric varices which may bleed (see Chapter 20). Often presents as haematemesis (vomiting fresh red blood), 'coffee ground' vomiting, or melaena (black tarry stool indicating partially digested blood from stomach). Less severe is a Mallory–Weis tear of the mucous membrane of the upper gastrointestinal tract caused by vomiting often secondary to alcohol ingestion. Alcohol can also be associated with gastric ulcers (erosion in membrane of stomach; see Chapter 19).
- *Pancreatitis*: acutely presents with severe abdominal pain radiating to the back, often precipitated by an alcohol binge (see Chapter 88). Additional features include fever, tachycardia, and nausea. Raised serum amylase/lipase is diagnostic (although amylase levels may be blunted in chronic pancreatitis). Can be life-threatening, requiring supportive care and fluid resuscitation. Manage in hospital acutely. Surgical intervention may be required for debridement of peripancreatic necrosis.
- *Hepatic encephalopathy.*
- *Spontaneous bacterial peritonitis*: acute bacterial infection of ascitic fluid.
- *Others*: severe alcohol intoxication (ethanol poisoning) can cause respiratory and central nervous depression. Surrogate alcohols (e.g. hand sanitiser, mouthwash) are sometimes consumed in the absence of commercially available alcohol, and owing to their especially high alcohol concentrations are particularly dangerous. Other substitutes such as antifreeze can cause methanol poisoning, presenting with abdominal pain, alterations in consciousness, and retinal toxicity.

Chronic presentations

These will merit outpatient referral for physician assessment (in the UK, usually via a general practitioner).

- *Alcoholic liver disease*: alcohol is one of the most common causes of chronic liver disease (the others being non-alcoholic fatty liver disease, NAFLD), viral hepatitis, autoimmune hepatitis, and idiopathic causes (see Chapters 23 and 43). There is a wide range of damage alcohol can cause to the liver, including inflammation, fibrosis, and cirrhosis. Severe alcohol damage can lead to portal venous hypertension and decompensation in liver synthetic function, including decreased plasma proteins and impaired clotting. End-stage liver disease may lead to hepatic encephalopathy, a picture of chronic confusion sometimes associated with asterixis (coarse shaking of the hands when the wrist is extended).

- *Cardiac disease*: there are a range of cardiac complications including arrhythmias (particularly atrial fibrillation, atrial flutter, and ventricular tachyarrhythmias; see Chapter 1). Alcoholic cardiomyopathy can present with dilation of heart muscle secondary to heavy chronic alcohol ingestion leading to heart failure (see Chapter 7). Alcohol is a risk factor for cardiovascular disease, synergistic with other risk factors (including smoking, obesity, hypertension, and increased cholesterol; see Chapters 5, 9, 14, and 46 for details of all these presentations).
- *Immune dysfunction*: alcohol is associated with bone marrow suppression and alteration in cytokine expression [3]. This may lead to immunosuppression and predispose to infections. Alcohol abuse is associated with increased risk of pneumonia (consider tuberculosis or mycobacterial infection if chronic and there is evidence of poor nutrition and accommodation; see Chapters 39 and 44), cellulitis (particularly if peripheral neuropathy and poor self-care), and spontaneous bacterial peritonitis in association with ascites.
- *Neurotoxicity*: alcohol has a plethora of neurotoxic effects. Central nervous system effects include global atrophic changes, frontal degeneration and change in personality, chronic subdural haemorrhage, Wernicke–Korsakoff syndrome (thiamine deficiency leading to triad of confusion, ataxia, and ophthalmoplegia), cerebellar degeneration (slurred speech, nystagmus, ataxia, hypotonia, intention tremor), reduction in seizure threshold, and withdrawal seizures. Hepatic encephalopathy may occur secondary to chronic liver disease. Peripherally, alcohol can cause a symmetrical distal peripheral neuropathy.
- *Cancer*: heavy alcohol intake is associated with increased risk of cancers of the mouth, pharynx, larynx, oesophagus, breast, bowel, and liver [4].

APPROACH TO THE PATIENT WITH SUSPECTED ALCOHOL MISUSE

A brief assessment of problematic alcohol use can be undertaken by using the CAGE questionnaire, which is a series of four yes/no questions.

1 Have you ever felt you needed to Cut down on your drinking?
2 Have people Annoyed you by criticising your drinking?
3 Have you ever felt Guilty about drinking?
4 Have you ever felt you needed a drink first thing in the morning (Eye-opener) to steady your nerves or to get rid of a hangover?

Two 'yes' answers indicates problematic alcohol use and should be investigated further.

CHAPTER 24

Further freely available validated questionnaires include the following.

- Alcohol Use Disorders Identification Test (AUDIT): provides a more detailed measure over the previous year with a score of 8/40 or above indicating harmful use [5].
- Severity of Alcohol Drinking Questionnaire (SADQ): rates the severity of dependence [6].
- Clinical Institute Withdrawal Assessment of Alcohol Scale, Revised (CIWA-Ar): assesses for presence of withdrawal symptoms (nausea/vomiting, tremor, sweating, anxiety, tactile/auditory/visual disturbances, headache, disorientation) and rates their severity [7,8].

History

Quantify the amount the individual is currently drinking. Enquiring about the daily pattern of drinking can be useful ('Tell me how much you drink on a typical day...'). Establish harmful use and dependence criteria ('Who has control – you or the drink?'). If appropriate, quantify severity of withdrawal using the CIWA-Ar. Ask about any comorbid cardiac or liver conditions that can exacerbate comorbid pathology (e.g. hepatitis B and C, NAFLD). Ask about the presence of risk factors for cardiovascular disease (obesity, raised cholesterol, hypertension). Enquire about smoking status and use of illicit drugs.

Physical examination

Examine for evidence of the following.

- Alcohol misuse: signs of alcohol intoxication or withdrawal, including tremor, smell of alcohol, Dupuytren's contracture.
- Evidence of organ disease:
  - Liver: clubbing, pallor, cachexia, unsteadiness, telangiectasia, jaundice, spider naevi, hepatomegaly, ascites.
  - Cardiac: displaced apex beat, heaves and thrills, anaemia.
- Evidence of decompensated hepatic function: signs of easy bruising, signs of low body albumin such as pitting oedema and ascites, splenomegaly, and caput medusae.

If there is evidence of chronic liver disease, ensure that the patient is referred to general medical services.

In cases of acute bleeding (haematemesis or malaena), measure blood pressure (noting for hypotension and a postural drop) and heart rate and oxygen saturations if available (see Chapter 20), resuscitate as necessary using the ABCDE approach, and ensure the patient is referred as an emergency to medical services.

Liver failure can be associated with hypoglycaemia, and therefore regular blood sugar monitoring may be required (symptoms of hypoglycaemia include suddenly feeling trembly, increased anxiety, irritability, hunger, and blurring of vision), with treatment as necessary (see Chapter 74).

Investigations

Blood tests

1 Full blood count to check for anaemia, low platelets, and neutropenia. Raised mean corpuscular volume (MCV) is a marker of chronic alcohol use (more than three months).
2 Haematinic studies (iron deficiency anaemia may indicate chronic gastrointestinal bleeding).
3 Urea and electrolytes.
4 Liver function tests including aspartate aminotransferase (AST) and alanine aminotransferase (ALT): an AST/ALT ratio >2 is suggestive of alcoholic hepatitis, rather than other causes of hepatitis (e.g. viral). Raised gamma-glutamyltransferase (GGT) is a marker of recent alcohol use (24 hours to two weeks).
5 Increased international normalised ratio (INR) and low albumin are tests of synthetic liver function and can help define the degree of hepatic failure.
6 C-reactive protein (CRP) if infection suspected.
7 Serum amylase or lipase if suspected pancreatitis (amylase can normalise in chronic pancreatitis). Testing for urine amylase may be useful in delayed presentations (hyperamylasuria occurs two to three days after an elevated serum level).
8 Serum ammonia if hepatic encephalopathy is a differential (liaise with laboratory before collection and deliver on ice).

Electrocardiogram

May show atrial fibrillation or flutter, evidence of cardiomyopathy (bizarre QRS complexes), or other arrhythmias. In case of an abnormal ECG, confirm haemodynamic stability and refer to general medical colleagues as appropriate.

Breathalyser

This is useful in detoxification settings. Wait until blood alcohol levels are in safe limits before commencing detoxification.

Urine drug sampling

May be useful in determining use of other drugs.

CHAPTER 24

Specialist investigations

Other tests often undertaken by general medical doctors include abdominal ultrasound (to quantify the degree of cirrhosis, for evidence of ascites, and for evidence of portal venous hypertension such as splenomegaly). A needle aspiration can help determine the cause of ascites: a serum ascites albumin gradient in excess of 11 g/L is indicative of ascites secondary to portal hypertension [9]. Antibiotic prophylaxis should be offered alongside needle aspiration if the patient has a history of hepatic encephalopathy or spontaneous bacterial peritonitis (please refer to local guidelines).

Gastroenterologists and surgeons may undertake gastroscopy to investigate and treat gastrointestinal bleeding. Imaging of the brain with either CT or MRI may be required to rule out subdural haemorrhage. MRI may show evidence of Wernicke–Korsakoff syndrome with mammillary body and thalamic hyperintensities.

If dilated cardiomyopathy secondary to alcohol use is suspected, an echocardiogram can help diagnose and quantify the extent of heart failure.

MANAGEMENT

Patients with alcohol misuse are at high risk of physical health complications. There should be a low threshold for seeking help from general medical colleagues.

Refer patients to emergency services in the following instances: signs of haemodynamic instability (low blood pressure, high pulse rate, low oxygen saturations), vomiting of blood or melaena, sudden change of consciousness or evidence of hepatic encephalopathy (confusion, obtundation, tremor), severe acute abdominal pain, seizures, evidence of sepsis, evidence of developing Wernicke–Korsakoff syndrome (confusion, ophthalmoplegia, ataxia), acute pancreatitis (generally managed conservatively but may require surgical intervention), severe alcohol withdrawal, or delirium tremens that cannot be safely managed in the psychiatric setting.

If there is evidence of chronic organ damage such as ascites on physical examination, anaemia without frank bleeding, unexplained lethargy or weight loss, or abnormal ECG, seek advice from general medical colleagues and arrange for an outpatient referral to gastroenterology.

Detoxification

Detoxification (when appropriate) is undertaken with long-acting benzodiazepine substitution therapy such as chlordiazepoxide or diazepam reduced over 5–14 days depending on setting, combined with parenteral thiamine (see section Nutrition). Dose and regimen are titrated to severity and can be fixed dose or symptom triggered as appropriate to knowledge and skills of your unit. Examples of fixed-dose regimens for moderate (SADQ score 16–30) and severe (SADQ score >30) alcohol dependence are respectively provided in Tables 24.1 and 24.2 as a guide. These example regimens are not intended to be prescriptive, and regimens should be tailored to the individual patient. Symptom-triggered therapy is generally used in patients without a history of

Table 24.1 Moderate alcohol dependence: example of fixed-dose chlordiazepoxide treatment regimen.

		Total daily dose (mg)
Day 1	20 mg q.d.s.	80
Day 2	15 mg q.d.s.	60
Day 3	10 mg q.d.s.	40
Day 4	5 mg q.d.s.	20
Day 5	5 mg b.d.	10

Table 24.2 Severe alcohol dependence: example of fixed-dose chlordiazepoxide treatment regimen.

		Total daily dose (mg)
Day 1	40 mg q.d.s. + 40 mg p.r.n.	200
Day 2	40 mg q.d.s.	160
Day 3	30 mg q.d.s.	120
Day 4	25 mg q.d.s.	100
Day 5	20 mg q.d.s.	80
Day 6	15 mg q.d.s.	60
Day 7	10 mg q.d.s.	40
Day 8	10 mg t.d.s.	30
Day 9	5 mg q.d.s.	20
Day 10	10 mg nocte	10

complications and should only be carried out by staff with experience of its delivery. In all detoxification regimens, monitor for signs of over-sedation, ataxia, and signs of undertreatment (i.e. withdrawal). Daily doses can be adjusted accordingly.

Nutrition

Input from dieticians may be required to support the nutritional needs of patients with advanced liver disease. Heavy alcohol use is associated with depletion of thiamine (vitamin B_1) and Wernicke–Korsakoff syndrome. Those with a history of heavy alcohol use should be prescribed prophylactic oral thiamine replacement therapy (300 mg daily). In detoxification settings, individuals with severe alcohol dependence (SADQ score >30 or alcohol consumption >30 units/day) and/or evidence of malnutrition should be prescribed parenteral (intramuscular or intravenous) thiamine as vitamin replacement due to inadequate enteral absorption of thiamine. Standard parenteral regimen is one pair

CHAPTER 24

of Pabrinex IMHP daily (containing thamine 250 mg/dose) for five days, followed by oral thiamine and/or vitamin B compound for as long as required (where diet is inadequate or alcohol consumption is resumed) [10]. Where parenteral thiamine is used, facilities for treating anaphylaxis should be available. If Wernicke's encephalopathy is suspected, the patient should be transferred to a medical unit where intravenous thiamine can be administered (at least two pairs of Pabrinex IVHP, i.e. four ampoules) three times daily for three to five days followed by one pair of ampoules once daily for a further three to five days, or longer (until no further response is seen) [10]. Patients with encephalopathy should be prescribed laxatives, aiming to achieve bowels opening three to four times daily (example prescription: lactulose 10 mL four times daily).

Relapse prevention

Acamprosate and supervised disulfiram are licensed in the UK for the treatment of alcohol dependence and may be offered in combination with psychosocial treatment [11]. Treatment should be initiated by specialist services. Naltrexone is also recommended as an adjunct in the treatment of moderate and severe alcohol dependence [11]. Further details are provided in the *Maudsley Prescribing Guidelines in Psychiatry* [12].

Liver transplant

In the UK, approximately 600–800 people receive liver transplants every year, with alcohol-related liver disease the most common precipitant [13]. Patients generally need to have demonstrated abstinence from alcohol for six months prior to the operation.

References

1. National Institute on Drug Abuse. Commonly used drugs charts. https://www.drugabuse.gov/drugs-abuse/commonly-abused-drugs-charts (accessed 5 May 2019).
2. UK Chief Medical Officers. UK Chief Medical Officers' low risk drinking guidelines. https://www.gov.uk/government/publications/alcohol-consumption-advice-on-low-risk-drinking (accessed 5 May 2019).
3. Cook RT. Alcohol abuse, alcoholism, and damage to the immune system: a review. *Alcohol Clin Exp Res* 1998;22(9):1927–1942.
4. Bagnardi V, Rota M, Botteri E, et al. Alcohol consumption and site-specific cancer risk: a comprehensive dose-response meta-analysis. *Br J Cancer* 2015;112(3):580–593.
5. World Health Organization. Alcohol Use Disorders Identification Test (AUDIT). https://www.drugabuse.gov/sites/default/files/files/AUDIT.pdf (accessed 5 May 2019).
6. SMART. Severity of Alcohol Dependence Questionaire (SADQ-C). https://www.smartcjs.org.uk/wp-content/uploads/2015/07/SADQ.pdf (accessed 5 May 2019).
7. Sullivan JT, Sykora K, Schneiderman J, et al. Assessment of alcohol withdrawal: the revised clinical institute withdrawal assessment for alcohol scale (CIWA-Ar). *Br J Addict* 1989;84(11):1353–1357.
8. Clinical Institute Withdrawal Assessment of Alcohol Scale, Revised (CIWA-Ar). https://umem.org/files/uploads/1104212257_CIWA-Ar.pdf (accessed 5 May 2019).
9. Runyon BA, Montano AA, Akriviadis EA, et al. The serum–ascites albumin gradient is superior to the exudate–transudate concept in the differential-diagnosis of ascites. *Ann Intern Med* 1992;117(3):215–220.
10. Lingford-Hughes AR, Welch S, Peters L, et al. BAP updated guidelines: evidence-based guidelines for the pharmacological management of substance abuse, harmful use, addiction and comorbidity: recommendations from BAP. *J Psychopharmacol* 2012;26(7):899–952.
11. National Institute for Health and Care Excellence. *Alcohol-use Disorders: Diagnosis, Assessment and Management of Harmful Drinking and Alcohol Dependence.* Clinical Guideline CG115. London: NICE, 2011. https://www.nice.org.uk/guidance/cg115 (accessed 5 May 2019).
12. Taylor DM, Barnes TRE, Young AH. *The Maudsley Prescribing Guidelines in Psychiatry*, 13th edn. Chichester: Wiley Blackwell, 2018.
13. National Health Service. Transplant Activity Report 2017–18. https://www.organdonation.nhs.uk/helping-you-to-decide/about-organ-donation/statistics-about-organ-donation/transplant-activity-report/ (accessed 5 May 2019).

Unintentional Weight Loss

Mary Denholm, John O'Donohue

Clinically significant weight loss is defined as loss of more than 5% of a patient's baseline body weight over a period of 6–12 months [1]. Unintentional weight loss that is progressive may be a sign of either significant physical or mental illness [2]. Unintentional weight loss is often associated with specific conditions (Box 25.1), but is also a general feature of ageing [3]. Weight loss is an important prognostic indicator of increased mortality in both the general population [4] and certain patient groups, for example people with chronic cardiorespiratory disease or nursing home residents [5]. A malignant cause of unexplained weight loss is found in 15–37% of patients [6,7]. Many serious illnesses are associated with the syndrome of *cachexia*, featuring a loss of muscle mass sometimes accompanied by a loss of adipose tissue, combined with a systemic inflammatory response [8]. For example, cancer cachexia, pulmonary cachexia, and cardiac cachexia are all well-recognised syndromes [9,10]. In older patients, loss of muscle mass may lead to the syndrome of *sarcopenia*, also associated with weight loss. This is characterised by loss of muscle mass and strength with consequent reductions in functional ability/performance. It can be an important contributing factor to falls in this population [11].

In addition to eating disorders, individuals with other serious mental illness (SMI) may be at increased risk of weight loss and malnutrition, particularly if requiring inpatient care [12] and in those with coexisting substance abuse [13]. This has associated implications for physical health and increased mortality risk [14]. This risk is particularly pronounced in older patients [15]. Indeed, patients with dementia treated with acetylcholinesterase inhibitors are at increased risk of weight loss, over and above being a vulnerable population at baseline [16]. Unintentional weight loss may also be observed in patients who discontinue long-term treatment with antipsychotics (e.g. chlorpromazine and haloperidol) [17]. Significant life events including bereavement can also cause weight loss alongside psychological symptoms [18]. Weight loss is common in cancer

The Maudsley Practice Guidelines for Physical Health Conditions in Psychiatry, First Edition.
David M. Taylor, Fiona Gaughran, and Toby Pillinger.
© 2021 John Wiley & Sons Ltd. Published 2021 by John Wiley & Sons Ltd.

Box 25.1 Common causes of weight loss in the general and psychiatric patient population

Gastrointestinal disease

- Malabsorption (e.g. coeliac disease, pancreatic insufficiency)
- Inflammatory bowel disease (e.g. Crohn's disease, ulcerative colitis)
- Peptic ulcer disease

Malignancy

- Haematological malignancy (e.g. lymphoma, leukaemia)
- Solid tumours, particularly gastrointestinal and lung cancers

Endocrine causes

- Hyperthyroidism
- Diabetes mellitus: acute presentation of type 1 diabetes (weight gain a more common presenting feature for type 2), incorrect use of/omitting insulin treatment
- Adrenal causes: primary adrenal insufficiency (e.g. Addison's disease)

Chronic systemic disease

- Chronic cardiac disease (e.g. heart failure)
- Chronic lung disease (e.g. chronic obstructive pulmonary disease)
- Chronic/end-stage renal failure

Rheumatological/connective tissue diseases

- Rheumatoid arthritis
- Giant cell arteritis

Infection

- HIV
- Tuberculosis: can be a sign of active disease or reactivation of previous disease
- Hepatitis B and C
- Parasitic/helminth infections

Neurological disease

- Dementia
- Stroke
- Parkinson's disease/Lewy body dementia (impaired cognition and physical factors, e.g. dysphagia)

Psychiatric conditions

- Depression (particularly in the elderly/nursing home residents)
- Anxiety
- Eating disorders (weight loss distinguished as being intentional)
- As part of clinical spectrum of altered behaviours in serious mental illness

Medication

- Thyroxine replacement for hypothyroidism
- Anti-seizure medications (e.g. topiramate)
- GLP-1 agonists (e.g. exenatide) used in management of diabetes
- Acetylcholinesterase inhibitors used in the treatment of dementia (e.g. donepezil, galantamine, rivastigmine)
- Over-the-counter remedies (e.g. St John's Wort)

Substance abuse

- Alcohol
- Recreational drugs (e.g. cocaine, amphetamines, cannabis)
- Tobacco

patients at presentation [19,20]. Cancer diagnoses are often delayed in the SMI population, and this group are known to have poorer cancer outcomes compared with the general population [19].

DIAGNOSTIC PRINCIPLES

History

- Record and assess amount of weight loss, time frame, and whether progressive/ongoing.
- Patient's weight patterns over previous years: stable or fluctuating.
- Constitutional symptoms (e.g. night sweats, fatigue, fevers).
- Evaluate for any intentional weight loss (e.g. dieting, increased exercise regimes, and evidence of disordered eating behaviours).
- Screen for low mood/depression.
- Determine if the patient has noticed any new swellings/lymphadenopathy.
- Symptoms of hyperthyroidism: palpitations, sweating, tremor.
- Symptoms of adrenal insufficiency: nausea, vomiting, significant lethargy and fatigue.
- Respiratory symptoms: increasing breathlessness, chronic cough, haemoptysis.
- Abdominal pain, distension, nausea and vomiting, early satiety.
- Rectal bleeding or melaena, change in bowel habit, steatorrhoea.
- Extraintestinal manifestations of inflammatory bowel disease/coexisting conditions (e.g. cholangitis, uveitis, skin complaints, arthritis, synovitis).
- Medication history (see Box 25.1).
- Comprehensive social history:
  - recreational drugs
  - alcohol and smoking

- accommodation
- travel history
- sexual history.
- Issues with purchasing or accessing food/any financial constraints.
- Problems with physical or mental capacity to coordinate or make meals.

Examination

- General: ill-fitting clothes.
- Mouth: candidiasis, stomatitis (iron or B vitamin deficiencies).
- Neck for goitre (hyperthyroidism).
- Lymphadenopathy: neck nodes, axillae, groin (malignancy or tuberculosis).
- Cardiovascular and respiratory examination (evidence of chronic pulmonary disease or cardiac failure).
- Abdominal examination:
  - abdominal masses
  - distension/presence of ascites
  - tenderness
  - hepatomegaly, splenomegaly
  - extraintestinal manifestations of inflammatory bowel disease (e.g. pyoderma gangrenosum, erythema nodosum).
- Neurological examination: features of Parkinson's disease/Lewy body dementia, tardive dyskinesia, signs of bulbar/pseudobulbar palsy (motor neurone disease), sensory, motor or speech deficit to suggest previous stroke, peripheral neuropathy (malignant paraneoplastic syndromes, e.g. small cell lung cancer). Screening assessment of cognition if concerns regarding dementia.

Investigations

- Blood tests:
  - full blood count
  - urea and creatinine
  - electrolytes (sodium, potassium, calcium, magnesium, phosphate, especially if concerns regarding refeeding syndrome)
  - haematinics including B_{12}, folate, iron studies
  - liver function tests
  - thyroid function tests
  - C-reactive protein
  - fasting glucose, HbA_{1c}
  - HIV/hepatitis B and C serology
  - if concerns over Addison's, consider a 9 a.m. cortisol with or without proceeding to short synacthen test (discussion with general medical colleagues first is recommended).
- Urinalysis (haematuria, glucose).
- Chest X-ray if concerns regarding underlying chest pathology.

MANAGEMENT

Management will depend on the underlying cause.

- Correction of endocrine abnormalities, e.g. thyroid function, management of diabetes, steroid replacement in Addison's disease.
- Identification and management of malignancy.
- Optimisation and management of underlying chronic illnesses and psychiatric conditions.
- Assessment and management of substance abuse and its sequelae.

General points

- Dietician review (inpatient or community) should be considered for accurate dietetic assessment and advice about the optimal dietary management.
- Refeeding syndrome may occur with rapid correction of weight loss, especially if more than 10% or body weight has been lost. It results from rapid flux of electrolytes into cells from the circulation and may cause profound biochemical derangements including hypokalaemia, hypophosphataemia, hypomagnesaemia, and occasionally hypocalcaemia. Regular monitoring of electrolytes and blood sugars may be required under the guidance of a dietician to recognise and avoid this.
- Thiamine (vitamin B_1) deficiency may also be present in malnourished individuals. If commencing feeding in a thiamine-depleted patient, further depletion could result in Wernicke's encephalopathy and Korsakov's syndrome. Oral supplementation with thiamine 300 mg once daily and one to two Vitamin B Compound Strong tablets three times daily may be indicated. Parenteral delivery of B vitamins may be required in patients with inadequate enteral absorption of thiamine (see Chapter 24).
- Control of symptoms due to underlying conditions (e.g. nausea and vomiting, constipation, and breathlessness) can help significantly in promoting oral intake.
- If there is any concern over safety of swallowing, then a speech and language therapy assessment should be obtained.

References

1. Wong CJ. Involuntary weight loss. *Med Clin North Am* 2014;98:625–643.
2. Malhi GS, Mann JJ. Depression. *Lancet* 2018;392:2299–2312.
3. Moriguti JC, Moriguti EK, Ferriolli E, et al. Involuntary weight loss in elderly individuals: assessment and treatment. *Sao Paulo Med J* 2001;119:72–77.
4. Sahyoun NR, Serdula MK, Galuska DA, et al. The epidemiology of recent involuntary weight loss in the United States population. *J Nutr Health Aging* 2004;8:510–517.
5. Morley JE, Kraenzle D. Causes of weight loss in a community nursing home. *J Am Geriatr Soc* 1994;42:583–585.
6. Hernández JL, Riancho JA, Matorras P, González-Macías J. Clinical evaluation for cancer in patients with involuntary weight loss without specific symptoms. *Am J Med* 2003;114:631–637.
7. Thompson MP, Morris LK. Unexplained weight loss in the ambulatory elderly. *J Am Geriatr Soc* 1991;39:497–500.
8. Evans WJ, Morley JE, Argilés J, et al. Cachexia: a new definition. *Clin Nutr* 2008;27:793–799.
9. Kotler DP. Cachexia. *Ann Intern Med* 2000;133:622–634.
10. Graul AI, Stringer M, Sorbera L. Cachexia. *Drugs Today (Barc)* 2016;52:519–529.
11. Beaudart C, McCloskey E, Bruyère O, et al. Sarcopenia in daily practice: assessment and management. *BMC Geriatr* 2016;16:170.

12. Haga T, Ito K, Ono M, et al. Underweight and hypoalbuminemia as risk indicators for mortality among psychiatric patients with medical comorbidities. *Psychiatry Clin Neurosci* 2017;71:807–812.
13. Jeynes KD, Gibson EL. The importance of nutrition in aiding recovery from substance use disorders: a review. *Drug Alcohol Depend* 2017;179:229–239.
14. Haga T, Ito K, Sakashita K, et al. Risk factors for death from psychiatric hospital-acquired pneumonia. *Intern Med* 2018;57:2473–2478.
15. Kvamme J-M, Grønli O, Florholmen J, Jacobsen BK. Risk of malnutrition is associated with mental health symptoms in community living elderly men and women: the Tromsø Study. *BMC Psychiatry* 2011;11:112.
16. Soysal P, Isik AT, Stubbs B, et al. Acetylcholinesterase inhibitors are associated with weight loss in older people with dementia: a systematic review and meta-analysis. *J Neurol Neurosurg Psychiatry* 2016;87:1368–1374.
17. Mikkelsen EJ, Albert LG, Upadhyaya A. Neuroleptic-withdrawal cachexia. *N Engl J Med* 1988;318:929.
18. Parkes CM. Bereavement in adult life. *BMJ* 1998;316:856–859.
19. Howard LM, Barley EA, Davies E, et al. Cancer diagnosis in people with severe mental illness: practical and ethical issues. *Lancet Oncol* 2010;11:797–804.
20. Zhu R, Liu Z, Jiao R, et al. Updates on the pathogenesis of advanced lung cancer-induced cachexia. *Thorac Cancer* 2019;10:8–16.

Dry Mouth

Enrico D'Ambrosio, Andrea Falsetti, Stephen Challacombe

Xerostomia is defined as the subjective sensation of oral dryness, which a patient will typically describe as a dry mouth [1]. Hyposalivation is defined as the objective reduction in the volume of saliva secreted measured with sialometry [2]. Approximately 20% of the adult population complain of xerostomia, though not all have salivary gland hypofunction [3]. Common causes of dry mouth are summarised in Box 26.1 [4–6]. Specific considerations for patients with a psychiatric disorder include a psychiatric medication review, with attention to drugs with a marked anticholinergic action (see http://www.medichec.com). Such drugs typically reduce salivary flow by approximately 30%, and their effects are additive [7]. Thus, any patient on two or more xerostomic medications (with a resultant reduction in salivary flow of up to 60%) may experience a significant degree of hyposalivation and resultant dry mouth [7]. While patients with depression may present with medication-induced salivary hypofunction, depression is itself independently associated with dry mouth [5]. Chronic systemic conditions associated with xerostomia (e.g. Sjögren's syndrome and systemic lupus erythematosus) may be associated with psychiatric comorbidity. Parotid gland hypertrophy as a consequence of bulimia nervosa may result in impaired salivary secretion.

Box 26.1 Common causes of dry mouth

Medication (non-psychiatric)

Xerostomia

- Beta-blockers
- Bronchodilators (e.g. tiotropium)
- Calcium channel blockers (e.g. verapamil)

The Maudsley Practice Guidelines for Physical Health Conditions in Psychiatry, First Edition.
David M. Taylor, Fiona Gaughran, and Toby Pillinger.
© 2021 John Wiley & Sons Ltd. Published 2021 by John Wiley & Sons Ltd.

- Muscle relaxants (e.g. baclofen)
- Ophthalmologic drugs (e.g. brimonidine)
- Opiates

Hyposalivation

- Anticholinergics (e.g. atropine)
- Antihypertensives (e.g. clonidine)
- Anti-Parkinsonism drugs (e.g. rotigotine)
- Bisphosphonates (e.g. alendronate)
- Diuretics (e.g. thiazides)

Medication (psychiatric)

Xerostomia

- Anticonvulsants (e.g. gabapentin)
- Benzodiazepines (e.g. lorazepam)
- Benzodiazepine-related drugs (e.g. zolpidem)

Hyposalivation

- Antidepressants (e.g. tricyclics)
- Antipsychotics (e.g. quetiapine)
- Mood stabilisers (e.g. lithium)

Recreational drugs

Hyposalivation

- Cannabis
- Methamphetamine (e.g. MDMA)
- Cocaine

Systemic disorders

Xerostomia

- Burning mouth syndrome
- Fibromyalgia
- Chronic renal failure
- Endocrine disorders (e.g. diabetes mellitus)

Hyposalivation

- Chronic inflammatory disorders (e.g. Sjögren's syndrome)

Effects of treatment

Hyposalivation

- Radiotherapy of head and neck cancer

Other

Xerostomia

- Ageing
- Alcohol
- Mouth breathing
- Tobacco
- Oral infection (e.g. candidiasis/gingivitis)

Psychiatric disorders

Hyposalivation

- Eating disorders
- Autonomic activation associated with panic, anxiety and depression

DIAGNOSTIC PRINCIPLES

History and examination

After establishing the duration and severity of xerostomia, history should be directed to establish potential underlying causes. For example, nasal obstruction resulting in mouth breathing can cause dry mouth, similarly poor fluid intake and poor self-care resulting in dehydration. A past medical history for rheumatoid conditions may raise suspicion for Sjögren's syndrome. Take a thorough medication history, focusing on the drugs listed in Box 26.1 and calculate the anticholinergic burden using http://www.medichec.com. A mental state examination may identify comorbid anxiety or depression resulting in autonomic hyperactivity and dry mouth. Examine the patient's mouth for evidence of candidiasis or gingivitis. Examine under the tongue to check for masses blocking salivary excretion. Check the parotid glands for swelling. Investigations will be guided by the identification of any potential underlying conditions, although generally diagnosis is a clinical one. The Clinical Oral Dryness Score (CODS) is a useful scale used to grade oral dryness [8]. The scoring system includes three levels of severity (mild, moderate, and severe dryness) and can guide the clinician in the choice of treatment [1].

MANAGEMENT

Reversible causes such as dehydration, infection, and nasal congestion leading to mouth breathing should be addressed, alongside any psychiatric comorbidity that may be leading to autonomic overactivity. Psychiatric medications may be responsible for hyposalivation, although the risk profile with different drugs is variable [9–13]. Nevertheless, rationalising pharmacotherapy may be key to providing symptomatic relief. In patients who are well established on an efficacious antipsychotic or antidepressant regimen and where there is a reluctance to change medication, consider dose reduction.

Non-pharmacological therapy for dry mouth may involve lifestyle modification, such as avoiding alcohol and caffeine [14]. Betel nut, citric acid, and red pepper can stimulate salivary secretion [2]. Regular sips of water during meals can facilitate chewing and swallowing. Saliva substitutes are available, including gums, gels, and sprays. Patients can also try natural lubricants, namely two drops of edible oil in the mouth every hour [1]. Dry mouth is associated with dental caries, so referral to a dentist may be required.

Sialogogic drugs are medications designed to stimulate salivary secretion. Pilocarpine and cevimeline (the latter not licensed in the UK) have been shown to be efficient in Sjögren's syndrome; however, their role in treating dry mouth in patients on psychiatric medications has not been well explored [15] and side effects, especially with pilocarpine, can be considerable. Bethanechol has been studied in the treatment of dry mouth in patients taking antidepressant and antipsychotic drugs resulting in symptomatic improvement [2,16,17].

Pilocarpine is a non-selective muscarinic agonist with a relatively high affinity for muscarinic receptors in the central nervous system. It is effective and well tolerated, administered at a dose of 5 mg four times a day [18]. It is contraindicated in patients with asthma, hypertension, and glaucoma. Cevimeline, a specific agonist of the M3 muscarinic receptor, is prescribed at a dose of 30 mg three times daily [19]. Because of its high selectivity, the use of cevimeline is associated with fewer neurological, cardiac, and gastrointestinal side effects when compared with pilocarpine. Bethanechol is a carbamic ester of β-methylcholine resistant to cholinesterase with a long duration of action that stimulates M3 receptors. It is effective at a dose of 25 mg three times daily [20]. It can cause lacrimation, frequent urination, diarrhoea, and nausea.

References

1. Piali D, Challacombe SJ. Dry mouth and clinical oral dryness scoring systems. *Prim Dent J* 2016;5:77–79.
2. Miranda-Rius J, Brunet-Llobet L, Lahor-Soler E, Farré M. Salivary secretory disorders, inducing drugs, and clinical management. *Int J Med Sci* 2015;12:811–824.
3. Furness S, Worthington HV, Bryan G, et al. Interventions for the management of dry mouth: topical therapies. *Cochrane Database Syst Rev* 2011;(12):CD008934.
4. Ying Joanna ND, Thomson WM. Dry mouth: an overview. *Singapore Dent J* 2015;36:12–17.
5. Saleh J, Figueiredo MAZ, Cherubini K, Salum FG. Salivary hypofunction: an update on aetiology, diagnosis and therapeutics. *Arch Oral Biol* 2015;60(2):242–255.
6. von Bültzingslöwen I, Sollecito TP, Fox PC, et al. Salivary dysfunction associated with systemic diseases: systematic review and clinical management recommendations. *Oral Surg Oral Med Oral Pathol Oral Radiol Endod* 2007;103(Suppl):S57.e1–e15.
7. Singh ML, Papas A. Oral implications of polypharmacy in the elderly. *Dent Clin North Am* 2014;58(4):783–796.
8. Osailan SM, Pramanik R, Shirlaw P, et al. Clinical assessment of oral dryness: development of a scoring system related to salivary flow and mucosal wetness. *Oral Surg Oral Med Oral Pathol Oral Radiol* 2012;114(5):597–603.
9. Wolff A, Joshi RK, Ekström J, et al A guide to medications inducing salivary gland dysfunction, xerostomia, and subjective sialorrhea: a systematic review sponsored by the World Workshop on Oral Medicine VI. *Drugs R D* 2017;17:1–28.
10. Marques LO, Lima MS, Soares BG. Trifluoperazine for schizophrenia. *Cochrane Database Syst Rev* 2004;(1):CD003545.
11. Kreinin A, Epshtein S, Sheinkman A, Tell E. Sulpiride addition for the treatment of clozapine-induced hypersalivation: preliminary study. *Isr J Psychiatry Relat Sci* 2005;42(1):61–63.
12. Lancaster SG, Gonzalez JP. Lofepramine: a review of its pharmacodynamic and pharmacokinetic properties, and therapeutic efficacy in depressive illness. *Drugs* 1989;37(2):123–140.

13. Szabadi E, Tavernor S. Hypo- and hypersalivation induced by psychoactive drugs: Incidence, mechanisms and therapeutic implications. *CNS Drugs* 1999;11:449–466.
14. Villa A, Connell CL, Abati S. Diagnosis and management of xerostomia and hyposalivation. *Ther Clin Risk Manag* 2014;11:45–51.
15. Swager LWM, Morgan SK. Psychotropic-induced dry mouth: don't overlook this potentially serious side effect. *Curr Psychiatry* 2011;10(12):54–58.
16. Everett HC. The use of bethanechol chloride with tricyclic antidepressants. *Am J Psychiatry* 1975;132(11):1202–1204.
17. Schubert DSP. Use of bethanechol chloride with phenothiazines: a case report. *Am J Psychiatry* 1979;136(1):110–111.
18. Wu CH, Hsieh SC, Lee KL, et al. Pilocarpine hydrochloride for the treatment of xerostomia in patients with Sjögren's sydrome in Taiwan: a double-blind, placebo-controlled trial. *J Formos Med Assoc* 2006;105(10):796–803.
19. Leung KCM, McMillan AS, Wong MC, et al. The efficacy of cevimeline hydrochloride in the treatment of xerostomia in Sjögren's syndrome in southern Chinese patients: a randomised double-blind, placebo-controlled crossover study. *Clin Rheumatol* 2008;27(4):429–436.
20. Kavitha M, Mubeen K, Vijaylakshmi KR. A study on evaluation of efficacy of bethanechol in the management of chemoradiation-induced xerostomia in oral cancer patients. *J Oral Maxillofac Pathol* 2017;21:459–460.

CHAPTER 26

Hypersalivation

Enrico D'Ambrosio, Andrea Falsetti, Toby Pillinger,
Stephen Challacombe

Hypersalivation, sialorrhoea, ptyalism, and excessive drooling are interchangeable terms to describe excess production or decreased clearance of saliva from the mouth. Unstimulated whole saliva (UWS) flow rates have wide interindividual variability [1]. Although the diagnosis is mainly based on symptoms, a UWS rate higher than 0.8 mL/min measured with sialometry is indicative of hypersalivation [2]. Common causes of hypersalivation are summarised in Box 27.1 [3–5]. The mechanisms by which different drugs induce hypersalivation are multiple, and for some agents poorly defined. They include direct agonism of muscarinic acetylcholine receptors (e.g. clozapine), indirect muscarinic agonism via acetylcholinesterase inhibition (e.g. rivastigmine), blockade of α_2-adrenergic receptors (e.g. clozapine), dopamine antagonism leading to extrapyramidal side effects such as orofacial dyskinesia and thus impaired clearance of saliva (all antipsychotics), and sedation leading to reduced clearance of saliva [3]. Hypersalivation is not only socially embarrassing and affects quality of life but may also increase risk of choking and aspiration pneumonia.

DIAGNOSTIC PRINCIPLES

History and examination

Enquire about episodes of hypersalivation during the day and at night, for example waking up with a choking sensation, or noticing that the pillow is wet in the morning. A comprehensive drug history is recommended (see Box 27.1), although in the psychiatric population the causative agent may be clear (e.g. hypersalivation in a patient recently started on clozapine). The age of the patient should be considered, as elderly patients may have altered positioning of the head and neck and/or dysphagia that

The Maudsley Practice Guidelines for Physical Health Conditions in Psychiatry, First Edition.
David M. Taylor, Fiona Gaughran, and Toby Pillinger.

Box 27.1 Common causes of hypersalivation

Medication (non-psychiatric)

- Adrenergic antagonists (e.g. ephedrine)
- Antibiotics (e.g. doxycycline)
- Direct cholinergics (e.g. pilocarpine)
- Poisons and toxins (e.g. mercury, insecticides)

Medication (psychiatric)

- Acetylcholinesterase inhibitors (e.g. rivastigmine)
- Anticonvulsants
- Antipsychotics
- Stimulants (e.g. modafinil)

Recreational drug

- Phencyclidine (PCP)
- Ketamine

Increased production

- Gastro-oesophageal reflux disease
- Infection (e.g. rabies)
- Oral inflammation
- Pregnancy

Impaired clearance

- Anatomical (e.g. macroglossia)
- Neuromuscular/sensory dysfunction (e.g. cerebral palsy, Down's syndrome, Parkinson's disease, amyotrophic lateral sclerosis, dysphagia)
- Positional problems of the head/neck (e.g. in elderly)

---

compromise clearance of saliva. If aetiology is unclear, enquire about past medical history of gastro-oesophageal reflux disease, any orthodontic complaints or historical interventions, and any past/recent dental/gingival infections. A social history should include quantification of alcohol and illicit drug use. Examination of the oral cavity may be indicated, examining for evidence of gingival or dental infection. In the absence of infection, further investigations are not indicated; diagnosis of hypersalivation is a clinical one.

MANAGEMENT

If a clear reversible cause for hypersalivation is identified, such as poor oral hygiene, then appropriate referral to the relevant specialist should be made (e.g. a dentist). Non-pharmacological management of hypersalivation includes using chewing gum to increase swallowing, sleeping with extra pillows at night (at least two) to reduce risk of aspiration, and placing a towel on the pillow to prevent soaking of clothes.

Several classes of psychiatric medication cause salivary dysfunction (see Box 27.1), although the risk profile is variable [4]. Since the hypersalivatory effects of some treatments may be dose-related, in patients who are well established on an efficacious antipsychotic regimen and where there is a reluctance to change medication, consider dose reduction.

Clozapine-induced hypersalivation is well recognised, generally occurring early on in treatment and likely to be dose-related [6]. A number of pharmacological agents are available to treat sialorrhoea associated with clozapine (Table 27.1); the evidence base supporting different agents is variable and treatment often based on clinical experience. Hyoscine (scopolamine) hydrobromide is probably the most commonly prescribed first-line agent for clozapine-induced hypersalivation. A recent randomised controlled trial observed a reduction in the severity of hypersalivation with oral hyoscine hydrobromide 0.3 mg once daily [7]. It is generally used as an oral tablet (0.3 mg up to three times daily; in cases of predominantly nocturnal hypersalivation, doses of up to 0.9 mg at night can be trialed, sucked or chewed for local effect) or as a transdermal patch 1.5 mg per 72 hours. Clinicians should monitor for emergence of anticholinergic side effects, and where patients are already experiencing such side effects (especially constipation), use of hyoscine or indeed any other anticholinergic agent is not recommended. In this setting, metoclopramide is a reasonable alternative; a recent double-blind randomised controlled trial observed that metoclopramide (dose 10–30 mg/day) significantly improved clozapine-induced nocturnal hypersalivation [8]. There is also some evidence from China to support the use of antihistamines (e.g. diphenhydramine) [9]. Since there is some evidence that amisulpride/sulpiride augmentation can improve psychotic symptoms in patients with only a partial response to clozapine [10,11], addition of amisulpride/sulpiride in such patients who also present with hypersalivation may be considered [12–15]. Use of atropine eye drops (as a mouthwash) and botulinum toxin injections into the parotid salivary glands is an attractive strategy owing to their local

Table 27.1 Drug treatments for hypersalivation.

Treatment	Dose	Comments
Antimuscarinics		
Amitriptyline [17,18]	25–100 mg/day	Limited literature to support
Atropine [19,20]	1% eye drops: three drops up to t.d.s. (or just at night if predominantly nocturnal hypersalivation). Use as mouthwash: put three drops in small amount of water, swill, then spit out	Contraindicated in narrow-angle glaucoma, bladder obstruction, and gastrointestinal motility disorders. Although significant systemic absorption unlikely when used as described, still monitor for anticholinergic side effects
Benzatropine + terazosin [21]	2 mg/day (benzatropine) 2 mg/day (terazosin)	Combination shown to be better than either drug alone. Be wary of hypotension with terazosin (α_1 antagonist)
Glycopyrrolate [22–25]	0.5–4 mg b.d.	RCT-level evidence to support its efficacy over placebo and biperiden (another anticholinergic agent)

(continued)

CHAPTER 27

Table 27.1 (Continued)

Treatment	Dose	Comments
Hyoscine hydrobromide [7,26]	Oral up to 300 μg t.d.s. or transdermal patch (1.5 mg/72 h). If predominant nocturnal hypersalivation can trial up to 900 μg at night. Suck tablets to obtain local effect	Competitive muscarinic antagonist. Contraindicated in patients with severe constipation and paralytic ileus, pyloric stenosis, prostatic hyperplasia, and glaucoma. As with all anticholinergic agents, not advised in patients already experiencing anticholinergic side effects (e.g. constipation)
Ipratropium nasal spray (0.03 or 0.06%) [27–29]	Two sprays 0.06% sublingually three times daily or one spray 0.03% intranasally daily	Non-selective muscarinic receptor antagonist used in respiratory diseases. Limited evidence in literature including a negative RCT [29]. However, minimal side effects mean that a trial may be considered
Oxybutynin [30]	5–10 mg/day	Anticholinergic agent used for the treatment of urinary incontinence and overactive bladder syndrome. Very limited evidence (single case report) [30]
Pirenzepine [31,32]	50–150 mg/day	Anticholinergic with M1–M4 receptor antagonist action that does not cross the blood–brain barrier. The only RCT examining its efficacy was negative [32]
Propantheline [33]	7.5 mg/day	One positive and one negative RCT. Monitor for constipation
Adrenoceptor agonists		
Clonidine [34]	0.1–0.2 mg patch weekly or oral 0.1 mg/day	Presynaptic partial α_2 agonist used in hypertension treatment. Addition to clozapine can lead to a worsening of postural hypotension. May exacerbate depression and psychosis. Limited data to support use
Guanfacine [35]	1 mg/day	Presynaptic α_2 agonist structurally similar to clonidine. Single case report. Can cause postural hypotension
Lofexidine [36]	0.2 mg twice daily	Presynaptic α_2 agonist used to treat hypertension and opioid withdrawal. Single case report. May exacerbate depression and psychosis
Others		
Amisulpride [12,13]	100–400 mg/day	RCT level of evidence of efficacy versus placebo and moclobemide
Botulinum toxin [37,38]	Bilateral parotid gland injections, 150 IU into each gland	Evidence base from treatment of hypersalivation associated with neurological disorders. Case-report level of evidence in context of clozapine use
Bupropion [39]	100–150 mg/day	Noradrenaline/dopamine receptor antagonist antidepressant also used in smoking cessation. Lowers seizure threshold. Only single case report to support use
Metoclopramide [8]	10–30 mg/day	Supported by double-blind placebo-controlled RCT; use is generally well tolerated
Moclobemide [40]	150–300 mg/day	Effective in a small open label study
Sulpiride [14,15]	150–300 mg/day	Evidence of efficacy from a small RCT and supported by a Cochrane review

RCT, randomised controlled trial.

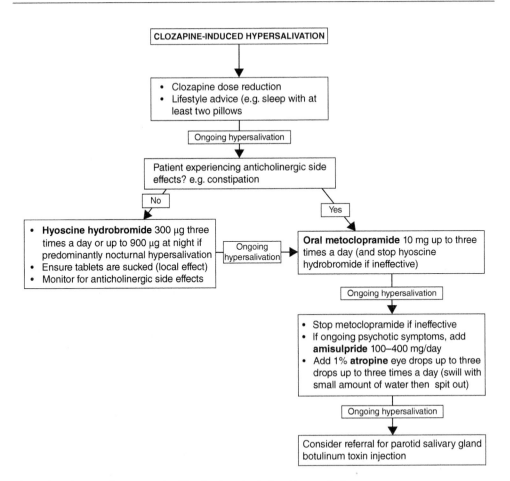

CHAPTER 27

Figure 27.1 Suggested treatment algorithm for clozapine-induced hypersalivation.

action, thus avoiding/reducing the risk of systemic side effects. However, atropine use should be avoided (or at least supervised) in the context of chaotic or self-harming behavior (i.e. where there is risk of overdose) [16] and it is recognised that there may be logistical barriers to arranging botulinum toxin injections (e.g. requiring a referral to interventional radiology). A suggested management algorithm for clozapine-induced hypersalivation is presented in Figure 27.1; however, trials of various agents may be required.

References

1. Proctor GB. The physiology of salivary secretion. *Periodontol 2000* 2016;70(1):11–25.
2. Edgar WM. Saliva and dental-health: clinical implications of saliva. Report of a consensus meeting. *Br Dent J* 1990;169(3–4):96–98.
3. Miranda-Rius J, Brunet-Llobet L, Lahor-Soler E, Farre M. Salivary secretory disorders, inducing drugs, and clinical management. *Int J Med Sci* 2015;12(10):811–824.
4. Wolff A, Joshi RK, Ekstrom J, et al. A guide to medications inducing salivary gland dysfunction, xerostomia, and subjective sialorrhea: a systematic review sponsored by the World Workshop on Oral Medicine VI. *Drugs R D* 2017;17(1):1–28.
5. von Bultzingslöwen I, Sollecito TP, Fox PC, et al. Salivary dysfunction associated with systemic diseases: systematic review and clinical management recommendations. *Oral Surg Oral Med Oral Pathol Oral Radiol Endod* 2007;103(Suppl):S57.e1–e15.

6. Praharaj SK, Arora M, Gandotra S. Clozapine-induced sialorrhea: pathophysiology and management strategies. *Psychopharmacology* 2006;185(3):265–273.

7. Segev A, Evans A, Hodsoll J, et al. Hyoscine for clozapine-induced hypersalivation: a double-blind, randomized, placebo-controlled cross-over trial. *Int Clin Psychopharmacol* 2019;34(2):101–107.

8. Kreinin A, Miodownik C, Mirkin V, et al. Double-blind, randomized, placebo-controlled trial of metoclopramide for hypersalivation associated with clozapine. *J Clin Psychopharmacol* 2016;36(3):200–205.

9. Chen SY, Ravindran G, Zhang Q, et al. Treatment strategies for clozapine-induced sialorrhea: a systematic review and meta-analysis. *CNS Drugs* 2019;33(3):225–238.

10. Shiloh R, Zemishlany Z, Aizenberg D, et al. Sulpiride augmentation in people with schizophrenia partially responsive to clozapine. A double-blind, placebo-controlled study. *Br J Psychiatry* 1997;171:569–573.

11. Munro J, Matthiasson P, Osborne S, et al. Amisulpride augmentation of clozapine: an open non-randomized study in patients with schizophrenia partially responsive to clozapine. *Acta Psychiatr Scand* 2004;110(4):292–298.

12. Kreinin A, Miodownik C, Sokolik S, et al. Amisulpride versus moclobemide in treatment of clozapine-induced hypersalivation. *World J Biol Psychiatry* 2011;12(8):620–626.

13. Kreinin A, Novitski D, Weizman A. Amisulpride treatment of clozapine-induced hypersalivation in schizophrenia patients: a randomized, double-blind, placebo-controlled cross-over study. *Int Clin Psychopharmacol* 2006;21(2):99–103.

14. Kreinin A, Epshtein S, Sheinkman A, Tell E. Sulpiride addition for the treatment of clozapine-induced hypersalivation: preliminary study. *Isr J Psychiatry Relat Sci* 2005;42(1):61–63.

15. Wang JJ, Omori IM, Fenton M, Soares B. Sulpiride augmentation for schizophrenia. *Schizophr Bull* 2010;36(2):229–230.

16. Stellpflug SJ, Cole JB, Isaacson BA, et al. Massive atropine eye drop ingestion treated with high-dose physostigmine to avoid intubation. *West J Emerg Med* 2012;13(1):77–79.

17. Copp PJ, Lament R, Tennent TG. Amitriptyline in clozapine-induced sialorrhoea. *Br J Psychiatry* 1991;159:166.

18. Praharaj SK, Arora M. Amitriptyline for clozapine-induced nocturnal enuresis and sialorrhoea. *Br J Clin Pharmacol* 2007;63(1):128–129.

19. Antonello C, Tessier P. Clozapine and sialorrhea: a new intervention for this bothersome and potentially dangerous side effect. *J Psychiatry Neurosci* 1999;24(3):250.

20. Van der Poorten T, De Hert M. The sublingual use of atropine in the treatment of clozapine-induced sialorrhea: a systematic review. *Clin Case Rep* 2019;7(11):2108–2113.

21. Reinstein MJ, Sirotovskaya LA, Chasanov MA, et al. Comparative efficacy and tolerability of benzatropine and terazosin in the treatment of hypersalivation secondary to clozapine. *Clin Drug Invest* 1999;17(2):97–102.

22. Bird AM, Smith TL, Walton AE. Current treatment strategies for clozapine-induced sialorrhea. *Ann Pharmacother* 2011;45(5):667–675.

23. Blissit KT, Tillery E, Latham C, Pacheco-Perez J. Glycopyrrolate for treatment of clozapine-induced sialorrhea in adults. *Am J Health Syst Pharm* 2014;71(15):1282–1287.

24. Qurashi I, Chu S, Husain N, et al. Glycopyrrolate in comparison to hyoscine hydrobromide and placebo in the treatment of hypersalivation induced by clozapine (GOTHIC1): study protocol for a randomised controlled feasibility study. *Trials* 2016;17(1):553.

25. Robb AS, Lee RH, Cooper EB, et al. Glycopyrrolate for treatment of clozapine-induced sialorrhea in three adolescents. *J Child Adolesc Psychopharmacol* 2008;18(1):99–107.

26. Gaftanyuk O, Trestman RL. Scopolamine patch for clozapine-induced sialorrhea. *Psychiatr Serv* 2004;55(3):318.

27. Calderon J, Rubin E, Sobota WL. Potential use of ipatropium bromide for the treatment of clozapine-induced hypersalivation: a preliminary report. *Int Clin Psychopharmacol* 2000;15(1):49–52.

28. Freudenreich O, Beebe M, Goff DC. Clozapine-induced sialorrhea treated with sublingual ipratropium spray: a case series. *J Clin Psychopharmacol* 2004;24(1):98–100.

29. Sockalingam S, Shammi C, Remington G. Treatment of clozapine-induced hypersalivation with ipratropium bromide: a randomized, double-blind, placebo-controlled crossover study. *J Clin Psychiatry* 2009;70(8):1114–1119.

30. Leung JG, Puri NV, Jacobson MJ. Immediate-release oxybutynin for the treatment of clozapine-induced sialorrhea. *Ann Pharmacother* 2011;45(9):e45.

31. Fritze J, Elliger T. Pirenzepine for clozapine-induced hypersalivation. *Lancet* 1995;346(8981):1034.

32. Bai YM, Lin CC, Chen JY, Liu WC. Therapeutic effect of pirenzepine for clozapine-induced hypersalivation: a randomized, double-blind, placebo-controlled, cross-over study. *J Clin Psychopharmacol* 2001;21(6):608–611.

33. Syed Sheriff RJ, Au K, Cahill C, et al. Pharmacological interventions for clozapine-induced hypersalivation. *Schizophr Bull* 2008;34(4):611–612.

34. Grabowski J. Clonidine treatment of clozapine-induced hypersalivation. *J Clin Psychopharmacol* 1992;12(1):69–70.

35. Webber MA, Szwast SJ, Steadman TM, et al. Guanfacine treatment of clozapine-induced sialorrhea. *J Clin Psychopharmacol* 2004;24(6):675–676.

36. Corrigan FM, MacDonald S, Reynolds GP. Clozapine-induced hypersalivation and the alpha 2 adrenoceptor. *Br J Psychiatry* 1995;167(3):412.

37. Kahl KG, Hagenah J, Zapf S, et al. Botulinum toxin as an effective treatment of clozapine-induced hypersalivation. *Psychopharmacology* 2004;173(1–2):229–230.

38. Steinlechner S, Klein C, Moser A, et al. Botulinum toxin B as an effective and safe treatment for neuroleptic-induced sialorrhea. *Psychopharmacology* 2010;207(4):593–597.

39. Stern RG, Bellucci D, Cursi-Vogel N, et al. Clozapine-induced sialorrhea alleviated by bupropion: a case report. *Prog Neuropsychopharmacol Biol Psychiatry* 2009;33(8):1578–1580.

40. Kreinin A, Miodownik C, Libov I, et al. Moclobemide treatment of clozapine-induced hypersalivation: pilot open study. *Clin Neuropharmacol* 2009;32(3):151–153.

CHAPTER 27

Constipation

John Lally, Toby Pillinger, Kalliopi Vallianatou, Immo Weichert

Constipation is defined as infrequent and/or difficult defecation, characterised by excessive straining, hard stools (see the Bristol Stool Form Scale in Figure 28.1) [1], the sensation of incomplete evacuation, or the passage of fewer than three stools per week [2]. Constipation is either idiopathic or due to secondary causes (Box 28.1). Chronic idiopathic constipation has a pooled global prevalence of 14% [3]. There is increased

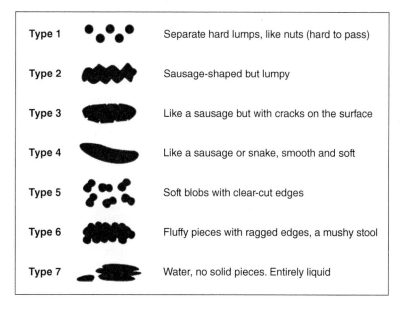

Type 1		Separate hard lumps, like nuts (hard to pass)
Type 2		Sausage-shaped but lumpy
Type 3		Like a sausage but with cracks on the surface
Type 4		Like a sausage or snake, smooth and soft
Type 5		Soft blobs with clear-cut edges
Type 6		Fluffy pieces with ragged edges, a mushy stool
Type 7		Water, no solid pieces. Entirely liquid

Figure 28.1 The Bristol Stool Form Scale. Source: adapted from Lewis and Heaton [1].

The Maudsley Practice Guidelines for Physical Health Conditions in Psychiatry, First Edition.
David M. Taylor, Fiona Gaughran, and Toby Pillinger.
© 2021 John Wiley & Sons Ltd. Published 2021 by John Wiley & Sons Ltd.

Box 28.1 Secondary causes of constipation

- Hypothyroidism (see Chapter 12)
- Electrolyte abnormalities (e.g. hypercalcaemia, hypokalaemia)
- Gastrointestinal obstruction (e.g. strictures or malignancy)
- Central neurological disorders (e.g. Parkinson's disease, multiple sclerosis)
- Peripheral neurological disorders (e.g. diabetic autonomic neuropathy)
- Irritable bowel syndrome (may be associated with constipation)
- Previous abdominal surgery (adhesions)
- Inflammatory bowel disease (strictures)
- Anorexia nervosa
- Pregnancy
- Learning disability
- Medication (see Box 28.2)

---

prevalence in the elderly, females, and those with a sedentary lifestyle [4]. Risk of constipation is increased in some psychiatric patient groups, in particular patients with schizophrenia and those with learning difficulties [5–7]. This can be related to psychiatric medication, decreased physical activity, and dietary factors [5,7].

The neural and hormonal control of colonic peristalsis is complex. Simplistically, serotonin, produced by enterochromaffin cells in response to gut wall distension by a food/stool bolus, is the major orchestrator of gut peristalsis and prompts enteric nerves to produce neurotransmitters such as acetylcholine and nitric oxide that respectively contract and relax gut wall smooth muscle in a coordinated fashion. Various drugs cause constipation by disrupting these neurochemical pathways (Box 28.2). Many psychiatric medications list constipation as a potential side effect, although for some agents this occurrence will be rare. Psychotropics where constipation is common include antidepressants (e.g. tricyclic antidepressants, paroxetine, and reboxetine) and antipsychotics with strong anticholinergic effects. There is also evidence that some 'first-generation' antipsychotics (e.g. haloperidol, flupentixol, and pimozide) increase risk of constipation despite not having strong anticholinergic effects [5]; this is potentially related to concurrently prescribed anticholinergic medication to manage extrapyramidal side effects.

Box 28.2 Medications that can cause constipation

- Some antihypertensive drugs, e.g. calcium channel blockers (reduce smooth muscle contractility)
- Any drugs with anticholinergic effects: antispasmodics, some antidepressants (tricyclics, paroxetine, reboxetine), anti-Parkinsonian drugs, older sedating antihistamines (e.g. chlorphenamine), antipsychotics (especially clozapine). Venlafaxine and monoamine oxidase inhibitors such as phenelzine and isocarboxazid also commonly cause constipation
- Serotonin antagonists (e.g. ondansetron)
- Diuretics
- Opioids
- Oral iron supplementation
- Calcium/aluminium antacids

Of all the antipsychotics, clozapine is associated with the highest risk of causing constipation; indeed, patients are three times more likely to be constipated when treated with clozapine compared with other antipsychotics [8]. Clozapine-treated patients have, as a group, colonic transit times that are four times longer than expected in the general adult population [9], with constipation affecting approximately one-third of patients [8]. This is believed to be secondary to a combination of anticholinergic, antihistaminergic, and anti-serotonergic properties of the drug, alongside its sedative effects and resultant sedentary behaviour which in itself increases risk of constipation [10]. Untreated constipation can lead to severe complications, including faecal impaction, colonic obstruction, bowel ischaemia and necrosis, perforation, and sepsis. The prevalence of life-threatening constipation with clozapine is 0.3%, and case fatality as high as 28% [11]. A Danish nationwide study reported a 0.8% incidence of hospital admission as a consequence of ileus in clozapine-treated patients [12]. Thus, constipation represents a greater threat to the physical health of patients who take clozapine compared with the risk of blood dyscrasias. Despite this, there is evidence that management of clozapine-induced constipation is poor in certain patient groups, in particular men [13].

DIAGNOSTIC PRINCIPLES

Through history and examination one should aim to determine the severity of constipation and identify any secondary causes. If the patient presents with severe abdominal pain, vomiting, fever, tachycardia, or hypotension, have a low threshold for transferring care to emergency services (see Chapters 72 and 88). When in doubt, discuss with general surgical/medical colleagues.

History

In the non-acute setting, a directed history should cover the following.

1 History of presenting complaint.
   a Define bowel habits prior to onset of constipation.
   b Define stool frequency, consistency, and size (see Figure 28.1). Note that diarrhoea may indicate constipation with overflow. On an inpatient ward, consider use of a stool chart.
   c Recent change in bowel habit may be a feature of gastrointestinal malignancy. Screen for other associated 'red flag' signs, symptoms, and investigation findings such as tenesmus (feeling of incomplete defecation), weight loss, gastrointestinal bleeding, and anaemia (see Chapters 15, 20, and 25 for more details on anaemia, gastrointestinal bleeding, and unexplained weight loss, respectively).
   d Document diet (including fluid intake) and amount of regular physical activity the patient engages in.
2 Past medical history: screen for disorders documented in Box 28.1.
3 Drug history: note laxative use and any potentially causative agents documented in Box 28.2.

Examination

Examination may be entirely normal. During abdominal examination, high-pitched 'tinkling' bowel sounds on auscultation may indicate obstruction. Digital rectal examination may be performed to identify a faecally loaded rectum, masses, abnormal sphincter function (ask the patient to squeeze during examination), blood in stool, or fissures/hemorrhoids.

Investigations

Investigations may not be required if symptoms are mild or there is a clear pharmacological precipitant. If there are concerns regarding a secondary cause of constipation (Box 28.1), the following tests should be considered:

1 full blood count (for anaemia or evidence of infection)
2 C-reactive protein (infection)
3 urea and electrolytes and bone profile (for evidence of dehydration, hypokalaemia, or hypercalcaemia)
4 HbA$_{1c}$
5 thyroid function tests (unless already performed in the last eight weeks)
6 if there is abdominal pain in a woman of childbearing age, perform a pregnancy test.

A plain abdominal X-ray may be indicated if obstruction is suspected; in a psychiatric setting this will require a referral to emergency or surgical services. Other investigations that may be performed by medical/surgical services in such a context include an erect chest X-ray (examining for air under the diaphragm in the context of bowel perforation) and computed tomography (CT) of the abdomen. Chronic constipation may require endoscopic investigation (flexible sigmoidoscopy/colonoscopy) to examine for strictures or masses. Endoscopy or CT pneumocolon is certainly indicated if the patient presents with any red flags for gastrointestinal malignancy; in patients who may be too frail or will not tolerate endoscopy, CT of the colon is an alternative option.

MANAGEMENT

Non-pharmacological and pharmacological management of constipation are described here. An algorithm describing an approach to clozapine-induced gastrointestinal hypomotility is provided in Figure 28.2.

Non-pharmacological

All patients with constipation should be provided with dietary advice [14]. This includes increasing water intake (2 L/day) and fibre intake (25–30 g/day). Dietary fibre may be in the form of fruit (where appropriate including the skin), vegetables, legumes, and bran. Note that the effects of a high-fibre diet may be seen in a few days but can take weeks. A referral to a dietician may be considered. Patients should also be encouraged to increase physical activity levels (see Chapter 10).

CHAPTER 28

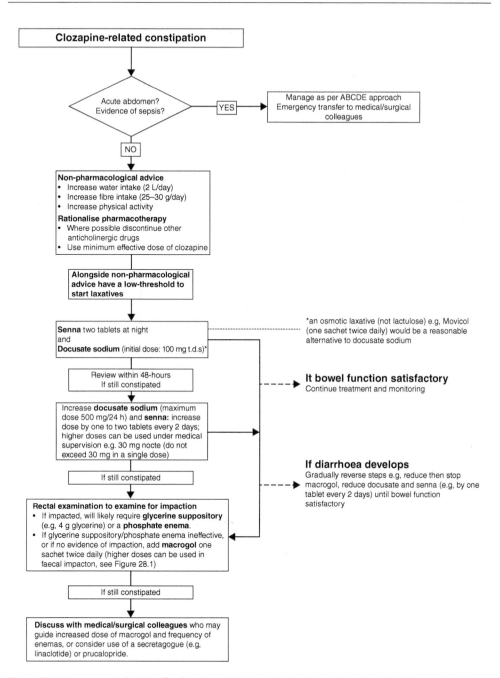

Clozapine-related constipation

Acute abdomen?
Evidence of sepsis?

YES → Manage as per ABCDE approach
Emergency transfer to medical/surgical colleagues

NO

Non-pharmacological advice
• Increase water intake (2 L/day)
• Increase fibre intake (25–30 g/day)
• Increase physical activity

Rationalise pharmacotherapy
• Where possible discontinue other anticholinergic drugs
• Use minimum effective dose of clozapine

Alongside non-pharmacological advice have a low-threshold to start laxatives

Senna two tablets at night
and
Docusate sodium (initial dose: 100 mg t.d.s)*

*an osmotic laxative (not lactulose) e.g, Movicol (one sachet twice daily) would be a reasonable alternative to docusate sodium

Review within 48-hours
If still constipated

It bowel function satisfactory
Continue treatment and monitoring

Increase **docusate sodium** (maximum dose 500 mg/24 h) and **senna:** increase dose by one to two tablets every 2 days; higher doses can be used under medical supervision e.g. 30 mg nocte (do not exceed 30 mg in a single dose)

If still constipated

If diarrhoea develops
Gradually reverse steps e.g, reduce then stop macrogol, reduce docusate and senna (e.g, by one tablet every 2 days) until bowel function satisfactory

Rectal examination to examine for impaction
• If impacted, will likely require **glycerine suppository** (e.g, 4 g glycerine) or a **phosphate enema**.
• If glycerine suppository/phosphate enema ineffective, or if no evidence of impaction, add **macrogol** one sachet twice daily (higher doses can be used in faecal impacton, see Figure 28.1)

If still constipated

Discuss with medical/surgical colleagues who may guide increased dose of macrogol and frequency of enemas, or consider use of a secretagogue (e.g, linaclotide) or prucalopride.

CHAPTER 28

Figure 28.2 Management algorithm for clozapine-related constipation. Source: based on the Porirua protocol (Every-Palmer et al. [9]).

Pharmacological

Where possible, rationalise use of medications that may be contributing to constipation. For psychiatric medications this might involve switching an antidepressant or antipsychotic to a treatment with lower anticholinergic burden. For example, avoid tricyclic antidepressants and consider switching to a selective serotonin reuptake inhibitor (apart from paroxetine), and consider switching antipsychotic treatment to agents such as aripiprazole, amisulpride, or risperidone. Where treatment cannot be switched, aim to use the minimum effective dose; this advice also applies to patients treated with clozapine. Liaise with primary care practitioners or medical colleagues if physical health medications are thought to be causative. For example, if oral iron supplementation is playing a role, consider if the patient is in fact iron deficient (and therefore needs supplementation), reducing the frequency of dosing, switching to an alternative iron salt, or switching to intravenous iron supplementation.

Laxatives

There are four main types of laxative, described in Box 28.3. For idiopathic constipation it is generally recommended to start with a bulk-forming laxative; note that this approach may be ineffective in clozapine-induced constipation (i.e. slow transit constipation; see section Special considerations with clozapine). If this is ineffective, an osmotic laxative can be tried instead of or as well as the bulk-forming laxative. Persistent constipation may require a stimulant laxative. It is essential to remember that long-term use of stimulant laxatives does not cause damage to, or impair functioning of, the bowel [15]. Persistent severe constipation may require use of glycerine suppositories (which helps to break down obstruction, with onset of efficacy in minutes) or a phosphate enema (onset of efficacy in minutes).

Box 28.3 Commonly used laxatives and their doses for treatment of idiopathic constipation in adults

Bulk-forming laxatives

Bulk-forming laxatives increase faecal mass and soften stool to stimulate a bowel motion. Onset of action is usually 48–72 hours. Examples include:

- Isphaghula husk (e.g. Fybogel), one sachet in water twice daily.
- Methylcellulose, three to six tablets twice daily.

Osmotic laxatives

Osmotic laxatives draw water into the bowel to soften stool. Onset of action is usually 24–72 hours. Examples include:

- Lactulose, dose adjusted according to response to 30–50 mL three times daily.
- Polyethylene glycol (also known as macrogol and Movicol). Dose for chronic constipation (non-proprietary 'full-strength sachets' or Movicol oral powder), one to three sachets daily. Dose for faecal impaction (non-proprietary 'full-strength sachets' or Movicol oral powder): four sachets on first day then increased in steps of two sachets daily up to a maximum of eight sachets daily (drink daily dose in 6 hours).

Emollient laxatives

Emollient laxatives are stool softeners. Onset of action is usually 24–72 hours. Examples include:

- Docusate sodium, up to 500 mg daily (as oral solution or capsule) in divided doses, adjusted according to response.

Stimulant laxatives

Stimulant laxatives stimulate the muscles of the gut lining and generally take 6–12 hours to work. Examples include:

- Senna, 7.5–15 mg once daily (usually at night) but higher doses may be prescribed under medical supervision (e.g. 45 mg in two to three divided doses; do not give more than 30 mg in a single dose).
- Bisacodyl, 10 mg once daily, increased up to 20 mg if necessary (usually at night).
- Sodium picosulfate, 5–10 mg once daily (usually at night).

Newer pharmacological agents

Lubiprostone (a prostaglandin E1 analogue) functions as an osmotic agent, acting on intestinal epithelial chloride channels to increase intestinal fluid secretion, and was previously licensed in the UK for management of chronic idiopathic constipation [16]. There is case-level evidence of its efficacy in the management of 'treatment-resistant constipation' associated with clozapine use [17]. However, lubiprostone (Amitiza) marketing in the UK was discontinued in 2018. Other secretagogues that are available include linaclotide (an oral guanylate cyclase C agonist licensed for the treatment of moderate to severe irritable bowel syndrome associated with constipation; dose 290 μg once daily) and plecanatide (also an oral guanylate cyclase C agonist licensed for treatment of chronic idiopathic constipation; dose 3 mg once daily). Neither linaclotide nor plecanatide have published evidence of efficacy in the treatment of clozapine-induced constipation, although absence of evidence is not evidence of absence [18]. Plecanatide is not currently available in the UK.

The prokinetic agent prucalopride is a selective 5-HT$_4$ receptor agonist that promotes gut peristalsis and thus gastrointestinal transit and can be used in chronic constipation when other laxatives fail to provide an adequate response (2 mg once daily). There is case-report level evidence supporting its use in the management of clozapine-induced constipation [19].

Opioid-induced constipation

Opioid-induced constipation (OIC) affects 40–90% of patients on long-term opioid therapy [20] but is also prominent in short-term use of opioid analgesics [21]. Osmotic laxatives (but not non-absorbable sugars like lactulose, which can ferment within the colon and exacerbate bloating and distension) and stimulants are first-line choices in the management of OIC [22]. Bulk-forming laxatives should be avoided due to an increased risk of bowel obstruction [23].

CHAPTER 28

Peripherally acting μ-opioid receptor antagonists (PAMORAs) such as naldemedine, naloxegol, and methylnaltrexone inhibit opioid binding in the gastrointestinal tract and as such decrease the constipating effects of opioids. Naloxegol and naldemedine should be used with caution alongside CYP3A4 inhibitors (e.g. fluvoxamine, diltiazem, verapamil, clarithromycin, systemic antifungals, and protease inhibitors) as resultant increased systemic levels of PAMORAs can antagonise the central effects of opioids and precipitate withdrawal. In such a scenario, the PAMORA dose may need to be reduced or indeed the drug stopped. As such, in patients with OIC who do not respond to standard laxatives and where PAMORAs are being considered, first discuss use with pharmacy, medical colleagues, or specialist pain services.

Special considerations with clozapine

The algorithm for management of clozapine-induced gastrointestinal hypomotility in Figure 28.2 is based on the Porirua protocol, a stepwise approach taken from the only prospective study of colonic transit time changes in clozapine-treated patients performed to date [9]. This pharmacological approach reduced colonic transit time in patients from a median of 110 hours at baseline to 62 hours and reduced prevalence of gastrointestinal hypomotility from 86% before treatment to 50% after treatment. General principles regarding management of clozapine-induced constipation are as follows.

- Pre-existing constipation should be managed prior to starting clozapine, i.e. provide lifestyle advice and start laxatives to ensure regular bowel motions before clozapine initiation.
- There is an argument that people taking clozapine should be offered prophylactic laxative treatment to prevent constipation (i.e. proactive rather than reactive treatment) [24].
- Patients receiving clozapine should recognise the importance of presenting to medical services if they become constipated.
- Prescribing clinicians should ask about clozapine-associated constipation at each clinical assessment [25].
- Where constipation occurs during clozapine initiation, a slow titration is recommended and use of the minimum effective dose (colonic transit times correlate with plasma clozapine levels) [9].
- Bulk-forming laxatives are not effective in slow-transit constipation and should therefore be avoided [26]. In contrast, stimulant laxatives should be used early. There are similarities between clozapine-induced and opioid-induced constipation in that they are both characterised by slow transit; therefore, osmotic laxatives such as macrogol (but not non-absorbable sugars such as lactulose; see preceding section) are a reasonable choice and can be considered early (alongside a stimulant laxative) instead of the emollient laxative docusate sodium (see Figure 28.2) [27].

When to refer to a specialist

Constipation can usually be managed by psychiatrists or in primary care, although a referral to medical/surgical colleagues may be necessary if investigations demonstrate a secondary cause, or if constipation persists despite the interventions described in this chapter. Early involvement of specialists may be necessary in the context of clozapine-induced gastrointestinal hypomotility.

References

1. Lewis SJ, Heaton KW. Stool form scale as a useful guide to intestinal transit time. *Gut* 1997;41:A122–A123.
2. Drossman DA. Functional gastrointestinal disorders: history, pathophysiology, clinical features and Rome IV. *Gastroenterology* 2016;150(6):1262–1279.
3. Suares NC, Ford AC. Prevalence of, and risk factors for, chronic idiopathic constipation in the community: systematic review and meta-analysis. *Am J Gastroenterol* 2011;106(9):1582–1591.
4. Sonnenberg A, Koch TR. Physician visits in the United States for constipation: 1958 to 1986. *Dig Dis Sci* 1989;34(4):606–611.
5. De Hert M, Dockx L, Bernagie C, et al. Prevalence and severity of antipsychotic related constipation in patients with schizophrenia: a retrospective descriptive study. *BMC Gastroenterol* 2011;11:17.
6. Jancar J, Speller CJ. Fatal intestinal obstruction in the mentally handicapped. *J Intellect Disabil Res* 1994;38(Pt 4):413–422.
7. Coleman J, Spurling G. Constipation in people with learning disability. *BMJ* 2010;340:c222.
8. Shirazi A, Stubbs B, Gomez L, et al. Prevalence and predictors of clozapine-associated constipation: a systematic review and meta-analysis. *Int J Mol Sci* 2016;17(6):863.
9. Every-Palmer S, Ellis PM, Nowitz M, et al. The Porirua protocol in the treatment of clozapine-induced gastrointestinal hypomotility and constipation: a pre- and post-treatment study. *CNS Drugs* 2017;31(1):75–85.
10. De Hert M, Hudyana H, Dockx L, et al. Second-generation antipsychotics and constipation: a review of the literature. *Eur Psychiatry* 2011;26(1):34–44.
11. Palmer SE, McLean RM, Ellis PM, Harrison-Woolrych M. Life-threatening clozapine-induced gastrointestinal hypomotility: an analysis of 102 cases. *J Clin Psychiatry* 2008;69(5):759–768.
12. Nielsen J, Meyer JM. Risk factors for ileus in patients with schizophrenia. *Schizophr Bull* 2012;38(3):592–598.
13. Bailey L, Varma S, Ahmad N, et al. Factors predicting use of laxatives in outpatients stabilized on clozapine. *Ther Adv Psychopharmacol* 2015;5(5):256–262.
14. Tramonte SM, Brand MB, Mulrow CD, et al. The treatment of chronic constipation in adults. A systematic review. *J Gen Intern Med* 1997;12(1):15–24.
15. Wald A. Is chronic use of stimulant laxatives harmful to the colon? *J Clin Gastroenterol* 2003;36(5):386–389.
16. National Institute for Health and Care Excellence. Lubiprostone for treating chronic idiopathic constipation. Technology appraisal guidance TA318. https://www.nice.org.uk/guidance/ta318.
17. Meyer JM, Cummings MA. Lubiprostone for treatment-resistant constipation associated with clozapine use. *Acta Psychiatr Scand* 2014;130(1):71–72.
18. Altman DG, Bland JM. Absence of evidence is not evidence of absence. *Aust Vet J* 1996;74(4):311.
19. Thomas N, Jain N, Connally F, et al. Prucalopride in clozapine-induced constipation. *Aust N Z J Psychiatry* 2018;52(8):804.
20. Chey WD, Webster L, Sostek M, et al. Naloxegol for opioid-induced constipation in patients with noncancer pain. *N Engl J Med* 2014;370(25):2387–2396.
21. Nilsson M, Poulsen JL, Brock C, et al. Opioid-induced bowel dysfunction in healthy volunteers assessed with questionnaires and MRI. *Eur J Gastroenterol Hepatol* 2016;28(5):514–524.
22. Farmer AD, Drewes AM, Chiarioni G, et al. Pathophysiology and management of opioid-induced constipation: European expert consensus statement. *United European Gastroenterol J* 2019;7(1):7–20.
23. Kumar L, Barker C, Emmanuel A. Opioid-induced constipation: pathophysiology, clinical consequences, and management. *Gastroenterol Res Pract* 2014;2014:141737.
24. Attard A, Iles A, Attard S, et al. Clozapine: why wait to start a laxative? *BJPsych Advances* 2019;25(6):377–386.
25. Cohen D, Bogers JP, van Dijk D, et al. Beyond white blood cell monitoring: screening in the initial phase of clozapine therapy. *J Clin Psychiatry* 2012;73(10):1307–1312.
26. Voderholzer WA, Schatke W, Muhldorfer BE, et al. Clinical response to dietary fiber treatment of chronic constipation. *Am J Gastroenterol* 1997;92(1):95–98.
27. Brandt LJ, Prather CM, Quigley EM, et al. Systematic review on the management of chronic constipation in North America. *Am J Gastroenterol* 2005;100(Suppl 1):S5–S21.

CHAPTER 28

Part 5

Renal and Urology

Urinary Retention

Atheeshaan Arumuham, Vimoshan Arumuham

Urinary retention describes the difficulty to voluntarily void urine, a presentation that may be acute or chronic. Acute urinary retention (AUR) is the most common urological emergency [1] and as such will form the predominant focus of this chapter. Causes of AUR include outflow obstruction (e.g. benign prostatic hyperplasia or BPH, urethral stricture, or infection causing inflammation) and neurological disorders (e.g. Parkinson's disease or diabetic neuropathy), with risk also increasing in postoperative and postpartum periods. AUR is up to 13 times more likely in males than females [2], with 86% of AUR episodes in the UK ascribed to men [3]. Within the general population, BPH is the most common cause of urinary retention [4].

Numerous drugs have been associated with urinary retention (Box 29.1) [5]. In particular, drugs with anticholinergic 'activity' pose a higher risk of precipitating retention. The reader is directed to www.medichec.com, a web-based application that provides an 'anticholinergic score' for individual drugs [6].

URINARY RETENTION AND SERIOUS MENTAL ILLNESS

Psychiatric medication represents a key cause of AUR in patients with serious mental illness (SMI). Furthermore, the prevalence of type 2 diabetes is higher in psychiatric patients [7]. The resultant autonomic neuropathy can precipitate urinary retention.

Control of micturition involves coordination of the autonomic, peripheral, and central nervous systems. The bladder receives direct autonomic input, with adrenoreceptors in the detrusor and internal sphincter promoting storage, while muscarinic receptors in the detrusor muscle receiving cholinergic input induce contraction [8]. Both dopaminergic and serotonergic signalling pathways have been implicated in central control of urinary voiding [9]. It is thus little surprise that various psychiatric medications, with

The Maudsley Practice Guidelines for Physical Health Conditions in Psychiatry, First Edition.
David M. Taylor, Fiona Gaughran, and Toby Pillinger.
© 2021 John Wiley & Sons Ltd. Published 2021 by John Wiley & Sons Ltd.

> **Box 29.1** Drugs associated with urinary retention [5]
>
> Drugs with anticholinergic effects
>   Antipsychotics
>   Antidepressants
>   Antispasmodics
>   Anti-Parkinsonian agents
>   Atropine
>   Class I antiarrhythmic agents
>   Histamine H_1 receptor antagonists
>   Anticholinergics prescribed for treatment of overactive bladder, chronic obstructive pulmonary
>   disease, and asthma
> Analgesia (opioids, non-steroidal anti-inflammatory drugs)
> Benzodiazepines
> Calcium channel antagonists
> α-Adrenoreceptor agonists

their broad receptor-binding profiles, can cause urinary retention. This risk may be compounded when multiple treatments are co-prescribed.

Antipsychotics differ in terms of their anticholinergic activity, which may play a role in the relative associated risk of AUR. Inhibition of noradrenergic reuptake [10] and central serotonergic effects [11] have also been implicated in the mechanisms underlying antipsychotic-induced AUR. Retention has been reported with phenothiazines (e.g. chlorpromazine) [12], haloperidol [13], olanzapine [12], quetiapine [12], risperidone [12], and ziprasidone at high doses (likely secondary to inhibition of noradrenergic reuptake) [14].

Of all the different antidepressants, tricyclics are more commonly associated with urinary retention [5], in particular amitriptyline and imipramine [15]. Episodes of AUR have been reported with the selective serotonin reuptake inhibitors sertraline [16] and escitalopram [17], potentially owing to central serotonergic effects [11].

There are reports of clonazepam [18], diazepam [19], and alprazolam [20] causing urinary retention, the proposed mechanism being a relaxant effect on the detrusor muscle that prevents voiding contraction.

DIAGNOSTIC PRINCIPLES

In AUR, the patient is typically in great discomfort and prompt catheterisation is required. This will not generally be possible in a psychiatric environment and if AUR is suspected the patient will need to be transferred to acute medical or urological services. In chronic presentations there may be an opportunity to take a history and perform basic examinations that will strengthen a referral to urology. This will almost certainly be required if the patient is a psychiatric inpatient where a urology review is being requested.

History

1 History of presenting complaint
   a Onset (sudden or prolonged) and duration (minutes to hours or months to years).
   b Nature of symptoms (painful or painless).
   c Characterise micturition:
      i frequency
      ii urgency
      iii hesitancy
      iv strength of urinary stream
      v post-micturition dribbling
      vi nocturia.
   d Course of symptoms (worsening, improving, or fluctuating).
   e Associated symptoms:
      i fever may suggest urinary tract infection
      ii constipation can result in AUR
      iii recent trauma and neurological symptoms may suggest cauda equina.
2 Past medical history
   a BPH/prostate cancer.
   b Recurrent urinary tract infection (see Chapter 41).
   c Diabetes mellitus (see Chapter 11).
   d Surgical history/postpartum.
   e Pelvic malignancy.
3 Medication review: note any recent additions or dose changes (see Box 29.1).
4 Social history: history of recreational drug use.

Examination

1 Basic observations including temperature.
2 Abdominal examination: suprapubic tenderness, distension, and dullness to percussion.
3 Neurological examination: in context of comorbid type 2 diabetes mellitus, the presence of a peripheral neuropathy may herald broader neurological dysfunction (i.e. an autonomic neuropathy). Spinal cord compression must be excluded in the presence of focal neurological deficits (saddle anaesthesia, lower limb motor weakness, and sensory deficits).
4 With a chaperone, consider examination of external genitalia:
   a Males: phimosis, balanitis, discharge.
   b Females: prolapse, acute vulvovaginitis, discharge.
5 With a chaperone, consider digital rectal examination:
   a Males: is the prostate enlarged?
   b Males and females: is there a rectal mass? Is there faecal loading?

Investigations

1 Urinalysis:
   a protein and glucose (diabetes mellitus)
   b blood (infection, stones, malignancy, trauma)
   c nitrites and leucocytes (infection)
   d send sample for microscopy, culture and sensitivity.
2 Bloods:
   a full blood count (white cell count for evidence of infection)
   b renal function (acute and/or chronic kidney failure)
   c inflammatory markers (C-reactive protein for evidence of infection)
   d glucose and HbA_{1c} (diabetes mellitus).
3 For inpatients, a bedside bladder scan (ultrasound), if available, can be useful in monitoring retention.

MANAGEMENT

As already discussed, acute management of AUR will require transfer of the patient to acute medical/urological services. Once retention has been relieved, focus will turn to deducing and treating the precipitant (e.g. infection, BPH).

Psychiatric input is indicated as part of a multidisciplinary approach if psychiatric treatment is felt to be causative. This may involve rationalisation of treatment, such as dose reduction or switching treatment to an agent with less anticholinergic activity. The reader is directed to www.medichec.com which may be used to guide treatment rationalisation (i.e. defining which drugs have greater anticholinergic activity and may therefore need switching).

If the effects of psychiatric treatment were indirect but still related to a drug that one wishes to continue (e.g. clozapine causing constipation which in turn precipitated AUR), then a management plan that better targets the side effects of treatment is indicated (in this case laxatives; see Chapter 28).

References

1. Marshall JR, Haber J, Josephson EB. An evidence-based approach to emergency department management of acute urinary retention. *Emerg Med Pract* 2014;16(1):1–20; quiz 21.
2. Klarskov P, Andersen JT, Asmussen CF, et al. Acute urinary retention in women: a prospective study of 18 consecutive cases. *Scand J Urol Nephrol* 1987;21(1):29–31.
3. Cathcart P, van der Meulen J, Armitage J, Emberton M. Incidence of primary and recurrent acute urinary retention between 1998 and 2003 in England. *J Urol* 2006;176(1):200–204.
4. Rosenstein D, McAninch JW. Urologic emergencies. *Med Clin North Am* 2004;88(2):495–518.
5. Verhamme KMC, Sturkenboom MCJM, Stricker BHC, Bosch R. Drug-induced urinary retention: incidence, management and prevention. *Drug Saf* 2008;31(5):373–388.
6. Bishara D, Harwood D, Sauer J, Taylor DM. Anticholinergic effect on cognition (AEC) of drugs commonly used in older people. *Int J Geriatr Psychiatry* 2017;32(6):650–656.
7. Mitchell AJ, Vancampfort D, Sweers K, et al. Prevalence of metabolic syndrome and metabolic abnormalities in schizophrenia and related disorders: a systematic review and meta-analysis. *Schizophr Bull* 2013;39(2):306–318.
8. Ochodnicky P, Uvelius B, Andersson KE, Michel MC. Autonomic nervous control of the urinary bladder. *Acta Physiol (Oxf)* 2013;207(1):16–33.

CHAPTER 29

9. Fowler CJ, Griffiths D, de Groat WC. The neural control of micturition. *Nat Rev Neurosci* 2008;9(6):453–466.

10. Walker NF, Brinchmann K, Batura D. Linking the evidence between urinary retention and antipsychotic or antidepressant drugs: a systematic review. *Neurourol Urodynam* 2016;35(8):866–874.

11. Ramage AG. The role of central 5-hydroxytryptamine (5-HT, serotonin) receptors in the control of micturition. *Br J Pharmacol* 2006;147:S120–S131.

12. Tueth MJ. Emergencies caused by side-effects of psychiatric medications. *Am J Emerg Med* 1994;12(2):212–216.

13. Crawford GB, Meera AM, Quinn SJ, et al. Pharmacovigilance in hospice/palliative care: net effect of haloperidol for delirium. *J Palliat Med* 2013;16(11):1335–1341.

14. Xomalis D, Bozikas VP, Garyfallos G, et al. Urinary hesitancy and retention caused by ziprasidone. *Int Clin Psychopharmacol* 2006;21(1):71–72.

15. Degner D, Grohmann R, Kropp S, et al. Severe adverse drug reactions of antidepressants: results of the German multicenter drug surveillance program AMSP. *Pharmacopsychiatry* 2004;37(Suppl 1):S39–S45.

16. Lowenstein L, Mueller ER, Sharma S, FitzGerald MP. Urinary hesitancy and retention during treatment with sertraline. *Int Urogynecol J* 2007;18(7):827–829.

17. Ferentinos P, Margaritis D, Douzenis A. Escitalopram-associated acute urinary retention in elderly men with known or latent benign prostatic hyperplasia: a case series. *Clin Neuropharmacol* 2016;39(6):327–328.

18. Caksen H, Odabas D. Urinary retention due to clonazepam in a child with dyskinetic cerebral palsy. *J Emerg Med* 2004;26(2):244.

19. Maany I, Greenfield H, Dhopesh V, Woody G. Urinary retention as a possible complication of long-term diazepam abuse. *Am J Psychiatry* 1991;148(5):685.

20. Aykut DS, Uysal RAE. Acute urinary retention after alprazolam use: a case report. *Psychiatry Clin Psychopharmacol* 2018;28(2):220–221.

CHAPTER 29

Chapter 30

Urinary Incontinence
Atheeshaan Arumuham, Vimoshan Arumuham

Urinary incontinence is the involuntary and inappropriate voiding of urine. Although prevalence estimates vary depending on the population studied, in the USA the age-standardised prevalence in the general population is approximately 51% in women and 14% in men [1]. There are various types and causes of urinary incontinence as described in Table 30.1.

Some risk factors for urinary incontinence, such as obesity [2], smoking [3], and excessive alcohol intake [4], are increased in patients with serious mental illness [5–7] and may play a role in the increased rates of incontinence (compared with the general population) in some patients with schizophrenia [8] and major depressive disorder [9]. It has also been proposed that there may be an overlap in the neurobiological/chemical aetiology of urinary incontinence and some psychiatric conditions [9–11]. Detrusor overactivity and resultant urinary incontinence has historically been proposed as a symptom of schizophrenia owing to putative disruption of neural control of bladder voiding [10], and alterations in serotonergic signalling have been proposed as a cause of urinary incontinence in depression [9]. Indeed, the noradrenaline and serotonin reuptake inhibitor duloxetine can be effective in the treatment of stress incontinence [11].

Rates of incontinence are also increased in patients with dementia owing to several neurobiological factors (e.g. impaired sensory function to sense bladder fullness, impaired higher cortical function to provide inhibition of the desire to void) and environmental issues (e.g. poor access to the toilet, poor manual dexterity to undress) [12]. Of note, there is a bidirectional relationship between urinary incontinence and mental illness. Rates of anxiety and depression are increased in patients with pre-existing urinary incontinence [13], and comorbid depression increases severity of urinary incontinence in patients with overactive bladder [14].

The Maudsley Practice Guidelines for Physical Health Conditions in Psychiatry, First Edition.
David M. Taylor, Fiona Gaughran, and Toby Pillinger.
© 2021 John Wiley & Sons Ltd. Published 2021 by John Wiley & Sons Ltd.

Table 30.1 Types of urinary incontinence.

Incontinence type	Features	Causes
Stress	Urine leakage secondary to abrupt increase in intra-abdominal pressure (e.g. cough, sneeze, laugh), combined with weakness of pelvic floor muscles More common in older women	Weakening of pelvic floor muscles (e.g. following pregnancy) Anti-adrenergic drugs (e.g. some antipsychotics, antihypertensives/treatments for prostatic enlargement, e.g. doxazosin, tamsulosin) leading to reduced urethral sphincter tone
Urge	Involuntary voiding of urine, preceded by an urgent, irrepressible need to void Often termed 'overactive bladder' Prevalent in both genders, and more common in older age Accounts for 40–80% of male urinary incontinence [17]	Atrophic urethritis in postmenopausal women Enlarged prostate in men (e.g. BPH or prostatitis) or after prostate surgery Diuretics (including alcohol and caffeine) leading to rapid bladder filling may worsen urge incontinence Infection (see Chapter 41)
Mixed	A combination of both stress and urge incontinence	
Overflow	Urinary leaking secondary to urinary retention with bladder distension Either caused by structural abnormality occluding normal flow of urine, or weakness of the detrusor muscles Increased intra-abdominal pressure may lead to exacerbation of leaking, so can be misdiagnosed as stress incontinence	Structural abnormalities (e.g. prostate enlargement, urethral narrowing) Neuropathic denervation of detrusor (e.g. diabetes neuropathy, surgery) Any drugs that can cause urinary retention, leading to overflow (see Chapter 29)

BPH, benign prostatic hypertrophy.

Antipsychotics have the potential to cause urinary incontinence, although the course is typically sporadic and self-limiting [15,16]. However, there is a strong association between urinary incontinence and clozapine; nocturnal enuresis (bed wetting) has been reported in up to 41% of clozapine-treated patients [17–19]. The mechanisms by which antipsychotic-induced urinary incontinence occurs are not clearly defined owing to the multiple physiological systems involved in the normal storage and excretion of urine that can be affected by these drugs. Nevertheless, there are several proposed mechanisms, including dopamine blockade in the basal ganglia leading to bladder hyperactivity, anticholinergic effects on the bladder wall causing retention and overflow incontinence, and anti-adrenergic activity causing relaxation of the bladder outlet and stress incontinence [20–23]. For clozapine, it has been postulated that although its anticholinergic effect should cause urinary retention (see Chapter 29), its strong serotonergic activity inhibits parasympathetic control of micturition leading to enuresis [24].

Antidepressants, namely selective serotonin reuptake inhibitors (SSRIs), have been associated with urinary incontinence, although this evidence is limited to case reports and in most cases antidepressants were used in combination with either antipsychotics or benzodiazepines [25–27]. Evidence to suggest that antidepressants are associated with urinary incontinence is further undermined by duloxetine's efficacy in treating stress incontinence in women, putatively via increasing urethral sphincter tone [11]. Benzodiazepine use, especially in the elderly, has been associated with urinary incontinence [28].

DIAGNOSTIC PRINCIPLES

History

1 Determine the nature of urinary incontinence using the features of stress and urge incontinence described in Table 30.1 as a guide. Ask if the patient is experiencing nocturnal enuresis. Incontinence that occurs without warning may point towards overflow.
2 Determine the speed of onset of incontinence and if there was a temporal relationship with medication change/dose adjustments.
3 Associated symptoms:
   a If there is increased urinary frequency, ask about symptoms of infection (see Chapter 41).
   b In men, ask about other features of prostatic hypertrophy (e.g. increased urinary frequency, nocturia, difficulty starting urination, weak urine stream, dribbling at the end of urination, and inability to completely empty the bladder).
   c Enquire if there have been any concurrent neurological symptoms (e.g. weakness/sensory disturbance in the legs or difficulty walking).
   d Ask if the patient is constipated (which can contribute to urinary incontinence) [29].
4 Past medical history:
   a Diabetes mellitus: poorly controlled disease may lead to increased urinary frequency and increased risk of urinary tract infection.
   b Obstructive sleep apnoea: has been associated with overactive bladder and urge incontinence [30,31].
   c Previous spinal cord injury/surgery (all patients), previous prostate surgery in men.
5 Social history:
   a Alcohol and smoking history.
   b Recreational drug use: chronic ketamine use can lead to sclerotic changes within the bladder that reduce functional bladder capacity, leading to lower urinary tract symptoms that include incontinence.
6 Medication review (see Table 30.1).

Examination

Weigh the patient and calculate body mass index (see Chapter 14). If there is evidence of infection, check basic observations including pulse, blood pressure, respiratory rate, oxygen saturation, and temperature (see Chapters 41 and 72).

CHAPTER 30

Further examination may not be necessary. Abdominal examination may be indicated where retention and overflow are suspected (palpable bladder), and a neurological examination should be performed in patients with evidence of neurology.

Baseline investigations

In the psychiatric setting, the only laboratory investigation that will usually be performed in the context of urinary incontinence is urinalysis alongside sending urine for microscopy, culture, and sensitivity if infection is suspected (see Chapter 41). In inpatients where retention is suspected and potential hydronephrosis, check renal function.

Where there is diagnostic uncertainty and the patient is referred to urology, further investigations may include ultrasound examination of the kidneys, ureters, and bladder (e.g. examining for retention, obstruction, and hydronephrosis), a bladder stress test (where stress incontinence is suspected), measurement of post-void residual (where retention is suspected), and urodynamic testing.

MANAGEMENT

Management of urinary incontinence is dependent on the cause, and the provision of most such interventions is clearly beyond the remit of the psychiatrist. However, psychiatrists are well placed to recommend and facilitate some non-pharmacological interventions that may improve certain types of urinary incontinence and which can improve the physical health of patients more broadly. Furthermore, where psychotropic medications are implicated in the pathoaetiology of incontinence, the psychiatrist will play a central role in rationalising drug interventions. Also, treatment of comorbid anxiety and depression in patients with pre-existing urinary incontinence improves physical health outcomes in these individuals [13,14]. A suggested management algorithm for clozapine-induced nocturnal enuresis is provided in Figure 30.1.

Non-pharmacological interventions

1 Where psychotropic medications are implicated in urinary incontinence, one approach is simply to observe the progression of symptoms: episodes of incontinence may be transient and resolve spontaneously.
2 Simple lifestyle modifications can be suggested. In cases of nocturnal enuresis, suggest reducing fluid intake in the evening (e.g. nothing to drink after 6 p.m.). If caffeine/alcohol is related to episodes of incontinence, advise reducing the amount of caffeine/alcohol consumed or consider a trial of abstinence. If appropriate, recommend that the patient stops smoking (see Chapter 46) and loses weight (see Chapter 14). If the patient stops smoking, be aware that blood concentrations of some psychiatric drugs (e.g. olanzapine, clozapine, and tricyclic antidepressants) may be altered (see Chapter 46 for further information).

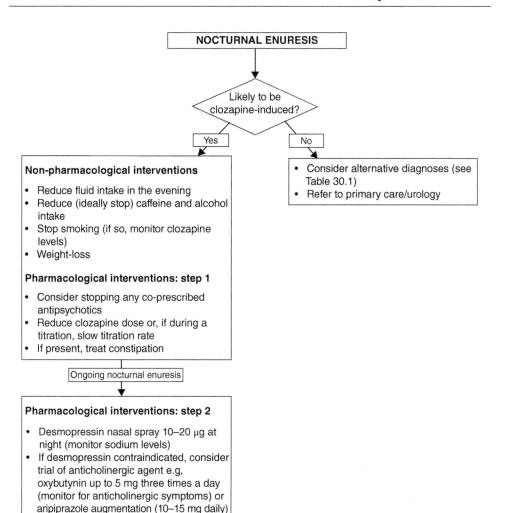

Figure 30.1 Suggested management of clozapine-induced nocturnal enuresis.

3 Some patients may need to be provided with absorbent pads or protective undergarments.

4 Pelvic floor/bladder training may be provided by specialist incontinence services, accessed either via primary care or urology [32].

Pharmacological interventions

1 Consider dose reduction/cessation of implicated psychotropic medications, having first weighed up the risks and benefits of such an action. If nocturnal enuresis occurs during a clozapine titration, consider the following: slow the rate of titration; take evening clozapine dose earlier (e.g. 6 p.m.) or, if tolerated, weight dose such that more is given in the morning; ideally stop any other co-prescribed antipsychotics.

CHAPTER 30

2 Treat comorbid constipation (see Chapter 28).

3 For perimenopausal women with stress/urge incontinence, consider use of topical vaginal oestrogen (see Chapter 63).

4 Duloxetine has been shown to be beneficial in the treatment of stress incontinence in women [11].

5 Men with benign prostatic hypertrophy may benefit from anti-adrenergic drugs (e.g. doxazosin, tamsulosin).

6 Anticholinergic agents such as oxybutynin, tolterodine, and darifenacin can be used in the treatment of urge incontinence as they reduce overactivity of bladder muscle and the feeling of urgency. However, caution should be taken in the prescription of such agents alongside psychotropic agents with their own anticholinergic effects; patients (especially those prescribed clozapine) should be monitored for the development of constipation among other anticholinergic symptoms (e.g. cognitive deficits). There is case report-level evidence to support the use of anticholinergic agents in the treatment of clozapine-induced nocturnal enuresis; in these reports, oral oxybutynin (up to 5 mg three times daily) [33] and oral trihexyphenidyl (up to 6 mg daily) [34] were reported as effective.

7 Desmopressin, which may be given orally, sublingually, or as a nasal spray, can be used to manage both urinary incontinence and nocturnal enuresis. There is case report-level evidence for the efficacy of desmopressin in the treatment of clozapine-induced nocturnal enuresis (most commonly given as a nasal spray 10–20 µg at night) [33,35–37]. However, patients should be monitored for the development of hyponatraemia [35]. Check sodium levels at baseline (before desmopressin initiation), and then the week and month following treatment initiation.

8 In terms of other pharmacological agents used in the management of clozapine-induced nocturnal enuresis, one study has observed efficacy of the adrenergic agonist ephedrine (150 mg/day) [38] and there is some evidence that aripiprazole augmentation (10–15 mg/day) can be effective [39]

When to refer to a specialist

Patients should be referred to primary care, urology, or a specialist incontinence service where incontinence is not clearly a consequence of psychotropic prescription, or where incontinence is persistent and chronic in nature despite attempts made to rationalise psychiatric medication. Beyond specialist investigations, urology colleagues will provide access to other treatment modalities for specific presentations, including surgical interventions.

References

1. Markland AD, Richter HE, Fwu CW, et al. Prevalence and trends of urinary incontinence in adults in the United States, 2001 to 2008. *J Urol* 2011;186(2):589–593.
2. Subak LL, Richter HE, Hunskaar S. Obesity and urinary incontinence: epidemiology and clinical research update. *J Urol* 2009;182(6 Suppl):S2–S7.
3. Tahtinen RM, Auvinen A, Cartwright R, et al. Smoking and bladder symptoms in women. *Obstet Gynecol* 2011;118(3):643–648.
4. Lee AH, Hirayama F. Is alcohol consumption associated with male urinary incontinence? *Low Urin Tract Symptoms* 2011;3(1):19–24.
5. Dickerson FB, Brown CH, Kreyenbuhl JA, et al. Obesity among individuals with serious mental illness. *Acta Psychiatr Scand* 2006;113(4):306–313.

CHAPTER 30

6. Lasser KE, Boyd JW, Woolhandler SJ, et al. Smoking and mental illness: a population-based prevalence study. *JAMA* 2000;284(20):2606–2610.

7. Petrakis IL, Gonzalez G, Rosenheck R, Krystal JH. Comorbidity of alcoholism and psychiatric disorders: an overview. *Alcohol Res Health* 2002;26(2):81–89.

8. Hsu WY, Muo CH, Ma SP, Kao CH. Association between schizophrenia and urinary incontinence: a population-based study. *Psychiatry Res* 2017;248:35–39.

9. Zorn BH, Montgomery H, Pieper K, et al. Urinary incontinence and depression. *J Urol* 1999;162(1):82–84.

10. Bonney WW, Gupta S, Hunter DR, Arndt S. Bladder dysfunction in schizophrenia. *Schizophr Res* 1997;25(3):243–249.

11. Jost WH, Marsalek P. Duloxetine in the treatment of stress urinary incontinence. *Ther Clin Risk Manag* 2005;1(4):259–264.

12. Sakakibara R, Uchiyama T, Yamanishi T, Kishi M. Dementia and lower urinary dysfunction: with a reference to anticholinergic use in elderly population. *Int J Urol* 2008;15(9):778–788.

13. Vrijens D, Drossaerts J, van Koeveringe G, et al. Affective symptoms and the overactive bladder: a systematic review. *J Psychosom Res* 2015;78(2):95–108.

14. Lai HH, Shen BX, Rawal A, Vetter J. The relationship between depression and overactive bladder/urinary incontinence symptoms in the clinical OAB population. *BMC Urol* 2016;16:60.

15. Berrios GE. Temporary urinary incontinence in the acute psychiatric patient without delirium or dementia. *Br J Psychiatry* 1986;149:224–227.

16. Ambrosini PJ, Nurnberg HG. Enuresis and incontinence occurring with neuroleptics. *Am J Psychiatry* 1980;137(10):1278–1279.

17. Harrison-Woolrych M, Skegg K, Ashton J, et al. Nocturnal enuresis in patients taking clozapine, risperidone, olanzapine and quetiapine: comparative cohort study. *Br J Psychiatry* 2011;199(2):140–144.

18. Lin CC, Bai YM, Chen JY, et al. A retrospective study of clozapine and urinary incontinence in Chinese in-patients. *Acta Psychiatr Scand* 1999;100(2):158–161.

19. Yusufi B, Mukherjee S, Flanagan R, et al. Prevalence and nature of side effects during clozapine maintenance treatment and the relationship with clozapine dose and plasma concentration. *Int Clin Psychopharmacol* 2007;22(4):238–243.

20. Yoshimura N, Kuno S, Chancellor MB, et al. Dopaminergic mechanisms underlying bladder hyperactivity in rats with a unilateral 6-hydroxy-dopamine (6-OHDA) lesion of the nigrostriatal pathway. *Br J Pharmacol* 2003;139(8):1425–1432.

21. Barnes TR, Drake MJ, Paton C. Nocturnal enuresis with antipsychotic medication. *Br J Psychiatry* 2012;200(1):7–9.

22. Tsakiris P, Oelke M, Michel MC. Drug-induced urinary incontinence. *Drugs Aging* 2008;25(7):541–549.

23. Ambrosini PJ. A pharmacological paradigm for urinary incontinence and enuresis. *J Clin Psychopharmacol* 1984;4(5):247–253.

24. Torre DL, Isgro S, Muscatello MR, et al. Urinary incontinence in schizophrenic patients treated with atypical antipsychotics: urodynamic findings and therapeutic perspectives. *Int J Psychiatry Clin Pract* 2005;9(2):116–119.

25. Votolato NA, Stern S, Caputo RM. Serotonergic antidepressants and urinary incontinence. *Int Urogynecol J Pelvic Floor Dysfunct* 2000;11(6):386–388.

26. Verhamme KM, Sturkenboom MC, Stricker BH, Bosch R. Drug-induced urinary retention: incidence, management and prevention. *Drug Saf* 2008;31(5):373–388.

27. Carvalho AF, Sharma MS, Brunoni AR, et al. The safety, tolerability and risks associated with the use of newer generation antidepressant drugs: a critical review of the literature. *Psychother Psychosom* 2016;85(5):270–288.

28. Landi F, Cesari M, Russo A, et al. Benzodiazepines and the risk of urinary incontinence in frail older persons living in the community. *Clin Pharmacol Ther* 2002;72(6):729–734.

29. Wood LN, Anger JT. Urinary incontinence in women. *BMJ* 2014;349:g4531.

30. Ipekci T, Cetintas G, Celik O, et al. Continuous positive airway pressure therapy is associated with improvement in overactive bladder symptoms in women with obstructive sleep apnea syndrome. *Cent Eur J Urol* 2016;69(1):78–82.

31. Kemmer H, Mathes AM, Dilk O, et al. Obstructive sleep apnea syndrome is associated with overactive bladder and urgency incontinence in men. *Sleep* 2009;32(2):271–275.

32. Dumoulin C, Hay-Smith J. Pelvic floor muscle training versus no treatment for urinary incontinence in women. A Cochrane systematic review. *Eur J Phys Rehabil Med* 2008;44(1):47–63.

33. Lurie SN, Hosmer C. Oxybutynin and intranasal desmopressin for clozapine-induced urinary incontinence. *J Clin Psychiatry* 1997;58(9):404.

34. Frankenburg FR, Kando JC, Centorrino F, Gilbert JM. Bladder dysfunction associated with clozapine therapy. *J Clin Psychiatry* 1996;57(1):39–40.

35. Sarma S, Ward W, O'Brien J, Frost AD. Severe hyponatraemia associated with desmopressin nasal spray to treat clozapine-induced nocturnal enuresis. *Aust N Z J Psychiatry* 2005;39(10):949.

36. Steingard S. Use of desmopressin to treat clozapine-induced nocturnal enuresis. *J Clin Psychiatry* 1994;55(7):315–316.

37. Aronowitz JS, Safferman AZ, Lieberman JA. Management of clozapine-induced enuresis. *Am J Psychiatry* 1995;152(3):472.

38. Fuller MA, Borovicka MC, Jaskiw GE, et al. Clozapine-induced urinary incontinence: incidence and treatment with ephedrine. *J Clin Psychiatry* 1996;57(11):514–518.

39. Rocha FL, Hara C. Benefits of combining aripiprazole to clozapine: three case reports. *Prog Neuropsychopharmacol Biol Psychiatry* 2006;30(6):1167–1169.

CHAPTER 30

Polyuria

Atheeshaan Arumuham, Toby Pillinger, Benjamin Whitelaw

Polyuria in adults is defined as a urine output exceeding 3 L/day. It should be differentiated from other urinary complaints such as increased urinary frequency or nocturia, which are not associated with increased total urine output. Common causes of polyuria are shown in Table 31.1. Major causes that should be considered in patients with serious mental illness (SMI) include the glucose-induced osmotic diuresis of diabetes mellitus, psychogenic polydipsia, and nephrogenic diabetes insipidus in the context of lithium use. Use of diuretics may also be considered in individuals with eating disorders. Primary polydipsia is present in more than 20% of inpatients with chronic psychiatric conditions, and is commonly seen in individuals with schizophrenia, those with developmental disability, and anxiety disorders [1–3]. The underlying pathoaetiology is unclear.

Table 31.1 Causes of polyuria.

Cause	Mechanism
Osmotic diuresis (e.g. diabetes mellitus)	Water follows non-reabsorbed solute (e.g. glucose) across the kidney tubules
Primary polydipsia	Excessive water intake
Central diabetes insipidus	Deficient pituitary antidiuretic hormone (ADH) secretion
Nephrogenic diabetes insipidus	Normal ADH secretion but renal resistance to its water-retaining effect

The Maudsley Practice Guidelines for Physical Health Conditions in Psychiatry, First Edition.
David M. Taylor, Fiona Gaughran, and Toby Pillinger.
© 2021 John Wiley & Sons Ltd. Published 2021 by John Wiley & Sons Ltd.

DIAGNOSTIC PRINCIPLES

Key points for determining the aetiology of polyuria are shown in Box 31.1.

Box 31.1 Key points in determining the aetiology of polyuria

- Distinguish true polyuria from increased urinary frequency.
- Evaluate sense of thirst and determine how much the patient is drinking.
- Paired (obtained at the same time) blood and urine samples for osmolality are often very useful.
- Serum tests to exclude diabetes mellitus and hypercalcaemia (HbA$_{1c}$ and bone profile) are essential.

History

1 Clarify if there is increased volume of urine or increased frequency of urination.
2 Determine if there is associated polydipsia.
3 Screen for associated symptoms:
   a urinary symptoms that may point towards infection/prostatism
   b weight loss may point towards diabetes mellitus, malignancy, or tuberculosis.
4 Past medical history:
   a diabetes mellitus (osmotic diuresis)
   b head trauma or pituitary surgery (central diabetes insipidus)
   c history of any infiltrative conditions, e.g. sarcoid (central diabetes insipidus).
5 Social history:
   a alcohol inhibits pituitary secretion of antidiuretic hormone (ADH)
   b recreational drug use, e.g. 3,4-methylenedioxymethamphetamine (Ecstasy) increases secretion of ADH and impact on serotonergic pathway causes polydipsia.
6 Family history of polyuria/excessive water drinking.
7 Medication review (e.g. diuretics, lithium).

Examination

1 Assess fluid status: check pulse, capillary refill time, skin turgor, assess for dry mucous membranes. Perform lying and standing blood pressure assessing for postural hypotension (see Chapter 6).
2 Assess body habitus: obesity may point towards diabetes mellitus, cachexia may point towards malignancy, tuberculosis, or an eating disorder.
3 Skin examination: hyperpigmented/hypopigmented lesions, ulcers, or subcutaneous nodules may suggest sarcoidosis (see Chapter 60). Lymphadenopathy may herald malignancy or infiltrative disorders.

Investigations

Urine

1 History alone will often distinguish polyuria from frequency, but occasionally a 24-hour urine collection may be required. The practicality of such an investigation in a psychiatric setting will be dependent on the patient's mental state.

Box 31.2 Interpretation of paired urine/serum osmolalities and sodium levels in the context of polydipsia and diabetes insipidus

- A low plasma sodium concentration (<137 mmol/L) with a low urine osmolality (e.g. less than half the plasma osmolality) is usually indicative of water overload due to psychogenic polydipsia.
- A high-normal plasma sodium concentration (>142 mmol/L) in conjunction with a urine osmolality that is lower than plasma osmolality points toward diabetes insipidus.
- A normal plasma sodium concentration is not helpful in diagnosis but, if associated with a urine osmolality of more than 600 mosmol/kg, excludes a diagnosis of diabetes insipidus.

2 Urine dip examining for evidence of infection (if so, send to the laboratory for microscopy, culture, and sensitivity), proteinuria (if concern about renal failure or diabetes mellitus), glucose, and ketones.
3 Urine osmolality and sodium levels paired with plasma osmolality and sodium levels (see Box 31.2 for interpretation).

Blood

1 Renal function, specifically:
  a sodium levels (see Chapter 32)
  b potassium levels (hypokalaemia may point towards diuretic use; see Chapter 33)
  c urea levels to assess for degree of dehydration
  d creatinine levels to assess for evidence of renal failure (see Chapters 34 and 73).
2 Plasma osmolality paired with urine osmolality (see Box 31.2).
3 Serum calcium levels (hypercalcaemia can induce polyuria).
4 Fasting/random glucose and HbA_{1c} levels.
5 If appropriate, lithium levels.

The gold standard test to differentiate between primary polydipsia and central and nephrogenic diabetes insipidus is the water restriction test, followed by (if appropriate) administration of desmopressin. However, such tests should only be performed in a specialist clinic.

MANAGEMENT

Diabetes mellitus

Uncontrolled diabetes mellitus results in an osmotic diuresis. Treatment involves optimising glycaemic control (see Chapter 11 for more details).

Psychogenic polydipsia

Treatment principles involve the following.

1 Optimum management of the underlying psychiatric disorder.
2 Fluid restriction to 1–1.5 L/day.

CHAPTER 31

3 Cognitive behavioural techniques and reinforcement schedules [4,5]. Most behavioural intervention studies are reported in hospitalised patients, often requiring close monitoring and a substantial time commitment from staff.
4 Pharmacological interventions:
   a clozapine has shown benefit in case reports and prospective trials [5–7]
   b risperidone and olanzapine improved polydipsia in case reports, but prospective double-blind studies have not shown any benefit with olanzapine [8–10]
   c demeclocycline (a tetracycline antibiotic) has historically been prescribed for polydipsia, although it has not been demonstrated to be effective in double-blind, placebo-controlled trials [11].
5 Concomitantly giving loop diuretics (e.g. furosemide) to enhance water excretion may be necessary, although should be discussed with medical colleagues first.

Nephrogenic diabetes insipidus

Central diabetes insipidus (DI) is associated with deficient secretion of ADH. Nephrogenic DI is characterised by normal ADH secretion but varying degrees of renal resistance to its water-retaining effect. Nephrogenic DI is far more likely to be seen in psychiatric patients owing to the prescription of lithium. Polyuria due to impaired urinary concentrating ability occurs in up to 20% of patients chronically treated with lithium; an additional 30% have a subclinical impairment in concentrating ability. These adverse effects are mediated by lithium entry into the principal cells in the collecting tubule via the epithelial sodium channel [12]. At cytotoxic concentrations, lithium inhibits signalling pathways that involve glycogen synthase kinase type 3 β (GSK3β), resulting in dysfunction of the aquaporin-2 water channel [12]. GSK3β knockout mice have a reduced response to vasopressin administration [13]. The effect is thought to be dose dependent and is usually reversible in the short to medium term, but may be irreversible after long-term treatment (>15 years) [12]. Treatment should be carried out alongside input from medical colleagues (e.g. renal/endocrine) and pharmacy; general principles are as follows.

1 Dose reduction of lithium, if possible.
2 Low-sodium, low-protein diet [15].
3 Thiazide diuretics in combination with a low-sodium diet. A thiazide diuretic (e.g. hydrochlorothiazide 25 mg once or twice daily) acts by inducing mild volume depletion. As little as 1–1.5 kg weight loss can reduce urine output by more than 50% (e.g. from 10 L/day to below 3.5 L/day in a study of patients with nephrogenic DI on a severely sodium-restricted diet [9 mEq/day]) [16]. This effect is thought to be mediated by a hypovolaemia-induced increase in proximal sodium and water reabsorption, thereby diminishing water delivery to the ADH-sensitive sites in the collecting tubules and reducing urine output. However, thiazide diuretics can dramatically increase plasma lithium levels; use together with caution and check lithium levels regularly [17].
4 The potassium-sparing diuretic amiloride can be used to decrease urine volume [18], with evidence for benefit in combination with thiazide diuretics in the context of lithium use [19].

5 Non-steroidal anti-inflammatory drugs (NSAIDs) reduce urine output via inhibition of renal prostaglandin synthesis, thereby combating the antagonistic actions of prostaglandins on ADH function. The net effect in patients with DI may be a 25–50% reduction in urine output [20,21], a response that is partially additive to that of a thiazide diuretic [21]. Indomethacin has a greater effect than ibuprofen in increasing ADH's actions on the kidney. However, use of concomitant NSAIDs with lithium requires close monitoring of renal function tests and lithium levels; co-prescription unpredictably increases risk of lithium toxicity with potentially fatal consequences [22]. NSAID use will also likely require gastroprotection, especially if a selective serotonin reuptake inhibitor is co-prescribed (see Chapter 19).

6 Desmopressin (DDAVP) may be tried in patients who have persistent symptomatic polyuria after implementation of the above regimen, as there is likely only a partial rather than complete resistance to ADH in nephrogenic DI. One case report of a patient with lithium-induced nephrogenic DI suggested that benefit may be more likely if desmopressin is combined with an NSAID (although note cautions regarding concomitant lithium and NSAID use already documented) [23].

Central diabetes insipidus

Central DI is generally treated with desmopressin (either orally or as a nasal spray) two to three times per day. If desmopressin is omitted there is a risk of dehydration; there have been cases of patients dying due to omission of desmopressin for 48 hours [24]. Thus, ensuring regular desmopressin administration in such patients is essential.

References

1. de Leon J, Verghese C, Tracy JI, et al. Polydipsia and water intoxication in psychiatric patients: a review of the epidemiological literature. *Biol Psychiatry* 1994;35(6):408–419.
2. de Leon J. Polydipsia: a study in a long-term psychiatric unit. *Eur Arch Psychiatry Clin Neurosci* 2003;253(1):37–39.
3. Illowsky BP, Kirch DG. Polydipsia and hyponatremia in psychiatric patients. *Am J Psychiatry* 1988;145(6):675–683.
4. Bowen L, Glynn SM, Marshall BD Jr, et al. Successful behavioral treatment of polydipsia in a schizophrenic patient. *J Behav Ther Exp Psychiatry* 1990;21(1):53–61.
5. Costanzo ES, Antes LM, Christensen AJ. Behavioral and medical treatment of chronic polydipsia in a patient with schizophrenia and diabetes insipidus. *Psychosom Med* 2004;66(2):283–286.
6. Leadbetter RA, Shutty MS Jr. Differential effects of neuroleptic and clozapine on polydipsia and intermittent hyponatremia. *J Clin Psychiatry* 1994;55(Suppl B):110–113.
7. Lee HS, Kwon KY, Alphs LD, Meltzer HY. Effect of clozapine on psychogenic polydipsia in chronic schizophrenia. *J Clin Psychopharmacol* 1991;11(3):222–223.
8. Kruse D, Pantelis C, Rudd R, et al. Treatment of psychogenic polydipsia: comparison of risperidone and olanzapine, and the effects of an adjunctive angiotensin-II receptor blocking drug (irbesartan). *Aust N Z J Psychiatry* 2001;35(1):65–68.
9. Goldman MB, Hussain N. Absence of effect of olanzapine on primary polydipsia: results of a double-blind, randomized study. *J Clin Psychopharmacol* 2004;24(6):678–680.
10. Rao N, Venkatasubramanian G, Korpade V, et al. Risperidone treatment for polydipsia and hyponatremia in schizophrenia: a case report. *Turk Psikiyatri Derg* 2011;22(2):123–125.
11. Alexander RC, Karp BI, Thompson S, et al. A double blind, placebo-controlled trial of demeclocycline treatment of polydipsia-hyponatremia in chronically psychotic patients. *Biol Psychiatry* 1991;30(4):417–420.
12. Grunfeld JP, Rossier BC. Lithium nephrotoxicity revisited. *Nat Rev Nephrol* 2009;5(5):270–276.
13. Rao R, Patel S, Hao C, et al. GSK3beta mediates renal response to vasopressin by modulating adenylate cyclase activity. *J Am Soc Nephrol* 2010;21(3):428–437.
14. Bowen RC, Grof P, Grof E. Less frequent lithium administration and lower urine volume. *Am J Psychiatry* 1991;148(2):189–192.
15. Wesche D, Deen PM, Knoers NV. Congenital nephrogenic diabetes insipidus: the current state of affairs. *Pediatr Nephrol* 2012;27(12):2183–2204.

CHAPTER 31

16. Earley LE, Orloff J. The mechanism of antidiuresis associated with the administration of hydrochlorothiazide to patients with vasopressin-resistant diabetes insipidus. *J Clin Invest* 1962;41(11):1988–1997.

17. Kim GH, Lee JW, Oh YK, et al. Antidiuretic effect of hydrochlorothiazide in lithium-induced nephrogenic diabetes insipidus is associated with upregulation of aquaporin-2, Na-Cl co-transporter, and epithelial sodium channel. *J Am Soc Nephrol* 2004;15(11):2836–2843.

18. Batlle DC, Vonriotte AB, Gaviria M, Grupp M. Amelioration of polyuria by amiloride in patients receiving long-term lithium-therapy. *N Engl J Med* 1985;312(7):408–414.

19. Knoers N, Monnens LAH. Amiloride–hydrochlorothiazide versus indomethacin–hydrochlorothiazide in the treatment of nephrogenic diabetes insipidus. *J Pediatr* 1990;117(3):499–502.

20. Libber S, Harrison H, Spector D. Treatment of nephrogenic diabetes insipidus with prostaglandin synthesis inhibitors. *J Pediatr* 1986;108(2):305–311.

21. Monnens L, Jonkman A, Thomas C. Response to indomethacin and hydrochlorothiazide in nephrogenic diabetes insipidus. *Clin Sci* 1984;66(6):709–715.

22. New Zealand Medicines and Medical Devices Safety Authority. Drug interactions with lithium and therapeutic drug monitoring. *Prescriber Update* 2017;38(3):36–38. Available at https://www.medsafe.govt.nz/Profs/PUArticles/September2017/Lithium.htm

23. Stasior DS, Kikeri D, Duel B, Seifter JL. Nephrogenic diabetes insipidus responsive to indomethacin plus DDAVP. *N Engl J Med* 1991;324(12):850–851.

24. NHS England. Patient Safety Alert (Stage One: Warning). Risk of severe harm or death when desmopressin is omitted or delayed in patients with cranial diabetes insipidus. https://www.england.nhs.uk/patientsafety/wp-content/uploads/sites/32/2016/02/psa-desmopressin-080216.pdf (8 February 2016).

Sodium Derangement
Atheeshaan Arumuham, Peter Conlon

Dysnatraemia is defined as serum sodium levels of either less than 135 mmol/L (hyponatraemia) [1] or more than 145 mmol/L (hypernatraemia) [2]. Hyponatraemia is one of the most frequently encountered electrolyte imbalances encountered in medical practice [3]. Hypernatraemia is less common, with a reported incidence of 0.3% in general medical inpatients [4]. Both presentations, when severe, represent potentially life-threating medical emergencies, resulting in seizure, coma, and death.

Common causes of dysnatraemia are summarised in Table 32.1. The most significant risk factor for derangements in sodium levels is increasing age [5]. Psychiatric patients represent a vulnerable cohort for both hyponatraemia and hypernatraemia. For example, abuse of laxatives and diuretics in patients with eating disorders may result in excessive gastrointestinal sodium losses [6,7]. These patients may also present with hypodipsia; compounding gastrointestinal losses with severe dehydration can result in either a rise or fall in serum sodium levels. Several psychiatric drugs, including antidepressants (especially selective serotonin reuptake inhibitors, SSRIs), antipsychotics, and mood stabilisers, can cause syndrome of inappropriate antidiuretic hormone secretion (SIADH) resulting in hyponatraemia [8–17]. Nephrogenic diabetes insipidus, which occurs in up to 40% of patients prescribed lithium [18], can result in hypernatraemia; the reader is directed to Chapter 31 for further details on on polyuria. Furthermore, patients with serious forms of mental illness may present with psychogenic polydipsia, thus leaving them vulnerable to electrolyte imbalances [13]. Crucially, electrolyte imbalance itself may manifest as an organic cause of psychiatric symptoms such as depression and anxiety [19].

The Maudsley Practice Guidelines for Physical Health Conditions in Psychiatry, First Edition.
David M. Taylor, Fiona Gaughran, and Toby Pillinger.

Table 32.1 Common causes of hyponatraemia and hypernatraemia.

	Hyponatraemia	Hypernatraemia
Hypovolaemic	Cerebral salt wasting (e.g. head injury, intracranial haemorrhage) Diuretics Gastrointestinal losses (diarrhoea/vomiting) Primary (Addison's), secondary (pituitary failure), and tertiary (hypothalamic failure) mineralocorticoid deficiency Osmotic diuresis (e.g. diabetic ketoacidosis) Renal tubular acidosis 'Third-spacing' (bowel obstruction/burns)	Diuretics Gastrointestinal losses (diarrhoea/vomiting) Osmotic diuresis NB These presentations involve both a reduction in total body water and sodium, but with a relatively greater reduction in total body water
Euvolaemic	3,4-Methylenedioxymethamphetamine (Ecstasy) consumption Beer potomania Glucocorticoid deficiency Hypothyroidism Psychogenic polydipsia Syndrome of inappropriate antidiuretic hormone secretion (SIADH) Water intoxication	Diabetes insipidus (nephrogenic or central) Hypodipsia
Hypervolaemic	Congestive cardiac failure Cirrhosis Nephrotic syndrome Renal failure (acute/chronic)	Excess intravenous administration of sodium-containing fluids Mineralocorticoid excess (e.g. Cushing's, hyperaldosteronism)

DIAGNOSTIC PRINCIPLES

History

Dysnatraemia is often asymptomatic, with symptoms generally only occurring in severe derangement. However, identifying precipitating factors is key to guiding management, and thus a detailed history and examination is necessary.

Aim to cover the following when exploring the history of the presenting complaint.

- Quantify recent water/fluid intake.
- Presence of thirst and/or a reduction in urine output.
- Recent diarrhoea, vomiting, or constipation.
- Weight loss or other red flags for malignancy, e.g. change in bowel habit, dysphagia (malignancy is associated with SIADH).
- Assess for features of adrenal insufficiency such as hyperpigmentation, postural hypotension. (If there are acute concerns about Addison's disease, patients should be seen and reviewed in the accident and emergency department.)
- The presence of neurological symptoms is suggestive of severe alterations in sodium levels, and include lethargy, headache, dizziness, confusion, decreased consciousness, and seizures.

A past medical and psychiatric history should screen for comorbid conditions that may be associated with dysnatraemia, including thyroid dysfunction, congestive cardiac failure, chronic kidney disease, cirrhosis, diabetes mellitus, and malignancy. Psychogenic polydipsia can occur in the setting of serious mental illness.

A comprehensive drug history should screen for medications commonly associated with derangements in sodium levels. These include diuretics, laxatives, steroids, and psychotropic or anticonvulsant drugs. A Danish register-based study of over 600,000 individuals compared risk of hyponatraemia in those prescribed and not prescribed antidepressants [20]. Risk of hyponatraemia was increased with virtually all antidepressants examined (amitriptyline, clomipramine, nortriptyline, citalopram, escitalopram, fluoxetine, paroxetine, sertraline, duloxetine, venlafaxine, and mirtazapine); only mianserin did not increase risk. The strongest association between hyponatraemia and antidepressants was found in SSRIs, with highest risk within the first two weeks of treatment. These findings are complemented by a systematic review of the available literature published in 2014 which observed that risk of hyponatraemia during antidepressant treatment was highest with SSRIs and venlafaxine and lower with mirtazapine [21]. It was also observed that risk of antidepressant-associated hyponatraemia increased with age and co-prescription of a thiazide diuretic.

Social history should screen for recreational drug use such as 3,4-methylenedioxymethamphetamine (Ecstasy) consumption and quantify alcohol intake (screening for beer potomania).

Examination

- Assess level of consciousness. If there are concerns regarding reduced consciousness, manage as per the ABCDE approach and transfer care to the emergency services (see Chapter 78).
- Check basic observations, assessing heart rate, blood pressure, respiratory rate, and oxygen saturation. Hypotension or orthostatic hypotension should raise concerns for hypovolaemia. Also check finger-prick blood glucose (may identify hyperglycaemia in context of diabetic ketoacidosis).
- Derangements in sodium are most commonly associated with regulation of water balance rather than a derangement in sodium per se, so determining the fluid status of the patient can provide rapid insight into the underlying pathoaetiology (see Table 32.1). As such, assess if the patient is hypovolaemic, euvolaemic, or hypervolaemic. Features of hypovolaemia include tachycardia, postural hypotension, prolonged capillary refill time, reduced skin turgor, and dry mucous membranes. Features of hypervolaemia can include peripheral oedema, raised jugular venous pressure, and bibasal crackles on lung auscultation (pulmonary oedema).
- Cachexia may indicate underlying malignancy or an eating disorder.
- Perform an abdominal examination to assess for bowel obstruction/constipation, or for evidence of liver dysfunction. Chapter 24 describes an appropriate examination where alcohol abuse is suspected.
- If appropriate, perform a thyroid examination (see Chapter 12).

CHAPTER 32

Investigations

Bloods

- A general rule: when presented with any electrolyte abnormality, repeat the test. As such, take repeat blood for electrolytes (sodium, potassium), alongside urea and creatinine. Creatinine levels will provide insight into renal function.
- Check serum lipid and protein levels; severely raised triglyceride and protein levels can occasionally be responsible for incorrect laboratory calculation of sodium levels (pseudohyponatraemia).
- Check serum calcium (hypercalcaemia can induce diabetes insipidus and polydipsia).
- Check HbA_{1c} to screen for diabetes mellitus.
- Check lithium levels if appropriate.
- Check brain natriuretic peptide levels if heart failure is suspected.
- Perform liver function tests.
- Checking serum osmolality paired with urine osmolality and sodium levels can provide insight into the underlying aetiology of dysnatraemia. Interpretation of paired urine/serum osmolalities in the setting of water overload and diabetes insipidus is discussed further in Chapter 31. SIADH is characterised by reduced plasma osmolality (<275 mosmol/kg), increased urine osmolality (>100 mosmol/kg), and raised urinary sodium levels (>20 mmol/L). An early morning urine osmolality (after fasting for six to eight hours) is useful for diagnosing diabetes insipidus; if the urine osmolality is greater than 400 mosmol/kg, it excludes severe diabetes insipidus.

Urine

- History can often distinguish polyuria from increased urinary frequency, but occasionally a 24-hour urine collection may be needed. Where diabetes insipidus is suspected, give the patient two collection jars as they may produce in excess of 8 L of urine. The practicality of such an investigation will depend on a patient's mental state.
- Perform a urine dip examining for proteinuria (if concerns about renal failure or diabetes mellitus), glucose, and ketones.
- As already discussed, consider testing urine osmolality and sodium levels, paired with serum osmolality and sodium levels.

MANAGEMENT

Hyponatraemia

It is recommended that management of acute hyponatraemia, severe hyponatraemia (<120 mmol/L), or symptomatic hyponatraemia occurs in a general medical setting [3]. These patients will require careful monitoring of electrolytes, controlled use of fluid resuscitation or diuresis, and management of the underlying pathology. When in doubt regarding the appropriate setting for a patient's management, discuss with medical colleagues.

Mild hyponatraemia in stable patients may be managed in a psychiatric setting according to the clinician's experience. Any degree of hyponatraemia should prompt a medication review, and rationalisation of treatments performed where one or more agents are implicated. Where antidepressant treatment is necessary in the setting of hyponatraemia, strongly consider stopping concurrent use of thiazide diuretics (after consultation with medical colleagues). Compared with other antidepressants, mirtazapine and mianserin have lower hyponatraemia risk profiles. Alternatives are agomelatine or bupropion.

In patients with chronic hyponatraemia in association with underlying conditions (i.e. liver, heart, or kidney failure), referral to corresponding specialties may be of benefit in elucidating how these patients can be managed within mental health teams or whether they require specialist assessment. Psychogenic polydipsia may be managed using psychoeducation, fluid restriction, and treatment of the underlying psychiatric disorder. There is evidence that clozapine improves polydipsia [22].

Hypernatraemia

The most common cause of hypernatraemia is secondary to gastrointestinal losses or excessive use of diuretics [23]. Where intravenous replacement of fluids is required, the patient should be transferred to a general medical hospital; uncontrolled correction can result in cerebral oedema [24]. If nephrogenic diabetes insipidus is suspected secondary to lithium, it is important that the patient is given free access to water. Management of nephrogenic diabetes insipidus is covered in Chapter 31.

References

1. Henry DA. In the clinic: hyponatremia. *Ann Intern Med* 2015;163(3):ITC1–19.
2. Muhsin SA, Mount DB. Diagnosis and treatment of hypernatremia. *Best Pract Res Clin Endocrinol Metab* 2016;30(2):189–203.
3. Spasovski G, Vanholder R, Allolio B, et al. Clinical practice guideline on diagnosis and treatment of hyponatraemia. *Intensive Care Med* 2014;40(3):320–331.
4. Long CA, Marin P, Bayer AJ, et al. Hypernatraemia in an adult in-patient population. *Postgrad Med J* 1991;67(789):643–645.
5. Chan TY. Drug-induced syndrome of inappropriate antidiuretic hormone secretion. Causes, diagnosis and management. *Drugs Aging* 1997;11(1):27–44.
6. Mascolo M, Chu ES, Mehler PS. Abuse and clinical value of diuretics in eating disorders therapeutic applications. *Int J Eat Disord* 2011;44(3):200–202.
7. Tozzi F, Thornton LM, Mitchell J, et al. Features associated with laxative abuse in individuals with eating disorders. *Psychosom Med* 2006;68(3):470–477.
8. Letmaier M, Painold A, Holl AK, et al. Hyponatraemia during psychopharmacological treatment: results of a drug surveillance programme. *Int J Neuropsychopharmacol* 2012;15(6):739–748.
9. Lien YH. Antidepressants and hyponatremia. *Am J Med* 2018;131(1):7–8.
10. Wilkinson TJ, Begg EJ, Winter AC, Sainsbury R. Incidence and risk factors for hyponatraemia following treatment with fluoxetine or paroxetine in elderly people. *Br J Clin Pharmacol* 1999;47(2):211–217.
11. Peterson JC, Pollack RW, Mahoney JJ, Fuller TJ. Inappropriate antidiuretic hormone secondary to a monamine oxidase inhibitor. *JAMA* 1978;239(14):1422–1423.
12. Kimelman N, Albert SG. Phenothiazine-induced hyponatremia in the elderly. *Gerontology* 1984;30(2):132–136.
13. Spigset O, Hedenmalm K. Hyponatraemia and the syndrome of inappropriate antidiuretic hormone secretion (SIADH) induced by psychotropic drugs. *Drug Saf* 1995;12(3):209–225.
14. Peck V, Shenkman L. Haloperidol-induced syndrome of inappropriate secretion of antidiuretic hormone. *Clin Pharmacol Ther* 1979;26(4):442–444.

CHAPTER 32

15. Van Amelsvoort T, Bakshi R, Devaux CB, Schwabe S. Hyponatremia associated with carbamazepine and oxcarbazepine therapy: a review. *Epilepsia* 1994;35(1):181–188.
16. Miyaoka T, Seno H, Itoga M, et al. Contribution of sodium valproate to the syndrome of inappropriate secretion of antidiuretic hormone. *Int Clin Psychopharmacol* 2001;16(1):59–61.
17. Mewasingh L, Aylett S, Kirkham F, Stanhope R. Hyponatraemia associated with lamotrigine in cranial diabetes insipidus. *Lancet* 2000;356(9230):656.
18. Grunfeld JP, Rossier BC. Lithium nephrotoxicity revisited. *Nat Rev Nephrol* 2009;5(5):270–276.
19. Gehi MM, Rosenthal RH, Fizette NB, et al. Psychiatric manifestations of hyponatremia. *Psychosomatics* 1981;22(9):739–743.
20. Leth-Moller KB, Hansen AH, Torstensson M, et al. Antidepressants and the risk of hyponatremia: a Danish register-based population study. *BMJ Open* 2016;6(5):e011200.
21. De Picker L, Van den Eede F, Dumont G, et al. Antidepressants and the risk of hyponatremia: a class-by-class review of literature. *Psychosomatics* 2014;55(6):536–547.
22. Kirino S, Sakuma M, Misawa F, et al. Relationship between polydipsia and antipsychotics: a systematic review of clinical studies and case reports. *Prog Neuropsychopharmacol Biol Psychiatry* 2020;96:109756.
23. Pfennig CL, Slovis CM. Sodium disorders in the emergency department: a review of hyponatremia and hypernatremia. *Emerg Med Pract* 2012;14(10):1–26.
24. Adrogue HJ, Madias NE. Hypernatremia. *N Engl J Med* 2000;342(20):1493–1499.

CHAPTER 32

Potassium Derangement

Ellis Onwordi, Peter Conlon

Derangements in potassium levels are common in the general medical patient population. Hypokalaemia occurs in approximately 2–3% of outpatients [1] and 20% of inpatients [2] while hyperkalaemia occurs in 0.2–0.7% of outpatients [1] and 1.4% of inpatients [3]. Rates of potassium abnormalities in patients with serious mental illness (SMI) are poorly defined. However, psychiatric patients represent a vulnerable cohort for renal disease that increases risk of hyperkalaemia (see Chapters 34 and 73). Furthermore, rhabdomyolysis, which can occur in the context of physical restraint or neuroleptic malignant or serotonin syndrome, can also result in hyperkalaemia. Some psychiatric disorders predispose to hypokalaemia owing to insufficient dietary potassium (e.g. in patients with eating disorders, catatonia, stupor, dementia, severe negative symptoms, or alcohol dependence). Severe derangements in potassium levels are medical emergencies owing to the associated risk of cardiac arrhythmia and arrest. Where patients are prescribed psychiatric medications that prolong the QT interval (see Chapter 3), derangements in potassium levels further increase the risk of torsade de pointes [4].

HYPERKALAEMIA

While there is no universally accepted definition of abnormally elevated extracellular potassium levels (hyperkalaemia), it is often defined as a serum potassium concentration of 5.5 mmol/L or greater [5,6]. It can be categorised as mild (5.5–5.9 mmol/L), moderate (6.0–6.4 mmol/L), and severe (≥6.5 mmol/L) [5]. As shown in Box 33.1, hyperkalaemia is caused by one or a combination of excessive potassium intake, reduced renal

The Maudsley Practice Guidelines for Physical Health Conditions in Psychiatry, First Edition.
David M. Taylor, Fiona Gaughran, and Toby Pillinger.

Box 33.1 Common causes of raised potassium [8]

Excessive intake

- Dietary (foods high in potassium, e.g. bananas, dried fruit)
- Excessive iatrogenic potassium supplementation or use of potassium-containing laxatives (e.g. Movicol and Fybogel)
- Red blood cell transfusion
- Pica

Insufficient excretion

- Acute kidney injury (AKI; see Chapter 73)
- Chronic kidney disease (CKD; see Chapter 34)
- Decreased renal blood flow (AKI/CKD, cirrhosis, congestive heart failure)
- Drugs: angiotensin-converting enzyme inhibitors, angiotensin receptor blockers, non-steroidal anti-inflammatories, spironolactone
- Primary renal tubular disorders:
  - Sickle cell disease
  - Obstructive uropathy
  - Amyloidosis
  - Systemic lupus erythematosus
  - Tubular defects
- Hypoaldosteronism (e.g. Addison's)

Transcellular shift

- Insulin deficiency or resistance
- Metabolic acidosis
- Medications (e.g. beta-blockers, digoxin)
- Cell breakdown (e.g. rhabdomyolysis, haemolysis)
- Genetic (e.g. hyperkalaemic periodic paralysis)

---

potassium excretion, or transcellular potassium shifts [7]. Pseudohyperkalaemia is where laboratory test results erroneously report hyperkalaemia; the most common cause is haemolysis of blood cells owing to poor blood-drawing/handling technique or samples being left for prolonged periods before being analysed.

Diagnostic principles

Severe hyperkalaemia is a medical emergency. When a potassium level of ≥6.0mmol/L is recorded in a psychiatric inpatient setting, the patient should be immediately assessed using the ABC approach with an ECG performed. In an outpatient setting, and in the absence of facilities to allow appropriate clinical assessment, the patient will likely require assessment in an Accident and Emergency department. If possible, check previous blood test results; chronic hyperkalaemia is generally better tolerated that an acute rise in potassium.

History

1 Symptoms:
   a Many patients are asymptomatic. Severe hyperkalaemia can be associated with weakness, flaccid paralysis, and paraesthesia. Arrhythmia may be accompanied by palpitations, shortness of breath, and chest pain.
   b Screen for symptoms indicative of an underlying pathoaetiology, e.g. recent diarrhoea/vomiting if concerns regarding volume depletion, or fatigue, weight loss, and abdominal pain that may accompany Addison's disease.
2 Past medical history: screen for chronic kidney disease. If patients are receiving dialysis, determine the time since last dialysis, any recent complications during dialysis (e.g. insufficient duration), or non-compliance with dialysis or a low-potassium diet.
3 Drug history (see Box 33.1).

Examination

1 Check basic observations, assessing heart rate, blood pressure, respiratory rate, and oxygen saturation. Also check finger-prick blood glucose.
2 Assess volume status and examine for potential causes of acute kidney injury (AKI)/chronic kidney disease (CKD) (see Chapters 34 and 73). If creatinine is raised, the patient is a poor historian, previously not known to services, and with an unclear past medical history, examine for evidence of dialysis access (central venous catheter, peritoneal dialysis catheter, arteriovenous fistula). Assess for features of adrenal insufficiency (e.g. hyperpigmentation, postural hypotension).
3 Perform a cardiac examination for evidence of arrhythmia or cardiac failure (e.g. pulmonary oedema).

Investigations

1 Bloods that are generally available in a psychiatric setting:
   a repeat serum potassium (rule out pseudohyperkalaemia)
   b urea, electrolytes, and creatinine
   c creatine kinase (if rhabdomyolysis, neuroleptic malignant syndrome, or serotonin syndrome suspected)
   d morning (9 a.m.) cortisol if suspicion of Addison's (hyponatraemia alongside hyperkalaemia may be indicative of adrenal insufficiency).*
2 Perform an ECG in all patients with potassium in excess of 6.0 mmol/L. ECG features of hyperkalaemia include:
   a tented T waves (larger than R wave in more than one lead)
   b flattened/absent P waves
   c prolonged PR interval (>200 ms)
   d ST depression
   e widened QRS complex (>120 ms)

---

*If there are acute concerns about Addison's, patients should be seen and reviewed in the accident and emergency department.

f QRS complexes merging with T waves ('sine-wave' pattern)
g sinus bradycardia
h ventricular tachycardia.

A widened QRS complex, sine-wave pattern, bradycardia, and ventricular tachycardia are associated with a high risk of cardiac arrest. Of note, even in the presence of severe hyperkalaemia, ECG changes may not occur. Thus, a normal ECG does not mean that escalation of care is not indicated. However, the presence of ECG changes should prompt urgent action.

Management [9]

The principles of the treatment of hyperkalaemia are as follows [10].

1 Protect the heart.
2 Shift potassium into cells.
3 Remove potassium from the body.
4 Assess medications. Most cases of hyperkalaemia result from use of angiotensin-converting enzyme inhibitors, angiotensin receptor blockers, or spironolactone. Assess dietary potassium intake and advise low potassium diet (no bananas, oranges, orange juice, or tomatoes).
5 Monitor potassium over time.
6 Prevent recurrence.

Realistically, only mild hyperkalaemia without ECG changes can be managed in a psychiatric setting, and any treatment should be guided by the skillset of the clinician and available facilities. To reiterate, patients with more advanced hyperkalaemia and/or associated ECG changes must be managed as a medical emergency and referred urgently to acute medical colleagues. In a psychiatric setting this will likely involve calling an ambulance. When in doubt, discuss with general medical colleagues.

The exchange resin oral calcium resonium (15 g q.d.s.), which shifts potassium across the intestinal wall, can be used to remove potassium from the body. Glucose/insulin intravenous infusion (50 mL 50% glucose containing 5–10 units of short-acting insulin over 15 minutes) and nebulised salbutamol (10–20 mg) shift potassium into cells. Of these three options, only oral calcium resonium is likely to be available in an inpatient psychiatric setting. Such an intervention may be considered in patients with mild hyperkalaemia while also treating/managing the underlying precipitant (e.g. stopping a causative drug; see Box 33.1).

Intravenous calcium salts (calcium chloride or calcium gluconate) antagonise cardiac membrane excitability and thus protect the heart. This intervention, alongside other interventions such as sodium bicarbonate infusion if the patient is acidotic and haemodialysis, may be considered by medical colleagues.

HYPOKALAEMIA

Hypokalaemia is the most common electrolyte disturbance in general medical patients [11]. It is defined as a serum potassium concentration below 3.5 mmol/L [12]. It can be categorised as mild (3.0–3.5 mmol/L), moderate (2.5–3.0 mmol/L), and severe (<2.5 mmol/L) [10]. As shown in Box 33.2, hypokalaemia is caused by one or a combination

Box 33.2 Causes of reduced serum potassium [8]

Insufficient intake

- Anorexia
- Bulimia
- Starvation
- Dementia
- Alcohol excess
- Total parenteral nutrition

Excessive losses

- Medications:
  - Diuretics
  - Laxative abuse
  - Enemas
  - Corticosteroids
- Gastrointestinal losses
  - Vomiting
  - Diarrhoea
  - Villous adenoma
  - Intestinal fistula
  - Ileostomy
- Renal losses
  - Osmotic diuresis
  - Mineralocorticoid excess
  - Renal tubular acidosis
  - Polydipsia
  - Intrinsic renal transport defects
- Endocrine
  - Cushing's syndrome
  - Hyperaldosteronism
  - Conn's syndrome
- Primary renal tubular disorders
  - Sickle cell disease
  - Obstructive uropathy
  - Amyloidosis
  - Systemic lupus erythematosus
  - Hereditary tubular defects
- Dialysis (haemodialysis using a low potassium dialysate, peritoneal dialysis)
- Hypomagnesaemia

Transcellular shift

- Medication, e.g. insulin, β_2 agonists (e.g. salbutamol)
- Refeeding syndrome
- Increased β_2 adrenergic stimulation:
  - Head injury
  - Delirium tremens
  - Myocardial ischaemia
  - Hypothermia
- Thyrotoxicosis
- Alkalosis
- Genetic (e.g. familial hypokalaemic periodic paralysis)

of excessive potassium loss, cellular shift of potassium out of the blood into cells, and decreased potassium intake. Most cases are due to medication and gastrointestinal disease (e.g. diarrhoea).

Diagnostic principles

History

1 Symptoms:
   a Mild hypokalaemia is generally asymptomatic; however, as hypokalaemia becomes more pronounced, patients can develop generalised weakness, fatigue, cramps, paraesthesia, and constipation.
   b In severe hypokalaemia, cardiac arrhythmia, ascending paralysis, tetany, respiratory failure, ileus, and rhabdomyolysis may occur.
   c Screen for signs or symptoms associated with causative pathology, e.g. diarrhoea/vomiting of gastroenteritis, presence of purging behaviour in the context of an eating disorder, evidence of thyrotoxicosis or of alcohol dependence.
2 Document past medical history for conditions associated with hypokalaemia (see Table 2). Furthermore, enquire as to a history of cardiovascular disease: the probability of symptoms associated with hypokalaemia increases in the presence of pre-existing heart disease [12].
3 Drug history (see Box 33.2).
4 Social history: define quantity and frequency of alcohol consumption.

Examination

1 Check basic observations, assessing heart rate, blood pressure, respiratory rate, and oxygen saturation.
2 Perform a general examination assessing for cachexia (insufficient oral intake of potassium) or features of purging behaviour in eating disorders (e.g. calluses/scars on fingers).
3 If appropriate, perform a thyroid examination if concerns regarding thyrotoxicosis (see Chapter 12). Chapter 24 describes an appropriate examination where alcohol abuse is suspected.
4 Perform a cardiac examination for evidence of arrhythmia or cardiac failure (e.g. pulmonary oedema).

Investigations

1 Consider performing the following blood tests.
   a Repeat urea, electrolytes (sodium and potassium), and creatinine to confirm hypokalaemia.
   b Also check serum magnesium (hypomagnesaemia is associated with hypokalaemia; low levels of both magnesium and potassium increase risk of cardiac arrhythmia) and thyroid function tests if concerns regarding thyrotoxicosis.

2 Perform an ECG in all patients with potassium below 3.5 mmol/L. ECG changes may be absent, but severe hypokalaemia may be associated with U waves (a small deflection immediately following the T wave, usually in the same direction as the T wave), T-wave flattening, or ST segment changes.

Management

Treatment is guided by the extent of hypokalaemia, the presence of symptoms, and associated ECG changes. The principles of treatment of hypokalaemia are as follows.

1 Replace potassium.
2 Identify and address underlying cause.
3 Prevent recurrence.

Stable patients with mild hypokalaemia typically require only oral potassium replacement therapy with potassium chloride, which may be provided in a psychiatric setting. Effervescent tablets (e.g. Sando-K), which each contain 12 mmol of potassium and 8 mmol of chloride, are preferable over modified-release tablets (e.g. SlowK) which may cause gastric irritation. For plasma potassium levels of 3.0–3.5 mmol/L, an appropriate starting dose is Sando-K two tablets three times daily, accompanied by twice-weekly monitoring of potassium. Once plasma potassium levels are stable or if potassium is above 4.5 mmol/L, reassess need for supplementation. Regardless of the preparation of potassium used (different countries may use different products), a dose of 20 mmol/day of potassium in oral form is generally sufficient for the prevention of hypokalaemia, and 40–100 mmol/day enough for its treatment [13]. It would be unwise to manage plasma potassium levels of 2.5–2.9 mmol/L using oral potassium preparations as these patients typically have a total body deficit of potassium of between 100 and 200 mmol and will likely require intravenous supplementation. It is recommended that these patients are discussed with medical colleagues to assess need for intravenous potassium replacement. Severe hypokalaemia (<2.5 mmol/L) or any degree of hypokalaemia with associated ECG changes should prompt urgent medical referral for intravenous supplementation.

Efforts should also be made to identify and address the underlying cause of hypokalaemia. This may be obvious in the case of malnutrition or diarrhoea/vomiting. Medications such as loop/thiazide diuretics may be implicated and need review, although changes to such treatment should not be attempted without prior discussion with medical colleagues. For persistent hypokalaemia, a diet high in potassium may be necessary (i.e. rich in bananas, oranges, and tomatoes).

References

1. Liamis G, Rodenburg EM, Hofman A, et al. Electrolyte disorders in community subjects: prevalence and risk factors. *Am J Med* 2013;126(3):256–263.
2. Paice BJ, Paterson KR, Onyanga-Omara F, et al. Record linkage study of hypokalaemia in hospitalized patients. *Postgrad Med J* 1986;62(725):187–191.
3. Paice B, Gray JM, McBride D, et al. Hyperkalaemia in patients in hospital. *BMJ* 1983;286(6372):1189–1192.

4. Drew BJ, Ackerman MJ, Funk M, et al. Prevention of torsade de pointes in hospital settings: a scientific statement from the American Heart Association and the American College of Cardiology Foundation. *J Am Coll Cardiol*. 2010;55(9):934–947.

5. Soar J, Perkins GD, Abbas G, et al. European Resuscitation Council Guidelines for Resuscitation 2010 Section 8. Cardiac arrest in special circumstances: Electrolyte abnormalities, poisoning, drowning, accidental hypothermia, hyperthermia, asthma, anaphylaxis, cardiac surgery, trauma, pregnancy, electrocution. *Resuscitation* 2010;81(10):1400–1433.

6. Nyirenda MJ, Tang JI, Padfield PL, Seckl JR. Hyperkalaemia. *BMJ* 2009;339:b4114.

7. Evans KJ, Greenberg A. Hyperkalemia: a review. *J Intensive Care Med* 2005;20(5):272–290.

8. Viera AJ, Wouk N. Potassium disorders: hypokalemia and hyperkalemia. *Am Fam Physician* 2015;92(6):487–495.

9. Alfonzo A, Soar J, MacTier R, et al. Treatment of acute hyperkalaemia in adults. UK Renal Association: Clinical Practice Guidelines. Final revision March 2014. https://renal.org/wp-content/uploads/2017/06/hyperkalaemia-guideline-1.pdf

10. Alfonzo AV, Isles C, Geddes C, Deighan C. Potassium disorders: clinical spectrum and emergency management. *Resuscitation* 2006;70(1):10–25.

11. Rastegar A, Soleimani M. Hypokalaemia and hyperkalaemia. *Postgrad Med J* 2001;77(914):759–764.

12. Gennari FJ. Hypokalemia. *N Engl J Med* 1998;339(7):451–458.

13. Cohn JN, Kowey PR, Whelton PK, Prisant LM. New guidelines for potassium replacement in clinical practice: a contemporary review by the National Council on Potassium in Clinical Practice. *Arch Intern Med* 2000;160(16):2429–2436.

Chronic Kidney Disease

Ellis Onwordi, Toby Pillinger, Anne Connolly, Peter Conlon

Chronic kidney disease (CKD) is defined as deterioration in kidney function or kidney damage lasting for at least three months [1]. Deterioration in kidney function is often identified as a reduction in glomerular filtration rate (GFR), usually estimated from blood creatinine (eGFR). eGFR is calculated from serum creatine, race, sex, and age; if eGFR is not provided by a laboratory, there are several online calculators.* From the eGFR, patients can be categorised into one of five stages of CKD (Table 34.1). Damage to the kidney may be identified indirectly by identification of blood or albumin (available from urine dipstick or laboratory measurement) in the urine. End-stage renal disease is CKD requiring dialysis or transplantation.

CKD represents a heterogeneous group of disorders, with many causes (Box 34.1). It is common, with a global mean prevalence (accounting for all stages of the disease) of 13.4% [2]. Compared with the general population, there is a higher prevalence of CKD in patients with severe mental illness (SMI), in particular schizophrenia and bipolar affective disorder [3–6]. This is likely secondary to increased rates of physical comorbidity associated with development of CKD such as diabetes mellitus and hypertension [7–10], as well as the nephrotoxic effects of some psychiatric drugs. Most notably, lithium is directly nephrotoxic [11], although case reports suggest that direct nephrotoxicity can (rarely) occur with other psychotropic agents [12–17]. Furthermore, the anticholinergic effects of some psychiatric drugs can cause urinary retention which, via

---

*Estimated glomerular filtration rate can be determined using various equations, including the Cockcroft–Gault formula (an online calculator is available at https://www.mdcalc.com/creatinine-clearance-cockcroft-gault-equation) or the Chronic Kidney Disease Epidemiology Collaboration (CKD-EPI) formula (https://www.kidney.org/professionals/kdoqi/gfr_calculator). Note that the CKD-EPI formula is more accurate; however, the Cockcroft–Gault formula should usually be used to determine appropriate drug doses since this is the formula used in the literature to calculate most (but not all) current dose recommendations.

The Maudsley Practice Guidelines for Physical Health Conditions in Psychiatry, First Edition. David M. Taylor, Fiona Gaughran, and Toby Pillinger.

Table 34.1 Stages of chronic kidney disease based on glomerular filtration rate (GFR) and degree of albuminuria (albumin excretion rate, AER) [1].

GFR stages	GFR (mL/min per 1.73 m²)	Interpretation
G1	≥90	Normal
G2	60–89	Mildly decreased
G3a	45–59	Mildly to moderately decreased
G3b	30–44	Moderately to severely decreased
G4	15–29	Severely decreased
G5	<15	Kidney failure ('5D' if treated with dialysis)
Albuminuria stages	AER (mg/day)	
A1	<30	Normal to mildly increased
A2	30–300	Moderately increased
A3	>300	Severely increased

hydronephrosis, may damage the kidneys [18,19]. Of note, the relationship between CKD and psychiatric disorders is bidirectional. For example, patients with CKD undergoing renal replacement therapy exhibit high rates of depression and anxiety [20,21].

CKD is associated with increased all-cause mortality, although the leading cause of death in this group is cardiovascular disease [22–24]. CKD is also associated with a number of other complications which reflect diminished endocrine and/or exocrine function. These include, depending on the severity of CKD, increased risk of acute kidney injury (see Chapter 73), anaemia (secondary to reduced renal erythropoietin synthesis capacity), hypertension, dyslipidaemia, mineral bone disorders, metabolic acidosis, electrolyte abnormalities most notably hyperphosphataemia and hyperkalaemia (see Chapter 33), hyperparathyroidism, infection, uraemia (symptoms/complications of which can include pruritis, restless legs syndrome, sleep disturbance, fatigue, sexual dysfunction, anorexia and cachexia, bleeding, pericarditis, and encephalopathy), thyroid dysfunction (see Chapter 12), and increased risk of drug toxicity owing to accumulation of renally excreted agents [1,25–27].

There are various clinical scenarios in which a psychiatric practitioner may need to consider CKD as part of the holistic care they provide patients. The first scenario, usually encountered in an inpatient setting, is determining whether a patient with raised serum creatinine is presenting with an acute or a chronic kidney injury, as this will determine the urgency with which subsequent investigations are performed. The second scenario, again generally encountered in an inpatient setting, is dealing with the complications of CKD, such as electrolyte disturbance or the accumulation of renally excreted drugs such as lithium. The third scenario, which occurs in both inpatient and outpatient settings, is supporting patients with established CKD to reduce the risk of worsening renal disease via control of risk factors such as smoking, hypertension, and diabetes mellitus. The fourth scenario, again pertinent to all clinical

---

Box 34.1 Causes of chronic kidney disease

Diabetes mellitus

- Hypertension
- Obesity
- Obstructive uropathy
- Glomerulonephritis
- Chronic interstitial nephritis
- Polycystic kidney disease
- Autoimmune disease
- Genetic
- Malignancy

Infections (examples)

- Human immunodeficiency virus
- Hepatitis B and C
- Malaria
- Schistosomiasis
- Leptospirosis
- Hantavirus
- Scrub typhus

Drug toxicity (examples)

- Lithium
- Non-steroidal anti-inflammatory drugs
- Chemotherapy
- Proton pump inhibitors
- Antimicrobial agents
- Some herbal medicines (e.g. *Aristolochia* species)

---

settings, is appropriate prescription of psychiatric medication in the context of CKD, be that drugs that are directly nephrotoxic (lithium) or those indirectly nephrotoxic (e.g. metabolic effects of some antipsychotics and mood stabilisers), drugs that are predominantly renally excreted and thus may accumulate (e.g. lithium, sulpiride, and amisulpride), or drugs with side effects that may be amplified in the context of reduced renal excretion (e.g. sedative effects of benzodiazepines or anticholinergic effects of tricyclic antidepressants).

DIAGNOSTIC PRINCIPLES

Promptly determining whether a blood test result represents an acute or chronic deterioration in kidney function is paramount. As such, it is recommended that previous blood test results, where available, are checked early. The reader is directed to Chapter 73 on acute kidney injury where such a presentation is suspected.

History

Chronic kidney disease is usually asymptomatic, with signs and symptoms only arising in later stages of illness in the context of the complications detailed previously. However, non-specific symptoms such as lethargy, nausea and vomiting, anorexia, and pruritis may occur, and some symptoms may point to specific renal/urinary pathology, such as loin pain, haematuria, changes in urinary frequency, and frothy urine.

In terms of past medical history, other than determining if there is pre-existing CKD, enquire about the presence of other comorbidities and risk factors for CKD (see Box 34.1). Scrutinise medication lists for any agents that are associated with kidney damage (see Box 34.1), for drugs that may accumulate in the context of renal dysfunction, and for drugs that may be harmful in CKD (e.g. metformin owing to risk of lactic acidosis; use is contraindicated when GFR <30 mL/min). In terms of drug accumulation, psychiatric medications to be particularly aware of are lithium, amisulpride, and sulpiride; however, the reader should be aware that a number of psychiatric drugs and their active metabolites can accumulate in CKD [28]. Take a family history for CKD and polycystic kidney disease, and a social history for smoking, alcohol intake, and recreational drug use; complications of the latter include glomerulonephritis and amyloidosis in intravenous drug users, renal failure secondary to rhabdomyolysis with use of cocaine and amphetamines for example, and renal artery atherosclerosis with cocaine use [29].

Examination

The purpose of examination is to rule out complications secondary to CKD, and if aetiology is unclear to identify potential causes. A set of basic observations including blood pressure may identify comorbid hypertension, and low oxygen saturation may indicate pulmonary oedema. Abdominal, cardiac, and respiratory examinations should be performed. General inspection may provide evidence of fluid overload (shortness of breath, peripheral oedema), anaemia (conjunctival pallor), or the accumulation of certain drugs (e.g. tremor in context of lithium). Cardiac and respiratory examination will again screen for evidence of fluid overload (raised jugular venous pressure, crackles on auscultation of the lungs). Abdominal examination should inspect for masses, which may indicate polycystic kidney disease, or for a distended bladder in a male patient in chronic urinary retention. General inspection may identify features of other systemic illnesses associated with CKD (e.g. rheumatological disease).

Investigations

The following tests may be considered by a psychiatric team and will aid in ruling out acute life-threatening presentations that may accompany CKD (e.g. hyperkalaemia), but will also strengthen a referral to renal colleagues, especially if the aetiology of the CKD has not previously been investigated.

Bloods

- Urea, electrolytes (sodium and potassium), creatinine, and eGFR.
- Bone profile (check phosphate levels).
- Liver function.
- Full blood count (anaemia).
- HIV, hepatitis B and C (potential causes of CKD).
- HbA_{1c} (diabetes mellitus).
- Autoimmune profile (autoimmune cause suspected).
- If appropriate, plasma levels of drugs that accumulate in renal failure (e.g. lithium, amisulpride, and sulpiride).

Urine

- Dip urine for proteinuria and haematuria.
- Measure urinary albumin and calculate the albumin/creatinine ratio.
- Consider sending urine for microscopy (casts).

ECG

Examine for consequences (e.g. hyperkalaemia) or causes (e.g. left ventricular hypertrophy of hypertension) of CKD.

Imaging and other specialist investigations

If this is a new presentation of CKD with no previous investigations, consider referring the patient for an ultrasound of the kidney and urinary tract, examining for any structural abnormalities. If appropriate, renal physicians may request/perform specialist investigations such as MRI of the kidneys (examining for renal artery stenosis) and potentially renal biopsy if aetiology of CKD remains unclear

MANAGEMENT

Specific management of CKD is clearly beyond the remit of the psychiatrist; however, as already described, there are various clinical scenarios in which a psychiatric practitioner may need to consider CKD as part of the holistic care they provide their patient. The reader is directed to Chapter 73 on acute kidney injury where such a presentation is suspected, or indeed acute-on-chronic injury (where a renal insult occurs in the setting of already chronically impaired renal function). The reader is also directed to Chapter 33 on potassium disturbance, which provides advice on appropriate management of hyperkalaemia.

The general principles of management of CKD are summarised in Box 34.2. In the UK, patients with CKD stage 4 or above are generally managed in secondary care, with regular follow-up to monitor for progression of disease. Specialist renal input should

> **Box 34.2** General principles of chronic kidney disease management
>
> - Manage reversible causes of renal impairment, e.g. nephrotoxic drugs (especially non-steroidal anti-inflammatory drugs), decreased perfusion, urinary tract obstruction
> - Control risk factors, e.g. glycaemic control in diabetes, blood pressure control in hypertension, smoking cessation
> - Manage complications, e.g. anaemia, but this should be managed with secondary care input. People with stage 3, 4 or 5 CKD are at increased risk of influenza and should be immunised (see Chapter 40)

also be sought where hereditary renal disease is suspected, or for persistent CKD-associated complications such as recurrent hyperkalaemia or recalcitrant hypertension.

Regardless of the cause of CKD, all patients should have risk factors for CKD and broader cardiovascular risk factors aggressively managed, including control of weight gain, hypertension, hypercholesterolaemia, and diabetes mellitus, and referral for smoking cessation. Psychiatrists may be in a unique position to facilitate management of these comorbidities and risk factors, particularly in patients who engage poorly with primary or secondary (renal) care. Thus, rationalisation of psychiatric medication may be indicated, switching to agents with fewer metabolic side effects (see Chapter 14) [30], as well as providing the patient with information on smoking cessation (see Chapter 46) and diet.

It is generally wise to assume mild renal impairment in all patients above 65 years of age, and to adjust prescribing practice accordingly until blood test results are available. A summary of considerations when prescribing antidepressants, antipsychotics, mood stabilisers, anxiolytics/hypnotics, and anti-dementia drugs in the context of CKD is provided in Table 34.2; the reader is directed to the latest edition of the *Maudsley Prescribing Guidelines in Psychiatry* for further information on individual drugs [31]. General principles when prescribing psychiatric medications in CKD are as follows.

1 Psychotropic and other medications should be rationalised to minimise the risk of direct nephrotoxicity. Decisions to continue lithium treatment (especially when GFR drops below 60 mL/min per 1.73 m²) should be made following a risk–benefit multidisciplinary discussion involving both renal and psychiatric practitioners, alongside the patient. Drugs with anticholinergic effects should be used cautiously, given the risk of urinary retention. As a rule, advice from renal physicians/specialist pharmacists should be sought where psychiatric prescription is being considered in a patient with moderate/severe CKD or end-stage renal failure (ESRF).
2 There is a risk of drug accumulation (including accumulation of active metabolites) [28] in patients with CKD. As such, drugs that are substantially renally excreted (e.g. lithium, amisulpride, sulpiride) should be used with caution (see Table 34.2), and as a rule all medications should be started at a low dose and up-titrated slowly, ideally with plasma level monitoring. Furthermore, long-acting preparations such as antipsychotic depots, which are hard to titrate safely in the context of changing renal function, should be avoided.

Table 34.2 Special considerations when prescribing antidepressants, antipsychotics, mood stabilisers, anxiolytics and hypnotics, and anti-dementia drugs in the context of chronic kidney disease (CKD) [31].

Drug class	Special considerations	Dose adjustment required in moderate/severe CKD?	Reasonable choices in CKD
Antidepressants	Specific evidence for use in CKD with bupropion, citalopram, escitalopram, fluoxetine, paroxetine, and sertraline [34–39]; however, note recent evidence suggesting that sertraline's efficacy in CKD may be limited [40]. There is risk of urinary retention, sedation, and confusion with tricyclic antidepressants. Desvenlafaxine has also been associated with urinary retention	For many antidepressants no specific dose adjustments are recommended by manufacturers; however, a principle of starting at a low dose and increasing slowly is widely suggested. Some antidepressants have specific dosing advice by manufacturers or are contraindicated when GFR drops below a threshold. The reader is encouraged to review the summary of product characteristics for a given antidepressant prior to prescribing in patients with CKD, and is directed to the latest edition of the *Maudsley Prescribing Guidelines in Psychiatry* for further information on individual drugs [31]	Citalopram (although monitor for QTc prolongation)
Antipsychotics	Monitor anticholinergic, hypotensive, and sedative effects of antipsychotics. Avoid highly anticholinergic agents where possible. Consider metabolic side effects of some antipsychotics (in particular clozapine, olanzapine, quetiapine, risperidone, and paliperidone) which may indirectly increase risk of progressive CKD [30]. Where possible avoid using long-acting injectable formulations	Most antipsychotics can be used in severe CKD, although with all antipsychotics caution is advised (start with low dose and titrate). The reader is encouraged to review the summary of product characteristics for a given antipsychotic prior to prescribing in patients with CKD, and is directed to the latest edition of the *Maudsley Prescribing Guidelines in Psychiatry* for further information on individual drugs [31]. For paliperidone (where renal clearance is reduced by 71% in severe kidney disease), manufacturer recommendations are as follows: oral treatment contraindicated if GFR <10 mL/min, depot contraindicated if GFR <50 mL/min. Although not contraindicated in severe kidney disease, similar caution is recommended with risperidone. Amisulpride and sulpiride are principally excreted renally so should be avoided in ESRF. For less severe CKD, manufacturer recommendations are as follows: ■ Amisulpride: if GFR 30–60 mL/min, give 50% of dose; if GFR 10–30 mL/min, give 33% of dose ■ Sulpiride: if GFR 30–60 mL/min, give 70% normal dose; if GFR 10–30 mL/min, give 50% of dose	Low-dose olanzapine (although beware metabolic side effects) or haloperidol

CHAPTER 34

(continued)

294   The Maudsley Practice Guidelines for Physical Health Conditions in Psychiatry

Table 34.2 (Continued)

Drug class	Special considerations	Dose adjustment required in moderate/severe CKD?	Reasonable choices in CKD
Mood stabilisers	Long-term treatment with lithium may cause progressive irreversible impaired renal function, altered renal histology, nephrogenic diabetes insipidus (see Chapter 31), and nephrotic syndrome. Lithium causes CKD via chronic interstitial nephritis, glomerulonephritis, and formation of renal cysts Carbamazepine is associated with increased rates of CKD [5] Consider metabolic side effects of lithium and sodium valproate which may indirectly increase risk of progressive CKD	Apart from lithium, no specific dose adjustments are advised, although with all mood stabilisers caution is advised (start with small dose and titrate) Lithium is not only nephrotoxic but is also almost entirely renally excreted. As such, it is contraindicated in severe renal impairment (consider if continued prescription is appropriate when GFR <60 mL/min). Where a decision is made to continue lithium despite renal impairment, the following dose adjustments are recommended: ■ If GFR 10–50 mL/min, give 50–75% normal dose and monitor levels ■ If GFR <10 mL/min, give 25–50% normal dose and monitor levels	Low-dose lamotrigine with up-titration as required (if possible, with plasma concentration monitoring)
Anxiolytics and hypnotics	Monitor for excessive sedation	Caution advised with all agents: start with small dose and titrate	Lorazepam (as short-acting) and zopiclone
Anti-dementia drugs	N/A	No dose adjustment required with donepezil Start galantamine, memantine, and rivastigmine at low dose and titrate	No specific agent deemed to be superior in CKD

ESRF, end-stage renal failure; GFR, glomerular filtration rate.

3 Diminished drug clearance in CKD increases the risk of side effects with certain medications (e.g. sedation and confusion with benzodiazepines). Thus, as described, low doses of medication with cautious titration should be employed. Avoid drugs associated with QTc interval prolongation given the prevalence of electrolyte disturbance in CKD, and polypharmacy to minimise the risk of drug interactions and associated adverse effects.

End-stage renal failure

Management of ESRF can be particularly challenging in the context of SMI. Many ESRF patients require regular (usually three times weekly) haemodialysis at a dedicated unit or will receive self-administered home dialysis; fluctuations in mental state may impact ability to adhere to dialysis timetables with inevitable risk to physical health. Furthermore, these patients will be maintained on a 'renal' diet, which has considerable restrictions in water and potassium content; adhering to this regimen in the setting of poor mental health may be difficult. In such circumstances, a multidisciplinary decision will need to be made regarding what level of social care that individual requires. Where a patient has received a renal transplant, consideration must be given to potential interactions between immunosuppressant and psychiatric medication. For example, CYP3A4 inducers (e.g. carbamazepine and St John's Wort) can reduce concentrations of the immunosuppressant tacrolimus leading to transplant rejection [32,33]. Again, multidisciplinary working between psychiatry and renal colleagues is required to avoid potentially fatal complications.

References

1. Kidney Disease: Improving Global Outcomes (KDIGO) CKD Work Group. KDIGO 2012 Clinical Practice Guideline for the Evaluation and Management of Chronic Kidney Disease. *Kidney Int Suppl* 2013;3(1):1–150.
2. Hill NR, Fatoba ST, Oke JL, et al. Global prevalence of chronic kidney disease: a systematic review and meta-analysis. *PLoS One* 2016;11(7):e0158765.
3. Tzeng NS, Hsu YH, Ho SY, et al. Is schizophrenia associated with an increased risk of chronic kidney disease? A nationwide matched-cohort study. *BMJ Open* 2015;5(1):e006777.
4. Smith DJ, Martin D, McLean G, et al. Multimorbidity in bipolar disorder and undertreatment of cardiovascular disease: a cross sectional study. *BMC Med* 2013;11:263.
5. Kessing LV, Gerds TA, Feldt-Rasmussen B, et al. Use of lithium and anticonvulsants and the rate of chronic kidney disease: a nationwide population-based study. *JAMA Psychiatry* 2015;72(12):1182–1191.
6. Iwagami M, Mansfield KE, Hayes JF, et al. Severe mental illness and chronic kidney disease: a cross-sectional study in the United Kingdom. *Clin Epidemiol* 2018;10:421–429.
7. Osborn DPJ, Wright CA, Levy G, et al. Relative risk of diabetes, dyslipidaemia, hypertension and the metabolic syndrome in people with severe mental illnesses: Systematic review and metaanalysis. *BMC Psychiatry* 2008;8(1):84.
8. Mezuk B, Eaton WW, Albrecht S, Golden SH. Depression and type 2 diabetes over the lifespan: a meta-analysis. *Diabetes Care* 2008;31(12):2383–2390.
9. Perez-Pinar M, Mathur R, Foguet Q, et al. Cardiovascular risk factors among patients with schizophrenia, bipolar, depressive, anxiety, and personality disorders. *Eur Psychiatry* 2016;35:8–15.
10. Ayerbe L, Forgnone I, Addo J, et al. Hypertension risk and clinical care in patients with bipolar disorder or schizophrenia; a systematic review and meta-analysis. *J Affect Disord* 2018;225:665–670.
11. Markowitz GS, Radhakrishnan J, Kambham N, et al. Lithium nephrotoxicity: a progressive combined glomerular and tubulointerstitial nephropathy. *J Am Soc Nephrol* 2000;11(8):1439–1448.
12. Kanofsky JD, Woesner ME, Harris AZ, et al. A case of acute renal failure in a patient recently treated with clozapine and a review of previously reported cases. *Prim Care Companion CNS Disord* 2011;13(3):PCC.10br01091.
13. An NY, Lee J, Noh JS. A case of clozapine induced acute renal failure. *Psychiatry Investig* 2013;10(1):92–94.
14. Knights MJ, Finlay E. The effects of sodium valproate on the renal function of children with epilepsy. *Pediatr Nephrol* 2014;29(7):1131–1138.
15. Eguchi E, Shimazu K, Nishiguchi K, et al. Granulomatous interstitial nephritis associated with atypical drug-induced hypersensitivity syndrome induced by carbamazepine. *Clin Exp Nephrol* 2012;16(1):168–172.
16. He LY, Peng YM, Fu X, et al. Dibenzodiazepine derivative quetiapine- and olanzapine-induced chronic interstitial nephritis. *Renal Failure* 2013;35(5):657–659.
17. Onishi A, Yamamoto H, Akimoto T, et al. Reversible acute renal failure associated with clomipramine-induced interstitial nephritis. *Clin Exp Nephrol* 2007;11(3):241–243.
18. Semaan WE, Doyon J, Jolicoeur F, Duchesneau J. Dose-dependent urinary retention following olanzapine administration. *Ann Pharmacother* 2006;40(9):1693.
19. Novicki DE, Willscher MK. Case profile: anticholinergic-induced hydronephrosis. *Urology* 1979;13(3):324–325.
20. Hedayati SS, Finkelstein FO. Epidemiology, diagnosis, and management of depression in patients with CKD. *Am J Kidney Dis* 2009;54(4):741–752.
21. Pereira BDS, Fernandes NDS, de Melo NP, et al. Beyond quality of life: a cross sectional study on the mental health of patients with chronic kidney disease undergoing dialysis and their caregivers. *Health Qual Life Outcomes* 2017;15(1):74.
22. Perazella MA, Khan S. Increased mortality in chronic kidney disease: a call to action. *Am J Med Sci* 2006;331(3):150–153.
23. Sarnak MJ, Levey AS, Schoolwerth AC, et al. Kidney disease as a risk factor for development of cardiovascular disease: a statement from the American Heart Association councils on kidney in cardiovascular disease, high blood pressure research, clinical cardiology, and epidemiology and prevention. *Circulation* 2003;108(17):2154–2169.
24. Tonelli M, Wiebe N, Culleton B, et al. Chronic kidney disease and mortality risk: a systematic review. *J Am Soc Nephrol* 2006;17(7):2034–2047.

25. Bello AK, Alrukhaimi M, Ashuntantang GE, et al. Complications of chronic kidney disease: current state, knowledge gaps, and strategy for action. *Kidney Int Suppl* 2017;7(2):122–129.

26. Hsu CY, Ordonez JD, Chertow GM, et al. The risk of acute renal failure in patients with chronic kidney disease. *Kidney Int* 2008;74(1):101–107.

27. Thomas R, Kanso A, Sedor JR. Chronic kidney disease and its complications. *Prim Care* 2008;35(2):329–344, vii.

28. Nagler EV, Webster AC, Vanholder R, Zoccali C. Antidepressants for depression in stage 3–5 chronic kidney disease: a systematic review of pharmacokinetics, efficacy and safety with recommendations by European Renal Best Practice (ERBP). *Nephrol Dial Transplant* 2012;27(10):3736–3745.

29. Crowe AV, Howse M, Bell GM, Henry JA. Substance abuse and the kidney. *Q J Med* 2000;93(3):147–152.

30. Pillinger T, McCutcheon R, Vano L, et al. Comparative effects of 18 antipsychotics on metabolic function in patients with schizophrenia, predictors of metabolic dysregulation, and association with psychopathology: a systematic review and network meta-analysis. *Lancet Psychiatry* 2020;7(1):64–77.

31. Taylor DM, Barnes TRE, Young AH. The Maudsley Prescribing Guidelines in Psychiatry, 13th edn. Chichester: Wiley Blackwell, 2018.

32. Mai I, Stormer E, Bauer S, et al. Impact of St John's wort treatment on the pharmacokinetics of tacrolimus and mycophenolic acid in renal transplant patients. *Nephrol Dial Transplant* 2003;18(4):819–822.

33. Wada K, Takada M, Sakai M, et al. Drug interaction between tacrolimus and carbamazepine in a Japanese heart transplant recipient: a case report. *J Heart Lung Transpl* 2009;28(4):409–411.

34. Worrall SP, Almond MK, Dhillon S. Pharmacokinetics of bupropion and its metabolites in haemodialysis patients who smoke. A single dose study. *Nephron Clin Pract* 2004;97(3):c83–c89.

35. Joffe P, Larsen FS, Pedersen V, et al. Single-dose pharmacokinetics of citalopram in patients with moderate renal insufficiency or hepatic cirrhosis compared with healthy subjects. *Eur J Clin Pharmacol* 1998;54(3):237–242.

36. Yazici AE, Erdem P, Erdem A, et al. Efficacy and tolerability of escitalopram in depressed patients with end stage renal disease: an open placebo-controlled study. *Klin Psikofarmakol B* 2012;22(1):23–30.

37. Blumenfield M, Levy NB, Spinowitz B, et al. Fluoxetine in depressed patients on dialysis. *Int J Psychiat Med* 1997;27(1):71–80.

38. Doyle GD, Laher M, Kelly JG, et al. The pharmacokinetics of paroxetine in renal impairment. *Acta Psychiatr Scand* 1989;80:89–90.

39. Friedli K, Guirguis A, Almond M, et al. Sertraline versus placebo in patients with major depressive disorder undergoing hemodialysis: a randomized, controlled feasibility trial. *Clin J Am Soc Nephrol* 2017;12(2):280–286.

40. Hedayati SS, Gregg LP, Carmody T, et al. Effect of sertraline on depressive symptoms in patients with chronic kidney disease without dialysis dependence: the CAST randomized clinical trial. *JAMA* 2017;318(19):1876–1890.

CHAPTER 34

Part 6

Sexual and Reproductive Health

Sexual Dysfunction

Rudiger Pittrof

Sexual dysfunction (SD) describes difficulty experienced at any stage of sexual activity, including pleasure, desire, arousal, or orgasm. In the US general population, the prevalence of SD is estimated at 43% for women, and 31% for men [1]. Prevalence estimates are even higher in people with serious mental illness (SMI), with SD reported in 60–80% of individuals with anxiety, mood, or psychotic disorders [2–6]. The aetiology of SD is multifactorial, including psychological, physiological, and pharmacological precipitants [7], and a number of these precipitants are more prevalent in people with SMI. For example, rates of type 2 diabetes mellitus (T2DM), a major risk factor for SD (up to 75% of men with T2DM experience erectile dysfunction [8]), are increased in psychiatric patients [9,10]. Furthermore, SD is associated with use of serotonergic antidepressants, prolactin-inducing antipsychotics, mood stabilisers that lower testosterone, and anxiolytics [11]. SD is recognised to have a significant impact on the quality of life and ongoing mental distress of people with SMI [12], and contributes to poor psychotropic medication concordance [13,14]. Thus, identifying and addressing SD is a key part of holistic care provision.

ASSESSMENT OF A PATIENT WITH SEXUAL DYSFUNCTION

History

- Embarrassment and stigma associated with SD is a significant barrier to its discussion with healthcare professionals and thus identification [15]. Box 35.1 provides example phrases that a clinician may use to broach the subject.
- Consider using a questionnaire or rating scale, for example the Arizona Sexual Experiences Scale (ASEX) [16]. The ASEX assesses each of the following: strength of

The Maudsley Practice Guidelines for Physical Health Conditions in Psychiatry, First Edition.
David M. Taylor, Fiona Gaughran, and Toby Pillinger.
© 2021 John Wiley & Sons Ltd. Published 2021 by John Wiley & Sons Ltd.

Box 35.1 Normalising discussion about sexual dysfunction: example phrases and approaches

Example phrases

- 'Many men have problems with their sex life. Some stop wanting sex, some cannot get an erection, or sometimes their sperm comes too early or not at all. Many of my patients have these problems, so I ask everyone about this. Is this something that concerns you too?'
- 'Many women have problems with their sex life. Some stop wanting sex, some cannot get in the mood for sex, and many cannot achieve an orgasm. Many of my patients have these problems, so I ask everyone about this. Is this something that concerns you too?'

Notes

- Some psychiatric clinics employ pre-assessment psychotropic side-effect rating assessments. This can provide a convenient entry point to discussion about sexual dysfunction, for example 'On the side-effect assessment you ticked experiencing problems with sex. May men/women have problems with their sex life... [continue with example phrases above]'.
- As the clinician you may need to endure a few seconds of awkward silence after asking questions about sexual dysfunction. However, allowing a patient to talk about his or her sexual dysfunction is destigmatising, can improve self-esteem, and will facilitate future discussion. Framing any conversation in the context that most men and women report sexual dysfunction at some point in their lives helps to normalise experiences.

---

sex drive, ease of sexual arousal, for men the ability to get and maintain an erection, for women the ease with which the vagina becomes moist/wet during sex, the ability to reach orgasm, the satisfaction of orgasm.

- Assess the time frame over which sexual dysfunction has occurred. Erectile dysfunction that occurs gradually often points to problems with the blood supply or nerves supplying the penis, while a sudden loss of sexual desire or the ability to get erections is more causally suggestive of medication or psychological difficulties.
- As part of a discussion about SD, establish the extent to which SD is impacting quality of life, the patient's view on the aetiology of SD, treatments they have previously sought (e.g. from primary care or over the counter), and if they are considering stopping (or have stopped) their psychiatric medication.
- Take a past medical history for comorbid physical health complaints associated with SD. These include obesity, hypertension, hypercholesterolaemia, diabetes mellitus, Parkinson's disease, previous surgical treatments for prostate cancer/prostatic hypertrophy, and surgery/injury to pelvic area/spinal cord.
- Take a drug history assessing for medical and psychiatric drugs associated with SD (Figure 35.1 and Box 35.2). Polypharmacy increases the risk of SD [17].
- Take a social history assessing smoking status, alcohol use, and recreational drug use, all of which are associated with SD.
- Screen for stress, anxiety, or depressive symptoms that may be contributing to SD.

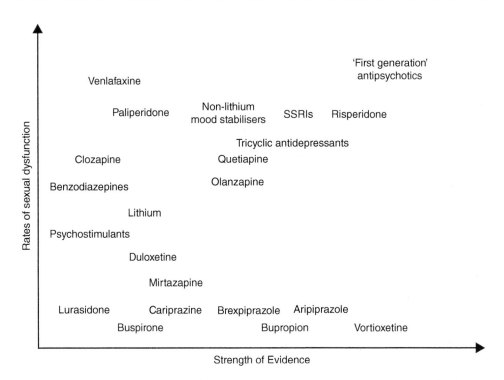

Figure 35.1 Approximate rates of sexual dysfunction with psychiatric drugs and associated strength of evidence. Source: adapted from Clayton et al. [11].

Examination and investigations

- Ask if the patient has noticed anything abnormal about their genitals. If the answer is yes, either offer to examine the patient or arrange an examination via primary care, a local sexual health clinic, gynaecology, or urology as appropriate.
- Perform a set of basic observations, noting for evidence of hypertension (see Chapter 5).
- Check prolactin levels and HbA_{1c} (see Chapters 11 and 13).

MANAGEMENT

Management of SD will of course depend on the underlying cause; non-pharmacological and pharmacological approaches are detailed in the following sections. Where SD improves there may be an increased risk of pregnancy and sexually transmitted infection (see Chapters 36 and 38).

Box 35.2 Medications and recreational drugs implicated in sexual dysfunction

General medical drugs

- Antihypertensives
- Diuretics
- Hormone treatments (e.g. 5α-reductase inhibitors versus benign prostatic hypertrophy)
- Contraceptive hormones
- Metformin
- Antihistamines

Psychiatric drugs (see Figure 35.1)

- Antipsychotics (although note large variation between different agents)
- Antidepressants: tricyclic antidepressants, selective serotonin reuptake inhibitors (SSRIs), serotonin/noradrenaline reuptake inhibitors (SNRIs), monoamine oxidase inhibitors
- Mood stabilisers: lithium, sodium valproate, lamotrigine, carbamazepine

Recreational drugs

- Practically all recreational drugs, including alcohol and nicotine

---

Non-pharmacological management

Where poor physical health is implicated in SD, there is evidence that weight loss [18], smoking cessation [19], a Mediterranean diet [20], and exercise [21] can improve sexual function (see Chapters 10, 14, and 46). Bearing in mind the cardiometabolic burden in people with SMI, we recommend that these lifestyle interventions are considered for all patients. The efficacy of such interventions in treating SD may have a psychological component; there is evidence that the placebo effect accounts for up to 70% of treatment response for SD in females and up to 50% of treatment response for erectile dysfunction [22]. Thus, any lifestyle interventions should be accompanied by motivational interviewing reinforcing their potential efficacy. Psychosexual therapy may be appropriate where physiological/pharmacological causes of SD are ruled out and where there is a clear psychological precipitant (e.g. previous sexual violence or childhood sexual abuse).

Pharmacological management

- The first step in pharmacological management is considering rationalisation of medication. Any changes to physical healthcare medication should be made in dialogue with either primary or secondary medical services. Pharmacological management of physiological causes of SD may also be indicated, for example diabetes mellitus and hypertension (see Chapters 5 and 11).
- Where psychiatric medication is implicated, the following should be considered.
  - For antidepressants, if patients have achieved full remission of depressive symptoms then dose reduction may be considered. Where switching antidepressants is considered, lower-risk antidepressants for SD include agomelatine, bupropion, mirtazapine, vilazodone, vortioxetine, and moclobemide [11].

- For antipsychotics, SD is often associated with hyperprolactinaemia, and the reader is directed to Chapter 13 on this topic. Essentially, either adjunctive aripiprazole [23] (except for with amisulpride treatment, where such an intervention tends to be ineffective) [24] or a switch to aripiprazole should be considered in patients with symptomatic antipsychotic-induced hyperprolactinaemia. Adjunctive aripiprazole in females with antipsychotic-induced hyperprolactinaemia has been shown to improve SD in 50% of cases [25], and aripiprazole in long-acting injectable formulation is associated with improved sexual functioning compared with paliperidone in both men and women [26]. However, antipsychotic-related SD may also be related to histamine receptor antagonism (increasing sedation), α_1-receptor antagonism (resulting in erectile dysfunction), and dopamine receptor antagonism (reducing motivation and reward). Thus, trialling an agent with less of a sedative profile and/or one with a lower preponderance to cause secondary negative symptoms may be considered (e.g. aripiprazole) [27].
- Where benzodiazepines are implicated, attempt slow reduction and cessation. Where mood stabilisers are implicated, a risk–benefit decision should be made regarding their continuation. Rates of SD with lithium may be reduced compared with other mood stabilisers, and thus a cross-titration to lithium may be considered [11].
- Phosphodiesterase inhibitors (e.g. sildenafil and tadalafil, among others) are effective treatments for erectile dysfunction [28] and considered so safe that, in the UK, sildenafil (Viagra Connect) can be bought over the counter without a prescription. Phosphodiesterase inhibitors have also been shown to be effective and well tolerated in patients with schizophrenia [29]. Side effects of phosphodiesterase inhibitors include headache, flushing, dyspepsia, blurred vision, and nasal congestion. Furthermore, prescribers should be aware that sildenafil can prolong the QTc and increases the risk of hypotension (see Chapter 3). Guidance on use of sildenafil is provided in Box 35.3.
- Bupropion is a noradrenaline/dopamine reuptake inhibitor. In the UK it is licensed for smoking cessation. At doses of 150–400 mg/day it has been used off-label for the treatment of hypoactive sexual desire disorder, with a Cochrane review concluding that 'for women with antidepressant-induced sexual dysfunction the addition of

---

Box 35.3 Guidance on use of sildenafil[a]

- Reassure that sildenafil is safe and commonly used, pointing to its availability over the counter as evidence of this.
- Sildenafil does not influence arousal, but will help the man, if aroused, to get and maintain an erection.
- Counsel the man to take half (25 mg) of a 50-mg tablet one hour before planned sexual activity. Absorption is delayed and reduced if taken with or after food. It works for about four hours. Counsel the patient not to take more than 50 mg/day. Most men only need 25 mg but, if necessary, the dose may be increased to 50 mg.
- In terms of common side effects, one in five men will get a headache, and one in five men will experience flushes.[a]

[a] Longer-acting phosphodiesterase inhibitors are available (e.g. tadalafil)

bupropion at higher doses (300 mg/day) appears to be the most promising approach studied so far' [28].

- In 2015, the US Food and Drug Administration (FDA) approved flibanserin as a treatment for hypoactive sexual desire disorder in premenopausal women, despite concern about suboptimal risk–benefit trade-offs [30]. A subsequent meta-analysis of five trials including 5914 women showed that use of flibanserin leads to only a small improvement in sexual functioning, and a more recent review found that flibanserin was as effective as cognitive behavioural therapy and mindfulness meditation training [30,31]. It is clearly not a 'female Viagra' even if its marketing tries to suggest this.
- Low testosterone is associated with poor sexual function. If hyperprolactinaemia is responsible for low testosterone, then hyperprolactinaemia should be addressed (see Chapter 13). There is evidence that transdermal testosterone is effective in women with SSRI/SNRI-emergent loss of libido (see also Chapter 63) and in men who continue to take serotonergic antidepressants with low or low-normal testosterone levels [32,33].

References

1. Laumann EO, Paik A, Rosen RC. Sexual dysfunction in the United States: prevalence and predictors. *JAMA* 1999;281(6):537–544.
2. Peuskens J, Sienaert P, De Hert M. Sexual dysfunction: the unspoken side effect of antipsychotics. *Eur Psychiatry* 1998;13(1 Suppl 1):23s–30s.
3. Rosen RC, Lane RM, Menza M. Effects of SSRIs on sexual function: a critical review. *J Clin Psychopharmacol* 1999;19(1):67–85.
4. Clayton AH, Pradko JF, Croft HA, et al. Prevalence of sexual dysfunction among newer antidepressants. *J Clin Psychiatry* 2002;63(4):357–366.
5. Osvath P, Fekete S, Voros V, Vitrai J. Sexual dysfunction among patients treated with antidepressants: a Hungarian retrospective study. *Eur Psychiatry* 2003;18(8):412–414.
6. Kaplan HS. Anxiety and sexual dysfunction. *J Clin Psychiatry* 1988;49(Suppl):21–25.
7. Lewis RW, Fugl-Meyer KS, Bosch R, et al. Epidemiology/risk factors of sexual dysfunction. *J Sex Med* 2004;1(1):35–39.
8. Hackett GI. Erectile dysfunction, diabetes and cardiovascular risk. *Br J Diabetes* 2016;16(2):52–57.
9. Ward M, Druss B. The epidemiology of diabetes in psychotic disorders. *Lancet Psychiatry* 2015;2(5):431–451.
10. Moulton CD, Pickup JC, Ismail K. The link between depression and diabetes: the search for shared mechanisms. *Lancet Diabetes Endocrinol* 2015;3(6):461–471.
11. Clayton AH, Alkis AR, Parikh NB, Votta JG. Sexual dysfunction due to psychotropic medications. *Psychiatr Clin North Am* 2016;39(3):427–463.
12. Kelly DL, Conley RR. Sexuality and schizophrenia: a review. *Schizophr Bull* 2004;30(4):767–779.
13. Rosenberg KP, Bleiberg KL, Koscis J, Gross C. A survey of sexual side effects among severely mentally ill patients taking psychotropic medications: impact on compliance. *J Sex Marital Ther* 2003;29(4):289–296.
14. Clayton A, Ramamurthy S. The impact of mental illness on sexual dysfunction. *Adv Psychosom Med* 2008;29:70–88.
15. Sarkadi A, Rosenqvist U. Contradictions in the medical encounter: female sexual dysfunction in primary care contacts. *Fam Pract* 2001;18(2):161–166.
16. McGahuey CA, Delgado PL, Gelenberg AJ. Assessment of sexual dysfunction using the Arizona Sexual Experiences Scale (ASEX) and implications for the treatment of depression. *Psychiatr Ann* 1999;29(1):39–45.
17. Hashimoto Y, Uno J, Miwa T, et al. Effects of antipsychotic polypharmacy on side-effects and concurrent use of medications in schizophrenic outpatients. *Psychiatry Clin Neurosci* 2012;66(5):405–410.
18. Theleritis C, Bonaccorso S, Habib N, et al. Sexual dysfunction and central obesity in patients with first episode psychosis. *Eur Psychiatry* 2017;42:1–7.
19. Biebel MG, Burnett AL, Sadeghi-Nejad H. Male sexual function and smoking. *Sex Med Rev* 2016;4(4):366–375.
20. Maiorino MI, Bellastella G, Caputo M, et al. Effects of Mediterranean diet on sexual function in people with newly diagnosed type 2 diabetes: The MEDITA trial. *J Diabetes Complications* 2016;30(8):1519–1524.
21. Lorenz TA, Meston CM. Exercise improves sexual function in women taking antidepressants: results from a randomized crossover trial. *Depress Anxiety* 2014;31(3):188–195.
22. Weinberger JM, Houman J, Caron AT, et al. Female sexual dysfunction and the placebo effect: a meta-analysis. *Obstet Gynecol Surv* 2018;73(12):685–686.
23. Meng M, Li W, Zhang S, et al. Using aripiprazole to reduce antipsychotic-induced hyperprolactinemia: meta-analysis of currently available randomized controlled trials. *Shanghai Arch Psychiatry* 2015;27(1):4–17.

24. Chen CK, Huang YS, Ree SC, Hsiao CC. Differential add-on effects of aripiprazole in resolving hyperprolactinemia induced by risperidone in comparison to benzamide antipsychotics. *Prog Neuropsychopharmacol Biol Psychiatry* 2010;34(8):1495–1499.

25. Kelly DL, Powell MM, Wehring HJ, et al. Adjunct aripiprazole reduces prolactin and prolactin-related adverse effects in premenopausal women with psychosis: results from the DAAMSEL clinical trial. *J Clin Psychopharmacol* 2018;38(4):317–326.

26. Potkin SG, Loze JY, Forray C, et al. Reduced sexual dysfunction with aripiprazole once-monthly versus paliperidone palmitate: results from QUALIFY. *Int Clin Psychopharmacol* 2017;32(3):147–154.

27. Knegtering H, van der Moolen AEGM, Castelein S, et al. What are the effects of antipsychotics on sexual dysfunctions and endocrine functioning? *Psychoneuroendocrinology* 2003;28:109–123.

28. Taylor MJ, Rudkin L, Bullemor-Day P, et al. Strategies for managing sexual dysfunction induced by antidepressant medication. *Cochrane Database Syst Rev* 2013;(5):CD003382.

29. Bacconi L, Gressier F. Efficacy and tolerance of PDE-5 in the treatment of erectile dysfunction in schizophrenic patients: A literature review. *Encephale* 2017;43(1):55–61.

30. Jaspers L, Feys F, Bramer WM, et al. Efficacy and safety of flibanserin for the treatment of hypoactive sexual desire disorder in women: a systematic review and meta-analysis. *JAMA Intern Med* 2016;176(4):453–462.

31. Pyke RE, Clayton AH. Effect size in efficacy trials of women with decreased sexual desire. *Sex Med Rev* 2018;6(3):358–366.

32. Montejo AL, Montejo L, Navarro-Cremades F. Sexual side-effects of antidepressant and antipsychotic drugs. *Curr Opin Psychiatry* 2015;28(6):418–423.

33. Amiaz R, Pope HG Jr, Mahne T, et al. Testosterone gel replacement improves sexual function in depressed men taking serotonergic antidepressants: a randomized, placebo-controlled clinical trial. *J Sex Marital Ther* 2011;37(4):243–254.

CHAPTER 35

Contraception
Neha Pathak, Usha Kumar

Mental illness contributes to several adverse reproductive health outcomes including increased risk of unintended pregnancy [1]. Thus, pregnancy planning and contraception counselling for people with serious mental illness (SMI) should form a key part of holistic care provision. However, contraception screening in mental health settings is often suboptimal [2,3]. This is despite the additional reproductive vulnerabilities associated with mental illness, including teratogenicity of certain psychotropic medications (see Chapter 62); higher rates of risky sexual behaviour, coercive sex, and sexually transmitted infections (see Chapter 38) [4]; and higher prevalence of contraceptive non-use, misuse, and discontinuation [1]. The association between poor mental health and unintended pregnancy is bidirectional, with unintended pregnancy a risk factor for perinatal depression [5]. The mental health implications of unintended pregnancy go beyond that of the mother's; unplanned pregnancy where the child is not wanted increases risk of schizophrenia in that child [6].

In the UK, the National Institute for Health and Care Excellence (NICE) advises that clinicians engage in conversations about contraception and pregnancy with all women of present or future childbearing potential who have a new, existing, or past mental health diagnosis [7]. This conversation should cover contraception and pregnancy planning; the effects of pregnancy and childbirth on mental health; and how mental health and associated treatment may affect the woman, fetus, or baby. This chapter should equip mental healthcare providers with the core knowledge to discuss contraception and pregnancy planning with people with SMI. The reader is also directed to the complementary Chapter 62 on pregnancy.

The Maudsley Practice Guidelines for Physical Health Conditions in Psychiatry, First Edition.
David M. Taylor, Fiona Gaughran, and Toby Pillinger.
© 2021 John Wiley & Sons Ltd. Published 2021 by John Wiley & Sons Ltd.

CLINICAL APPROACH

Contraceptive counselling should be performed opportunistically at primary care consultations, antenatal/postnatal appointments, mental health appointments, and during psychiatric inpatient admissions. As part of an assessment, aim to cover the following.

- Establish current need for contraception including emergency contraception on day of assessment. As part of this discussion, define current risk of pregnancy (including date of last sexual intercourse), any pregnancy plans, partner history, and contraception currently used.
- Determine contraceptive preferences: types currently and previously used, reasons for stopping previous types, any preferred choice, any concerns about specific types.
- Take a past medical and surgical history, drug history (with allergy status), obstetric history, gynaecological history (in women record last menstrual period and any menstrual problems), family history of venous thromboembolism, and social history (smoking status, alcohol and substance misuse, domestic violence).
- If the patient might be pregnant, perform a pregnancy test. Note that pregnancy cannot be excluded using a urinary test until 21 days or more after last unprotected sexual intercourse. Check blood pressure and calculate body mass index (BMI), the results of which may contribute to contraceptive decision-making.

CONTRACEPTIVE OPTIONS

Table 36.1 provides a description of the different contraceptive options available. The Faculty of Sexual and Reproductive Healthcare (FSRH) provides more detailed guidance and regularly publishes statements based on new evidence [8]. Broadly, there are three group of contraceptives.

1 *Methods not dependent on the user*: the patient does not need to remember taking or using the contraceptive. These drugs include long-acting reversible contraceptives (LARCs) and sterilisation. LARCs are the most effective types of contraception and are defined as methods administered less than once per menstrual cycle or month.
2 *User-dependent methods*: the patient must remember to use the contraceptive regularly or during sex, resulting in greater variation in efficacy. These are less suited to chaotic lifestyles.
3 *Emergency contraception*: contraception is used after unprotected sex or if the contraception used has failed. The most effective method is the copper intrauterine device (IUD), which can be inserted up to five days after first unprotected sexual intercourse (UPSI) in a menstrual cycle or up to five days after the earliest likely date of ovulation (whichever is later). Oral methods include ulipristal acetate or levonorgestrel pills which can be used, respectively, up to 120 hours and 72 hours post UPSI; ulipristal acetate is the more effective of the two.

Table 36.1 Contraception options.

Methods not dependent on the user

Long-acting reversible contraceptives (LARCs)

Subdermal implants	*Pregnancy rate*: <1 in 1000 users in 1 year
	What: small flexible rod releasing progestogen under the skin of the upper arm inserted in a simple procedure under local anaesthetic
	How: inhibits ovulation, thickens cervical mucus, thins the endometrium
	Advantages: not user-dependent, lasts for 3 years but can be removed sooner, no impact on fertility
	Disadvantages: can cause irregular bleeding or amenorrhoea, involves procedure, effectiveness reduced by liver enzyme inducers
Injectables	*Pregnancy rate*: <1 in 100 users in 1 year with perfect use (6 in 100 users in 1 year with typical use)
	What: progestogen injection 13 weekly (intramuscular Depo Provera/subcutaneous Sayana Press) or eight weekly (Noristerat); Sayana Press injection can be self-administered
	How: inhibits ovulation, thickens cervical mucus, thins the endometrium
	Advantages: no need to do anything for the duration, can stop heavy painful periods
	Disadvantages: periods may stop/be irregular/last longer, delayed return of fertility, weight gain, need to remember to repeat injections at regular intervals
Intrauterine systems	*Pregnancy rate*: <1 in 100 users in 1 year
	What: small T-shaped plastic device inserted into the uterus (a short procedure when awake) that releases progestogen
	How: thins the endometrium, thickens cervical mucus
	Advantages: not user-dependent, lasts for 3–5 years depending on the type; periods usually become lighter, shorter and less painful; no impact on fertility
	Disadvantages: periods may stop/be irregular/light spotting may occur, insertion may be uncomfortable and carries a small risk of infection/uterine perforation, small increased risk of ectopic pregnancy in the unlikely event of a pregnancy
Copper intrauterine device	*Pregnancy rate*: <1 in 100 users in 1 year
	What: small T-shaped plastic and copper device inserted into the uterus (a short procedure when awake)
	How: prevents egg and sperm meeting (fertilisation), makes endometrium unfavourable for implantation
	Advantages: works immediately, can be used as emergency contraception, works for 5–10 years depending on type but can be removed sooner, not user-dependent, no impact on fertility, hormone-free
	Disadvantages: periods may become heavier, longer, or more painful; insertion may be uncomfortable and carries a small risk of bleeding, infection, and uterine perforation; small increased risk of ectopic pregnancy in the unlikely event of a pregnancy

CHAPTER 36

(*continued*)

Table 36.1 (Continued)

Methods not dependent on the user

Sterilisation	
Male	*Pregnancy rate*: 1 in 2000 users in 1 year
	What: vas deferens are cut, sealed, or tied (irreversible)
	How: stops fertilisation
	Advantages: permanent, under local anaesthetic
	Disadvantages: can take at least 8 weeks to become effective, may experience testicular pain post procedure
Female	*Pregnancy rate*: 1 in 200 users in 1 year
	What: fallopian tubes are cut, sealed or blocked in an operation
	How: stops fertilisation
	Advantages: permanent, not easily reversed, periods unaffected
	Disadvantages: operative and anaesthetic risk, small increased risk of ectopic pregnancy

User-dependent methods

Combined hormonal contraception	*Pregnancy rate*: <1 in 100 users in 1 year if used perfectly (9 in 100 users in 1 year with typical use)
	What: pill, transdermal patch, or vaginal ring releasing oestrogen and progestogen
	How: inhibits ovulation, thickens cervical mucus, thins the endometrium
	Advantages: periods can become lighter and less painful, reduced risk of certain cancers (ovarian/endometrial/colon), can improve acne, no impact on fertility
	Disadvantages: user must remember to take pill (daily) or change patch (weekly)/ring (3-weekly); small risk of thromboembolism, breast cancer, cervical cancer; can have side effects, e.g. headache, nausea, mood change (especially in adolescents), breast tenderness; effectiveness reduced by liver enzyme inducers
Progestogen-only pill	*Pregnancy rate*: <1 in 100 users in 1 year if used perfectly (9 in 100 users in 1 year with typical use)
	What: pill containing progestogen to be taken daily with no break
	How: thickens cervical mucus, can inhibit ovulation
	Advantages: useful alternative if contraindication to oestrogen, can improve painful periods
	Disadvantages: periods may stop/become lighter, irregular or more frequent/last longer; may get premenstrual syndrome (PMS)-type side effects; ineffective if taken >3 hours or >12 hours late depending on which type; effectiveness reduced by liver enzyme inducers
Male condoms	*Pregnancy rate*: 2 in 100 users in 1 year if used perfectly (18 in 100 users with typical use)
	What: thin barrier placed over erect penis
	How: stops sperm entering the vagina
	Advantages: widely available, protects from sexually transmitted infections, no serious side effects, hormone-free
	Disadvantages: can fall off, split or easily spill semen if removed incorrectly, interrupts sex
Female condoms	*Pregnancy rate*: 5 in 100 users in 1 year if used perfectly (21 in 100 users with typical use)
	What: thin silicone barrier that loosely lines the vagina
	How: stops sperm entering the vagina
	Advantages: can be inserted before sex, can help protect from sexually transmitted infections, no serious side effects
	Disadvantages: not as widely available as male condoms, may get pushed into vagina during sexual intercourse

Table 36.1 (Continued)

Methods not dependent on the user

Diaphragm/cap with spermicide	*Pregnancy rate*: 6 in 100 users in 1 year if used perfectly (12 in 100 users with typical use)
	What: flexible latex or silicone device inserted into the vagina
	How: covers the cervix to prevent sperm entering the uterus
	Advantages: can be inserted before sex, no serious side effects
	Disadvantages: need extra spermicide if having sex more than once, can take time to learn to use effectively
Fertility awareness methods	*Pregnancy rate*: 1 in 100 users in 1 year with perfect use (24 in 100 users with typical use)
	What: combines fertility indicators such as basal body temperature and cervical secretions to determine when safe to have sex
	How: avoiding sex at fertile times of the menstrual cycle
	Advantages: no serious side effects
	Disadvantages: need high motivation to keep daily records, takes time to learn to use effectively, sex must be planned

Emergency contraception

Copper intrauterine device	*Pregnancy rate*: <1 in 1000 users; most effective emergency method
	What: small T-shaped plastic and copper device inserted into the uterus (a short procedure when awake) to be inserted up to 5 days post first unprotected sexual intercourse (UPSI) in a menstrual cycle or up to 5 days after the earliest likely date of ovulation (whichever is later)
	How: prevents fertilisation and/or implantation
	Advantages: most effective method, provides ongoing contraception, not affected by body mass index (BMI) or other drugs
	Disadvantages: periods may become heavier, longer, or more painful; insertion may be uncomfortable and carries a small risk of infection, bleeding, and uterine perforation; small increased risk of ectopic pregnancy if it fails
Ulipristal acetate	*Pregnancy rate*: second most effective emergency method, 1–2 in 100 users
	What: tablet containing ulipristal acetate to be taken within 120 hours of first UPSI
	How: delays/inhibits ovulation
	Advantages: no procedure, more effective than levonorgestrel, no serious side effects, can use more than once per cycle
	Disadvantages: ineffective after ovulation has occurred; effectiveness may be reduced by liver enzyme inducers; must wait 5 days before using other hormonal contraception; may experience nausea, vomiting, headaches, or painful/altered next period
Levonorgestrel	*Pregnancy rate*: up to 3 in 100 users
	What: tablet containing a type of progestogen to be taken within 72 hours of UPSI
	How: delays/inhibits ovulation
	Advantages: no procedure, can start other contraceptives immediately, no serious side effects, can use more than once per cycle
	Disadvantages: ineffective after ovulation has occurred; effectiveness may be reduced by liver enzyme inducers or weight >70 kg/BMI >26 kg/m^2; may experience nausea, vomiting, headaches, or painful/altered next period

CHAPTER 36

The UK Medical Eligibility Criteria (UKMEC) is a freely available and easy-to-use tool designed to help clinicians determine which contraceptives are safe for patients based on their comorbid medical conditions [9]. Medical conditions considered by the UKMEC include ischaemic heart disease and cardiovascular risk factors; venous thromboembolism and risk factors; neurological conditions (e.g. migraine, epilepsy); breast and reproductive tract conditions; endocrine conditions (e.g. type 2 diabetes mellitus, thyroid disease); infectious disease status (e.g. human immuno-deficiency or tuberculosis infection), gastrointestinal disease; rheumatological dis-ease; and reproductive history. History of depression is also included in the UKMEC assessment. Comorbid conditions are ranked on a scale of 1–4 based on their suitability in association with individual contraceptive methods; 1 indicates that the condition has no restriction for use of that contraceptive method, and 4 indicates that the condition represents an unacceptable health risk if that contra-ceptive method is used. It is recommended that the UKMEC is consulted before making contraceptive decisions.

Patient information leaflets for different contraceptive methods are available online through the Family Planning Association [10]. Patients should be advised how long they need to use additional contraception such as condoms before their chosen contra-ception becomes effective and be given a plan for follow-up.

ETHICAL AND LEGAL CONSIDERATIONS

Contraceptive decisions should be non-coercive and autonomous. In people with SMI, loss of capacity may be temporary and/or improve with treatment. Ulysses contracts can apply to contraceptive decisions, where a woman gives informed consent when she is most stable and indicates that she wants her consent to remain valid if she later becomes unwell [11].

Under English law, 'Gillick competence' means that children under the age of 16 are able to consent to his or her own medical treatment without parental involvement or consent [12]. Fraser guidelines are specific to contraception, abortion, and sexual health interventions [13]. In this case, advice and treatment can be given to under 16-year-olds, provided:

- he or she has sufficient maturity and intelligence to understand the nature and impli-cations of the proposed treatment
- he or she cannot be persuaded to tell his or her parents or to allow the doctor to tell them
- he or she is very likely to begin or continue having sexual intercourse with or without contraceptive treatment
- his or her physical or mental health is likely to suffer unless he or she receives the advice or treatment
- the advice or treatment is in his or her best interests.

WHEN TO REFER

Referral to sexual/reproductive health specialists may be indicated for complex contraceptive decisions (e.g. in the context of multiple comorbidities) or for complex LARC procedures (e.g. failed IUD insertions in primary care). It is beneficial to patients for psychiatric services to work closely with sexual and reproductive health services to provide timely and effective contraception.

SPECIAL CONSIDERATIONS IN PATIENTS WITH SERIOUS MENTAL ILLNESS

Contraception and mood

Table 36.2 details factors specific to mental health disorders that may influence contraceptive decisions. Although there are anecdotal reports of hormonal contraception's association with emotional lability, most studies have failed to show evidence that this method of contraception negatively impacts mood (including in women with depressive or bipolar affective disorders), although there is evidence that adolescents may be vulnerable to contraception-related mood disturbance [14–16].

Table 36.2 Specific considerations regarding contraception in people with serious mental illness.

Mental illness	Issues to consider
Bipolar affective disorder	Impulsivity and risky sexual behaviour associated with mania
	Mood stabilisers resulting in drug interactions and teratogenicity
Psychotic disorders	Paranoia associated with indwelling contraception
	Antipsychotic-induced hyperprolactinaemia and resultant amenorrhoea or oligomenorrhoea associated with perception of infertility
	Cardiovascular disease, obesity, and smoking are contraindications to combined hormonal contraception
	Mood stabilisers as adjuncts resulting in drug interactions and teratogenicity
Anxiety and depression	Heightened negative perceptions of contraception and its impact on mood
	Impact of fluctuating or low motivation on user-dependent contraceptive methods (condoms, pills, patches, rings)
Eating disorders	Weight gain concerns
	Amenorrhoea and a perception of infertility
Substance misuse disorders	High risk of unplanned pregnancy, risk of fetal exposure to alcohol, drugs, tobacco

CHAPTER 36

Contraception and cardiometabolic disease

Increased rates of cardiovascular disease, obesity, and smoking in patients with SMI are an important consideration in contraceptive decision-making and are a contraindication to use of combined hormonal contraception. Of note, injectable contraceptives are the contraceptive type most associated with weight gain, typically in younger patients who are already overweight.

Contraception and fertility

Progestogen-only injectable contraception can delay fertility by up to one year. There is no evidence of an association between infertility and other types of contraception. For amenorrhoeic patients (e.g. people with eating disorders), return of ovulation and therefore fertility precedes return of a first period; thus being on effective contraception before this is essential to avoid unwanted pregnancy.

Contraception and psychiatric medication

Sexually active women of reproductive age who are taking known teratogenic drugs or drugs with potential teratogenic effects must use highly effective contraception, such as a copper IUD, levonorgestrel intrauterine system (LNG-IUS), or progestogen-only implant. A pregnancy prevention plan should be in place to ensure there is no risk of conception. The reader is directed to Chapter 62 for further information on the teratogenic potential of different psychiatric drugs.

Clinicians should be aware of potential interactions between contraceptives and psychiatric drugs. For example, psychiatric drugs that are CYP3A4 inducers (e.g. carbamazepine and St John's Wort) reduce the bioavailability and hence contraceptive efficacy of combined hormonal contraceptives, the progestogen-only pill, and the subdermal implant both during use and for up to 28 days after stopping enzyme-inducer treatment. Thus, patients on enzyme inducers should be encouraged to use intrauterine contraception or injectables. Conversely, combined hormonal contraceptives increase plasma clozapine concentrations; where co-prescribed, monitor for clozapine-related side effects and monitor plasma levels [17]. Where there are concerns regarding potential drug interactions between contraceptives and other prescribed medication, discussion with pharmacy colleagues is recommended.

References

1. Seeman MV, Ross R. Prescribing contraceptives for women with schizophrenia. *J Psychiatr Pract* 2011;17(4):258–269.
2. Coverdale JH, Aruffo JF. Aids and family-planning counseling of psychiatrically ill women in community mental-health clinics. *Community Ment Health J* 1992;28(1):13–20.
3. Zacher J, Peterson J, Lempicki K, Zaror P. Comparing current practices of screening for pregnancy and contraceptive use in female veterans of child-bearing age prescribed psychotropic medications in a mental health versus a women's health clinic. *Ment Health Clin* 2013;3(2):71–77.
4. Field N, Prah P, Mercer CH, et al. Are depression and poor sexual health neglected comorbidities? Evidence from a population sample. *BMJ Open* 2016;6(3):e010521.
5. Yanikkerem E, Ay S, Piro N. Planned and unplanned pregnancy: effects on health practice and depression during pregnancy. *J Obstet Gynaecol Res* 2013;39(1):180–187.

6. Myhrman A, Rantakallio P, Isohanni M, et al. Unwantedness of a pregnancy and schizophrenia in the child. *Br J Psychiatry* 1996;169(5):637–640.

7. National Institute for Health and Care Excellence. *Antenatal and Postnatal Mental Health: Clinical Management and Service Guidance.* Clinical Guideline CG192. London: NICE, 2014. https://www.nice.org.uk/guidance/cg192

8. Faculty of Sexual and Reproductive Healthcare of the Royal College of Obstetricians and Gynaecologists. Standards and Guidance, 2020. https://www.fsrh.org/standards-and-guidance/

9. Faculty of Sexual and Reproductive Healthcare of the Royal College of Obstetricians and Gynaecologists. UK Medical Eligibility Criteria For Contraceptive Use, 2016. https://www.fsrh.org/standards-and-guidance/documents/ukmec-2016/

10. Family Planning Association (FPA). Leaflet and booklet downloads: contraceptive methods. https://www.fpa.org.uk/professionals/resources/leaflet-and-booklet-downloads

11. Miller LJ. Sexuality, reproduction, and family planning in women with schizophrenia. *Schizophr Bull* 1997;23(4):623–635.

12. Great Britain. England. Court of Appeal, Civil Division. *Gillick v. West Norfolk and Wisbech Area Health Authority.* Engl Law Rep. 1984 Dec 19;1985(1):533–559.

13. Wheeler R. Gillick or Fraser? A plea for consistency over competence in children. *BMJ* 2006;332(7545):807.

14. Pagano HP, Zapata LB, Berry-Bibee EN, et al. Safety of hormonal contraception and intrauterine devices among women with depressive and bipolar disorders: a systematic review. *Contraception* 2016;94(6):641–649.

15. Worly BL, Gur TL, Schaffir J. The relationship between progestin hormonal contraception and depression: a systematic review. *Contraception* 2018;97(6):478–489.

16. de Wit AE, Booij SH, Giltay EJ, et al. Association of use of oral contraceptives with depressive symptoms among adolescents and young women. *JAMA Psychiatry* 2020;77(1):52–59.

17. Bookholt DE, Bogers JP. Oral contraceptives raise plasma clozapine concentrations. *J Clin Psychopharmacol* 2014;34(3):389–390.

CHAPTER 36

Infertility

Rudiger Pittrof

In the UK, one in eight women and one in ten men aged 16–74 years experience infertility, defined as unsuccessfully attempting to conceive for a year or longer [1]. Infertility data in people with serious mental illness (SMI) are scarce. However, a prospective cohort study drawing on the entire Danish population born after 1950 showed that people with SMI have significantly lower first-child fertility rates compared with the general population [2]. Furthermore, compared with the general population, women with psychotic illness are less likely to receive fertility treatment, and fertility treatment in this group is less successful [3].

ADDRESSING INFERTILITY IN PSYCHIATRIC PRACTICE

Psychiatric practitioners are well positioned to help their patients address fertility concerns, facilitate onward referral, and provide support during a time associated with significant psychological distress [4]. In the UK, if a heterosexual couple has regular (every two to three days) unprotected sex for one year without conception, then clinical assessment and investigation for infertility are indicated [5]. Fertility declines with age and if the woman is aged 36 years or older, referral should not be delayed.

As part of a conversation, assess the importance of having children for the patient, and discuss any concerns that patient may have about their ability to cope in pregnancy or as a parent. Confirm that the couple are engaging in sufficient sex; anything less than once a week dramatically reduces the risk of conception. Simple pre-conception advice can also be provided (Box 37.1). Undertake a medication review, assessing for any drugs that may pose a risk to an unborn child (see Chapter 62) and for any drugs that may be contributing to sexual dysfunction (see Chapter 35). Check prolactin levels if sexual dysfunction is suspected. Based on these assessments, rationalisation of

---

Box 37.1 Pre-conception advice [5]

- Sexual intercourse every two to three days optimises the chance of pregnancy.
- Women who are trying to become pregnant should not drink more than 1–2 units of alcohol per week and avoid episodes of intoxication.
- Women who smoke should be informed that this is likely to reduce their fertility. Passive smoking is also likely to reduce likelihood of conception. Where appropriate refer to smoking cessation services (see Chapter 46).
- Women who have a body mass index (BMI) over 30 kg/m² should be informed that they are likely to take longer to conceive. Similarly, men with a BMI over 30 kg/m² are likely to have reduced fertility. Thus, where appropriate, advise weight loss (see Chapter 14).
- Women with a BMI under 19 kg/m² and who have irregular menstruation or are not menstruating should be advised that increasing body weight is likely to improve their chances of conception.

---

psychiatric medication may be indicated. This information should be included in any onward referrals to primary/secondary care.

ONWARD REFERRAL AND FURTHER TESTS FOR INFERTILITY

Initial tests for infertility can be performed in primary care. For the man, this involves semen analysis, and for the woman a mid-luteal phase progesterone level to confirm ovulation (blood test taken seven days before expected period). In the UK, onward referral for people presenting with infertility vary between health authorities and should be directed by primary care [5].

INFERTILITY TREATMENTS

There are three main types of fertility treatment: medical, surgical, and assisted conception. Medical treatment involves the use of drugs to induce ovulation (e.g. clomifene) and surgical treatment may be indicated for women with fallopian tube obstruction/ endometriosis or for men with epididymal obstruction. Assisted conception describes means of conception other than via normal coitus. This includes intrauterine insemination (where sperm is placed in the woman's uterus using a fine plastic tube) and *in vitro* fertilisation (where one or more eggs are retrieved from the woman and mixed with the man's sperm; the resultant embryo is then injected into the uterus via the cervix).

References

1. Datta J, Palmer MJ, Tanton C, et al. Prevalence of infertility and help seeking among 15 000 women and men. *Hum Reprod* 2016;31(9):2108–2118.
2. Laursen TM, Munk-Olsen T. Reproductive patterns in psychotic patients. *Schizophr Res* 2010;121(1–3):234–240.
3. Ebdrup NH, Assens M, Hougaard CO, et al. Assisted reproductive technology (ART) treatment in women with schizophrenia or related psychotic disorder: a national cohort study. *Eur J Obstet Gynecol Reprod Biol* 2014;177:115–120.
4. Nachtigall RD, Becker G, Wozny M. The effects of gender-specific diagnosis on men's and women's response to infertility. *Fertil Steril* 1992;57(1):113–121.
5. National Institute for Health and Care Excellence. *Fertility Problems: Assessment and Treatment*. Clinical Guideline CG156. London: NICE, 2013. Available at https://www.nice.org.uk/guidance/cg156

Sexually Transmitted Infection
Harriet Le Voir, Rudiger Pittrof

There are several shared risk factors for sexually transmitted infection (STI) and serious mental illness (SMI), including low socioeconomic status, abuse (e.g. childhood and/or sexual abuse), and recreational drug use [1–5]. Risk of STI is further increased in people who at times lack capacity to make decisions about sexual activity (e.g. negotiation of condom use). This chapter outlines an approach to history taking, diagnosis, and management of STIs in the SMI population. The reader is also directed to complementary chapters on contraception (Chapter 36), sexual dysfunction (Chapter 35), pregnancy (Chapter 62), and human immunodeficiency virus (HIV; Chapter 45).

HISTORY

When taking an STI history, the clinician should be sensitive to the patient's previous sexual experiences that may be contributing to poor mental health (e.g. in the context of same-sex relationships that are not culturally approved or a history of sexual abuse). Furthermore, capacity to consent to STI testing will need to be considered in some patients. Patients may be surprised to be asked about their sex life; clear explanations about the rationale for such a discussion will provide reassurance. Assessment of STI risk should take place in the context of broader discussions about sexual dysfunction and contraception.

Typical symptoms of common STIs are presented in Table 38.1. To enquire about such symptoms, use a phrase such as 'Do you have any genital symptoms you are concerned about, for example discharge, abnormal bleeding, pain when passing urine, or ulcers?' To enquire whether a male patient has had sex with another man, use a phrase such as 'About one in ten men have had sex with another man in the past. Have you ever had sex with a man?' Box 38.1 provides a series of questions that assess risk of a

The Maudsley Practice Guidelines for Physical Health Conditions in Psychiatry, First Edition.
David M. Taylor, Fiona Gaughran, and Toby Pillinger.
© 2021 John Wiley & Sons Ltd. Published 2021 by John Wiley & Sons Ltd.

Table 38.1 Symptoms of sexually transmitted infections.

Symptoms	Aetiology
Discharge, dysuria, testicular/pelvic pain	*Chlamydia trachomatis, Neisseria gonorrhoeae, Trichomonas vaginalis, Mycoplasma genitalium*
Wart-like lesions	Human papillomavirus
Blisters and ulcers	Herpes simplex virus, *Treponema pallidum* (syphilis)
Rectal symptoms	*Chlamydia trachomatis* (and lymphogranuloma venereum subtype), *Neisseria gonorrhoeae*, herpes simplex virus
Rash	*Treponema pallidum* (syphilis), HIV

Box 38.1 Identifying risk of blood-borne virus sexual transmission

Answering yes to any of the following questions should indicate testing for HIV and hepatitis B/C.

- Have you had sex with someone who has HIV or hepatitis?
- Have you had sex with someone who injects drugs, or do you inject drugs?
- Have you had sex with someone who is born outside Europe/Australasia/North America?
- Have you paid for sex or been paid for sex?
- Have you had sex with men (if male) or bisexual men (if female)?

---

sexually transmitted blood-borne virus infection (HIV and hepatis B and C). Forensic examination may be indicated where non-consensual sex has taken place in the last seven days. In this scenario, discussion with a local sexual assault centre is indicated.

STI TESTING IN PSYCHIATRY

In certain areas, home testing kits for STI (including HIV) can be ordered online (e.g. in London, via www.shl.uk). Such kits may be appropriate for patients reluctant to attend sexual health clinics. However, home testing kits may not be practical or appropriate for all patients owing to logistical barriers such as the need for online registration and relaying test results back via text message. HIV and syphilis testing should already be routinely performed in psychiatric practice. For patients with systemic symptoms consider repeating syphilis, HIV (rash and/or flu-like symptoms), and hepatitis B/C testing (fatigue, jaundice, itching, nausea/vomiting). If testing for STIs other than HIV and syphilis is required in a patient who is unable to attend a sexual health clinic, then discussion with local sexual health services is recommended. For an inpatient with symptoms suggestive of an STI who may lack capacity to consent to STI testing, a risk–benefit decision regarding investigation/treatment will need to be made. This will weigh up the immediate benefits of treatment (symptomatic relief and reduction in long-term poor physical health) against the potential distress to the patient in terms of attending a

---

Box 38.2 Screening tests recommended for STI based on presenting complaint

Symptomatic male

- First-void urine sample for *Chlamydia trachomatis* and *Neisseria gonorrhoeae* gonorrhoea (combined test), *Mycoplasma genitalium*, and *Trichomonas vaginalis*: total of three samples required for nucleic acid amplification tests (NAATs)
- Microscopy, culture, and sensitivity of urethral discharge
- Syphilis and HIV blood tests

Symptomatic female

- Vaginal swab for *C. trachomatis*, *N. gonorrhoeae*, and *T. vaginalis* NAATs
- Microscopy, culture, and sensitivity for *N. gonorrhoeae* culture
- Syphilis and HIV blood tests

Genital ulcers

- Herpes simplex virus and syphilis swab for polymerase chain reaction (PCR)
- *C. trachomatis* and *N. gonorrhoeae* swab for NAATs
- Syphilis and HIV blood tests

Rectal symptoms

- *C. trachomatis* and *N. gonorrhoeae* swab for NAATs
- Herpes simplex virus swab for PCR
- Syphilis and HIV blood tests

HIV screening test (fourth-generation antibody and antigen), syphilis antibody, hepatitis B core antibody, and HCV antibody are recommended for all patients who have had unprotected sex. Discussion with the local laboratory to identify which serology blood bottles are required is advised to avoid rejected samples.

CHAPTER 38

sexual health clinic and/or the necessary associated investigations. Box 38.2 describes the investigations indicated depending on presenting complaint, and Box 38.3 the appropriate time frame for STI testing based on date of last sexual contact.

DETERMINING URGENCY OF CLINICAL ACTION/REFERRAL

1 Symptoms/results/presentations that require urgent action (same day):
  a Any genital injury or anything causing severe pain, particularly acute scrotal or pelvic pain; erections that are painful or persist for longer than two hours; and genital ulcers in the presence of neurological symptoms/acute psychiatric symptoms (which could indicate herpes encephalitis; see Chapter 81).
  b Where HIV post-exposure prophylaxis is indicated (if a man who is presumed to be HIV negative has had unprotected receptive anal sex in the last 72 hours). Please see Chapter 45.

> **Box 38.3** When to perform STI testing based on date of last sexual contact
>
> ### Chlamydia and gonorrhoea
>
> - Two weeks after unprotected sex
>
> ### HIV
>
> - Four weeks after unprotected sex if blood test, *or*
> - Three months after unprotected sex with saliva/finger-prick test
>
> ### Syphilis
>
> - Three months after unprotected sex
> - Two weeks after genital ulcer symptoms if initial test negative
>
> ### Hepatitis
>
> - Three months after unprotected sex
>
> Sexual health screening is advised every three months if regular changes of partner

   c A new positive HIV or syphilis test should always be discussed with local sexual health services within 24 hours to assess urgency of need for assessment and treatment.

2 Symptoms that need to be discussed with local sexual health services within three days: genital or anal ulcers or blisters, penile discharge, or anything that is distressing the patient.

3 Symptoms that can await discussion with a local sexual health clinic for up to two weeks if immediate discussion is impractical (e.g. if acutely unwell on a psychiatric ward): genital skin problems that are not ulcers, rectal or vaginal discharge that is not distressing, blood in semen, scrotal masses, long-term pelvic or scrotal pain, rectal pain that is not distressing, and mild rectal bleeding.

REFERRAL TO SEXUAL HEALTH SERVICES

Discussion with local sexual health services is recommended if a patient requires an STI test or treatment. Men who have sex with men, those who are involved in transactional sex (e.g. sex for money, drugs, food, or shelter), and those who have been a victim of sexual violence should also be seen by sexual health services. Ask a health adviser from the sexual health service to speak directly to the patient on the phone to arrange/offer a meeting. If possible and appropriate, offer to go with the patient to the meeting, as attending sexual health services can be daunting.

   There are many services available within a sexual health clinic: human papillomavirus (HPV) vaccination for men who have sex with men, hepatitis A and B vaccination, information about HIV pre- and post-exposure prophylaxis (see Chapter 45), counselling and training relating to risk reduction, condom use, safer recreational drug use in the context of sex, safer dating, and sexuality.

Treatment of STI

In the case of a positive STI test, best practice is for the patient to be reviewed by sexual health services who will guide appropriate management. Current first-line treatment options are outlined in Table 38.2, although treatment regimens are regularly updated (see www.bashh.org) and should be guided by local protocols.

Contact tracing is important to prevent both complications in the partner and re-infection. Where available, health advisors in a sexual health clinic are best placed to provide this service. Anonymous contact tracing for partner notification of infection can also be carried out by sexual health services, with consent from the patient.

Table 38.2 Typical treatment regimens for sexually transmitted infections.

Infection	Typical first-line treatment	Alternative treatment
Chlamydia trachomatis	Oral doxycycline[a] 100 mg b.d. for 7 days	Oral azithromycin 1 g stat, then 500 mg o.d. for 2 days (3 days total)
Symptomatic rectal *Chlamydia*	Oral doxycycline 100 mg b.d. for 21 days until LGV status known	
Neisseria gonorrhoeae	Ceftriaxone 1 g i.m. stat	Oral options possible with guidance from culture results
Trichomonas vaginalis	Oral metronidazole 400 mg b.d. for 5 days	Oral metronidazole 2 g stat (not in pregnancy)
Mycoplasma genitalium	Discuss with local sexual health clinic	
Genital herpes simplex virus	Oral aciclovir 400 mg t.d.s. for 5 days, salt water bathing, simple analgesia, urgent medical assessment if unable to pass urine or neurological symptoms	
Genital warts (human papillomavirus)	Cryotherapy/topical podophyllotoxin/topical imiquimod: discuss with sexual health services. Delay of less than four weeks does not impact treatment efficacy	
Syphilis	Dependent on stage of infection relating to serology (RPR), symptoms, and history of previous syphilis treatment. Usually either penicillin-based intramuscular injection or oral doxycycline	
HIV	See Chapter 45. Discussion with HIV service required. CD4 count required to help guide urgency of clinical state for HIV team	

[a] Doxycycline should not be used in pregnant women (see Chapter 62).
LGV, lymphogranuloma venereum; RPR, rapid plasma reagin.

CHAPTER 38

References

1. Huang SY, Hung JH, Hu LY, et al. Risk of sexually transmitted infections following depressive disorder: a nationwide population-based cohort study. *Medicine (Baltimore)* 2018;97(43):e12539.

2. World Health Organization Executive Board, 124th Session. HIV/AIDS and mental health: report by the Secretariat. EB124/6, 20 November 2008. https://apps.who.int/iris/handle/10665/2107

3. Magidson JF, Blashill AJ, Wall MM, et al. Relationship between psychiatric disorders and sexually transmitted diseases in a nationally representative sample. *J Psychosom Res* 2014;76(4):322–328.

4. Petrak J, Byrne A, Baker M. The association between abuse in childhood and STD/HIV risk behaviours in female genitourinary (GU) clinic attendees. *Sex Transm Infect* 2000;76(6):457–461.

5. Whooley MA, Simon GE. Primary care: managing depression in medical outpatients. *N Engl J Med* 2000;343(26):1942–1950.

Part 7

Infectious Diseases

Pneumonia

Emma McGuire, Loren Bailey, Peter Saunders, Meera Chand

Pneumonia is an infection of the lungs that results in acute lower respiratory symptoms, including cough and difficulty in breathing, which may be accompanied by fever. There may be new focal chest signs on examination and if chest X-ray is performed there is new shadowing which cannot be ascribed to any other cause (e.g. pulmonary oedema or infarction) [1].

Pneumonia can be broadly categorised as community-acquired pneumonia (CAP) or hospital-acquired pneumonia (HAP), the latter occurring after 48 hours of hospitalisation or within two weeks of discharge from hospital [1]. Pneumonia acquired in long-term care facilities may be caused by either community or healthcare-associated respiratory pathogens. Psychiatric hospital-acquired pneumonia (PHAP) is defined as pneumonia that occurs during psychiatric hospitalisation. PHAP is associated with significant mortality, estimated at 21.3%, and is reported to account for 9.5–18% of deaths in psychiatric hospitals [2–4].

CAP can be caused by bacteria or viruses (Box 39.1). Whilst a small number of pathogens account for most pneumonia, causes vary significantly with age, with pneumococcal pneumonia, influenza, and aspiration pneumonia predominating in the elderly [5]. There is also seasonal variation, particularly evident in viral causes, either alone or in association with bacterial co-infection. In the context of immunosuppression (HIV infection, steroids, post transplantation) the range of organisms causing pneumonia is broader. Consideration should also be given to non-infective mimics of pneumonia, including pulmonary oedema, pulmonary embolism, lung cancer, and vasculitic or connective tissue disease.

At the time of writing this book, coronavirus disease 2019 (COVID-19), an infectious disease caused by severe acute respiratory syndrome coronavirus 2 (SARS-CoV-2), has resulted in an ongoing pandemic [6], with the elderly and individuals with comorbidities such as respiratory and cardiovascular disease at increased risk of severe disease and death [7].

The Maudsley Practice Guidelines for Physical Health Conditions in Psychiatry, First Edition.
David M. Taylor, Fiona Gaughran, and Toby Pillinger.
© 2021 John Wiley & Sons Ltd. Published 2021 by John Wiley & Sons Ltd.

Box 39.1 Common causative organisms of pneumonia

Community-acquired pneumonia

Bacteria (common)

Streptococcus pneumoniae
Haemophilus influenzae
Staphylococcus aureus (including MRSA)
Streptococcus pyogenes
Moraxella catarrhalis
Klebsiella pneumoniae
Mycoplasma pneumoniae
Legionella spp.
Chlamydophila pneumoniae
Mycobacterium tuberculosis

Bacteria (less common; consider depending on setting and exposures)

Chlamydia psittaci
Q fever
Endemic mycoses

Viruses

Influenza A and B
Parainfluenza
Respiratory syncytial virus
Human metapneumovirus
Adenoviruses
Seasonal coronaviruses (e.g. MERS Co-V)
Severe acute respiratory syndrome coronavirus 2 (SARS-CoV-2)

Hospital-acquired pneumonia

Staphylococcus aureus (including MRSA)
Gram-negative organisms such as *Pseudomonas* spp., Enterobacteriaceae and *Acinetobacter* spp.

Aspiration pneumonia

Multifactorial: chemical injury ± mixed upper respiratory tract bacteria, commonly including anaerobes

Immunocompromise

In addition to conventional causes of CAP:
Atypical mycobacteria
Nocardia spp.
Cytomegalovirus
Pneumocystis jirovecii
Aspergillus spp. and other moulds
Cryptococcus spp.

MRSA, methicillin-resistant *Staphylococcus aureus*; MERS Co-V, Middle Eastern respiratory syndrome-related coronavirus.

PNEUMONIA AND SERIOUS MENTAL ILLNESS

Patients with serious mental illness (SMI) and pneumonia are more likely to present late and have higher rates of admission to the intensive care unit (ICU) and mortality [8–11]. Indeed, in schizophrenia, patients are seven times more likely to die as a consequence of pneumonia or influenza compared with the general population [12]. There is a higher prevalence of smoking, substance abuse, and obesity among patients with SMI, all of which are independently associated with worse outcomes in pneumonia (see Chapters 24 and 46) [7]. There may also be reduced respiratory reserve due to nutritional deficiency and poorer control of pulmonary comorbidities such as asthma and chronic obstructive pulmonary disease (COPD) (see Chapters 47 and 48) [13]. There is a higher prevalence of HIV among patients with SMI which is associated with increased severity and frequency of CAP, as well as opportunistic infections (see Chapter 45) [14,15]. Rates of homelessness, incarceration, and vitamin D deficiency are disproportionately high among patients with SMI, all of which are risk factors for tuberculosis (TB; see Chapter 44) [16–19]. In the general population, individuals at highest risk for severe disease and death from COVID-19 infection include people aged over 60 years, those who smoke, and those with underlying conditions such as obesity, hypertension, diabetes, cardiovascular disease, chronic respiratory disease, and cancer [7,20]. Owing to increased multimorbidity and rates of smoking, patients with serious mental illness represent a vulnerable population for developing severe COVID-19 infection.

Psychotropic medications may also elevate the risk of respiratory complications including aspiration pneumonia (see Chapter 27) [9,11,21,22]. In particular, clozapine is associated with increased risk of pneumonia, which may be related not only to increased risk of salivary aspiration, but also its immunosuppressive effects [23,24].

DIAGNOSTIC PRINCIPLES

History

1 Typical symptoms include fever, cough, difficulty in breathing, and pleuritic chest pain.
2 Atypical presentations include confusion, gastrointestinal symptoms (e.g. diarrhoea, abdominal pain), headache, myalgia, or rash.
3 Elderly or immunosuppressed patients may be afebrile and may present with atypical features.
4 Coryzal symptoms suggestive of viral infection include sore throat, runny nose, and myalgia.
5 Take note of any TB risk factors and symptoms: homelessness, incarceration, migration, personal history of TB, contact with a known case of TB, or prolonged fever, weight loss, or night sweats.
6 Symptoms of COVID-19 include fever, cough, fatigue, myalgia, shortness of breath, loss of smell and taste, and diarrhoea.

CHAPTER 39

7 Take a travel history (discuss with an infection specialist or microbiologist if there is a history of recent foreign travel).
8 Medication history, including psychiatric treatments associated with hypersalivation and therefore potential aspiration, e.g. clozapine (see Chapter 27); note any allergies to antibiotics.
9 Past medical history, including:
    a respiratory disease such as asthma, COPD, interstitial lung disease
    b immunosuppression such as HIV, steroid use, bone marrow or solid organ transplantation
    c chronic cardiac, renal or hepatic failure or diabetes mellitus.
10 Social history, including:
    a smoking
    b alcohol intake
    c recreational drug use
    d homelessness
    e incarceration.

Examination

1 Check observations, including temperature, respiratory rate, blood pressure, and pulse oximetry. Consider scoring these with a clinical warning system such as the National Early Warning Score (NEWS) 2 [25].
2 Assess for the presence of septic shock and manage accordingly (see Chapter 72).
3 Assess fluid status: indicators of volume deficit include thirst, hypotension, dry skin or mucous membranes, reduced skin turgor, sunken eyes.
4 Assess nutritional status: indicators include weight, thin skin or hair, muscle wasting, nail changes, bruising, oedema.
5 Palpate the chest for tactile fremitus (may be increased in pneumonia or decreased if there is a pleural effusion), and for chest expansion (may be unilaterally reduced in pneumonia).
6 Percuss the chest for dullness (pneumonia or effusion) or hyper-resonance (pneumothorax or emphysema).
7 Auscultate the chest for signs of pneumonia (bronchial breathing, crackles, increased vocal resonance) or pleural effusion (reduced breath sounds, friction rub). Note that pneumonia may be complicated by parapneumonic effusion or empyema.

Investigations

Recommended investigations for pneumonia in community-based patients and general medical hospital-based patients are documented in Table 39.1. Additional investigations may be indicated in immunocompromise or following recent travel; liaise with an infectious disease specialist or microbiologist. Causative organisms of pneumonia in psychiatric inpatients may differ from those in general medical inpatients. At present, there is no specific guidance for management of PHAP and we would recommend tailoring investigations to the severity of the presentation, and if necessary following discussion with general medical services.

Table 39.1 Recommended investigations for pneumonia in patients being managed in the community or in hospital.

Investigation	Community setting	Hospital setting
Chest X-ray	Not necessary unless diagnosis is in doubt or underlying pathology such as lung cancer is suspected	Recommended
Blood tests: Full blood count (FBC) Urea and electrolytes Liver function tests C-reactive protein	Consider FBC is recommended in patients taking clozapine, mianserin, mirtazapine, or carbamazepine to assess for neutropenia	Recommended FBC is recommended in patients taking clozapine, mianserin, mirtazapine, or carbamazepine to assess for neutropenia
Pulse oximetry	Consider	Recommended at diagnosis and regularly if clinically indicated (consider medical admission if not available)
Sputum culture	Recommended for moderate or severe pneumonia Consider in mild pneumonia not responding to empirical antibiotics	Recommended, ideally prior to antibiotic therapy
Blood culture	Not routinely recommended	Recommended if available, ideally prior to antibiotic therapy
Urine pneumococcal antigen	Not routinely recommended	Recommended in moderate to severe CAP
Urine *Legionella* antigen[a]	Not routinely recommended	Recommended in severe CAP Consider in moderate CAP
Sputum AFB[a]	Consider if risk factors or suspicion of tuberculosis	Consider if risk factors or suspicion of tuberculosis[b]
Viral PCR on nose or throat swab	Not routinely recommended; however refer to local policy if COVID-19 is suspected	Recommended in influenza season or on clinical suspicion such as coryzal symptoms[b] Refer to local policy if COVID-19 is suspected
HIV test	Consider for all patients	Consider for all patients
Clozapine levels	Consider for all patients taking clozapine (see section Pharmacological considerations in SMI patients)	

[a] Consider discussion with an infection specialist if atypical clinical features are present or if tuberculosis is suspected (see section History).
[b] If tuberculosis, influenza or COVID-19 are suspected in hospitalised patients, remember to isolate according to local policy and use personal protective equipment (PPE) whilst awaiting investigation results.
AFB, acid-fast bacilli; HIV, human immunodeficiency virus; PCR, polymerase chain reaction.
Source: adapted from National Institute for Health and Care Excellence [1] and Lim et al. [26].

MANAGEMENT

- For CAP, assess the severity using clinical judgement, supported by the CURB-65 score (Table 39.2) [27]. Alternative clinical risk scoring systems include the Pneumonia Severity Index (PSI) [28].
- Severity of pneumonia will guide clinical management (Table 39.3) [1,26].
- In PHAP, predictors of mortality include age over 65, body mass index less than 18.5 kg/m², and bilateral pneumonic infiltration [2].
- Individuals at highest risk for severe disease and death from COVID-19 infection include people aged over 60 years, those who smoke, and those with underlying conditions such as obesity, hypertension, diabetes, cardiovascular disease, chronic respiratory disease, and cancer.

Non-pharmacological

- Advise patients to rest and drink plenty of fluids, and encourage smoking cessation (see Chapter 46).
- Repeat chest X-ray after about six weeks to assess for resolution of radiological changes and rule out underlying malignancy [26].
- Arrange vaccination in accordance with national guidance. In the UK, pneumococcal and influenza vaccination is advised after recovery from pneumonia if the patient is over 65 years old, a smoker, a long-term facility resident, or has a chronic medical condition (cardiac disease, respiratory disease, liver disease, renal failure, diabetes, alcoholism, or immunosuppression) [29]. Patients with SMI are at higher risk than others of pneumococcal disease, but in the UK are not yet recognised as a high-risk group in current immunisation policies [30]. We recommend that where key risk factors for pneumococcal disease are identified in patients with SMI (e.g. smoking, diabetes) that vaccination is offered.
- For inpatients with pneumonia:

Table 39.2 CURB-65 scoring for severity of community-acquired pneumonia [27].

Clinical feature	Details	Points
Confusion	AMTS ≤ 8/10 or new disorientation in person, place or time	1
Uraemia[a]	Urea >7 mmol/L	1
Respiratory rate	≥30 breaths/minute	1
Blood pressure	Systolic <90 mmHg or diastolic ≤60 mmHg	1
Age ≥65 years		1

[a] For hospitalised patients.
AMTS, abbreviated mental test score.

Table 39.3 Guidelines on management of CAP by severity, in the UK general population.[a]

Severity	Mortality	Treatment site	Preferred treatment	Alternative treatment
Low (CURB-65: 0–1)	<3%	Home-based care	Amoxicillin	Doxycycline, or Clarithromycin
Moderate (CURB-65: 2)	3–15%	Consider hospital-based care	Amoxicillin and clarithromycin, or Benzylpenicillin and clarithromycin	Doxycycline, or Levofloxacin, or Moxifloxacin
High (CURB-65: 3–5)	>15%	Hospital-based care Consider critical care review	Co-amoxiclav and clarithromycin	Benzylpenicillin *and either* Levofloxacin *or* Ciprofloxacin *or* Clarithromycin *and either* Cefuroxime *or* Cefotaxime *or* Ceftriaxone

[a] Antibiotic prescribing guidelines are for reference only and will differ between different geographic areas. Clinicians should consult local and national guidance.
Source: adapted from National Institute for Health and Care Excellence [1] and Lim et al. [26].

- If COVID-19, influenza, TB, or travel-related infections are suspected, isolate according to local policy and use personal protective equipment (PPE) whilst awaiting investigation results (refer to local policy).
- Patients requiring oxygen therapy to maintain their target saturations should be considered for transfer to a medical ward (target saturations are generally 94–98%, or 88–92% in those at risk of hypercapnic respiratory failure) [26].
- For outpatients with suspected COVID-19, follow local/national policy regarding self-isolation and further management.

Pharmacological

- Review allergy status before prescribing antibiotics.
- Empiric antibiotic choice will depend on the clinical diagnosis (CAP, HAP, or aspiration pneumonia).
- Refer to local antimicrobial prescribing guidelines which take into account the geographically variable prevalence and antimicrobial resistance of respiratory pathogens. National UK recommendations for the treatment of CAP are provided in Table 39.3 [31]. North American readers are directed to the Infectious Diseases Society of America/American Thoracic Society consensus guidelines on the management of CAP [32].
- Use oral antibiotics when possible for mild to moderate pneumonia. If intravenous antibiotics are required, consider transfer to a general medical ward.
- Duration for CAP: five days for low severity, seven to ten days for moderate to severe [1].
- Duration for HAP: five days [1].

CHAPTER 39

- Consider venous thromboembolism prophylaxis in all inpatients with pneumonia who are not fully mobile [26].
- Steroids are not indicated in CAP [1].
- Consider oseltamivir during influenza season for patients with evidence of lower respiratory tract infection and/or underlying medical conditions (see Chapter 40) [33].

Pharmacological considerations in SMI patients

- Abrupt smoking cessation can affect psychiatric medication levels (such as clozapine), so consider therapeutic drug monitoring (see Chapter 46) [34].
- Clozapine levels can rise during acute infection, and therefore close monitoring of plasma levels and dose reduction may be required [35].
- Ciprofloxacin and erythromycin may cause a rise in clozapine levels and increased risk of toxicity, so monitoring of plasma levels is recommended [36,37].
- Macrolides and quinolones may cause QTc prolongation: consider ECG monitoring if prescribed alongside other medications that prolong QTc (see Chapter 3) [38].
- Neuropsychiatric side effects of quinolones include insomnia (common), and anxiety, depression, hallucinations, and confusion (rare) [38].
- Neuropsychiatric side effects of macrolides include insomnia (common) and anxiety (uncommon) [38].
- Prescription of psychotropic medication (including clozapine) can generally continue in patients with pneumonia (including patients with COVID-19); however, as previously described doses may need to be reviewed. There are of course caveats to this advice, for example considering stopping predominantly renally excreted drugs such as lithium in the context of acute kidney injury (see Chapter 73). Where prescribing decisions are unclear, seek multidisciplinary input from general medical colleagues and pharmacy.
- Signs and symptoms of pneumonia (including influenza and COVID-19) can mimic those seen in severe clozapine-associated complications such as neutropenic sepsis and myocarditis; thus, screening for these presentations in patients receiving clozapine is recommended (see Chapters 8, 16, and 72).

When to refer to a medical subspecialty

- Advise patients that symptoms should steadily improve, although the rate of improvement will vary, and some symptoms are quicker to resolve than others [1]:
  - in general, symptoms should start to improve within three days
  - after one week, fever should have resolved
  - after four weeks, sputum production should have substantially reduced
  - after three months, most symptoms should have resolved, although fatigue may persist
  - most patients will feel back to normal after six months.
- When to seek local microbiology advice:
  - in suspected TB (see Chapter 44)

- in suspected COVID-19
- in patients who are immunosuppressed
- in patients who have recently travelled abroad
- in patients who are failing to improve on empiric treatment
- discuss positive test results to appropriately narrow antimicrobial therapy.
- When to seek medical advice (e.g. respiratory input):
  - if pneumonia is severe or complicated by respiratory failure (such as failure to meet target saturations without oxygen)
  - if there is evidence of more severe disease, such as an elevated NEWS 2 score or features of septic shock
  - in those with multiple medical comorbidities
  - if there is suspicion of malignancy or other underlying lung disease.
- Seek HIV specialist advice when managing infections in HIV-positive patients (see Chapter 45).

References

1. National Institute for Health and Care Excellence. *Pneumonia in Adults: Diagnosis and Management*. Clinical Guideline CG191. London: NICE, 2014. Av ailable at https://www.nice.org.uk/guidance/cg191

2. Haga T, Ito K, Sakashita K, et al. Risk factors for death from psychiatric hospital-acquired pneumonia. *Intern Med* 2018;57(17):2473–2478.

3. Hewer W, Rössler W, Fätkenheuer B, Löffler W. Mortality among patients in psychiatric hospitals in Germany. *Acta Psychiatr Scand* 1995;91:174–179.

4. Barnosa S, Sequeira M, Castro S, et al. Causes of death in an acute psychiatric inpatient unit of a Portuguese general hospital. *Acta Med Port* 2016;29(7–8):468–475.

5. Stupka J, Mortensen E, Anzueto A, Restrepo M. Community-acquired pneumonia in elderly patients. *Aging Health* 2009;5(6):763–774.

6. World Health Organization. Coronavirus disease (COVID-19) pandemic. Country and technical guidance. https://www.who.int/emergencies/diseases/novel-coronavirus-2019 (accessed 24 May 2020).

7. World Health Organization. Report of the WHO-China Joint Mission on Coronavirus Disease 2019 (COVID-19). https://www.who.int/docs/default-source/coronaviruse/who-china-joint-mission-on-covid-19-final-report.pdf

8. Brown S, Kim M, Mitchell C, Inskip H. Twenty-five-year mortality of a community cohort with schizophrenia. *Br J Psychiatry* 2010;196:116–121.

9. Chen YH, Lin HC, Lin HC. Poor clinical outcomes among pneumonia patients with schizophrenia. *Schizophr Bull* 2011;37(5):1088–1094.

10. Crump C, Winkleby M, Sundquist K, Sunquist J. Comorbidities and mortality in persons with schizophrenia: a Swedish national cohort study. *Am J Psychiatry* 2013;170:324–333.

11. Laursen TM, Nordentoft M, Mortensen PB. Excess early mortality in schizophrenia. *Annu Rev Clin Psychol* 2014;10:425–448.

12. Olfson M, Gerhard T, Huang C, et al. Premature mortality among adults with schizophrenia in the United States. *JAMA Psychiatry* 2015;72(12):1172–1181.

13. Filik R, Sipos A, Kehoe PG, et al. The cardiovascular and respiratory health of people with schizophrenia. *Acta Psychiatr Scand* 2006;113(4):298–305.

14. Rosenberg SD, Goodman LA, Osher FC, et al. Prevalence of HIV, hepatitis B, and hepatitis C in people with severe mental illness. *Am J Public Health* 2001;91:31–37.

15. Singh D, Berkman A, Bresnahan M. Seroprevalence and HIV-associated factors among adults with severe mental illness: a vulnerable population. *S Afr Med J* 2009;99(7):523–527.

16. Birmingham L. The mental health of prisoners. *Adv Psychiatr Treat* 2003;9:191–201.

17. Rees S. *Mental ill health in the adult single homeless population: a review of the literature*. London: Crisis, Public Health Resource Unit, 2009. Available at https://www.crisis.org.uk/media/20611/crisis_mental_ill_health_2009.pdf

18. Public Health England. *Tuberculosis in England: 2019 report*. London: PHE, 2019. Available at https://assets.publishing.service.gov.uk/government/uploads/system/uploads/attachment_data/file/821334/Tuberculosis_in_England-annual_report_2019.pdf

19. Lally J, Gardner-Sood P, Firdosi M, et al. Clinical correlates of vitamin D deficiency in established psychosis. *BMC Psychiatry* 2016;16:76.

20. World Health Organization. WHO Statement: tobacco use and COVID-19. https://www.who.int/news-room/detail/11-05-2020-who-statement-tobacco-use-and-covid-19

21. Herzig SJ, LaSalvia MT, Naidus E, et al. Antipsychotics and the risk of aspiration pneumonia in individuals hospitalised for non-psychiatric conditions: a cohort study. *J Am Geriatr Soc* 2007;65(12):2580–2586.

CHAPTER 39

22. Gurrera RJ, Parlee AC, Perry NL. Aspiration pneumonia: an underappreciated risk of clozapine treatment. *J Clin Psychopharmacol* 2016;36(2):174–176.

23. Stoecker ZR, George WT, O'Brien JB, et al. Clozapine usage increases the incidence of pneumonia compared with risperidone and the general population: a retrospective comparison of clozapine, risperidone, and the general population in a single hospital over 25 months. *Int Clin Psychopharmacol* 2017;32(3):155–160.

24. Hung GC, Liu HC, Yang SY, et al. Antipsychotic re-exposure and recurrent pneumonia in schizophrenia: a nested case-control study. *J Clin Psychiatry* 2016;77(1):60–66.

25. Royal College of Physicians. *National Early Warning Score (NEWS) 2: Standardising the assessment of acute-illness severity in the NHS.* Updated report of a working party. London: RCP, 2017.

26. Lim WS, Baudouin SV, George RC et al. BTS guidelines for the management of community acquired pneumonia in adults: update 2009. *Thorax* 2009;64(Suppl 3): iii1–iii55.

27. Lim WS, van der Eerden MM, Laing R, et al. Defining community acquired pneumonia severity on presentation to hospital: an international derivation and validation study. *Thorax* 2003;58(5):377–382.

28. Fine MJ, Auble TE, Yealy DM, et al. A prediction rule to identify low-risk patients with community-acquired pneumonia. *N Engl J Med* 1997;336(4):243–250.

29. Department of Health. *Immunisation Against Infectious Disease: The Green Book.* Chapter 25: Pneumococcal. https://www.gov.uk/government/publications/pneumococcal-the-green-book-chapter-25

30. Seminog OO, Goldacre MJ. Risk of pneumonia and pneumococcal disease in people with severe mental illness: English record linkage studies. *Thorax* 2013;68(2):171–176.

31. Woodhead M, Blasi F, Ewig S, et al. Guidelines for the management of adult lower respiratory tract infections: summary. *Clin Microbiol Infect* 2011;17(Suppl 6):1–24.

32. Mandell LA, Wunderink RG, Anzueto A, et al. Infectious Diseases Society of America/American Thoracic Society consensus guidelines on the management of community-acquired pneumonia in adults. *Clin Infect Dis* 2007;44(Suppl 2):S27–S72.

33. Public Health England. *Guidance on use of antiviral agents for the treatment and prophylaxis of seasonal influenza.* Version 10.0. London: PHE, September 2019. Available at https://assets.publishing.service.gov.uk/government/uploads/system/uploads/attachment_data/file/833572/PHE_guidance_antivirals_influenza_201920.pdf

34. Cormac I, Brown A, Creasy S, et al. A retrospective evaluation of the impact of total smoking cessation on psychiatric inpatients taking clozapine. *Acta Psychiatr Scand* 2010;121:393–397.

35. Clark SR, Warren NS, Kim G, et al. Elevated clozapine levels associated with infection: a systematic review. *Schizophr Res* 2018;192:50–56.

36. Raaska K, Neuvonen PJ. Ciprofloxacin increases serum clozapine and N-desmethylclozapine: a study in patients with schizophrenia. *Eur J Clin Pharmacol* 2000;56(8):585–589.

37. Cohen LG, Chesley S, Eugenio L, et al. Erythromycin-induced clozapine toxic reaction. *Arch Intern Med* 1996;156(6):675–677.

38. Joint Formulary Committee. *British National Formulary*, 76th edn. London: BMJ Group and Pharmaceutical Press, 2018.

Influenza

Anna Riddell, Eithne MacMahon

Influenza viruses cause both upper and lower respiratory tract infections. There are three types of influenza virus responsible: A, B, and C. Influenza A and B cause seasonal epidemics and are responsible for the morbidity and mortality associated with influenza. Influenza A also causes pandemics: when a new influenza A virus pandemic strain emerges, fewer people in the population have pre-existing immunity, leading to many more cases of influenza and a greater number of severe cases. Influenza C generally causes milder disease.

Influenza tends to pass from person to person via coughing and sneezing; this expels infectious particles which are then inhaled by another person [1]. Contact with surfaces contaminated with infectious particles is another important mode of transmission [1]. The median time taken between exposure to influenza virus and onset of symptoms (the incubation period) is 1.4 days but can be up to 4 days [2].

In temperate climates, influenza tends to occur seasonally during the colder winter months [3]. In tropical climates, the seasonality of influenza is less predictable but may be associated with months of higher rainfall [3]. Influenza is unusual out of 'flu season' but should be considered in travellers recently returned from an area with circulating influenza.

The severity of illness from influenza infection ranges from mild to severe. In the UK, it is estimated that an average of 600 people a year die from complications of flu, although during severe seasons this can increase dramatically, with 13,000 influenza-attributable deaths recorded in the UK in 2008–2009 [4].

Various patient groups are vulnerable to severe influenza infection, summarised in Box 40.1. Owing to increased multimorbidity and institutionalisation, patients with serious mental illness represent a vulnerable population.

The Maudsley Practice Guidelines for Physical Health Conditions in Psychiatry, First Edition.
David M. Taylor, Fiona Gaughran, and Toby Pillinger.
© 2021 John Wiley & Sons Ltd. Published 2021 by John Wiley & Sons Ltd.

Box 40.1 Risk factors for severe influenza infection

- Pregnancy (including two weeks postpartum)
- Children under six months
- Elderly over 65 years
- Chronic disease: diabetes mellitus; cardiovascular, respiratory, renal, liver, or neurological disease; asplenia or splenic dysfunction
- Immunocompromised state (due to either underlying disease or immunosuppressive therapy)
- Morbid obesity (BMI >40 kg/m^2)

DIAGNOSTIC PRINCIPLES

History

1 Symptoms are variable and inconsistent, but the classic infection often includes sudden-onset illness with fever, cough, headache, myalgia, extreme fatigue, sore throat, and runny nose.
2 Record any work that may increase exposure to influenza, e.g. healthcare or travel to an area with circulating influenza.
3 Past medical history:
   a malignancy
   b immunocompromised state (including immunosuppressive therapy, transplantation, chemotherapy, recent treatment for leukaemia or lymphoma, HIV, hyposplenism, asplenia)
   c chronic respiratory, heart, renal, liver, or neurological disease
   d diabetes mellitus
   e pregnancy.
4 Travel history (including contact with a healthcare facility abroad).
5 Social history, with attention to smoking status and residence with people who may be vulnerable to influenza infection.

Examination

1 Check for signs of sepsis and systemic shock: assess temperature, heart rate, blood pressure, and Glasgow Coma Scale (GCS) score (see Chapter 72).
2 Respiratory examination: check oxygen saturations; look for evidence of respiratory distress and signs of lower respiratory tract infection suggestive of influenza pneumonia or super-added bacterial infection.
3 Cardiovascular examination to assess for exacerbation of heart disease or pulmonary oedema.
4 Calculate body mass index (BMI): obesity is a risk factor for increased disease severity and mortality in infected individuals [5].

Investigations

No investigations may be required for a community-based patient where there are no risk factors for complicated influenza. However, in more severe cases and/or in at-risk individuals, the following tests may be requested.

1 Bloods:
  a full blood count with differential white cell count
  b renal function
  c liver function
  d clotting
  e C-reactive protein
  f blood glucose measurement
  g throat and nose swab for respiratory viral polymerase chain reaction (PCR)
  h throat swab for microscopy, bacterial culture, and sensitivity.
2 Consider chest X-ray to assess for consolidation or pulmonary oedema, if appropriate (although where these are suspected, referral to general medical colleagues is recommended).
3 Although unlikely to be immediately available in a psychiatric setting, 'point-of-care' testing for influenza A/B virus from a nasal swab is now available in some general medical hospitals [6]. The new molecular point-of-care tests have high sensitivity and specificity, with results in less than half an hour, thereby facilitating appropriate treatment of infected individuals and avoiding inappropriate treatment of non-infected individuals.

MANAGEMENT

- In patients where no risk factors for complicated influenza are identified, rest and antipyretics (e.g. paracetamol) are recommended.
- Time off work may be advisable depending on symptoms and to prevent onward spread of infection.
- The patient should be warned that the duration of symptoms is approximately one week, and that full recovery with return to normal activities may take even longer.
- Patients should be informed about simple measures to prevent onward transmission (Box 40.2).

Box 40.2 Techniques to avoid influenza and prevent onward transmission

- **Catch it**: Cover mouth and nose when coughing or sneezing
- **Bin it**: Dispose of used tissues
- **Kill it**: Wash hands

CHAPTER 40

Pharmacological treatment

- Patients with risk factors for severe infection (see Box 40.1) should be given pharmacological treatment. This should be started immediately if influenza is circulating or there is a high index of suspicion while waiting for test results.
- The neuraminidase inhibitors oseltamivir (oral 75 mg twice daily for five days) and zanamivir (inhalation 10 mg twice daily for five days) are the only effective available pharmacological therapies for influenza virus infection in the UK (Table 40.1) [7].
- Inhaled zanamivir is contraindicated in patients with underlying airways disease. Newer neuraminidase inhibitors are being developed. Therapy with neuraminidase inhibitors should be initiated as soon as possible after the start of symptoms as the greatest benefits of therapy have been observed if taken within the first 48 hours after development of symptoms [8].
- The main benefits of neuraminidase inhibitor therapy are to reduce the duration of symptoms and to reduce severity of illness [8].

Interactions with psychiatric medications

- The neuraminidase inhibitors are well tolerated with few drug interactions.
- There are no reported interactions of neuraminidase inhibitors with psychiatric medications.
- As the neuraminidase inhibitors are renally excreted, elevated plasma concentrations of oseltamivir in patients with renal dysfunction have been observed. Dose reduction is therefore recommended in those patients with a creatinine clearance of less than 30 mL/min [9].

When to refer to a specialist

- If severely unwell (e.g. hypotension, tachycardia, respiratory distress), the patient should be admitted to general medial hospital for monitoring and further investigations. Oseltamivir should be commenced, and additional broad-spectrum antibiotics considered. Discussion with an infectious diseases specialist is recommended.
- If the patient has already been taking oseltamivir or zanamivir as post-exposure prophylaxis (see following section) and they develop symptoms suggestive of influenza, change delivered dose to reflect treatment rather than prophylaxis (i.e. treatment is given twice rather than once daily). In the community consider a review in

Table 40.1 Pharmacological treatment and prophylaxis of influenza in adults.

Neuraminidase inhibitor	Mode of administration	Dose for treatment	Dose for prophylaxis
Oseltamivir	Oral (tablet)	75 mg twice daily for 5 days	75 mg once daily for 10 days
Zanamivir	Inhaler[a]	10 mg twice daily for 5 days	10 mg once daily for 10 days

[a] Intravenous preparation is available but only after discussion with an infectious diseases specialist.

primary care, or in severe cases a review in the emergency department, followed by discussion with an infectious diseases specialist. In severe cases, admission to the intensive care department may be required.

PREVENTING SPREAD OF INFLUENZA

- Strict infection control is key to preventing the spread of influenza in healthcare settings. Staff with influenza should not be at work. Patients and staff should adopt good hand hygiene practice: 'catch it, bin it, kill it' (see Box 40.2). Either alcohol sanitisers or soap and water are appropriate for washing hands.
- Patients should avoid vulnerable individuals if unwell (see Box 40.1).
- On inpatient wards, infection control measures should include isolation rooms to prevent nosocomial transmission, and ideally nursing should involve use of gloves, masks, and aprons/gowns.

Post-exposure prophylaxis

- Prompt pharmacological prophylaxis is advised for patients with risk factors for severe infection (see Box 40.1) who have been exposed to a confirmed case of influenza, or when influenza infection is circulating locally.
- In the UK, oseltamivir (oral 75 mg once daily for 10 days post exposure) or zanamivir (inhalation 10 mg once daily for up to 28 days) may be offered (see Table 40.1).
- In a hospital/residential setting, consider offering all inpatient contacts prophylaxis, regardless of vaccination history.

Pre-exposure prophylaxis: vaccination

- Influenza vaccines contains both influenza A virus subtypes (H1N1 and H3N2) and B virus strain(s).
- Vaccination offers significant additional individual protection and benefit in long-stay facilities and should be offered to all at-risk individuals over six months of age (see Box 40.1), and to individuals who are in frequent contact with those who are at risk (e.g. household contacts and healthcare providers).
- Vaccination is the most important intervention available to reduce the risk of acquiring influenza, providing protection against the anticipated seasonal circulating strains.
- In the UK, the reader is directed to the influenza chapter in *The Green Book*, which provides the latest information on vaccines and vaccine procedures [10].
- The World Health Organization (WHO) manages a twice-yearly meeting where the content of the influenza vaccine for the forthcoming season is decided based on global surveillance data of the viruses circulating the season before [11]. The vaccine content is based on prediction of the strains likely to be circulating the following season and for this reason can sometimes be mismatched, leading to lower efficacy. However, vaccination reduces the severity of influenza illness, hospitalisations, and deaths from influenza [12].

CHAPTER 40

- Annual re-vaccination is required.
- All staff should receive annual vaccination for personal protection and to minimise nosocomial transmission.

References

1. Killingley B, Nguyen-Van-Tam J. Routes of influenza transmission. *Influenza Other Respir Viruses* 2013;7(Suppl 2):42–51.
2. Lessler J, Reich NG, Brookmeyer R, et al. Incubation periods of acute respiratory viral infections: a systematic review. *Lancet Infect Dis* 2009;9(5):291–300.
3. Tamerius JD, Shaman J, Alonso WJ, et al. Environmental predictors of seasonal influenza epidemics across temperate and tropical climates. *PLoS Pathog* 2013;9(3):e1003194.
4. Green HK, Andrews N, Fleming D, et al. Mortality attributable to influenza in England and Wales prior to, during and after the 2009 pandemic. *PLoS One* 2013;8(12):e79360.
5. Sun Y, Wang Q, Yang G, et al. Weight and prognosis for influenza A(H1N1)pdm09 infection during the pandemic period between 2009 and 2011: a systematic review of observational studies with meta-analysis. *Infect Dis (Lond)* 2016;48(11–12):813–822.
6. World Health Organization. WHO recommendations on the use of rapid testing for influenza diagnosis. https://www.who.int/influenza/resources/documents/RapidTestInfluenza_WebVersion.pdf (accessed 11 November 2019).
7. National Institute for Health and Care Excellence. *Amantadine, Oseltamivir and Zanamivir for the Treatment of Influenza.* Technology Appraisal Guidance TA168. London: NICE, 2009. https://www.nice.org.uk/Guidance/TA168
8. Moscona A. Neuraminidase inhibitors for influenza. *N Engl J Med* 2005;353:1363–1373.
9. He G, Massarella J, Ward P. Clinical pharmacokinetics of the prodrug oseltamivir and its active metabolite Ro 64-0802. *Clin Pharmacokinet* 1999;37(6):471–484.
10. Public Health England. Influenza: The Green Book, chapter 19. Influenza immunisation information including updates for public health professionals. https://www.gov.uk/government/publications/influenza-the-green-book-chapter-19 (accessed 1 August 2019).
11. Ziegler T, Mamahit A, Cox NJ. 65 years of influenza surveillance by a World Health Organization-coordinated global network. *Influenza Other Respir Viruses* 2018;12(5):558–565.
12. Arriola C, Garg S, Anderson EJ, et al. Influenza vaccination modifies disease severity among community-dwelling adults hospitalized with influenza. *Clin Infect Dis* 2017;65(8):1289–1297.

Chapter 41

Urinary Tract Infection

Sian Cooper, Conor Maguire

Urinary tract infection (UTI) is caused by microorganism growth in the urine. It can be classified as uncomplicated or complicated. Uncomplicated UTI describes an infection of the lower urinary tract, i.e. urethra and/or bladder ('cystitis'), while complicated UTI describes infection of the urinary tract that may ascend to the kidney (pyelonephritis) or prostate, accompanied by systemic features of infection (e.g. fever and rigors), pelvic/renal-angle pain, and potentially sepsis (see Chapter 72). Recurrent UTI is defined as a UTI that reoccurs with a new causative organism, whereas relapsed UTI is defined by re-infection with the same organism. UTI is most commonly caused by bacteria (Box 41.1). While a small number of pathogens account for most infections, in immunosuppression the range of organisms causing UTI is broader.

Box 41.1 Common causative organisms of urinary tract infections in the UK

Community acquired

Escherichia coli
Enterobacteriaceae (including *Klesbsiella* spp. and *Proteus* spp.)
Enterococci
Staphylococcus saprophyticus

Healthcare associated

Pseudomonas
Methicillin-resistant *Staphylococcus aureus* (MRSA)
Extended-spectrum beta-lactamase (ESBL)-producing Enterobacteriaceae
Carbapenem-resistant Enterobacteriaceae (CRE)

The Maudsley Practice Guidelines for Physical Health Conditions in Psychiatry, First Edition.
David M. Taylor, Fiona Gaughran, and Toby Pillinger.
© 2021 John Wiley & Sons Ltd. Published 2021 by John Wiley & Sons Ltd.

Asymptomatic pyuria (elevated number of white blood cells in the urine in the absence of urinary symptoms) and asymptomatic bacteriuria (isolation of bacteria consistent with UTI in the absence of urinary symptoms) is commonly observed. Indeed, on urine testing, pyuria has been recorded in up to 45% of chronically disabled or incontinent adults, and up to 90% of individuals living in nursing homes [1]. Prevalence of asymptomatic bacteriuria is highly variable, and increases with age, in postmenopausal women, and in those with type 2 diabetes mellitus [2]. In people living in healthcare facilities, asymptomatic bacteriuria has been observed in 25–50% of women and 5–21% of men, with no associated increase in mortality or morbidity if left untreated [3]. Bacteriuria is seen in up to 100% of patients with chronic indwelling catheters [2]. In many patient groups, asymptomatic pyuria/bacteriuria in the absence of symptoms or signs of sepsis does not require antibiotic treatment (e.g. premenopausal non-pregnant women; diabetic women; elderly institutionalised men and women; and patients with indwelling urethral catheters) [4]. However, treatment of asymptomatic pyuria/bacteriuria is indicated in pregnant women and patients who have recently undergone a traumatic urological procedure (e.g. transurethral resection of the prostate). Asymptomatic pyuria/bacteriuria in patients with neutropenia (see Chapter 16) or in those who are otherwise immunosuppressed should be discussed with microbiology.

URINARY TRACT INFECTION AND SERIOUS MENTAL ILLNESS

Positive urinalysis for leucocytes/nitrites has been observed in up to 21% of psychiatric inpatients with psychosis, over ten times the prevalence seen in the general population [5]. Patients with serious mental illness are at increased risk of infection compared with the general population [6], and are more likely to present with comorbidities such as diabetes mellitus that increase risk of UTI. For example, young men with type 2 diabetes are four times more likely to have a UTI compared with non-diabetic individuals [7].

DIAGNOSTIC PRINCIPLES

History

Presenting complaint

Typical symptoms of UTI are increased urinary frequency, dysuria, urgency, haematuria, and suprapubic pain. Complicated infections may be heralded by fever, rigors, and flank pain. Patients with poor verbal communication may present with non-specific symptoms such as lethargy or confusion. Older adults or immunosuppressed patients may be afebrile and can present with atypical features (e.g. acute confusion; see Chapter 50) [8].

History and examination are vital in screening for differential diagnoses, which include acute appendicitis, diverticulitis, cholecystitis (see Chapter 88), salpingitis, ruptured ovarian cyst, or ectopic pregnancy (see Chapter 87).

Past medical history

Consider the following:

- pregnancy or menopause
- known structural abnormalities of the urological tract such as urinary stones, chronic urinary retention, long-term urinary catheterisation
- recent instrumentation of the urinary tract
- conditions that predispose to neurological dysregulation of bladder function (e.g. multiple sclerosis, Parkinson's disease, diabetic neuropathy)
- recent inpatient admission (increased risk of drug-resistant infection)
- immunosuppression such as HIV, steroid use, bone marrow or solid organ transplantation, poorly controlled diabetes
- chronic cardiac, renal, or hepatic failure (risk of decompensation in context of intercurrent UTI)
- sexual/gynaecological history including sexually transmitted infections (see Chapter 38).

Drug history

Review all medications including treatments associated with urinary stasis/retention (such as psychiatric drugs with anticholinergic activity) or those that may cause neutropenia (see Chapter 16). Record any antibiotic allergies.

Social history

Ascertain smoking status, alcohol intake, the use of recreational drugs, and housing circumstance (i.e. if homeless).

Examination

- Check observations, including temperature, respiratory rate, blood pressure, and pulse oximetry. Consider scoring these with a clinical warning system such as NEWS 2 [9].
- Assess for the presence of sepsis and manage accordingly (see Chapter 72).
- Assess fluid status (indicators of volume deficit: thirst, hypotension, dry skin or mucous membranes, reduced skin turgor, sunken eyes); dehydration may be an indicator for admission for intravenous fluids.
- Palpate the abdomen for suprapubic and flank tenderness/dullness.
- Consider a chaperoned pelvic examination for cervical motion tenderness in sexually active women to investigate possible pelvic inflammatory disease. Amongst male patients, a chaperoned digital rectal examination may be indicated to aid a diagnosis of prostatitis.

Investigations

Recommended investigations for UTI in community-based patients and general medical hospital-based patients are documented in Table 41.1. Additional investigations may be indicated in the immunocompromised (e.g. requiring broader infection screen

Table 41.1 Recommended investigations for UTI in patients being managed in the community or in hospital.

Investigation	Community setting	Hospital setting
Urinalysis	Recommended	Recommended
Mid-stream urine (MSU) for cultures	Recommended if leucocytes/nitrites positive on urinalysis or resistant organism suspected	Recommended if leucocytes/nitrites positive on urinalysis or resistant organism suspected
Blood tests: Full blood count (FBC) Urea and electrolytes C-reactive protein	Consider FBC is recommended in patients taking clozapine, mianserin, mirtazapine, or carbamazepine to assess for neutropenia	Recommended FBC is recommended in patients taking clozapine, mianserin, mirtazapine, or carbamazepine to assess for neutropenia
Pulse oximetry	Consider	Recommended at diagnosis and regularly if clinically indicated
Blood culture	Not routinely recommended	Recommended if signs of sepsis, ideally prior to antibiotic therapy
Urine pregnancy test	To exclude ectopic pregnancy and guide antibiotic choice	To exclude ectopic pregnancy and guide antibiotic choice
Ultrasound urinary tract	Not routinely recommended	Recommended if adverse features
HIV test	Consider	Consider
Clozapine levels	Consider for all patients taking clozapine (see section Pharmacological considerations in serious mental illness)	

Source: adapted from National Institute for Health and Care Excellence [10].

such as tuberculosis cultures), patients with recurrent UTIs (may require imaging of the urinary tract), or in patients where resistant organisms have previously been cultured (discussion with an infectious disease specialist or microbiologist is recommended). At present, there is no specific guidance for management of psychiatric hospital-associated UTI, and we would recommend tailoring investigations to the severity of the presentation, and if necessary following discussion with general medical services.

Urinalysis should be performed on a mid-stream clean-catch urine (MSU) sample to assess for the presence of nitrites and leucocyte esterase. Although a positive urinalysis is not diagnostic of a UTI, treat empirically with antibiotics if the patient is symptomatic and nitrites or leucocytes (pyuria) are present on urinalysis. It should be noted that some microorganisms do not produce nitrites. Absence of pyuria likely indicates an alternative diagnosis (Table 41.2).

Growth of greater than 10^5 organisms per millilitre in a fresh MSU sample is diagnostic of UTI in a symptomatic patient [11]. If fewer organisms grow but significant pyuria is observed (>20 white blood cells per mm^3), this still may be regarded as an indication to treat. When in doubt, discuss with a microbiologist [12]. Send the sample for micros-

Table 41.2 Determining likelihood of urinary tract infection based on urinalysis [12].

Leucocyte esterase	Nitrite	Interpretation
Negative	Negative	UTI unlikely
Positive	Negative	UTI moderately likely
Negative or positive	Positive	UTI highly likely

copy, culture and sensitivity to document the organism and antimicrobial therapy options, especially in patients who are male, pregnant, immunosuppressed, or presenting with recurrent infections. If the patient has a catheter, urinalysis is not helpful. However, microscopy, culture and sensitivity may still be performed, labelling the sample clearly as a catheter specimen. Similarly, the elderly may have 'symptomless bacteriuria' due to ageing changes, including incomplete bladder emptying, prostatic hypertrophy in men, and postmenopausal oestrogen loss in women, which may not require treatment.

Blood tests are generally not necessary in the outpatient setting unless the patient has specific signs or symptoms (sepsis, urinary retention, dehydration). For women of child-bearing age, consider a pregnancy test as this is relevant for management and antibiotic choice.

Imaging of the abdomen (e.g. ultrasound) is not indicated unless the patient requires hospitalisation, persistence of symptoms beyond 48–72 hours, recurrence within a short period of time, or if urine outflow obstruction is suspected. The role of imaging is to establish a potential structural cause of UTI, or complication such as abscess formation secondary to infection.

MANAGEMENT

Non-pharmacological

- Advise patients to drink plenty of fluids.
- Give paracetamol to reduce fever if no contraindications.
- There is insufficient evidence to recommend cranberry juice [3].
- For inpatients with carbapenem-resistant Enterobacteriaceae, isolate according to local policy.

Pharmacological

- Review allergy status before prescribing antibiotics.
- Empiric antibiotic choice will depend on the clinical diagnosis (community-acquired or hospital-associated disease).
- Refer to local antimicrobial prescribing guidelines that consider the geographically variable prevalence and antimicrobial resistance of urinary pathogens. National

Institute for Health and Care Excellence (NICE) guidance on common antibiotics for the treatment of UTI is provided in Table 41.3.

- Long-term catheterisation is often associated with colonisation by antibiotic-resistant organisms such as *Pseudomonas* [13]. Where treatment is required, discussion with microbiology is advised.
- Use oral antibiotics where possible for uncomplicated UTI. If intravenous antibiotics are required, consider transfer to a general medical ward.
- For non-pregnant women with no adverse features (i.e. no evidence of complicated UTI), consider a 'watchful waiting' approach whereby a back-up antibiotic prescription is provided that can be started if there is no improvement in symptoms after 48 hours.
- Duration of treatment should be three days for uncomplicated UTIs in women and seven days in men or pregnant women [10].
- Consider venous thromboembolism prophylaxis in all inpatients with UTI who are not fully mobile (see Chapter 18).

Table 41.3 Common antibiotic regimens for uncomplicated urinary tract infection in the UK.[a]

Antibiotic class	Antibiotic example	Considerations	Interactions with psychotropics
Antimetabolite	Trimethoprim 200 mg b.d. (p.o.)	Contraindicated in pregnancy, reduce dose in renal impairment	May increase risk of bone marrow aplasia if given with bone marrow suppressants
Antimetabolite	Nitrofurantoin 50 mg q.d.s. (p.o.)	Contraindicated if eGFR <45 mL/min; caution if anaemia, diabetes mellitus, electrolyte imbalance, vitamin B (particularly folate) deficiency. Considered safe in pregnancy, excreted in breast milk	None documented
Quinolone	Ciprofloxacin 250–500 mg (p.o.) b.d.	Avoid in pregnancy and breastfeeding, risk of articular damage, renal failure	Lowers seizure threshold, risk of 'psychiatric complications', CYP1A2 inhibitor
β-Lactam	Co-amoxiclav 625 mg t.d.s.	Avoid in pregnancy and breastfeeding unless essential, caution in renal and hepatic impairment	None documented
β-Lactam	Amoxicillin 250–500 mg (p.o.) t.d.s.	Use for asymptomatic bacteriuria in pregnancy, reduce dose in renal failure	None documented
β-Lactam	Cephalosporins, e.g. cefalexin 250 mg q.d.s./500 mg b.d.	No evidence of teratogenicity, excreted in breast milk	None documented

[a] Non-pregnant women should be treated for three days, men and pregnant women for seven days. Consult local antimicrobial guidelines as resistance patterns can vary.
eGFR, estimated glomerular filtration rate.

Pharmacological considerations in serious mental illness

- Abrupt smoking cessation can alter psychiatric medication levels (such as clozapine), so consider therapeutic drug monitoring (see Chapter 46).
- Clozapine levels can rise during acute infection, and therefore close monitoring of plasma levels and dose reduction may be required [14].
- Ciprofloxacin and erythromycin may cause a rise in clozapine levels and increased risk of toxicity, so monitoring of plasma levels is recommended [15].
- Macrolides and quinolones may cause QTc prolongation, so consider ECG monitoring if prescribed alongside other medications that prolong QTc (see Chapter 3).
- Neuropsychiatric side effects of quinolones include insomnia (common), and anxiety, depression, hallucinations, and confusion (rare).
- Neuropsychiatric side effects of macrolides include insomnia (common) and anxiety (uncommon).

Pregnant women (see also Chapter 62)

Prompt treatment of UTI is mandatory in pregnancy due to greater risk of complications, such as pyelonephritis or premature labour [16]. Send an MSU sample to microbiology before commencing antimicrobials; if a group B *Streptococcus* is isolated, inform antenatal services. Refer to local antimicrobial prescribing guidelines, although a reasonable first-line prescription would be nitrofurantoin 100 mg modified release twice daily for seven days.

When to refer to a medical subspecialty

- Advise patients that symptoms should steadily improve, although the rate of improvement will vary, and some symptoms are quicker to resolve than others. In general, symptoms should start to improve within 48 hours.
- When to seek local microbiology advice:
  - with suspected resistant organisms
  - in patients who are immunosuppressed
  - in patients who are failing to improve on empiric treatment.
- When to seek acute medical advice:
  - If there is evidence of more severe disease, such as an elevated NEWS 2 score or features of septic shock
  - if oral treatment is not possible and/or the patient is dehydrated
  - in those with multiple medical comorbidities
  - if there is suspicion of structural urological disease or obstruction.
- Seek HIV specialist advice when managing infections in HIV-positive patients (see Chapter 45).

Routine referral to urology for recurrent UTIs is indicated in:

- recurrent UTIs in men [17]
- suspected urinary tract structural abnormality (e.g. previous surgery or trauma, calculi, symptoms of fistula)

- obstructive symptoms, such as those attributable to prostatic hypertrophy
- previous abdominal or pelvic malignancy
- unusual pathogens cultured such as *Proteus* or *Yersinia*
- persistent bacteriuria despite antimicrobials
- immunocompromise, diabetes mellitus
- persistent microscopic haematuria in men, proteinuria.

Urgent referral (two-week wait) to urology services is indicated:

- if urological cancer is suspected (persistent haematuria, recurrent unexplained UTI)
- age over 45 years with unexplained visible haematuria without UTI or persistent haematuria after successful treatment of UTI
- age over 60 years with unexplained microscopic haematuria and lower urinary tract symptoms or elevated white cell count on blood test [18].

References

1. Detweiler K, Mayers D, Fletcher SG. Bacteriuria and urinary tract infections in the elderly. *Urol Clin North Am* 2015;42(4):561–568.
2. Nicolle LE. The paradigm shift to non-treatment of asymptomatic bacteriuria. *Pathogens.* 2016;5(2):38.
3. Jepson RG, Williams G, Craig JC. Cranberries for preventing urinary tract infections. *Cochrane Database Syst Rev* 2012;(10):CD001321.
4. Nicolle LE, Bradley S, Colgan R, et al. Infectious Diseases Society of America guidelines for the diagnosis and treatment of asymptomatic bacteriuria in adults. *Clin Infect Dis* 2005;40(5):643–654.
5. Graham KL, Carson CM, Ezeoke A, et al. Urinary tract infections in acute psychosis. *J Clin Psychiatry* 2014;75(4):379–385.
6. Pankiewicz-Dulacz M, Stenager E, Chen M, Stenager E. Incidence rates and risk of hospital registered infections among schizophrenia patients before and after onset of illness: a population-based nationwide register study. *J Clin Med.* 2018;7(12):485.
7. Hirji I, Guo ZC, Andersson SW, et al. Incidence of urinary tract infection among patients with type 2 diabetes in the UK General Practice Research Database (GPRD). *J Diabetes Complications* 2012;26(6):513–516.
8. Gavazzi G, Krause KH. Ageing and infection. *Lancet Infect Dis* 2002;2(11):659–666.
9. Royal College of Physicians. National Early Warning Score (NEWS) 2. https://www.rcplondon.ac.uk/projects/outputs/national-early-warning-score-news-2 (accessed 22 April 2019).
10. National Institute for Health and Care Excellence. *Urinary Tract Infections in Adults.* Quality Standard QS90. London: NICE, 2015. https://www.nice.org.uk/guidance/qs90/chapter/Quality-statement-5-Antibiotic-treatment-for-asymptomatic-adults-with-catheters-and-nonpregnant-women
11. Public Health England. Investigation of urine. https://www.gov.uk/government/publications/smi-b-41-investigation-of-urine
12. Public Health England. Diagnosis of urinary tract infections:quick reference guide. https://www.gov.uk/government/consultations/diagnosis-of-urinary-tract-infections-quick-reference-guide
13. Sabir N, Ikram A, Zaman G, et al. Bacterial biofilm-based catheter-associated urinary tract infections: causative pathogens and antibiotic resistance. *Am J Infect Control* 2017;45(10):1101–1105.
14. Clark SR, Warren NS, Kim G, et al. Elevated clozapine levels associated with infection: a systematic review. *Schizophr Res* 2018;192:50–56.
15. Cohen LG, Chesley S, Eugenio L, et al. Erythromycin-induced clozapine toxic reaction. *Arch Intern Med* 1996;156(6):675–677.
16. Juthani-Mehta M, Drickamer MA, Towle V, et al. Nursing home practitioner survey of diagnostic criteria for urinary tract infections. *J Am Geriatr Soc* 2005;53(11):1986–1990.
17. National Institute for Health and Care Excellence. Lower urinary tract infection in men. Clinical Knowledge Summary. https://cks.nice.org.uk/urinary-tract-infection-lower-men#!topicSummary
18. National Institute for Health and Care Excellence. Urological cancers: recognition and referral. Clinical Knowledge Summary. https://cks.nice.org.uk/urological-cancers-recognition-and-referral#!scenario

Gastroenteritis

Maria Krutikov, Luke Snell

Gastroenteritis is a transient infection of the bowel with a virus, bacterium, or parasite. It is characterised by sudden-onset diarrhoea, with or without vomiting [1]. Some forms are highly contagious (e.g. norovirus). Food poisoning is a form of gastroenteritis caused by ingestion of contaminated food, often with acute and severe symptoms. Gastroenteritis is associated with significant mortality rates, especially in low- and middle-income countries, with children particularly vulnerable. Indeed, according to the Centers for Disease Control, viral gastroenteritis accounts for approximately 200,000 childhood deaths per year worldwide [2].

The main causes and associated presentations of gastroenteritis in high/middle income countries are outlined in Table 42.1. Rotavirus and adenovirus are the most common causes in children, while norovirus is a frequent cause in adults. In general medical hospitals, gastroenteritis is most commonly caused by norovirus, *Clostridium difficile* (if recent antibiotics), and *Escherichia coli*. Data in psychiatric units are not yet available. In sexually active individuals who have anal sexual intercourse, especially men who have sex with men, *Shigella flexneri* and giardiasis are common causes of infection (see Chapter 38). Parasitic infections are usually related to travel but can be associated with unclean water supply [1,3–5].

DIAGNOSTIC PRINCIPLES

History

Presenting complaint

Ask about the following:

- frequency of bowel motions, duration of symptoms
- stool consistency and colour including presence of blood or mucus

Table 42.1 Common causes of gastroenteritis.

Organism	Presentation	Incubation period	Common sources	Highest risk group/ setting
Viruses				
Norovirus	Vomiting, watery diarrhoea, fever, muscle aches	24–48 hours	Shellfish, prepared foods, vegetables, fruits, close contacts	Healthcare settings, schools, cruise ships
Rotavirus	Fever, vomiting and diarrhoea	10–72 hours	Faecally contaminated water or food	Infants under age 5, winter seasonal pattern
Adenovirus	Diarrhoea, conjunctival and respiratory infection	10–72 hours	Faecally contaminated water/food	Children
Bacteria				
Campylobacter spp.	Fever, crampy abdominal pain, vomiting, diarrhoea, muscle aches	1–3 days	Undercooked meat (especially poultry), unpasteurised milk	Contact with young animals, travel to resource-limited settings
Enterohaemorrhagic *Escherichia coli*	Bloody diarrhoea, abdominal cramps	1–8 days	Contaminated food, especially undercooked meat	Contact with infected animals, healthcare settings and nursing homes
Non-typhoidal *Salmonella*	Watery bloody diarrhoea, abdominal cramps, fever, headache, rarely septic joint	1–3 days	Poultry, eggs, meat, fish, unpasteurised milk	Travel to resource-limited settings, contact with animals, immunosuppressed
Shigella spp.	Bloody diarrhoea, cramps, fever	1–3 days	Contaminated water, raw vegetables	Sexual transmission, daycare centres, travel to resource-limited settings
Clostridium difficile	Cramping abdominal pain and distension, fever, foul-smelling diarrhoea	N/A	Antibiotic use	Recent antibiotics, hospitalisation, gastric acid suppression
Listeria monocytogenes	Fever, watery diarrhoea, nausea, vomiting, headache, joint pains	1–10 days	Soft cheeses, processed meats, pates, unwashed fruit	Pregnancy, immunocompromise, children, adults >65 years
Staphylococcus aureus	Nausea, vomiting and abdominal	1–6 hours	Prepared food	Eating from buffet/ prepared food
Bacillus cereus	Nausea and profuse vomiting	1–6 hours	Rice, meat	Eating from buffet/ prepared food
Parasites				
Giardia lamblia	Acute and chronic diarrhoea with abdominal cramps, bloating and flatulence	7–14 days	Faecally contaminated food or water	Travellers, sexual transmission, swimming pools, daycare centres
Cryptosporidium parvum	Abdominal cramping and bloating, weight loss, watery diarrhoea, fever, weight loss	2–28 days	Vegetables, fruit, unpasteurised milk	Immunosuppression, swimming pool use, animal exposure
Entamoeba histolytica (amoebiasis)	Usually mild but can cause blood and mucus in stool with fevers. Rarely, extra-intestinal amoebic abscesses (e.g. liver)	1–3 weeks	Faecally contaminated food or water	Travel to resource-limited settings, sexual transmission

- vomiting, haematemesis (see gastrointestinal bleeding Chapter 20)
- fever
- abdominal pain (location, quality, duration, exacerbating and relieving factors)
- any associated symptoms (e.g. weight loss, muscle aches, conjunctivitis, joint swelling)
- food consumed over 24 hours preceding symptoms, with focus especially on unpasteurised dairy products or uncooked meat or fish, unwashed vegetables, eating at a buffet
- any affected contacts
- exposure to animals and contact with fresh water.

Past medical history

History of inflammatory bowel disease, immunosuppression, other bowel pathology, and HIV and hepatitis status.

Medication history

Enquire about use of opiates (constipation and overflow diarrhoea), laxatives, and proton pump inhibitors (increased risk of *Clostridium difficile*). Metformin can cause gastrointestinal side effects, and in acute kidney injury (secondary to dehydration) is associated with lactic acidosis; therefore, consider withholding metformin during severe episodes of gastroenteritis [6]. Gastric hypomotility may be seen with clozapine [7], for which overflow diarrhoea may be a presenting complaint (see Chapter 28).

Social history

Sexual history, travel within the last six months, recreational drug use, and alcohol intake.

Examination

- Observations: temperature, blood pressure, heart rate, and respiratory rate.
- Fluid status: check mucous membranes and skin turgor, capillary refill time, and hypotension (Table 42.2).

Table 42.2 Clinical features of dehydration.

	Mild dehydration	Moderate dehydration	Severe dehydration
Symptoms	Light-headedness, anorexia, nausea, fatigue	Nausea, headache, dizziness, fatigue, muscle cramps	Apathy, weakness, confusion leading to loss of consciousness
Signs	Postural hypotension	Dry tongue, sunken eyes, reduced skin elasticity (turgor), postural hypotension, tachycardia, oliguria	Tachycardia, hypotension (systolic blood pressure <90 mmHg), capillary refill time >3 s, oliguria or anuria

- Examine abdomen: look for evidence of peritonism with rebound tenderness or guarding (see Chapter 88), palpate for areas of tenderness, and auscultate for presence of bowel sounds or borborygmic or high-pitched sounds suggestive of bowel obstruction.

Investigations

Investigations may not be required, especially if the infection is mild and risk of complications is low. Most causes of gastroenteritis are self-limiting and do not require antimicrobial therapy.

If symptoms are persistent or there are signs of dehydration, consider performing blood tests to quantify degree of inflammatory response (C-reactive protein and white cell count) and to check electrolytes and renal function (sodium, potassium, urea, and creatinine). These results may guide whether a patient requires a general medical review.

It is recommended that stool samples are sent if there is [1]:

- presence of blood or pus in stool
- immunosuppression
- history of recent hospitalisation or antibiotic use
- persistent diarrhoea
- recent travel to resource-poor setting
- as part of outbreak or cluster of cases.

What to send

- Send stool in specimen pot. Advise patient to pass the stool into a clean empty plastic food container and ensure urine has not mixed with stool.
- In all cases send two samples, one to virology for viral nucleic acid detection and one to microbiology for faecal microscopy, culture, and sensitivity.
- If recent antibiotic use, then also send a separate sample to microbiology for *Clostridium difficile* testing.
- If recent travel, sexual anal intercourse, or symptoms lasting more than 10 days, send a separate sample to microbiology for microscopy (ova, cysts, and parasites).

MANAGEMENT

In most patients, gastroenteritis is a self-limiting illness that does not require specific therapy, and management is usually supportive.

Non-pharmacological

Hospital inpatients with suspected gastroenteritis should be isolated as soon as symptoms are reported. This should ideally be in a separate room with access to their own toilet facilities until symptoms have resolved. All staff and visitors should wear gloves and plastic aprons when entering the room. Ensure hand-washing with soap and water on removal of protective equipment when leaving the room and hands should subsequently be cleaned with alcohol hand rub (at least 60–95% ethanol or isopropanol).

The patient should be given strict instructions on hand hygiene and the importance of washing hands with soap and water after using the toilet. If more than one case is suspected within one healthcare facility, this should be discussed with the responsible infection control practitioner [1,8].

Pharmacological

Anti-diarrhoeal drugs (e.g. loperamide)

Not usually advised but may be used if symptoms are persistent and mild. Do not prescribe if the patient has fevers or blood or mucus in stools, or if the patient has confirmed shigellosis or verotoxin-producing *E. coli* 0157 [1,8,9].

Anti-emetics

Not usually advised, but can be used for symptomatic relief (see Chapter 21).

Antibiotics

Not usually advised as most cases of gastroenteritis are viral, and even when bacterial in aetiology, infections are usually self-limiting. Discussion with microbiology is always recommended if antibiotic treatment is being considered, and decisions may be guided by culture results. Table 42.3 provides examples of aetiologies where treatment may be considered, and antibiotics that may be prescribed.

Table 42.3 Examples of antibiotic treatments for bacterial gastroenteritis according to pathogen [1,9].

Pathogen	Indication to treat	Antibiotics
Campylobacter	Severe symptoms, non-resolving (>1 week), immunocompromise	Erythromycin Ciprofloxacin[a]
Non-typhoidal *Salmonella*	Age >50, history of valvular or endovascular abnormality	Ciprofloxacin
Shigella	Severe disease, immunocompromise, bloody diarrhoea	Ciprofloxacin Azithromycin
Entamoeba histolytica	Treatment recommended in all cases	Discuss with microbiologist
Giardia lamblia	Treatment recommended in all cases	Metronidazole[b]

[a] Ciprofloxacin lowers seizure threshold, is associated with 'psychiatric complications', and is a CYP1A2 inhibitor.
[b] Metronidazole can be associated with depression, and (rarely) psychosis.

When to refer

Patients with evidence of evolving sepsis (see Chapter 72), severe dehydration/hypovol-aemia, or an acute abdomen (see Chapter 88) should be discussed with medical/surgical colleagues as appropriate and transferred to the accident and emergency department.

Absolute indications for emergency admission to hospital

- Signs or symptoms of shock/sepsis or severe dehydration (see Table 42.2).
- Severe vomiting so unable to retain oral fluids.

Consider assessment in a general medical hospital if:

- age over 65 (higher risk of complications)
- severe abdominal pain and tenderness
- bloody diarrhoea
- faecal incontinence
- diarrhoea lasting more than 10 days
- recent foreign travel
- comorbid medical conditions/treatments that increase risk of severe disease (e.g. immunodeficiency or immunosuppression, diabetes mellitus, chronic renal, liver, respiratory, or cardiac disease).

When to report to local Health Protection Unit (UK guidance)

Urgent notification (same day by telephone) is indicated in cases of infectious bloody diarrhoea, haemolytic uraemic syndrome, and cholera. Routine notification (written within three days) is indicated in cases of food poisoning. The UK reader is directed to local contact details found on the Public Health England website [10].

References

1. National Institute for Health and Care Excellence. Gastroenteritis. Clinical Knowledge Summary. https://cks.nice.org.uk/gastroenteritis#!topicSummary
2. Monroe SS. Control and prevention of viral gastroenteritis. *Emerg Infect Dis* 2011;17(8):1347–1348.
3. Tam CC, O'Brien SJ, Tompkins DS, et al. Changes in causes of acute gastroenteritis in the United Kingdom over 15 years: microbiologic findings from 2 prospective, population-based studies of infectious intestinal disease. *Clin Infect Dis* 2012;54(9):1275–1286.
4. Bresee JS, Marcus R, Venezia RA, et al. The etiology of severe acute gastroenteritis among adults visiting emergency departments in the United States. *J Infect Dis* 2012;205(9):1374–1381.
5. Marder EP, Cieslak PR, Cronquist AB, et al. Incidence and trends of infections with pathogens transmitted commonly through food and the effect of increasing use of culture-independent diagnostic tests on surveillance: foodborne diseases active surveillance network, 10 US sites, 2013–2016. *MMWR Morbid Mortal Wkly Rep* 2017;66(15):397–403.
6. El-Hennawy AS, Jacob S, Mahmood AK. Metformin-associated lactic acidosis precipitated by diarrhea. *Am J Ther* 2007;14(4):403–405.
7. Palmer SE, McLean RM, Ellis PM, Harrison-Woolrych M. Life-threatening clozapine-induced gastrointestinal hypomotility: an analysis of 102 cases. *J Clin Psychiatry* 2008;69(5):759–768.
8. Riddle MS, DuPont HL, Connor BA. ACG Clinical Guideline: diagnosis, treatment, and prevention of acute diarrheal infections in adults. *Am J Gastroenterol* 2016;111(5):602–622.
9. Public Health England. Summary of antimicrobial prescribing guidance: managing common infections. https://www.gov.uk/government/publications/managing-common-infections-guidance-for-primary-care
10. Public Health England. Notifiable diseases and causative organisms: how to report. May 2010. https://www.gov.uk/guidance/notifiable-diseases-and-causative-organisms-how-to-report#laboratories-report-notifiable-organisms-causative-agents

Viral Hepatitis

Klara Doherty, Aisling Considine, Kosh Agarwal

There are several viruses that cause hepatitis, the most common being hepatitis A, B, and C. Most people recover from hepatitis A with no lasting liver damage, but hepatitis B and C can cause long-term liver disease and even liver cancer. As such, they form the focus of this chapter.

HEPATITIS B

Hepatitis B virus (HBV) is a highly infectious blood-borne virus that may be spontaneously cleared after acute infection or instead may develop into a chronic (carrier) state. Globally, mother-to-child transmission in the perinatal period is the most common route of acquisition and leads to a chronic carrier state in 90% of infants infected, making chronic HBV endemic in many parts of sub-Saharan Africa and Central and Southeast Asia [1,2]. In the UK, sex and intravenous drug use are the most significant routes of transmission [3]. In immunocompetent adults, 90–95% spontaneously clear acute HBV [4], although acute fulminant hepatitis can occur. Rates of HBV carriage amongst people with severe mental illness (SMI) is poorly studied but likely to be higher than in the general population [5].

Chronic HBV can progress to cirrhosis and hepatocellular carcinoma and current management is focused on halting progression towards liver damage (and preventing onward transmission) through lifelong pharmacological viral suppression. For those at risk of HBV, there is a highly effective vaccine. Thus, management in primary care and psychiatric care should focus on identifying those at risk of HBV and chronic HBV carriers.

The Maudsley Practice Guidelines for Physical Health Conditions in Psychiatry, First Edition.
David M. Taylor, Fiona Gaughran, and Toby Pillinger.
© 2021 John Wiley & Sons Ltd. Published 2021 by John Wiley & Sons Ltd.

Diagnostic principles

History

Acute HBV may present with jaundice, nausea, vomiting, abdominal pain, fever, malaise, arthralgia, maculopapular or urticarial skin rash, or (rarely) fulminant hepatitis with confusion and systemic inflammatory response. Chronic HBV may present with stigmata of chronic liver disease (CLD) or may also present with acute symptoms. However, both acute and chronic HBV are most commonly asymptomatic, so establishing risk factors for HBV infection to guide screening is key (Box 43.1) [1]. Obtaining a family history of viral hepatitis, liver cirrhosis, or hepatocellular carcinoma is also important to provide insight into risk for HBV and to guide further management [6].

Examination

Most patients will have a normal examination. There may however be evidence of CLD including finger clubbing, palmar erythema, asterixis, spider naevi, jaundice, and ascites. There may be evidence of routes of transmission such as tattoos or needle marks.

Investigations

Serology

HBV infection usually only becomes clinically apparent once complications develop, so proactive screening of all patients with risk factors for exposure is key (see Box 43.1). Screening uses serological markers summarised in Table 43.1.

Other investigations

While awaiting secondary care referral, consider requesting:

- liver function tests
- clotting screen
- alpha-fetoprotein

Box 43.1 Screening for hepatitis B [1]

- Birth, living, and/or healthcare work in an endemic country
- Sexual partner from endemic country
- Family members, children, sexual partners, and household contacts of HBV case
- Intravenous drug use or partner of intravenous drug user
- Sex workers
- Ten or more new sexual partners per year, especially if unprotected
- Medical or dental procedures abroad
- Tattooing, traditional circumcision or scarification, acupuncture
- Sharing razors and/or toothbrushes with known HBV case
- Clinical evidence of liver disease
- Deranged liver function tests
- If immunosuppressive therapy is due to commence
- Previous incarceration

Table 43.1 Interpretation of hepatitis B serology.

HBsAg (surface antigen)	Anti-HBs (surface antibody)	Anti-HBc (core antibody)	IgM anti-HBc (core IgM antibody)	Interpretation
–	+	–	–	Past immunisation[a]
–	+	+	–	Past infection with clearance of virus[b]
+	–	–	–	Early infection[c]
+	–	+	+	Acute infection[d]
–	+/–	+	+/–	Acute resolving infection[e]
+	–	+	–	Chronic carrier state[f]

[a] Titre must be >10 mIU/mL.
[b] Patient immune.
[c] 4–6 weeks from exposure.
[d] HBsAg disappears 24 weeks from exposure, anti-HBc IgM disappears 32 weeks from exposure.
[e] Anti-HBs appears from 32 weeks from exposure.
[f] Defined as HBsAg positive six months or more from exposure.

- blood-borne virus screen (hepatitis C antibody, hepatitis A IgG, hepatitis D antibody, HIV antibody)
- urea and electrolytes
- full blood count
- liver ultrasound if clinical evidence of liver disease.

Management

Acute

Patients with symptoms and exposure history consistent with acute HBV should be discussed with an on-call medical team and/or referred for acute medical assessment, especially if associated with deranged liver function tests and/or clotting. Signs of acute hepatic failure, such as acute confusion and systemic inflammatory response, requires urgent referral to secondary care. Acute HBV is a notifiable disease and Public Health England should be informed.

Chronic

Patients with confirmed chronic HBV should be referred to a specialist multidisciplinary team for monitoring and consideration of treatment. A referral letter should include documentation of evidence of CLD on history or examination, record of any family history of hepatocellular carcinoma, and results of serological tests and any other investigations that have been carried out including imaging.

Pharmacological therapy will normally be lifelong and is aimed at viral suppression to prevent hepatic complications and onward transmission. Commonly used antivirals in the UK include tenofovir and entecavir, which will be prescribed by the patient's specialist team.

Advice to patients

To limit hepatotoxicity
- Abstain from alcohol (accelerates hepatic complications in HBV).
- Use paracetamol within recommended limits.
- Maintain a healthy weight.
- Importance of full adherence to antiviral treatment.

To avoid transmission
- Do not donate blood or blood products.
- Avoid sharing razors or toothbrushes.
- Avoid sharing needles or drug-snorting paraphernalia.
- Use barrier protection for sexual encounters.

Patients can also be directed to information provided by the British Liver Trust (www.britishlivertrust.org.uk) and the Hepatitis B Positive Trust (www.hepbpositive.org.uk).

Prescribing in HBV and serious mental illness

Carbamazepine reduces levels of tenofovir, and therefore concurrent use is contraindicated. Otherwise, there are no expected drug–drug interactions between tenofovir and entecavir and commonly prescribed antipsychotics, antidepressants, and anxiolytics. When prescribing medication in a patient with chronic HBV it is worth considering hepatotoxicity of drugs, both in terms of direct hepatotoxic effects and indirect effects of drugs causing the metabolic syndrome. Any alterations in renal function and nephrotoxicity of any concomitant drugs should also be considered as both tenofovir and entecavir are renally cleared and would need dose reduction in renal impairment.

Prevention

Prevention involves the screening and vaccinating of those at risk of HBV (see Box 43.1). In the UK, three vaccine schedules of varying speeds are recommended by Public Health England and depend on the patient's exposure risk and likely compliance [1] (Table 43.2).

Pregnancy and breastfeeding

Chronic HBV in pregnancy requires management under a specialist team. Mothers will receive antiviral treatment in their final trimester to prevent vertical transmission and infants will require HBV immunoglobulin and immunisation immediately at birth [1]. Breastfeeding is safe if the child has completed immunoprophylaxis [7].

Table 43.2 HBV vaccine schedules.

	Injection date
Standard	0, 1 and 6 months
Rapid[a]	0, 1, 2 and 12 months
Ultra-rapid[a]	0, 1, and 3 weeks and 12 months

[a] Rapid vaccine schedules result in quicker immunity but lower antibody titres. Check HBs antibody titre at 4–12 weeks and give a booster if <10 mIU/mL.

HEPATITIS C

Hepatitis C virus (HCV) is a blood-borne virus most commonly acquired through intravenous drug use or unsafe medical/dental procedures [2], but may be acquired through any percutaneous blood exposure including sexually, perinatally, via intranasal drug use, or via contaminated blood products. In most cases, the virus is acquired asymptomatically [8]. In a minority it is spontaneously cleared [8]. After more than 20 years of infection, chronic HCV leads to the development of cirrhosis or hepatocellular carcinoma [8]. In the UK, there are 210,000 people known to be living with HCV, although there are undoubtedly many more unaware of their infection [9]. HCV is now a curable condition with direct-acting antiviral (DAA) regimens with high rates of viral eradication after 8–12 weeks of treatment [10].

Diagnostic principles

History and examination

One-third of patients who acquire HCV will have symptoms of acute infection such as fatigue, arthralgia, and jaundice [10]. Fulminant hepatitis, as possibly seen in HBV infection, is rare. Signs and symptoms of CLD are as described for HBV. Chronic HCV can also result in several extrahepatic manifestations including vasculitis, cryoglobulinaemia, and porphyria cutanea tarda.

Investigations

Screening
Proactive screening should occur in those at risk of HCV (Box 43.2). Screening involves HCV antibody testing followed by HCV RNA polymerase chain reaction (PCR) if appropriate (Figure 43.1).

Other investigations
Chronic HCV should be managed under a specialist team for consideration of curative treatment. While awaiting specialist assessment, full blood count, liver function tests, renal function, clotting screen, alpha-fetoprotein, full viral screen screen (hepatitis B surface antigen, HIV antibody), thyroid function tests, and liver ultrasound may be considered.

CHAPTER 43

Box 43.2 Screening for hepatitis C [1,3]

- Current or previous intravenous drug use
- Current or previous intranasal drug use
- Previous incarceration
- HIV-infected individuals
- Recipients of blood transfusion before 1991 or blood products before 1986
- Medical or dental treatment abroad in potentially unsterile conditions
- Tattooing, piercing, acupuncture, electrolysis, or semi-permanent make-up in potentially unsterile conditions
- Unprotected sex with someone with (known or suspected) chronic HCV
- Men who have sex with men
- Sharing a razor or toothbrush with someone with (known or suspected) chronic HCV
- Pregnant women
- Individuals with deranged liver functions tests
- Migrants from endemic countries

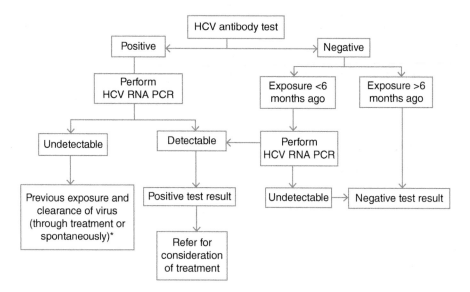

Figure 43.1 Hepatitis C testing algorithm. *Note that previous infection and clearance does not confer immunity to all HCV genotypes.

Management

Acute

Patients with signs and symptoms of acute HCV should be discussed with an on-call medical team and/or referred for acute medical assessment. HCV is a notifiable disease and Public Health England should be informed. Patients with acute HCV (prior to HCV antibody seroconversion) may be considered for curative treatment if viral

CHAPTER 43

levels do not clear spontaneously. Such patients should be referred to a specialist liver team as well.

Chronic

Patients with positive HCV RNA PCR should be referred to a specialist team for treatment and monitoring. The goal is sustained virological cure and will require regular blood monitoring to assess rate of viral clearance and to monitor side effects.

Several DAA regimens are used depending on HCV genotype and the patient's treatment history. Commonly used DAA regimens include elbasvir with grazoprevir, glecaprevir with pibrentasvir, ledipasvir with sofosbuvir, and sofosbuvir with velpatasvir.

Advice to patients

Patients should receive the same advice for limiting hepatotoxicity and avoiding transmission as described for patients with HBV. Patients should be advised that HCV is a curable disease. Sexual transmission of HCV is rare but is more common in patients with multiple partners, HIV co-infection, and other sexually transmitted infections [11]. Patients should be made aware that theoretically they could still acquire a different genotype of HCV after treatment or spontaneous clearance of the virus.

Treatment regimens may have teratogenic effects, so patients are advised to use two methods of contraception for the duration of DAA treatment ('double barrier'). Patients can be directed to information provided by the British Liver Trust (www.britishlivertrust.org.uk) and the Hepatitis C Trust (www.hepctrust.org.uk).

Prescribing in HCV and serious mental illness

As described for HBV, when prescribing psychiatric medication in a patient with HCV, consider the potential hepatotoxicity of drugs, both in terms of direct hepatotoxic effects and indirect effects of drugs causing the metabolic syndrome. Furthermore, plasma levels of both DAA and psychiatric drugs may be influenced by each other. For example, several of the DAA agents are metabolised by CYP3A4, which also metabolises various psychiatric agents. Some DAA regimens may be boosted with ritonavir, a CYP2D6 and CYP3A4 inhibitor but also a CYP2C9 inducer, which may therefore influence psychotropic drug levels. As such, monitoring of psychiatric drug plasma levels should be considered, and specialist advice sought prior to co-prescribing in the context of dual SMI and HCV treatment. Specialist treatment centres use the University of Liverpool website for guidance on DAA drug interactions (https://www.hep-druginteractions.org).

Prevention

If appropriate, patients should be signposted to local drug services with needle exchange facilities. Patients should also be offered vaccination against HBV and HAV (if not already immune) and be given lifestyle advice about avoiding HIV infection. There is no vaccine for HCV.

Pregnancy and breastfeeding

Vertical transmission of HCV is rare but more likely if the mother has high titres of HCV or is co-infected with HIV [12]. Breastfeeding is generally safe but mothers should refrain if there is broken skin around the nipples.

References

1. Public Health England. Hepatitis B: the green book, chapter 18. Hepatitis B immunisation information for public health professionals. https://www.gov.uk/government/publications/hepatitis-b-the-green-book-chapter-18
2. World Health Organization. *Global Hepatitis Report, 2017*. Geneva: WHO, 2017. Available at http://apps.who.int/iris/bitstream/10665/255016/1/9789241565455-eng.pdf?ua=1
3. British Association of Sexual Health and HIV. 2017 interim update of the 2015 BASHH National Guidelines for the Management of the Viral Hepatitides. Available at https://www.bashhguidelines.org/media/1161/viral-hepatitides-2017-update-18-12-17.pdf
4. Hyams KC. Risks of chronicity following acute hepatitis-B virus infection: a review. *Clin Infect Dis* 1995;20(4):992–1000.
5. Hughes E, Bassi S, Gilbody S, et al. Prevalence of HIV, hepatitis B, and hepatitis C in people with severe mental illness: a systematic review and meta-analysis. *Lancet Psychiatry* 2016;3(1):40–48.
6. Loomba R, Liu J, Yang HI, et al. Synergistic effects of family history of hepatocellular carcinoma and hepatitis B virus infection on risk for incident hepatocellular carcinoma. *Clin Gastroenterol Hepatol* 2013;11(12):1636–1645.e1-3.
7. Shi ZJ, Yang YB, Wang H, et al. Breastfeeding of newborns by mothers carrying hepatitis B virus: a meta-analysis and systematic review. *Arch Pediatr Adolesc Med* 2011;165(9):837–846.
8. Seeff LB. Natural history of hepatitis C. *Hepatology* 1997;26(3 Suppl 1):21S–28S.
9. Public Health England. *Hepatitis C in the UK. 2018 Report*. London: PHE, 2018. Available at http://www.hcvaction.org.uk/sites/default/files/resources/HCV_IN_THE_UK_2018_UK.pdf
10. Martin NK, Vickerman P, Grebely J, et al. Hepatitis C virus treatment for prevention among people who inject drugs: modeling treatment scale-up in the age of direct-acting antivirals. *Hepatology* 2013;58(5):1598–1609.
11. Terrault NA. Sexual activity as a risk factor for hepatitis C. *Hepatology* 2002;36(5 Suppl 1):S99–S105.
12. Yeung LTF, King SM, Roberts EA. Mother-to-infant transmission of hepatitis C virus. *Hepatology* 2001;34(2):223–229.

Tuberculosis

Sakib Rokadiya, Adrian R. Martineau

Tuberculosis (TB) is an airborne bacterial communicable disease caused by organisms of the *Mycobacterium tuberculosis* complex. The disease is characterised pathologically by necrotising granulomas. While most commonly affecting the lungs (approximately 85% of cases), *M. tuberculosis* can cause disease in almost any part of the body, including the skin, brain, and genitourinary tract [1].

TB is most commonly caused by the inhalation of aerosolised organisms from an infected host, but it only leads to symptomatic disease in a minority. Worldwide, around 1.7 billion people are estimated to be latently infected [2]. In asymptomatic individuals, latent *M. tuberculosis* is contained by the host immune system. However, these individuals can develop active TB in the future [3]; of patients with latent TB, around 10% develop active disease during their lifetime, approximately 5% within the first 18 months following exposure [4].

Patients with serious mental illness (SMI) are at higher risk of TB [5]. As shown in Box 44.1, patients with SMI are not only at increased risk of exposure (e.g. secondary to higher risk of homelessness), but are also at risk of progression of latent TB infection to active disease (e.g. secondary to comorbid HIV, diabetes mellitus, substance abuse, or malnutrition). Furthermore, patients with TB are at higher risk of psychiatric illness [5]; for example, the prevalence of comorbid depression in some TB populations is estimated at up to 72% [6]. There are several reasons for this association, including shared risk factors, the stress associated with infection, the psychiatric side effects of some treatments (e.g. psychosis associated with isoniazid therapy) [7], and even the direct effects of TB on the brain [5]. Other factors that can complicate TB treatment in patients with SMI include (i) poor treatment adherence in patients who present with chaotic behaviour and cognitive symptoms, which can lead to antimicrobial resistance and treatment failure; (ii) the risk of malabsorption of some TB medication in patients with eating disorders, leading to subtherapeutic treatment; and (iii) the potential use of

The Maudsley Practice Guidelines for Physical Health Conditions in Psychiatry, First Edition.
David M. Taylor, Fiona Gaughran, and Toby Pillinger.
© 2021 John Wiley & Sons Ltd. Published 2021 by John Wiley & Sons Ltd.

Box 44.1 Risk factors for the development of active tuberculosis[a]

Disease-related

Renal failure requiring dialysis [8]
Human immunodeficiency virus [9]
Diabetes mellitus [10]
Chronic obstructive pulmonary disease [11]
Recent tuberculosis infection
Malignancy [12]
Silicosis [13]

Medication-related

Tumour necrosis factor-α inhibitors (e.g. infliximab) [14]
Corticosteroids [15]
Transplant-related immunosuppression [16]

Exposure-related

Malnutrition [17]
Smoking [17]
Alcohol and substance abuse [17]
Overcrowding and poverty [17]

[a] Risk factors that are more prevalent in patients with serious mental illness are italicised.

---

high-dose glucocorticoids in patients with TB meningitis, which could exacerbate psychotic symptoms.

Management of TB is beyond the remit of the psychiatric practitioner; however, this chapter aims to improve practice in three domains: (i) identification of TB in psychiatric patients; (ii) understanding what TB treatment a given patient should be receiving; and (iii) awareness of potential TB–psychotropic drug interactions.

DIAGNOSTIC PRINCIPLES

A summary of an approach to the assessment of a patient with suspected TB is shown in Box 44.2. Suspected cases of TB should always be discussed with infectious diseases or respiratory colleagues.

History

1 TB symptoms are classically described as fever, cough, night sweats, and weight loss. With pulmonary involvement (85%), history may include dyspnoea, haemoptysis and cough. Constitutional symptoms such as lethargy, anorexia, and weight loss should be documented.

> **Box 44.2** An approach to the assessment of a patient with suspected tuberculosis
>
> **History**
>
> - Fever, cough, night sweats, and weight loss
> - Screen for symptoms of extrapulmonary TB
> - Past medical history: HIV, other systemic conditions particularly liver and renal conditions
> - Medication history
> - Travel and family history, with focus on potential TB contacts
> - Drug, alcohol and social history
>
> **Examination**
>
> - General examination specifically looking for weight loss and lymphadenopathy
> - Respiratory examination
>
> **Investigations**
>
> - Bloods including HIV test
> - Sputum (three samples) for microscopy, culture and sensitivity and acid-fast bacilli
> - Chest X-ray

2 TB can affect almost all other parts of the body and is often very difficult to diagnose, so a thorough systematic review of symptoms should take place.
   a Abdominal TB: abdominal pain, bloating and occasional ascites.
   b Central nervous system (CNS): headache, vomiting, and altered behaviour.
   c Genitourinary: 'sterile' pyuria (elevated white cells in urine without positive cultures), abdominal or back pain.
   d Lymph node TB: paratracheal, hilar, or superficial lymph nodes (often cervical) which can be tender/firm or be suppurative and discharging.
   e Musculoskeletal: back pain, arthritis, paraesthesia or dyaesthesia. Symptoms relate to bone/nerve involvement or abscess formation.
   f Optic: blurred vision.
   g Pericarditis: dyspnoea, peripheral oedema, atrial fibrillation.
   h Skin: any new skin lesions.
3 Medication history, specifically a change in medication or those medications that could interact with TB medications (see Table 44.1) and herbal or over-the-counter medications.
4 HIV infection, prior TB episodes, and consideration of TB mimics are essential (e.g. sarcoidosis, lymphoma, autoimmune disease, and malignancy).
5 Social history including TB exposure (including family history of TB), homelessness, incarceration, shelter-homes and travel to/from an area with endemic TB.

Examination

1 Examination is dependent on the organ system involved, although absence of signs does not exclude active TB.

Table 44.1 Common antituberculous agents and effects on psychiatric symptoms and medication [19–21].

Agent	Mechanism	Effects on psychotropic medicine and psychiatric side effects
Rifampicin	Potent inducer of CYP1A2, CYP2C9, CYP2C19, CYP3A4 and glucuronidation	May reduce plasma levels of various antidepressants, antipsychotics, mood stabilisers, hypnotics, and methadone. Documented effects of rifampicin reducing plasma levels of nortriptyline, sertraline, haloperidol, risperidone, clozapine, and methadone [5]
Isoniazid	Weak monoamine oxidase inhibitor, inhibits CYP2C19 and CYP3A	Co-prescription of selective serotonin reuptake inhibitors (SSRIs) is a relative contraindication due to theoretically increased risk of serotonin syndrome (although there are no described cases of serotonin syndrome in patients co-prescribed SSRIs and isoniazid/linezolid). Risk of increased plasma levels of psychiatric drugs metabolised by CYP2C19 and CYP3A (documented toxicity with carbamazepine [22] increases benzodiazepine levels) [23]. Isoniazid can be associated with acute psychosis [7]
Pyrazinamide	Not fully understood	No clear psychiatric drug interactions. Hepatotoxic: requires close monitoring of liver function tests
Ethambutol	Inhibits arabinosyl transferase	No clear psychiatric drug interactions. Renally excreted, therefore may require caution if used in patients with renal failure (e.g. in context of lithium use)

2 General examination may identify fever, muscle wastage, lymphadenopathy (including suppurative lesions), raised jugular venous pressure (pericarditis), and skin lesions (e.g. erythema nodosum).

3 Decreased air entry or 'crackles' in the lungs may be auscultated with pulmonary TB.

4 Systematic examination of the cardiovascular, musculoskeletal, and dermatological systems should be conducted.

Investigations

1 Bloods:

a Full blood count (evidence of anaemia, leucocytosis or eosinophilia).

b Renal function (renal failure).

c Liver function tests (baseline tests before treatment, alcohol misuse).

d Blood film and lactate dehydrogenase (help rule out lymphoma).

e Clotting screen.

f Autoimmune screen.

g HIV antibody test (co-infection has poorer TB outcomes).

h Hepatitis B and C serology (co-infection has poorer TB outcomes).

i Syphilis serology.

j Vitamin D levels.

k Interferon gamma release assay (IGRA). Note that these tests are only used to diagnose latent TB infection: a negative IGRA does not rule out active TB, and a positive IGRA cannot distinguish latent from active TB. Therefore, they should only be requested by an infectious diseases/respiratory specialist due to difficulty in their interpretation.

2 Three sputum samples for microscopy, culture and sensitivity and acid-fast bacilli (AFB) smear and culture, ideally on three separate mornings.

3 Chest X-ray to identify lymphadenopathy, cavitating/miliary lesions, evidence of pericardial TB, or evidence of presumed active pulmonary TB (parenchymal or pleural disease).

4 CT scan of the thorax and/or abdomen and pelvis may be useful but will be requested by infectious diseases/respiratory specialists if necessary.

MANAGEMENT

Those patients in whom there is a high index of suspicion for active TB should be immediately referred to infectious diseases/respiratory specialists before waiting for the results of requested investigations.

Non-pharmacological therapy

1 Infection control:
   a In a general practice/outpatient setting, a patient considered to have active pulmonary TB should be urgently referred to TB services due to concerns of infection control. If possible, the patient should be given an FFP3 mask and asked to wear it whilst at home and to self-isolate until seen by an infection/respiratory specialist.
   b Specific care should be taken to ask about any children/neonates at home and the patient should be asked to refrain from close contact until assessed.
   c Minimise the number and duration of visits a person makes to the outpatient department whilst they are still infectious.
   d In an inpatient setting, ideally patients suspected of having active pulmonary TB should be in respiratory isolation until reviewed by a specialty clinician. The hospital infection control team should be informed.

2 Explore any anxiety associated with TB diagnosis, alongside any stigmatised beliefs or myths surrounding TB infection. The treatment of tuberculosis lasts at least six months, and hence a strong, trusting doctor–patient relationship should be fostered early; in patients with SMI, a psychiatric practitioner can support medical colleagues in maintaining that relationship.

3 Use of TB specialist nurses and a multidisciplinary approach in patients with complex care needs is encouraged [18].

Pharmacological therapy

1 Antitubercular treatment (ATT) should only be initiated by an infectious diseases/respiratory specialist. Where possible, drug therapy is targeted based on drug susceptibility testing and treatment options and duration are dependent on site of

CHAPTER 44

Table 44.2 Common major and minor side effects of the most common antituberculous drugs [21].

Agent	Adverse effects	Management
Minor adverse effects		
Rifampicin	Flu-like symptoms	Continue and reassure
	Orange urine	Continue and reassure
	Abdominal discomfort, nausea	Take medication at night, or after a light meal with small sips of water. If symptoms persist or there is vomiting or bleeding, treat as major effect (see below)
Isoniazid	Paraesthesia	Pyridoxine 50 mg once daily
	Somnolence	Advise to take at bedtime
	Pruritis	Prescribe antihistamines
Pyrazinamide	Arthralgia	Prescribe simple analgesia
	Hyperuricaemia	Low-purine diet and prescribe acetylsalicylic acid
	Abdominal discomfort, nausea	Take medication at night, or after a light meal with small sips of water. If symptoms persist or there is vomiting or bleeding, treat as major effect (see below)
Major adverse effects		
Rifampicin	Shock, purpura, acute kidney injury, skin rash, jaundice, confusion	*Stop* medication and seek expert advice
Isoniazid	Jaundice, acute liver injury, skin rash, confusion	*Stop* medication and seek expert advice
Pyrazinamide	Acute liver injury, acute kidney injury, skin rash, confusion	*Stop* medication and seek expert advice
Ethambutol	Visual disturbance, confusion	*Stop* medication and seek expert advice

TB and comorbidities (e.g. liver/renal disease). There is the risk of interactions between ATT and psychiatric treatment (Table 44.1). A multidisciplinary approach is recommended, including the TB physician, psychiatric practitioner, pharmacist, and patient. Furthermore, engagement between TB clinical nurse specialists and psychiatric teams (including care coordinators) will ensure the patient is provided with appropriate support, and side effects of treatment are minimised (Table 44.2).

2 Typical regimens for drug-sensitive active pulmonary TB may include the following.
  a A regimen of rifampicin, isoniazid (with pyridoxine), ethambutol, and pyrazinamide may be offered for two months followed by four months of rifampicin and isoniazid (with pyridoxine) alone.
  b For patients with CNS involvement, a regimen of rifampicin, isoniazid (with pyridoxine), ethambutol, and pyrazinamide may be offered for two months followed by 10 months of rifampicin and isoniazid (with pyridoxine) alone. Patients with

CNS involvement should be offered high-dose corticosteroids, tapered within the first six weeks and other steroid-sparing agents may be used to negate the risk of steroid-induced psychosis [18].

3 Awareness of common side effects of first-line ATT should encourage prompt communication with the infection/respiratory team coordinating TB care (see Table 44.2).

When to refer to a specialist

If TB is suspected in a patient, then immediate discussion with infectious diseases or respiratory colleagues is required. TB is generally managed in secondary care; however, if patients are tolerating their initial medication well with limited side effects, often they can continue in primary care with the support of TB specialist nurses. As already detailed, if there are concerns surrounding non-adherence and side effects, then referral to secondary services is appropriate.

References

1. Furin J, Cox H, Pai M. Tuberculosis. *Lancet* 2019;393(10181):1642–1656.
2. Houben RMGJ, Dodd PJ. The global burden of latent tuberculosis infection: a re-estimation using mathematical modelling. *PLoS Med* 2016;13(10):e1002152.
3. Zumla A, Raviglione M, Hafner R, von Reyn CF. Tuberculosis. *N Engl J Med* 2013;368(8):745–755.
4. Vynnycky E, Fine PE. The natural history of tuberculosis: the implications of age-dependent risks of disease and the role of reinfection. *Epidemiol Infect* 1997;119(2):183–201.
5. Doherty AM, Kelly J, McDonald C, et al. A review of the interplay between tuberculosis and mental health. *Gen Hosp Psychiatry* 2013;35(4):398–406.
6. Aamir S, Aisha. Co-morbid anxiety and depression among pulmonary tuberculosis patients. *J Coll Physicians Surg Pak* 2010;20(10):703–704.
7. Alao AO, Yolles JC. Isoniazid-induced psychosis. *Ann Pharmacother* 1998;32(9):889–891.
8. Dobler CC, McDonald SP, Marks GB. Risk of tuberculosis in dialysis patients: a nationwide cohort study. *PLoS One* 2011;6(12):e29563.
9. Aaron L, Saadoun D, Calatroni I, et al. Tuberculosis in HIV-infected patients: a comprehensive review. *Clin Microbiol Infect* 2004;10(5):388–398.
10. Dooley KE, Chaisson RE. Tuberculosis and diabetes mellitus: convergence of two epidemics. *Lancet Infect Dis* 2009;9(12):737–746.
11. Inghammar M, Ekbom A, Engstrom G, et al. COPD and the risk of tuberculosis - a population-based cohort study. *PLoS One* 2010;5(4):e10138.
12. Kamboj M, Sepkowitz KA. The risk of tuberculosis in patients with cancer. *Clin Infect Dis* 2006;42(11):1592–1595.
13. Rees D, Murray J. Silica, silicosis and tuberculosis. *Int J Tuberc Lung Dis* 2007;11(5):474–484.
14. Keane J, Gershon S, Wise RP, et al. Tuberculosis associated with infliximab, a tumor necrosis factor (alpha)-neutralizing agent. *N Engl J Med* 2001;345(15):1098–1104.
15. Lee CH, Kim K, Hyun MK, et al. Use of inhaled corticosteroids and the risk of tuberculosis. *Thorax* 2013;68(12):1105–1112.
16. Singh N, Paterson DL. *Mycobacterium tuberculosis* infection in solid-organ transplant recipients: impact and implications for management. *Clin Infect Dis* 1998;27(5):1266–1277.
17. Lienhardt C. From exposure to disease: the role of environmental factors in susceptibility to and development of tuberculosis. *Epidemiol Rev* 2001;23(2):288–301.
18. National Institute for Health and Care Excellence. *Tuberculosis: Clinical Diagnosis and Management of Tuberculosis, and Measures for its Prevention and Control*. Clinical Guideline CG117. London: NICE, 2011. Available at https://www.nice.org.uk/guidance/cg117
19. Pachi A, Bratis D, Moussas G, Tselebis A. Psychiatric morbidity and other factors affecting treatment adherence in pulmonary tuberculosis patients. *Tuberc Res Treat* 2013;2013:489865.
20. Trenton AJ, Currier GW. Treatment of comorbid tuberculosis and depression. *Prim Care Companion J Clin Psychiatry* 2001;3(6):236–243.
21. Arbex MA, Varella MDL, de Siqueira HR, de Mello FAF. Antituberculosis drugs: drug interactions, adverse effects, and use in special situations. Part 1: First-line drugs. *J Bras Pneumol* 2010;36(5):626–640.
22. Wright JM, Stokes EF, Sweeney VP. Isoniazid-induced carbamazepine toxicity and vice-versa. *N Engl J Med* 1982;307(21):1325–1327.
23. Ochs HR, Greenblatt DJ, Roberts GM, Dengler HJ. Diazepam interaction with antituberculosis drugs. *Clin Pharmacol Ther* 1981;29(5):671–678.

CHAPTER 44

Chapter 45

Human Immunodeficiency Virus

Rebecca Marcus, Jessica Gaddie, Toby Pillinger,
Ben Spencer, Kalliopi Vallianatou, Rudiger Pittrof

Human immunodeficiency virus (HIV) is an infectious disease caused by a retrovirus that infects and replicates in human lymphocytes and macrophages. This progressively weakens the immune system, ultimately resulting in susceptibility to opportunistic and other infections, as well as certain malignancies.

There is a complex relationship between HIV infection and psychiatric conditions. Compared with the general population, the prevalence of HIV infection is four times higher in those with mental illness, and risk of HIV infection increases with psychiatric symptom severity [1]. Furthermore, in people living with HIV (PLWHIV), there is increased prevalence of neuropsychiatric disorders. For example, depression has a lifetime prevalence of 22–45% in PLWHIV [2,3]. Substance misuse and addiction is more common in PLWHIV, who also experience higher levels of suicidal ideation and have higher suicide rates compared with the general population [4]. The mechanisms underlying this relationship are multifactorial, including shared risk factors (e.g. low socioeconomic status and recreational drug use) [5], the direct neuropathological effects of HIV infection [6], and the psychological stress associated with the stigma of HIV diagnosis [7]. The combination of mental illness and HIV infection can compound difficulties in HIV diagnosis, access to and retention in care, and adherence to antiretroviral therapy (ART). For example, compared with HIV patients without a diagnosis of depression, patients with comorbid HIV and depression experience delays to accessing ART and have worse ART adherence [8,9]. Indeed, treatment of psychiatric comorbidity has been shown to increase the likelihood of HIV patients receiving ART [10].

In the UK, PLWHIV have a normal life expectancy if given appropriate treatment. ART is recommended from diagnosis of HIV with few exceptions, and people with a persistently undetectable HIV viral load on ART are unable to transmit HIV even without using condoms.

The Maudsley Practice Guidelines for Physical Health Conditions in Psychiatry, First Edition.
David M. Taylor, Fiona Gaughran, and Toby Pillinger.
© 2021 John Wiley & Sons Ltd. Published 2021 by John Wiley & Sons Ltd.

This chapter briefly covers the psychological impact of HIV, the effect of HIV on the central nervous system (CNS), the neuropsychiatric side effects of ART, and significant interactions between ART and psychiatric medications.

TESTING FOR HIV

Risk factors for HIV are documented in Box 45.1. In the UK, annual HIV testing in people who inject drugs is recommended [11]. In addition to this, HIV testing is recommended for all medical admissions and for general practice registrations where local prevalence exceeds 2 in 1000 [11]. Testing should be routine when investigating dementia and cognitive impairment [12]. Always consider HIV testing in patients presenting with psychiatric illness, given the increased prevalence of HIV in patients with mental disorders [1]. The British HIV Association provides useful guidance on testing for HIV in patients who lack capacity to consent [11].

Box 45.1 Risk factors for HIV

- Unprotected anal sex in men who have sex with men with a person of unknown HIV status/HIV positive and with a detectable viral load
- Unprotected vaginal or anal heterosexual sex with a person from an at-risk population such as high-risk country outside Europe, Australasia, and North America, or HIV positive with a detectable viral load
- Needle sharing with an HIV-positive person

The results of a fourth-generation HIV test, which detects both HIV antibodies and p24 antigen (a structural protein that comprises most of the HIV viral core), is reliable at four weeks post exposure, picking up 95% of infections [13]. In the UK, clinicians from a local sexual health clinic can support psychiatric practitioners in giving or explaining the diagnosis. Furthermore, if the patient is HIV positive, post-test discussions regarding treatment and partner notification/testing will be carried out by the local genitourinary medicine/HIV department.

HIV AND THE CENTRAL NERVOUS SYSTEM

HIV infection can directly affect the CNS (Box 45.2). A spectrum of cognitive impairments, collectively referred to as HIV-associated neurocognitive disorders (HAND), is recognised among PLWHIV [6]. Depending on severity of presentation, this ranges from asymptomatic neurocognitive impairment to HIV-associated dementia (HAD). Thus, in the early stages of HAND, patients may present with difficulty concentrating and memory impairment. As the disease progresses, there may be psychomotor retardation

---

> **Box 45.2** Effects of HIV infection on the central nervous system
>
> **Direct effects of HIV**
>
> - Aseptic meningitis: typical meningitic presentation (see Chapter 81) with negative bacterial cultures. May be seen at time of seroconversion
> - HIV-associated neurocognitive disorder [6]: exists on a scale defined by severity, from asymptomatic neurocognitive impairment, mild neurocognitive disorder to HIV-associated dementia. May be associated with motor dysfunction (HIV-associated motor-cognitive disorder) [15]
> - Vacuolar myelopathy: associated with advanced HIV infection. Presents with ataxic gait, slowly progressive spastic paraparesis, dorsal column-type sensory loss, incontinence, and erectile dysfunction
>
> **Opportunistic infections**
>
> - Cerebral toxoplasmosis: may present with psychiatric symptoms
> - Cryptococcal meningitis: may present with psychiatric symptoms
> - Progressive multifocal leukoencephalopathy: a demyelinating disease of the CNS due to infection by the John Cunningham (JC) virus
> - Tuberculous meningitis: people living with HIV are at increased risk of all forms of extrapulmonary tuberculosis, including tuberculous meningitis (see Chapter 44).
> - Neurosyphilis: progression to neurosyphilis is more common in HIV co-infection and can be asymptomatic, often for several years
>
> **Malignancy**
>
> - Primary CNS lymphoma: considered to be secondary to ineffective immunoregulation of Epstein–Barr virus

in association with irritability and depressive symptoms. HAD, if untreated, may progress to a bedridden state with mutism and incontinence. The mainstay of treatment is the suppression of virus replication in the brain (i.e. ART). Although the introduction of ART has reduced the incidence and prevalence of HAD, the incidence and prevalence of milder forms of HAND have not reduced over recent years [14]. Beyond its direct effects, HIV-associated immunosuppression can lead to opportunistic intracranial infections (e.g. cryptococcal meningitis) which may present with neuropsychiatric symptoms, and malignancy (e.g. primary CNS lymphoma).

ANTIRETROVIRAL THERAPY

First-line ART usually comprises three different antiretroviral medications, given once daily (Table 45.1) [16]. Adherence of at least 95% is usually needed to ensure drug resistance does not develop [17]. As drug resistance may develop on some ART regimens after only a few missed doses, it is vital that ART is accurately prescribed and that support is given to patients to adhere to HIV treatment, with specialist advice sought in the case of multiple missed doses.

Table 45.1 Antiretrovirals: classes, examples, and mechanisms of action.

Class of antiretroviral	Examples	Mechanism of action
Nucleoside and nucleotide reverse transcriptase inhibitors (NRTIs)	Abacavir, didanosine, lamivudine, tenofovir	Blocks viral replication by inhibiting viral reverse transcriptase activity
Non-nucleoside reverse transcriptase inhibitors (NNRTIs)	Efavirenz[a], etravirine, doravirine[a], rilpivirine[a], nevirapine	Blocks viral replication by inhibiting viral reverse transcriptase activity
Protease inhibitors	Atazanavir, darunavir, indinavir, ritonavir	Inhibits viral maturation resulting in production of non-infectious virions
Integrase inhibitors	Dolutegravir[a], elvitegravir, raltegravir	Inhibits integration of viral DNA into the genome of the host cell
Fusion inhibitors	Enfuvirtide	Blocks cell virus entry
Co-receptor antagonists	Maraviroc	Blocks cell virus entry

[a] Risk of neurological and psychiatric side effects.

Pre- and post-exposure prophylaxis

Post-exposure prophylaxis (PEP) is ART taken for a month that can reduce the risk of acquiring HIV after presumed HIV exposure. PEP is usually indicated if a man (who is assumed to be HIV negative) has had unprotected receptive anal sex in the last 72 hours. These patients need to be discussed as soon as possible with local sexual health services. Pre-exposure prophylaxis is ART taken by people who do not have HIV but are at risk of contracting HIV [18].

CNS side effects of ART

CNS side effects of the widely used non-nucleoside reverse transcriptase inhibitor (NNRTI) efavirenz are well documented and include dizziness, sedation, loss of concentration, abnormal dreams, sleep disturbance, depression, and anxiety. Indeed, psychiatric events are reported in 25–60% of patients taking efavirenz, and therefore its prescription is not recommended in patients with established psychiatric comorbidity [19]. Other NNRTIs, such as rilpivirine and doravirine, are also associated with neurological and psychiatric side effects. The newer and widely used integrase inhibitor dolutegravir has also been linked with neuropsychiatric symptoms, including insomnia, sedation, and depression [20]. Depression and suicidal ideation have occasionally been reported in association with integrase inhibitors, primarily in patients with psychiatric comorbidity [20]. Where there are concerns regarding the potential psychiatric side effects of ART, discussion with the patient's HIV clinical team is recommended.

Interactions between ART and psychotropics [21,22]

The interactions between ART and psychotropic treatment can be complex (Table 45.2). Decisions regarding appropriate and complementary HIV and psychiatric treatments

Table 45.2 Potential psychotropic–antiretroviral therapy interactions.

	Nucleoside and nucleotide reverse transcriptase inhibitors (NRTIs)	Non-nucleoside reverse transcriptase inhibitors (NNRTIs)	Protease inhibitors (PIs)	Fusion inhibitors	Co-receptor antagonists
Antipsychotics	No clinically significant interactions expected.	Risk of QTc prolongation with efavirenz and rilpivirine: caution advised Efavirenz and nevirapine are CYP3A4 inducers, so levels of aripiprazole, cariprazine, lurasidone, olanzapine, quetiapine, pimozide may be reduced (seek further advice)	Quetiapine, lurasidone and pimozide contraindicated in the UK (in the USA, reduce original dose to one-sixth) Aripiprazole, cariprazine, brexpiprazole dose reduction required. Risperidone and other substrates of CYP3A4 and/or 2D6 levels possibly increased; start low, titrate to response, monitor for adverse effects Olanzapine levels reduced by ritonavir, tipranavir/ritonavir; increase dose if needed QTc prolongation risk with saquinavir, atazanavir, darunavir, ritonavir, lopinavir	Elvitegravir with cobicistat: inhibition of CYP3A4 and 2D6 by the latter; advice as with PIs	No clinically significant interactions expected
Clozapine	Risk of haematological adverse effects with zidovudine (neutropenia, leucopenia)	QTc prolongation with some NNRTIs, as above Clozapine levels possibly reduced by efavirenz, nevirapine, etravirine owing to CYP3A4 effects (monitor levels and response)	Clozapine levels may be increased or reduced with ritonavir; therapeutic drug monitoring advised Risk of QTc prolongation (see above), avoid use with saquinavir	Elvitegravir with cobicistat: clozapine concentrations may be increased (inhibition of CYP3A4 and 2D6 by cobicistat), monitor clozapine levels and adverse effects	No clinically significant interactions expected
Mood stabilisers	Lithium and tenofovir are eliminated by the kidney. Monitor renal function as both nephrotoxic Valproate (glucuronosyltransferase inhibitor) increases zidovudine levels; liver toxicity reported with combination Carbamazepine (CYP3A4 and 1A2 inducer) reduces levels of tenofovir; use contraindicated	Most NNRTIs not recommended with carbamazepine (CYP3A4, 1A2 inducer) as levels of NNRTIs may be reduced	Complex interactions with carbamazepine and PIs: consider alternative or seek further advice Lamotrigine (metabolised via glucuronidation) reduced by atazanavir/ritonavir, darunavir, lopinavir and tripanavir; may need to increase lamotrigine dose (and consider lamotrigine therapeutic drug monitoring) Valproate levels possibly reduced by ritonavir via enhanced glucuronidation; valproate may increase lopinavir levels, so monitor for adverse effects	Carbamazepine (CYP3A4 and 1A2 inducer) use contraindicated, dose of dolutegravir requires adjustment with carbamazepine Monitor valproate levels and virological response	No clinically significant interactions expected

(continued)

Table 45.2 (Continued)

	Nucleoside and nucleotide reverse transcriptase inhibitors (NRTIs)	Non-nucleoside reverse transcriptase inhibitors (NNRTIs)	Protease inhibitors (PIs)	Fusion inhibitors	Co-receptor antagonists
Antidepressants	No clinically significant interactions expected	Efavirenz and nevirapine are CYP3A4 and 2B6 inducers; levels of sertraline, trazodone, bupropion, citalopram, and escitalopram may be reduced; titrate dose as per response Etravirine (weak 3A4 inducer and weak 2C19 inhibitor) may increase citalopram concentration, so monitor response and side effects including for QTc prolongation QTc prolongation with rilpivirine and efavirenz: caution with citalopram, escitalopram, and TCAs	Risk of QTc prolongation with citalopram, escitalopram, trazodone, TCAs, and saquinavir (contraindicated with the first two), atazanavir, darunavir, ritonavir and lopinavir TCA levels may be increased by ritonavir and tripanavir, so start low, use minimum effective dose SSRIs: fluvoxamine levels possibly increased, start low and titrate based on clinical response; levels of sertraline and paroxetine possibly decreased by darunavir, so dose based on response Mirtazapine, trazodone: start low, increase based on response and side effects; Venlafaxine: titrate dose as per response and side effects; modified-release venlafaxine preferred to limit P-glycoprotein interactions	Elvitegravir with cobicistat as booster: start low and titrate dose to response with SSRIs, TCAs, trazodone Fluvoxamine may affect elvitegravir levels; avoid use	No clinically significant interactions expected
Hypnotics	No clinically significant interactions expected	Alprazolam, diazepam, midazolam, triazolam, clonazepam levels reduced by nevirapine, efavirenz but caution with efavirenz as increased levels also possible Lorazepam not affected	Alprazolam, clonazepam, diazepam, triazolam, oral midazolam levels increased. Alternatives: lorazepam, oxazepam, temazepam Zopiclone, zolpidem dose reduction may be required	Elvitegravir with cobicistat as booster: advice as with PIs	No clinically significant interactions expected

should be made following a multidisciplinary discussion, ideally involving the HIV-clinician, psychiatrist, pharmacist, and patient. The HIV Liverpool drug interactions website is a comprehensive resource that may also be used to screen for potential drug interactions (www.hiv-druginteractions.org).

ART–psychotropic interactions: influence on plasma levels

Certain ART agents are cytochrome P450 enzyme inducers (e.g. the NNRTIs efavirenz and nevirapine) and this can result in reduced levels of some psychotropics and increases risk of psychiatric treatment failure. Conversely, antiretroviral agents that are CYP450 enzyme inhibitors (e.g. protease inhibitors such as ritonavir and lopinavir) can increase plasma levels of psychotropics and thus psychotropic-associated adverse effects or toxicity.

Increased hepatic clearance of antiretroviral agents by some psychotropics may result in ART failure (e.g. by carbamazepine, a potent enzyme inducer), while reduced hepatic clearance (e.g. by the potent enzyme inhibitors fluvoxamine, fluoxetine, and paroxetine) can increase ART-associated adverse effects.

Predicting the result of drug–drug interactions can be difficult, as some antiretroviral agents simultaneously inhibit some CYP450 enzymes while inducing others. For example, ritonavir is a CYP2D6 and CYP3A4 inhibitor but a CYP2C9 inducer. Furthermore, antiretrovirals may affect the metabolism of drugs via other pathways, for example by inhibiting or inducing glucuronosyltransferase or P-glycoprotein (a drug efflux protein). As such, dose adjustments may be required and, where appropriate, therapeutic drug monitoring of psychotropics employed to guide dosing. Advanced HIV also increases the risk of developing extrapyramidal side effects with antipsychotics, which should be reflected in the type and dose of antipsychotic prescribed [23].

ART–psychotropic interactions: influence on adverse effect profiles

Pharmacodynamic interactions between ART and psychotropics can lead to compound adverse effects. The protease inhibitors atazanavir, saquinavir, lopinavir, ritonavir, and tipranavir and the NNRTIs efavirenz and rilpivirine are associated with QTc prolongation. Thus, risk of arrhythmias may be increased with concurrent use of psychotropics that similarly prolong the QTc interval (see Chapter 3). Enhanced ECG monitoring, or rationalisation of psychiatric/ART treatment, may therefore be indicated. ART is also associated with development of the metabolic syndrome, which may compound the metabolic effects of many psychotropics and increase the risk of cardiovascular disease. Enhanced metabolic monitoring may therefore be indicated. Some antiretroviral agents (in particular the nucleoside reverse transcriptase inhibitor zidovudine) and HIV itself result in myelosuppression. When combined with psychotropics with myelosuppressant side effects (see Chapter 16), a low threshold for checking the white cell count is recommended (e.g. in the case of a sore throat). Finally, HIV is an independent risk factor for low bone mineral density, increasing the risk of osteoporosis and fractures. ART and concomitant prolactin-elevating antipsychotics further increase this risk (see Chapter 13). Gastro-oesophageal reflux is common in patients with serious mental illness [24]. Clinicians should be aware that concurrent use of gastric acid supressants (e.g. proton pump inhibitors) can alter antiretroviral pharmacokinetics and lead to treatment failure due to inadequate drug exposure [25].

Other treatment considerations

There may also be interactions between drugs used for prophylaxis against certain opportunistic infections and co-prescribed psychotropic medications. For example, pentamidine isetionate, used in the prophylaxis of *Pneumocystis* pneumonia, can prolong the QTc. This may influence the type and dose of psychotropic agent used (see Chapter 3).

References

1. Blank MB, Himelhoch SS, Balaji AB, et al. A multisite study of the prevalence of HIV with rapid testing in mental health settings. *Am J Public Health* 2014;104(12):2377–2384.
2. Penzak SR, Reddy YS, Grimsley SR. Depression in patients with HIV infection. *Am J Health Syst Pharm* 2000;57(4):376–386.
3. Del Guerra FB, Fonseca JLI, Figueiredo VM, et al. Human immunodeficiency virus-associated depression: contributions of immuno-inflammatory, monoaminergic, neurodegenerative, and neurotrophic pathways. *J Neurovirol* 2013;19(4):314–327.
4. Croxford S, Kitching A, Desai S, et al. Mortality and causes of death in people diagnosed with HIV in the era of highly active antiretroviral therapy compared with the general population: an analysis of a national observational cohort. *Lancet Public Health* 2017;2(1):e35–e46.
5. Pellowski JA, Kalichman SC, Matthews KA, Adler N. A pandemic of the poor: social disadvantage and the U.S. HIV epidemic. *Am Psychol* 2013;68(4):197–209.
6. Antinori A, Arendt G, Becker JT, et al. Updated research nosology for HIV-associated neurocognitive disorders. *Neurology* 2007;69(18):1789–1799.
7. Travaglini LE, Himelhoch SS, Fang LJ. HIV stigma and its relation to mental, physical and social health among black women living with HIV/AIDS. *AIDS Behav* 2018;22(12):3783–3794.
8. Fairfield KM, Libman H, Davis RB, et al. Delays in protease inhibitor use in clinical practice. *J Gen Intern Med* 1999;14(7):395–401.
9. Gordillo V, del Amo J, Soriano V, Gonzalez-Lahoz J. Sociodemographic and psychological variables influencing adherence to antiretroviral therapy. *AIDS* 1999;13(13):1763–1769.
10. Himelhoch S, Moore RD, Treisman G, Gebo KA. Does the presence of a current psychiatric disorder in AIDS patients affect the initiation of antiretroviral treatment and duration of therapy? *J Acquir Immune Defic Syndr* 2004;37(4):1457–1463.
11. British HIV Association. *UK National Guidelines for HIV Testing 2008*. https://www.bhiva.org/file/RHNUJgIseDaML/GlinesHIVTest08.pdf
12. National Institute for Health and Care Excellence. *HIV Testing: Encouraging Uptake*. Quality Standard QS157. London: NICE, 2017. Available at https://www.nice.org.uk/guidance/qs157
13. Stafylis C, Klausner JD. Evaluation of two 4th generation point-of-care assays for the detection of human immunodeficiency virus infection. *PLoS One* 2017;12(8):e0183944.
14. Eggers C, Arendt G, Hahn K, et al. HIV-1-associated neurocognitive disorder: epidemiology, pathogenesis, diagnosis, and treatment. *J Neurol* 2017;264(8):1715–1727.
15. Robinson-Papp J, Byrd D, Mindt MR, et al. Motor function and human immunodeficiency virus-associated cognitive impairment in a highly active antiretroviral therapy-era cohort. *Arch Neurol* 2008;65(8):1096–1101.
16. World Health Organization. *Consolidated Guidelines on the Use of Antiretroviral Drugs for Treating and Preventing HIV Infection: Recommendations for a Public Health Approach*. Geneva: WHO, 2013.
17. Paterson DL, Swindells S, Mohr J, et al. Adherence to protease inhibitor therapy and outcomes in patients with HIV infection. *Ann Intern Med* 2000;133(1):21–30.
18. Grant RM, Lama JR, Anderson PL, et al. Preexposure chemoprophylaxis for HIV prevention in men who have sex with men. *N Engl J Med* 2010;363(27):2587–2599.
19. Apostolova N, Funes HA, Blas-Garcia A, et al. Efavirenz and the CNS: what we already know and questions that need to be answered. *J Antimicrob Chemother* 2015;70(10):2693–2708.
20. Department of Health and Human Services, Panel on Antiretroviral Guidelines for Adults and Adolescents. *AIDSinfo. Guidelines for the Use of Antiretroviral Agents in Adults and Adolescents with HIV*. Rockville, MD: DHHS, 2019. Available at http://www.aidsinfo.nih.gov/ContentFiles/AdultandAdolescentGL.pdf
21. British HIV Association. *BHIVA guidelines for the routine investigation and adult HIV-1-positive individuals*. Available at https://www.bhiva.org/file/DqZbRxfzlYtLg/Monitoring-Guidelines.pdf

22. World Health Organization. *Consolidated Guidelines on the Use of Antiretroviral Drugs for Treating and Preventing HIV Infection: Recommendations for a Public Health Approach*, 2nd edn. Geneva: WHO, 2016. Available at https://www.who.int/hiv/pub/arv/arv-2016/en/

23. Perry SW. Organic mental-disorders caused by HIV: update on early diagnosis and treatment. *Am J Psychiatry* 1990;147(6):696–710.

24. Martin-Merino E, Ruigomez A, Garcia Rodriguez LA, et al. Depression and treatment with antidepressants are associated with the development of gastro-oesophageal reflux disease. *Aliment Pharmacol Ther* 2010;31(10):1132–1140.

25. McCabe SM, Smith PF, Ma Q, Morse GD. Drug interactions between proton pump inhibitors and antiretroviral drugs. *Expert Opin Drug Metab Toxicol* 2007;3(2):197–207.

Part 8

Respiratory

Smoking Cessation

Harriet Quigley, Mary Yates, John Moxham

Tobacco smoking is two to three times more prevalent among individuals with serious mental illness (SMI) compared with the general population [1,2]. The strength of this association correlates with severity of mental disorder, with the highest smoking prevalence recorded in psychiatric inpatient units [1,3]. The number of mental health diagnoses also influences smoking prevalence; rates range from 18% for individuals with no mental health diagnosis to 61% amongst those diagnosed with three or more mental health disorders [4]. Smoking prevalence among individuals with SMI has remained unchanged over the past two decades, compared with the striking decline seen in the general population. Moreover, tobacco smokers with SMI display patterns of heavy smoking and severe nicotine dependence, and are less likely succeed in cessation attempts [5]. Tobacco smoking is the foremost preventable cause of death globally, affecting individuals with SMI disproportionately and contributing to significant reductions in life expectancy and quality of life. Smoking can also influence the efficacy of multiple medications used in the treatment of SMI through CYP1A2 induction, reducing plasma levels of some drugs. This effect is caused by polyaromatic hydrocarbons in tobacco smoke rather than nicotine. Doses may need to be reduced when someone stops smoking (Table 46.1).

IDENTIFYING THOSE WHO WANT TO STOP SMOKING AND DEGREE OF NICOTINE DEPENDENCE

Asking 'Do you smoke?' or 'Have you recently stopped smoking?' should be a routine part of history taking in the SMI population. In an inpatient setting, these questions should be asked at the earliest opportunity so that nicotine replacement therapy (NRT)

The Maudsley Practice Guidelines for Physical Health Conditions in Psychiatry, First Edition. David M. Taylor, Fiona Gaughran, and Toby Pillinger.

Table 46.1 Prescribing guidelines for psychiatric drugs during smoking cessation [8].

Drug	Effect of smoking	Action on stopping smoking	Action to be taken on smoking relapse
Agomelatine	Plasma levels reduced	Monitor closely. Dose may need to be reduced	Consider reintroducing previous smoking dose
Benzodiazepines	Plasma levels reduced by 0–50% (depends on drug and smoking status)	Monitor closely. Consider reducing dose by up to 25% over 1 week	Monitor closely. Consider restarting 'normal' smoking dose
Carbamazepine	Unclear, but smoking may reduce carbamazepine levels to a small extent	Monitor for changes in severity of adverse effects	Monitor plasma levels
Chlorpromazine	Plasma levels reduced. Varied estimates of exact effect	Monitor closely and consider dose reduction	Monitor closely, consider restarting previous smoking dose
Clozapine	Reduces plasma levels by 50%. Plasma level reduction may be greater in those receiving valproate	Take plasma level before stopping. On stopping, reduce dose gradually (over 1 week) until around 75% of original dose reached. Repeat plasma level 1 week after stopping. Consider further dose reductions	Take plasma level before restarting. Increase dose to previous smoking dose over one week. Repeat plasma level
Duloxetine	Plasma levels may be reduced by 50%	Monitor closely and consider dose reduction	Consider restarting previous smoking dose
Fluphenazine	Reduces plasma levels by up to 50%	On stopping, reduce dose by 25%. Monitor closely over following 4–8 weeks. Consider further dose reductions	On restarting, increase to previous dose
Fluvoxamine	Plasma levels decreased by around one-third	Monitor closely and consider dose reduction	Dose may need to be increased to previous level
Haloperidol	Reduces plasma levels by around 25–50%	Reduce dose by around 25%. Monitor closely. Consider further dose reductions	On restarting, increase to previous smoking dose
Mirtazapine	Unclear, but effect probably minimal	Monitor	Monitor
Olanzapine	Reduces plasma levels by up to 50%	Take plasma level before stopping. On stopping reduce dose by 25%. After 1 week repeat plasma level. Consider further dose reductions	Take plasma level before restarting. Increase dose to previous smoking dose after 1 week. Repeat plasma level
Trazadone	Around 25% reduction	Monitor for increased sedation. Consider dose reduction	Monitor closely. Consider increasing dose
Tricyclic antidepressants	Plasma levels reduced by 25–50%	Monitor closely. Consider reducing the dose by 10–25% over 1 week. Consider further dose reductions	Monitor closely. Consider restarting previous smoking dose
Zuclopenthixol	Unclear, but effect probably minimal	Monitor	Monitor

Table 46.2 Fagerström test for nicotine dependence.

How soon after waking do you smoke your first cigarette?

Within 5 minutes	3 points
5–30 minutes	2 points
31–60 minutes	1 point
>60 minutes	0 points

How many cigarettes do you smoke per day?

>31	3 points
21–30	2 points
11–20	1 point
<10	0 points

Results

High dependence	≥5 points
Moderate dependence	4 points
Low to moderate dependence	3 points
Low dependence	1–2 points

Source: adapted from Heatherton et al. [6].

can be rapidly made available. If an individual is interested in stopping smoking, then clarifying the degree of nicotine dependence may guide management. This can be achieved with the Fagerström test for nicotine dependence (Table 46.2) [6].

APPROACHES TO SMOKING CESSATION

Step 1: Providing 'very brief advice'

The National Centre for Smoking Cessation and Training (NCSCT), funded by the UK Department of Health, recommends the provision of 'very brief advice' (VBA) for smokers, which takes less than 30 seconds [7]. The recommendation is to use a simple statement advising that the best way to stop is with a combination of support and medication:

'Did you know the best way to stop is with support and treatment provided by a specialist stop smoking service? They can make it much easier to stop than doing it alone, would it be OK if I refer you to such a service?'

The goal of VBA, which does not directly tell individuals to stop smoking, is to avoid provoking feelings of anxiety or making smokers feel defensive, which may reduce the chances of successful cessation.

Step 2: Referring smokers for specialist support

Smokers who are interested in stopping smoking should be offered both behavioural support and access to medication that increases the chances of successfully stopping. This is best provided by a specialist 'stop smoking' advisor. All psychiatric hospitals should aim to provide an on-site stop smoking service. Community-based smokers should be directed to local smoking cessation services, if available. In the UK, the public health team in each local authority is responsible for providing specialist stop smoking support.

Behavioural support

Behavioural support involves either scheduled face-to-face or telephone consultations with a counsellor trained in smoking cessation. It typically involves weekly sessions for at least four weeks after the quit date and is normally combined with pharmacotherapy. Group behavioural support involves scheduled meetings in which people who smoke receive information, advice and encouragement and some form of behavioural intervention (e.g. cognitive behavioural therapy).

In the general population, meta-analyses of trials comparing multi-session intensive behavioural support with brief advice report odds ratios (ORs) for cessation of 1.56 [95% confidence interval (CI) 1.32–1.84] for individual support, 2.04 (95% CI 1.60–2.60) for group support, and 1.64 (95% CI 1.41–1.92) for telephone support [9,10]. It is not clear which components of behavioural support, such as motivational interviewing or cognitive behavioural therapy, are most effective. Group support appears more effective than one-to-one support, and studies suggest that support should involve multiple sessions [11]. In SMI there is evidence that behavioural support in combination with NRT is effective, but no strong evidence that tailored behavioural interventions are more effective than standard group therapy [12,13].

Step 3: Recognising and responding to nicotine withdrawal (nicotine replacement therapy)

Symptoms of nicotine withdrawal may begin as soon as the last cigarette has been finished, and peak after approximately two hours (Table 46.3). Symptoms of nicotine withdrawal are easily confused with those of an underlying mental disorder (including anxiety, irritability, poor concentration, depression), and should be treated with NRT or another cessation therapy (see steps 4 and 5). In the UK, NRT is available in eight different preparations, including transdermal patches, lozenges, gum, sublingual tablets, inhalators, nasal spray, mouth spray, and oral strips (Table 46.4). It is preferable if patients are given a choice, so they can decide which method of delivery suits them best. Heavily dependent smokers (those who smoke within 30 minutes of waking and smoke more than 20 cigarettes per day) should be advised to use two products, usually a patch plus another product of their choice.

The most effective method of managing tobacco withdrawal symptoms is with combination NRT (i.e. a patch and oral product; see Box 46.1) and intensive behavioural

Table 46.3 Nicotine withdrawal symptoms

Symptoms	Typical duration
Light-headedness	<2 days
Sleep disturbance	<2 weeks
Irritability, restlessness	<4 weeks
Difficulty in concentrating	<4 weeks
Depressed mood	<4 weeks
Constipation	<4 weeks
Mouth ulcers	<4 weeks
Urge to smoke	>10 weeks
Increased appetite/weight gain	>10 weeks

Table 46.4 Nicotine replacement therapy preparations and dose.

	Low to moderate dependence (Fagerström score 1–3)	Moderate to high dependence (Fagerström score ≥ 4)
Topical patch: 24-hour formulation (21 mg, 14 mg, 7 mg) 16-hour formulation (25 mg, 15 mg, 10 mg)	In moderate to high dependence consider using 21 mg (24-hour) or 25 mg (16-hour) patch	
Nasal spray (0.5 mg/ spray)	One spray in each nostril when craving, no more than twice an hour, maximum 64 sprays daily	
Oral spray (1 mg/spray)	One to two sprays when craving, no more than two sprays per episode, no more than four sprays per hour, maximum 64 sprays daily	
Lozenge (1 mg, 2 mg, 4 mg)[a]	One 1-mg lozenge hourly to prevent craving	One 2- or 4-mg lozenge hourly to prevent craving
Gum (2 mg, 4 mg, 6 mg)	One piece of 2 mg hourly to prevent craving	One piece of 4 mg or 6 mg hourly to prevent craving
Inhalator (15 mg)	No more than six 15-mg cartridges per day	
Sublingual tablet (2 mg)[a]	One to two tablets hourly to prevent craving	Two tablets hourly to prevent craving, no more than 40 tablets per day
Mouth strips (2.5 mg)	One strip of 2.5 mg hourly to prevent craving	One strip hourly to prevent craving, no more than 15 strips per day

[a] Efficacy of sublingual and buccal preparations is very user-dependent. Nicotine is only absorbed if product is rested against gum/stuck under tongue.

CHAPTER 46

> **Box 46.1** Examples of nicotine replacement regimens depending on degree of dependence
>
> - Low dependence (e.g. 1–10 cigarettes per day): gum 4 mg, maximum 15 daily; *or* inhalator two to four cartridges daily; *or* patch 14 mg (24-hour) daily
> - Moderate dependence (e.g. 11–20 cigarettes per day): consider combination NRT comprising (gum 6 mg, maximum 15 daily *or* inhalator six cartridges daily) *and* patch 21 mg (24-hour) daily
> - High dependence (e.g. 20+ cigarettes per day): consider combination NRT comprising (gum 6 mg, maximum 15 daily *or* inhalator six cartridges daily) *and* two patches 21 mg (24-hour) daily

support. Any risks associated with NRT are substantially outweighed by the well-established dangers of continued smoking [14]. The National Institute for Health and Care Excellence (NICE) recommends the use of NRT during periods of temporary abstinence and when attempting to cut down cigarette intake without any intention to quit. NRT can be prescribed for up to nine months if cravings persist beyond the initial 8–12 week treatment period. Long-term use of NRT is considered safe and effective [15]. All forms of NRT can be used by smokers aged 12 and over [8]. If the NRT dose is too high, the patient may experience nausea, dizziness, palpitations, or dysphoria. The lower limit for a fatal outcome is 0.5–1 g of nicotine, far less than the recommended prescribed doses even for highly dependent smokers [16]. In practice most smokers are undertreated with NRT.

Step 4: Pharmacological approaches to smoking cessation beyond nicotine replacement therapy

Varenicline

Varenicline is a nicotinic receptor partial agonist. It is given orally and is the most effective cessation pharmacotherapy in the general population (summary OR for 12-month continuous abstinence for varenicline relative to placebo is 3.22, 95% CI 2.43–4.27) [17]. It is first-line treatment for individuals who are motivated to stop smoking, and is licensed for smokers over the age of 18 and women who are not pregnant or breastfeeding. In a head-to-head trial, varenicline was found to be more effective than bupropion, nicotine patch, or placebo for helping people with or without a mental health diagnosis to stop smoking [18].

Before starting varenicline, the smoker usually sets a quit date that is between day 8 and 14 of treatment. The patient continues to smoke as usual during the first one to two weeks. If the patient cannot smoke (e.g. if they are an inpatient in a designated smoke-free hospital), then combination NRT for the first two weeks is an option. Patients are likely to experience reduced enjoyment from each cigarette. Common side effects include nausea, sleep disturbance, and vivid dreams. Sleep disturbance can be minimised by taking the second tablet in early evening rather than before bed. Nausea can be managed by taking the tablet with food. Varenicline has no known interactions with psychotropic medication. Changes in mood and behaviour have been reported and should be monitored for; however, a recent randomised placebo-controlled trial observed that neuropsychiatric adverse events were no more common in individuals receiving varenicline relative to nicotine patch or placebo [18].

CHAPTER 46

Box 46.2 Typical varenicline treatment regimen for smoking cessation
Week 1
Days 1–3: 0.5 mg twice a day (oral) Days 4–7: 0.5 mg twice a day (oral)
Weeks 2–12
Day 8 to end of treatment: 1 mg twice a day (oral)

Box 46.2 describes how varenicline is usually prescribed. Nicotine replacement can also be considered in the first two weeks of treatment. Varenicline is usually titrated over one week up to a dose of 1 mg twice daily (oral), which is taken for a further 11 weeks. A further 12 weeks may be prescribed in abstinent individuals to reduce risk of relapse.

Bupropion

Buproprion is a nicotinic receptor antagonist with dopaminergic and adrenergic actions. Its therapeutic effect may be inhibition of the effects of nicotine, relieving withdrawal, or reducing depressed mood [19].

In the general population, bupropion is as effective as single-formulation NRT in increasing long-term cessation, with pooled relative risk (RR) relative to placebo of 1.69 (95% CI 1.53–1.85) [19]. In SMI, a meta-analysis of three studies comparing bupropion with placebo, delivered with group therapy, confirmed superiority of treatment with bupropion (RR 4.18, 95% CI 1.30–13.42) [20–22]. Its effectiveness was also evident in two trials comparing a bupropion/NRT combination with NRT only, delivered alongside group therapy, with an RR for cessation of 2.34 (95% CI 1.12–4.91) [22,23].

Bupropion increases the risk of seizures, although at lower doses (e.g. 150–300 mg once daily) the increase in risk is minimal. Nevertheless, caution should be exercised when co-prescribing bupropion with tricyclic antidepressants and some antipsychotic agents, which similarly lower seizure thresholds. Bupropion is contraindicated in bipolar affective disorder. Its use has also been associated with low mood and suicidal thoughts, and it is thus recommended that individuals are monitored for adverse psychological reactions [24]. In the context of the contraindications to bupropion's use and its associated side-effect profile, typically varenicline is the preferred pharmacological agent alongside NRT to aid smoking cessation in the SMI population.

E-cigarettes

E-cigarettes are battery-powered devices that deliver nicotine via inhaled vapour. Devices come in many shapes and forms, sometimes resembling cigarettes, but others pens. They commonly comprise a battery-powered heating element, a cartridge

CHAPTER 46

containing a solution principally of nicotine in propylene glycol or glycerine, water (frequently with flavouring), and an atomiser that when heated vaporises the solution in the cartridge enabling the nicotine to be inhaled. However, it should be noted that some e-cigarettes do not contain nicotine. E-cigarettes can be disposable, rechargeable or refillable, using e-liquid or pre-filled capsules. E-liquids are available in different volumes, concentrations, and flavourings. Recent reports from Public Health England and the Royal College of Physicians have concluded that e-cigarettes appear to be effective when used by smokers as an aid to stop smoking [25,26]. E-cigarettes offer a much less harmful alternative to tobacco for dependent smokers [27]. To date, no e-cigarette has undergone the Medicines and Healthcare products Regulatory Agency (MHRA) licensing process and come to market. Thus, in the UK, e-cigarettes cannot currently be prescribed by clinicians, although patients can still be directed to their use.

In acute mental healthcare settings, disposable e-cigarettes are advised due to their ease of use. Pre-filled capsules are an increasingly popular choice in all other mental healthcare settings. It is recommended that heavily dependent smokers start off using 20 mg nicotine strength in their e-liquid. Supplement e-cigarettes with an NRT patch if withdrawal symptoms persist. As the smoker adjusts, they can reduce the strength of nicotine down to zero. Use of flavoured e-liquids is optional.

References

1. Meltzer H, Gill B, Petticrew M, Hinds K. *The prevalence of psychiatric morbidity among adults aged 16–64 living in institutions.* London: Office of Population Censuses and Surveys, 1995.
2. Lasser K, Boyd JW, Woolhandler S, et al. Smoking and mental illness: a population-based prevalence study. *JAMA* 2000; 284(20):2606–2610.
3. Farrell M, Howes S, Taylor C, et al. Substance misuse and psychiatric comorbidity: an overview of the OPCS National Psychiatric Morbidity Survey. *Addict Behav* 1998;23(6):909–918.
4. Eriksen M, Mackay J, Schluger N, et al. *The Tobacco Atlas,* 5th edn. Atlanta, GA: American Cancer Society, 2015.
5. Royal College of Physicians. Smoking and mental health. https://www.rcplondon.ac.uk/projects/outputs/smoking-and-mental-health
6. Heatherton TF, Kozlowski LT, Frecker RC, et al. Measuring the heaviness of smoking: using self-reported time to the first cigarette of the day and number of cigarettes smoked per day. *Br J Addict* 1989;84(7):791–799.
7. Stead LF, Buitrago D, Preciado N, et al. Physician advice for smoking cessation. *Cochrane Database Syst Rev* 2013;(5):CD000165.
8. Taylor DM, Barnes TRE, Young AH. *The Maudsley Prescribing Guidelines in Psychiatry,* 13th edn. Chichester: Wiley Blackwell, 2018.
9. Lancaster T, Stead LF. Individual behavioural counselling for smoking cessation. *Cochrane Database Syst Rev* 2017;(3):CD001292.
10. Stead LF, Carroll AJ, Lancaster T. Group behaviour therapy programmes for smoking cessation. *Cochrane Database Syst Rev* 2017; (3):CD001007.
11. McEwen A, West R, McRobbie H. Effectiveness of specialist group treatment for smoking cessation vs one-one treatment in primary care. *Addict Behav* 2006;31(9):1650–1660.
12. George TP, Ziedonis DM, Feingold A, et al. Nicotine transdermal patch and atypical antipsychotic medications for smoking cessation in schizophrenia. *Am J Psychiatry* 2000;157(11):1835–1842.
13. Baker A, Richmond R, Haile M, et al. A randomized controlled trial of a smoking cessation intervention among people with a psychotic disorder. *Am J Psychiatry* 2006;163(11):1934–1942.
14. National Institute for Health and Care Excellence. *Smoking: Harm Reduction.* Public Health Guideline PH45. London: NICE, 2013. Available at https://www.nice.org.uk/guidance/ph45
15. Shahab L, Dobbie F, Hiscock R, et al. Prevalence and impact of long-term use of nicotine replacement therapy in UK stop-smoking services: findings from the ELONS study. *Nicotine Tob Res* 2016;20(1):81–88.
16. Mayer B. How much nicotine kills a human? Tracing back the generally accepted lethal dose to dubious self-experiments in the nineteenth century. *Arch Toxicol* 2014;88(1):5–7.
17. Cahill K, Stead LF, Lancaster T. Nicotine receptor partial agonists for smoking cessation. *Cochrane Database Syst Rev* 2007;(1):CD006103.
18. Anthenelli RM, Benowitz NL, West R, et al. Neuropsychiatric safety and efficacy of varenicline, bupropion, and nicotine patch in smokers with and without psychiatric disorders (EAGLES): a double-blind, randomised, placebo-controlled clinical trial. *Lancet* 2016; 387(10037):2507–2520.
19. Hughes JR, Stead LF, Hartmann-Boyce J, et al. Antidepressants for smoking cessation. *Cochrane Database Syst Rev* 2014;(1):CD000031.

20. Banham L, Gilbody S. Smoking cessation in severe mental illness: what works? *Addiction* 2010;105(7):1176–1189.

21. Evins AE, Mays VK, Cather C, et al. A pilot trial of bupropion added to cognitive behavioral therapy for smoking cessation in schizophrenia. *Nicotine Tob Res* 2001;3(4):397–403.

22. George TP, Vessicchio JC, Sacco KA, et al. A placebo-controlled trial of bupropion combined with nicotine patch for smoking cessation in schizophrenia. *Biol Psychiatry* 2008;63(11):1092–1096.

23. Evins A, Cather C, Maravic M, et al. A 12-week double-blind, placebo-controlled study of bupropion SR added to high-dose dual nicotine replacement therapy for smoking cessation or reduction in schizophrenia. *J Clin Psychopharmacol* 2007;27(4):380–386.

24. Hartmann-Boyce J, Aveyard P. Drugs for smoking cessation. *BMJ* 2016;352:i571.

25. McNeill A, Brose LS, Calder R, et al. *Evidence review of e-cigarettes and heated tobacco products 2018. A report commissioned by Public Health England.* London: PHE, 2018.

26. Hajek P, Phillips-Waller A, Przulj D, et al. A randomized trial of e-cigarettes versus nicotine-replacement therapy. *N Engl J Med* 2019;380(7):629–637.

27. McNeill A, Brose LS, Calder R, et al. *E-cigarettes: an evidence update: A report commissioned by Public Health England.* London: PHE, 2015.

CHAPTER 46

Chronic Obstructive Pulmonary Disease

Mary Docherty, Jenny Docherty, Peter Saunders

Chronic obstructive pulmonary disease (COPD) is a lung disease characterised by fixed airflow obstruction that interferes with normal breathing resulting in symptoms of breathlessness and cough. Inflammation of the bronchial wall causes narrowing of the airways. The terms 'chronic bronchitis' and 'emphysema' are included within the COPD diagnosis and encompass patients with chronic sputum production with repeated infections and those whose predominant issue is breathlessness [1]. The most common causative agent in COPD is tobacco smoke [2]. COPD can occur in people who have not smoked, but 90% of those with COPD have or do smoke. Burning of biomass fuels and air pollution have been speculated as other potential causative agents.

COMMON CAUSES OF COPD IN THE GENERAL POPULATION AND PATIENTS WITH SERIOUS MENTAL ILLNESS

COPD is one of the leading preventable causes of death worldwide, with smoking being the largest contributor, although other environmental and occupational causes exist (Table 47.1). There is suspected significant under-diagnosis, with estimates of more than 3 million people in the UK currently having COPD but it being undiagnosed in about 2 million of these [3]. About 30,000 people each year in the UK die of complications related to COPD [4].

COPD is variable in presentation and severity. It is chronic, often progressive, and can present with recurrent exacerbations. Stopping exposure to noxious agents may slow or halt the progression of the disease, but once developed its only cure is lung transplantation [5]. Exacerbations are the second largest cause of emergency inpatient admissions in the UK. There is a significant associated inpatient mortality rate [4,6].

The Maudsley Practice Guidelines for Physical Health Conditions in Psychiatry, First Edition.
David M. Taylor, Fiona Gaughran, and Toby Pillinger.
© 2021 John Wiley & Sons Ltd. Published 2021 by John Wiley & Sons Ltd.

Table 47.1 Causes of COPD in the general population [13] and in those living with SMI.

General population	Individual with SMI
Smoking	
Tobacco, pipe, cigar, water pipe, and marijuana smokers Passive smoking [12] Smoking enhances effects of other risk factors (e.g. occupational exposure)	Higher rates of smoking and substance use than general population
Occupational exposure	
Dust, chemicals, noxious gases, and particles (coal, grains, silica, welding fume, isocyanates, and polycyclic aromatic hydrocarbons)	Association of SMI with social deprivation and poor living conditions
Air pollution	
Wood and coal burned in open fires and motor vehicle emissions in cities	
Genetics	
Homozygous α_1-antitrypsin deficiency accounts for <1% of COPD associated with accelerated development of COPD in smokers and non-smokers A significant familial risk of airflow obstruction has been reported in smoking siblings of people with severe COPD	

Individuals living with serious mental illness (SMI) exhibit a higher prevalence of COPD than the general population [7]. This increased risk of COPD is mainly attributable to smoking behaviours (see Chapter 46). Individuals with SMI are more likely to smoke than the general population and tend to smoke more than the average smoker [8]. Smoking of substances other than tobacco, such as marijuana and heroin, will also contribute to the risk of developing COPD.

Some research has suggested that use of antipsychotic drugs may predispose to smoking. Smoking may also mask some of the side effects of the drugs [9]. Socioeconomic status affects both the risk of developing COPD and worsened health outcomes [10]. Living conditions, occupational status, and recreational drug use may be associated with the pathogenesis of COPD. It is likely these risk factors are mediated directly or indirectly through smoking, although other mechanisms have not been excluded.

Individuals with SMI may aggregate multiple risk factors for COPD, such as smoking histories, childhood exposure to tobacco smoke, and social deprivation. In addition to cumulative risk factors, they may also have a number of comorbidities which can increase associated disability with COPD. Higher prevalence of obesity, sleep apnoea, and substance misuse can worsen respiratory function and quality of life [11].

THE ASTHMA–COPD OVERLAP

Asthma and COPD were previously considered separate disease entities, asthma being characterised by reversible airflow obstruction (see Chapter 48). A relatively new syndrome termed the 'asthma–COPD overlap syndrome' (ACOS) has been applied to the condition in which a person has clinical features of both asthma and COPD [14]. ACOS is characterised by persistent airflow limitation with several features usually associated with asthma, and several features usually associated with COPD. Diagnosis is made by comparing the respective clinical features to asthma and COPD diagnostic criteria [13]. If there are similar numbers of features of asthma and COPD, the diagnosis of ACOS should be considered [15].

Some patients with chronic asthma also develop airflow obstruction that can be irreversible (a consequence of airway remodelling), which is often indistinguishable from COPD. Patients with SMI may have an increased likelihood of under-diagnosis and untreated asthma due to systematic diagnosis and treatment gaps across physical health conditions [16]. The possibility of ACOS and an untreated asthmatic component should always be considered in this population.

DIAGNOSTIC PRINCIPLES

Individuals with SMI may not spontaneously present with symptoms of COPD. Insidious onset, normalisation of symptoms, and barriers to engagement with physical health services may all contribute to under-diagnosis in this population. Diagnosis may be opportunistic, and symptoms should be proactively asked about in any current smoker. Late presentation worsens prognosis because this progressive condition will inevitably be more severe at diagnosis.

History

Common symptoms include breathlessness, wheeze, chronic productive cough, reduced exercise tolerance, fatigue, and recurrent winter bronchitis. Onset and variability should be characterised. If there is diurnal variation and young age of onset, asthma or ACOS should be considered. The Medical Research Council (MRC) dyspnoea scale [17] can be used to assess breathlessness, grading degree of dsypnoea on a five-point scale from 1 (breathless only on strenuous exercise) to 5 (too breathless to leave house).

Systemic features may point to alternative comorbid pathologies, such as cancer, tuberculosis (TB; see Chapter 44), and cardiac failure. Waking at night with breathlessness, ankle swelling, chest pain, and haemoptysis should all prompt further investigation (see Chapters 7, 67, and 68).

Symptoms of anxiety and depression should be specifically enquired about. A list of differential diagnoses for COPD is presented in Box 47.1.

Medication history

Specific enquiry should be made about use of beta-blockers or non-steroidal anti-inflammatory drugs (NSAIDs), which can trigger bronchoconstriction [18]. Individuals with SMI may have anxiety disorders or side effects from antipsychotics (tachycardia or akathisia), all of which can be treated with beta-blockers. Alternatives should be sought if an asthma overlap diagnosis is suspected.

CHAPTER 47

> **Box 47.1** Differential diagnoses for COPD
>
> - Gastro-oeseophageal reflux disease
> - Foreign body aspiration
> - Aspiration
> - Heart failure
> - Interstitial lung disease
> - Malignancy
> - Ciliary dyskinesia
> - Dysfunctional breathing
> - Pertussis
> - *Pneumocystis* pneumonia and other HIV-related conditions

Family history

Particularly cardiac and respiratory disease.

Past medical history

Ask the patient about childhood respiratory infections, atopy, frequency of lower respiratory tract infections, TB vaccination, and whether attending for annual flu and pneumococcal vaccinations; also human immunodeficiency virus (HIV) screening and potential exposure to HIV (see Chapter 45).

Smoking history

Comprehensive history should be taken establishing duration, quantity, knowledge of smoking risks, and motivation to change.

Alcohol and substance use

Comprehensive history making detailed enquiry about alcohol quantity, features of dependence, type of prescribed and illicit substances used, and method of ingestion (see Chapter 24).

Social history

Enquire about occupation history including potential exposure to toxins, living conditions including cleanliness, and exposure to any additional allergens (e.g. pets).

Examination

1 Perform a general inspection for signs of smoking or substance use, breathlessness at rest or on minimal exertion, and evidence of weight loss, cachexia, muscle wasting or atrophy, anaemia or polycythaemia, and chest wall deformities.

2 Comprehensive respiratory examination: oxygen saturations, inspection for an expanded chest or wheezing, and auscultation for decreased breath sounds or abnormal breath sounds such as crackles or wheeze.
3 Comprehensive cardiovascular examination: peripheral or central cyanosis, peripheral oedema, raised jugular venous pressure, or signs of cor pulmonale.

Investigations

The diagnosis of COPD is based on signs and symptoms. Additional investigations may be performed to explore differential diagnoses or on presentation with complications due to the condition which may be present in the event of late diagnosis. Reasons for additional investigations (Table 47.2) include prominent systemic features, crackles, clubbing, cyanosis, chronic sputum production, unexplained restrictive spirometry, and history of recurrent pulmonary emboli.

Basic investigations at initial diagnostic evaluation include the following.

1 Bloods: full blood count (check for polycythaemia or normochromic normocytic, eosinophilia) and C-reactive protein (CRP).
2 Spirometry: performed at diagnosis and to monitor disease progression. For most people, routine spirometric reversibility testing is not needed as part of the diagnostic process. Spirometry shows obstructive pattern: forced expiratory volume in 1 s (FEV_1)/ forced vital capacity (FVC) ratio of under 70% with no bronchodilator reversibility.
3 Body mass index (BMI) documented.
4 Chest X-ray to exclude other pathology.

Table 47.2 Additional investigations that may be requested in patients with COPD.

Investigation	Rationale
Metabolic and endocrine function: renal, liver, thyroid and bone function HIV screen	Comprehensive assessment of physical health to support holistic management of a long-term condition and exclude other concurrent pathologies
Sputum culture	Identify organisms if sputum persistent and purulent
Serial home peak flow measurements	Exclude asthma
ECG and serum natriuretic peptide	To assess cardiac status if cardiac disease or pulmonary hypertension are suspected. Indications would include a history of cardiovascular disease, hypertension or hypoxia or clinical signs such as tachycardia, oedema, cyanosis, or features of cor pulmonale
Echocardiogram	To assess cardiac status if cardiac disease or pulmonary hypertension are suspected
Serum α_1-antitrypsin	To assess for α_1-antitrypsin deficiency if early onset, minimal smoking history, or family history
Transfer factor for carbon monoxide (TLCO)	To investigate symptoms that seem disproportionate to the spirometric impairment To assess suitability for lung volume reduction procedures

> **Box 47.2** Indications for referral to respiratory services in COPD [19] and information to include in a referral
>
> **Rationale for respiratory referral**
>
> - Diagnostic uncertainty
> - Suspected severe disease, e.g. FEV_1 <30% predicted
> - Request for second opinion
> - Onset of cor pulmonale
> - Assessment for oxygen therapy, long-term nebuliser therapy or oral corticosteroid therapy, pulmonary rehabilitation, lung transplantation, lung volume reduction procedure
> - Bullous lung disease
> - Rapid decline in FEV_1
> - Dysfunctional breathing
> - Early onset <40 years of age or family history of α_1-antitrypsin deficiency
> - Symptoms disproportionate to lung function deficit
> - Frequent infections
> - Haemoptysis
>
> **Information to include in referral**
>
> - Brief summary of symptoms and reason for referral, e.g. to address diagnostic uncertainty, for specialist input in context of other comorbid conditions, uncontrolled symptoms, treatment optimisation
> - Mental health diagnosis: brief summary of what that mental health diagnosis means for that individual, current level of symptomology and impact on daily functioning from symptoms
> - Any psychosocial issues that may impact on COPD control and treatment choice, e.g. concurrent substance use, social deprivation or isolation
> - Summary of any potential impact of mental health condition on (i) accessing and engaging with investigations and follow-up; (ii) concordance with recommended management; and (iii) contact details of the patient's care team (e.g. care coordinator, keyworker, family member, friend, or carer) and information if the appointment should be sent to any one in addition to the patient
> - Any reasonable adjustments needed for the patient when seen in specialty care, e.g. time or duration of appointment, carer/support worker in attendance

When to refer

Indications for referral to respiratory physicians include uncertainty regarding diagnosis, disease severity, need for specialist input to support early intervention, and optimising therapies (Box 47.2).

MANAGEMENT

Although it is unlikely that a psychiatric practitioner will be leading the management of COPD, they may still represent a key member of the multidisciplinary team, especially in reviewing symptoms (both acute and chronic) and concordance in patients who have poor engagement with medical services, and via smoking cessation teams that mental health services may provide.

CHAPTER 47

Once diagnosis of COPD is confirmed, the fundamentals of treatment are:

1 smoking cessation
2 pneumococcal and influenza vaccinations
3 pulmonary rehabilitation
4 co-develop a personalised self-management plan
5 optimise treatment for comorbidities including ischaemic heart disease.

Inhaled therapies should only be offered once the above interventions have been offered and if they are needed to relieve breathlessness or exercise limitation.

Non-pharmacological treatment

There is a robust evidence base on smoking cessation for individuals living with SMI (see Chapter 46) and supporting smoking cessation should be the priority of all management [20]. Furthermore, psychoeducation about the condition and how to support self-management are fundamental to safe care. Factors that could compromise respiratory function, such as over-sedation with hypnotics or uncontrolled delivery of oxygen in type 2 respiratory failure, should be communicated across all mental and physical healthcare plans. Education around the role of additional triggers, such as dust in the home environment or substance use, should also be delivered. If inhaled treatments are being used, the technique for using the delivery system should be regularly reviewed. Oral health should be reviewed regularly if the patient is prescribed inhaled corticosteroids. Weight should be monitored. COPD can present at different stages of severity and management will differ accordingly. As COPD is a chronic and progressive disease, a multidisciplinary approach is required addressing symptoms alongside social and psychological needs. Pulmonary rehabilitation should be adjusted to the needs of the patient.

COPD is independently associated with other psychiatric comorbidity including depression and anxiety, which can relate to the burden of living with a debilitating condition and synergistically interact with the disease symptoms (e.g. panic and anxiety symptoms and breathlessness). Mood should be enquired about. Complications of COPD include disability and impaired quality of life, affective disorders, cor pulmonale, frequent chest infections, secondary polycythaemia, type 2 respiratory failure, and lung cancer. Such complications, recurrent exacerbations, and uncontrolled symptoms should prompt specialist referral. Specialist input is also needed for oxygen therapy, non-invasive ventilation, management of cor pulmonale, pulmonary hypertension, and consideration of lung volume reduction [19].

Follow-up of COPD patients in the UK is often managed by primary care and by community respiratory teams. Recommendations about frequency and content of follow-up in primary care are provided in Table 47.3 [19]. American readers are directed to the American College of Physicians Guidelines [21].

Pharmacological therapy

Pharmacological approaches include inhaled and oral therapies. Specialist input may be prudent in selecting oral therapies, particularly consideration of corticosteroids which can exacerbate psychiatric symptoms. SMI and COPD can present with challenging

CHAPTER 47

Table 47.3 Recommended primary care follow-up in patients with COPD. Frequency of review may need to be increased in those with serious mental illness.

	Mild/moderate/severe (stages 1–3)	Very severe (stage 4)
Review frequency	At least annually	At least twice a year
Clinical assessment	Check smoking status and enquire as to whether patient wishes to stop smoking (see Chapter 46) Are symptoms well controlled? Assess degree of breathlessness, exercise tolerance, and frequency of COPD exacerbations Assess need for pulmonary rehabilitation Presence of complications, e.g. cor pulmonale Assess efficacy of drug treatment Assess inhaler technique Determine if there is a need for specialist referral	Check smoking status and enquire as to whether patient wishes to stop smoking (see Chapter 46) Are symptoms well controlled? Assess degree of breathlessness, exercise tolerance, and frequency of COPD exacerbations Presence of complications, e.g. cor pulmonale Assess need for pulmonary rehabilitation Assess need for oxygen therapy Assess nutrition Assess mental state (depression?) Assess efficacy of drug treatment Assess inhaler technique Determine if there is a need for specialist referral, pulmonary rehabilitation, or need for social services/occupational therapy input
Measurements to make	Spirometry (check FEV_1 and FVC) Calculate body mass index Calculate MRC dyspnoea scale [17]	Spirometry (check FEV_1 and FVC) Calculate body mass index Calculate MRC dyspnoea scale [17] Check oxygen saturation

Source: adapted from National Institute for Health and Care Excellence [19].

multimorbidity and a multidisciplinary approach is important. Some evidence has suggested increased respiratory-related morbidity and mortality in older-adult new users of serotonergic antidepressants, but a recent Cochrane systematic review found insufficient evidence to make definitive statements about the efficacy or safety of antidepressants for treating COPD-related depression [22].

Inhaled therapies include bronchodilators and inhaled corticosteroids (Table 47.4). Bronchodilators reduce breathlessness and improve exercise tolerance without producing large improvements in FEV_1. Care follows a stepped approach of short-acting β_2-agonists and short-acting muscarinic antagonists, long-acting formulations, inhaled corticosteroids, and inhaled combination therapy (comprising long-acting muscarinic antagonists, long-acting β_2-agonists and inhaled corticosteroids). Oral therapies and their indications are summarised in Table 47.5.

Principles of inhaled therapy prescribing

When prescribing an inhaled therapy, the choice of delivery system should be assessed by someone familiar with the devices, usually a practice nurse with a special interest, commonplace in primary care settings. Education on technique should occur at each review. If the person has an exceptionally good response to treatment, repeat spirometry

Table 47.4 Stepped inhaled pharmacological treatment of COPD [19].

Presentation	Treatment
Breathless and exercise limitation	Prescribe a short-acting β₂-agonist (SABA): salbutamol or terbutaline, or Short-acting muscarinic antagonist (SAMA): ipratropium bromide Either as required to relieve symptoms
Breathless or exacerbations despite SABA or SAMA	Prescribe either a long-acting β₂-agonist (LABA): salmeterol or formoterol, or Long-acting muscarinic antagonist (LAMA): tiotropium Stop SAMA
Breathless or exacerbations despite LABA	Consider changing to a LABA plus an inhaled corticosteroid (ICS) in a combination inhaler If an ICS is declined or not tolerated, consider a LAMA plus a LABA An ICS should not be used as monotherapy in COPD
Breathless or exacerbations despite LABA plus ICS	Add LAMA
Breathless or exacerbations despite LAMA	Consider adding a LABA plus an ICS (in a combination inhaler)

Table 47.5 Oral therapies for COPD [19].

Therapy	Indication and considerations
Oral corticosteroids	Long-term use not normally recommended. If unavoidable, ensure osteoporosis prophylaxis and close monitoring of mental state
Oral theophylline	Only indicated after trial of inhaled therapies or if unable to tolerate inhaled therapies. Potential for drug interactions (carbamazepine, SSRIs) and needs plasma level monitoring
Oral mucolytic therapy	Consider in people with a chronic cough productive of sputum. Only continue if symptomatic improvement
Oral prophylactic antibiotic therapy	Consider specialist input prior to commencing any long-term antibiotic therapy: azithromycin three times weekly is the most popular but can cause long-term hearing issues, tinnitus and QT prolongation
Oral phosphodiesterase-4 inhibitors	Roflumilast (Daxas) is recommended for treating COPD in adults with chronic bronchitis but only under specialist care and its use if often limited by its side-effect profile

SSRI, selective serotonin reuptake inhibitor.

and reconsider the diagnosis if the FEV₁/FVC ratio is 0.7 or greater. A short-acting β₂-agonist (as required) may be continued at all stages of COPD.

References

1. World Health Organization. Chronic obstructive pulmonary disease. https://www.who.int/respiratory/copd/en/ (accessed 22 February 2019).
2. Corlateanu A, Odajiu I, Botnaru V, Cemirtan S. From smoking to COPD: current approaches. *Pneumologia* 2016;65(1):20–23.
3. Nardini S, Annesi-Maesano I, Simoni M, et al. Accuracy of diagnosis of COPD and factors associated with misdiagnosis in primary care setting. E-DIAL (Early DIAgnosis of obstructive lung disease) study group. *Respir Med* 2018;143:61–66.

CHAPTER 47

4. Snell N, Strachan D, Hubbard R, et al. S32 Epidemiology of chronic obstructive pulmonary disease (COPD) in the UK: findings from the British Lung Foundation's 'Respiratory Health of the Nation' project. *Thorax* 2016;71(Suppl 3):A20.

5. Bai JW, Chen XX, Liu S, et al. Smoking cessation affects the natural history of COPD. *Int J Chron Obstruct Pulmon Dis* 2017;12:3323–3328.

6. Calderon-Larranaga A, Carney L, Soljak M, et al. Association of population and primary healthcare factors with hospital admission rates for chronic obstructive pulmonary disease in England: national cross-sectional study. *Thorax* 2011;66(3):191–196.

7. Zareifopoulos N, Bellou A, Spiropoulou A, Spiropoulos K. Prevalence of comorbid chronic obstructive pulmonary disease in individuals suffering from schizophrenia and bipolar disorder: a systematic review. *COPD* 2018;15(6):612–620.

8. Dickerson F, Stallings CR, Origoni AE, et al. Cigarette smoking among persons with schizophrenia or bipolar disorder in routine clinical settings, 1999–2011. *Psychiatr Serv* 2013;64(1):44–50.

9. Wium-Andersen MK, Orsted DD, Nordestgaard BG. Tobacco smoking is causally associated with antipsychotic medication use and schizophrenia, but not with antidepressant medication use or depression. *Int J Epidemiol* 2015;44(2):566–577.

10. Pleasants RA, Riley IL, Mannino DM. Defining and targeting health disparities in chronic obstructive pulmonary disease. *Int J Chron Obstruct Pulmon Dis* 2016;11(1):2475–2496.

11. Stubbs B, Vancampfort D, Veronese N, et al. The prevalence and predictors of obstructive sleep apnea in major depressive disorder, bipolar disorder and schizophrenia: a systematic review and meta-analysis. *J Affect Disord* 2016;197:259–267.

12. Hagstad S, Bjerg A, Ekerljung L, et al. Passive smoking exposure is associated with increased risk of COPD in never smokers. *Chest* 2014;145(6):1298–1304.

13. Global Initiative for Chronic Obstructive Lung Disease. *Global Strategy for the Diagnosis, Management, and Prevention of COPD.* https://goldcopd.org/gold-reports/

14. Leung JM, Sin DD. Asthma–COPD overlap syndrome: pathogenesis, clinical features, and therapeutic targets. *BMJ* 2017;358:j3772.

15. Postma DS, Rabe KF. The asthma–COPD overlap syndrome. *N Engl J Med* 2015;373(13):1241–1249.

16. Docherty M, Stubbs B, Gaughran F. Strategies to deal with comorbid physical illness in psychosis. *Epidemiol Psychiatr Sci* 2016;25(3):197–204.

17. Bestall JC, Paul EA, Garrod R, et al. Usefulness of the Medical Research Council (MRC) dyspnoea scale as a measure of disability in patients with chronic obstructive pulmonary disease. *Thorax* 1999;54(7):581–586.

18. Covar RA, Macomber BA, Szefler SJ. Medications as asthma triggers. *Immunol Allergy Clin North Am* 2005;25(1):169–190.

19. National Institute for Health and Care Excellence. *Chronic Obstructive Pulmonary Disease in Over 16s: Diagnosis and Management.* NICE Guideline NG115. London: NICE, 2018. Available at https://www.nice.org.uk/guidance/ng115

20. Peckham E, Brabyn S, Cook L, et al. Smoking cessation in severe mental ill health: what works? An updated systematic review and meta-analysis. *BMC Psychiatry.* 2017;17(1):252.

21. Qaseem A, Wilt TJ, Weinberger SE, et al. Diagnosis and management of stable chronic obstructive pulmonary disease: a clinical practice guideline update from the American College of Physicians, American College of Chest Physicians, American Thoracic Society, and European Respiratory Society. *Ann Intern Med* 2011;155(3):179–191.

22. Pollok J, van Agteren JE, Carson-Chahhoud KV. Pharmacological interventions for the treatment of depression in chronic obstructive pulmonary disease. *Cochrane Database Syst Rev* 2018;(12):CD012346.

CHAPTER 47

Asthma

Mary Docherty, Jenny Docherty, Peter Saunders

Asthma is an airway disease characterised by recurrent attacks of breathlessness and wheezing that can vary in severity and frequency [1]. Symptoms occur secondary to immune-mediated airway inflammation resulting in airway hyperresponsiveness and reversible bronchial constriction [2]. During an asthma attack the lining of the airways swell, causing them to narrow and reduce airflow with resultant gas trapping and poor ventilation. Asthma is extremely common. It can be a cause of premature death and reduced quality of life if undertreated. Poor engagement with healthcare and prescribed medication regimens are important factors in asthma-related deaths. There was a substantial increase in reported prevalence in the latter part of the twentieth century [3]. There are current concerns about both over- and under-diagnosis of the condition at a general population level [4–6].

CAUSES IN THE GENERAL POPULATION AND PEOPLE WITH SERIOUS MENTAL ILLNESS

The exact cause of asthma is still the subject of research, but both genetic and environmental factors are implicated. A significant proportion, but not all, asthma is attributed to atopy, an abnormal immune-mediated response to an irritant. There is a strong relationship with family history of atopy and development of asthma. Atopy and asthma can occur jointly or dependently in patients. Environmental factors implicated in the development of asthma include exposure to tobacco smoke, air pollution, and allergens. The relationship between obesity, diet and asthma has also been the subject of much research [7].

Exposure to environmental triggers of asthma may be more significant in individuals living with serious mental illness (SMI). High rates of smoking and exposure to passive

The Maudsley Practice Guidelines for Physical Health Conditions in Psychiatry, First Edition. David M. Taylor, Fiona Gaughran, and Toby Pillinger.
© 2021 John Wiley & Sons Ltd. Published 2021 by John Wiley & Sons Ltd.

smoking in family or in peer groups elevates this risk. Lack of access to and engagement with physical healthcare increases the risk of late presentations with poorly managed asthma and subsequent fixed airflow obstruction akin to that seen in chronic obstructive pulmonary disease (COPD; see Chapter 47). Asthma cross-over spectrums are relatedly highly plausible in individuals living with SMI due to concurrent risks of poorly controlled asthma and earlier onset of COPD related to smoking history, which is characterised by longer and heavier consumption than in the general population [8]. Individuals with SMI may aggregate multiple risk factors, such as smoking histories, childhood exposure to tobacco smoke, social deprivation, and poor living environments. In addition to cumulative risk factors, they may also have several comorbidities that can increase the risk of poorly controlled disease and associated disability. Higher prevalence of obesity, sleep apnoea, and substance misuse can worsen respiratory function and relatedly asthma control [9]. The importance of good disease management and medication concordance cannot be overstated in this population due to the association of poor engagement with care and asthma-related deaths.

There is an evolving evidence base regarding a potential immune relationship between SMI and asthma [10]. Asthma has been found to be associated with an increased risk of schizophrenia although causation has not been proven [11–13]. The mechanism between this possible increased risk has not been elucidated but tentative hypotheses relate to complex interactions between the immune system and the brain [14]. Several epidemiological studies have reported an increased risk for schizophrenia among those with autoimmune disorders and infections, suggesting a possible convergent neurobiological substrate between the conditions [15]. Recently, evidence of increased risk of bipolar disorder in children of individuals with asthma has been identified [16].

DIAGNOSTIC PRINCIPLES

Asthma is a clinical syndrome and its diagnosis is based on medical history, physical examination, measurement of airflow obstruction using spirometry with reversibility testing, and exclusion of alternative diagnoses that mimic asthma.

History

History of presenting complaint

Symptoms are a consequence of airway inflammation and bronchospasm, and include wheeze, cough, or breathlessness. Daily or seasonal variation of symptoms is characteristic with a classic worsening at night. There may be a personal or family history of atopic disorders. Exacerbation triggers include common allergens (e.g. house dust), cold weather, and tobacco smoke. Cleanliness of the home environment is important, and negative symptoms of schizophrenia and social deprivation both increase risk of self-neglect and the risk of worse asthma control in those with SMI. Risk of environmental triggers such as house dust, mould, and animal dander should be assessed.

Questions regarding age of mattress, damp in the home, and how often the home is cleaned should be asked. If employed, any variation in symptoms when not at work should be explored, which may point to occupational asthma. It is important to establish the presence of associated symptoms that may point to alternative diagnoses. Progressive worsening of symptoms or lack of variability could suggest asthma cross-over syndrome or COPD. There is a recognised relationship between gastro-oesophageal reflux disease (GORD) and asthma, including GORD presenting with asthma-like symptoms [17]. A careful history of reflux symptoms is important, especially if cough dominates (see Chapter 19). Additional symptoms such as persistent rhinitis or rash may suggest related eosinophilic disorders.

Past medical history

Childhood respiratory or cardiac conditions and episodes of winter bronchitis should be noted. If there is a history of respiratory conditions, record age of onset, frequency of symptoms, and any associated hospitalisations. A history of intensive care admission is a feature of importance as it usually indicates poor disease control and a higher risk of more severe attacks. A history of other risk factors such as tuberculosis exposure and human immunodeficiency virus (HIV) infection should be recorded (see Chapters 44 and 45) as should compliance with annual flu (see Chapter 40) and pneumococcal vaccinations.

Medication history

In patients with atopy, there may be a history of medication allergies. Specific enquiry should be made about use of beta-blockers or non-steroidal anti-inflammatory drugs (NSAIDs) as these can trigger bronchoconstriction. Individuals with SMI may have anxiety disorders or side effects from antipsychotics (tachycardia or akathisia), all of which can be treated with beta-blockers and alternatives should be sought if an asthma diagnosis is suspected. Caution should be exercised when prescribing melatonin, which has been associated with asthma exacerbations [18]. Some treatments for asthma, such as oral aminophylline, may prolong the cardiac QT interval and therefore must be prescribed with caution in those taking other QT-prolonging drugs such as antidepressants and antipsychotics (see Chapter 3).

Family history

History of atopy, asthma, and cardiac and respiratory conditions should be noted.

Social history

Smoking history should be comprehensive, establishing duration, quantity, knowledge of smoking risks, and motivation to change (see Chapter 46). Furthermore, alcohol intake should be quantified (assessing for features of dependence; see Chapter 24), and type of prescribed and illicit substances used and method of ingestion.

CHAPTER 48

Examination

Examination may be normal. Attention should be paid to physical health, including weight, nutritional status, chest wall abnormalities, stigmata of smoking, and signs of respiratory distress. Respiratory examination may identify an expiratory polyphonic wheeze. Cardiac and respiratory examination should explore other comorbid cardiac or respiratory conditions which could affect prognosis. A peak flow test should be considered a mandatory part of the examination of a patient with asthma and this should be compared to the predicted value for their age and height. Reduced peak flows are a good predictor of poor asthma control.

Investigations

There is variation in the UK's main clinical guidelines for diagnosis and management of asthma but recommendations should be brought in line in coming years [19]. No one symptom, sign, or test is diagnostic, and the predictive value of diagnostic tests is influenced by the context, the reference test used, and the thresholds applied. Tests include fractional exhaled nitric oxide, obstructive pattern on spirometry, bronchodilator reversibility test, peak flow variability, and direct bronchial challenge test with histamine or methacholine. The current National Institute for Health and Care Excellence (NICE) guideline suggests an algorithmic approach and the establishment of asthma diagnostic hubs to improve accuracy of diagnoses. It is recommended that in the absence of unequivocal evidence of asthma, a diagnosis should be suspected and initiation of treatment be monitored carefully and the diagnosis reviewed if there is no objective benefit [20].

When to refer

Referral to a medical subspecialty may vary by local provision and availability of investigations. Indications for referral include inconclusive first-line investigations, diagnostic uncertainty, the presence of other physical comorbidities, uncontrolled symptoms, or severity of exacerbations. Information communicated in the referral letter should include the following.

- Brief summary of symptoms and reason for referral, e.g. to address diagnostic uncertainty, for specialist input in the context of other comorbid conditions, or uncontrolled symptoms.
- Mental health diagnosis and a brief summary of what that diagnosis means for that individual, current level of symptomology, and impact on daily functioning from symptoms.
- Any psychosocial issues that may impact on asthma control and treatment choice, e.g. concurrent substance use, social deprivation, or isolation.
- Summary of the potential impact of the mental health condition on the patient's ability to access and engage with investigations and follow-up, and to comply with recommended management.

CHAPTER 48

- Contact details of the patient's care team (e.g. care coordinator, keyworker, family member, friend, or carer) and whether the appointment information should be sent to anyone in addition to the patient.
- Any reasonable adjustments needed for the patient when seen in specialty care, e.g. time or duration of appointment, carer/support worker in attendance.

MANAGEMENT

Asthma can be a life-threatening condition and poorly controlled asthma has a high mortality rate. NICE guidance recommends risk stratification to identify people who are at increased risk of poor outcomes. Individuals with SMI have greater risk factors for psychosocial problems and difficulties accessing and engaging with medical care and should be considered an at-risk cohort. They should be offered tailored support to help them understand and manage their condition. The patient's psychiatrist may not be the primary prescriber for asthma treatment but involvement in the care plan and awareness of prescribed treatments is essential. The mental health team can be an important ongoing source of support to the patient in respect of disease self-management, education, and concordance with prescribed treatment.

Non-pharmacological treatment

Pharmacological treatments are necessary for good asthma control, but a range of non-pharmacological approaches can improve their efficacy. These include identifying and removing triggers and supporting disease self-management and concordance with prescribed medication regimens. Smoking cessation should be a priority. Environmental triggers should be carefully addressed. If home visits are not feasible for medical services, support and collateral information from mental health teams may be instructive. Care plans should include any steps needed to support the patient to maintain a clean dust-free home including, as required, purchase of new mattress.

Support for self-management is essential and education should focus on ensuring the patient understands the risks and triggers for symptoms, what to do when they start, and when to seek medical help. This is normally provided as a written asthma self-management plan. Carers and key workers should be involved in the education. Adherence with therapy should be regularly and closely reviewed and support given. In the UK, community respiratory nurses and GP practice nurses are often the key people involved in providing this support and review, although community pharmacists also help in checking inhaler technique and providing education. A multidisciplinary team-based approach involving all providers is essential.

Uncontrolled asthma is characterised by three or more days a week with symptoms, three or more days a week requiring reliever therapy, and one or more nights awakening due to asthma symptoms [20]. Inhaler technique should be assessed at each review and if asthma is uncontrolled, review of triggers, home environment, change in smoking habits, and adherence to medication regimen should be carefully reviewed before

CHAPTER 48

medication adjustments are made. All patients taking inhaled corticosteroids should have regular oral health reviews and be aware of increased risk of pneumonia. Pneumococcal and influenza vaccinations should be offered.

Pharmacological treatment

Pharmacological treatment is stepped and involves combinations of maintenance and reliever (i.e. ad hoc) therapies. Inhaled corticosteroids are used as maintenance therapy and the lowest dose effective for control should be prescribed. Treatment should be regularly reviewed to ensure the lowest effective doses are being used (see Table 48.1 for a stepped approach).

There is a high incidence of affective comorbidity in those living with SMI and the use of reliever therapy can present as anxiety symptoms since they are usually β-receptor agonists. Anxiety-like symptoms can also be observed in response to several drugs and substances that may be used by individuals with SMI, including sympathomimetics, selective serotonin reuptake inhibitors and antipsychotics (akathisia), and caffeine and energy drinks. Combined, these can worsen anxiety symptoms and careful review may be required to unpick and address these issues.

Table 48.1 Stepped pharmacological treatment of asthma [20].

Presentation	Treatment
Infrequent, short-lived wheeze and normal lung function	Consider short-acting β-agonist (SABA) alone
Symptoms indicating need for maintenance therapy, e.g. asthma-related symptoms three or more times a week, or causing waking at night Asthma that is uncontrolled with a SABA alone	Inhaled corticosteroid (ICS) maintenance therapy
Asthma uncontrolled on low-dose ICS	Offer a leukotriene receptor antagonist (LTRA) in addition to ICS. Review response in 4–8 weeks
Asthma uncontrolled on low-dose ICS and an LRTA	Offer a long-acting β-agonist (LABA) in combination with the ICS, and review ongoing role of LTRA according to response
Asthma uncontrolled on low-dose ICS, LTRA and LABA	Consider switch to maintenance and reliever therapy (MART). This is a form of combined ICS and LABA treatment in a single inhaler, containing both ICS and a fast-acting LABA. It is used for both daily maintenance therapy and the relief of symptoms as required
Asthma uncontrolled on a MART regimen with a low maintenance ICS dose	Consider increasing the ICS to a moderate maintenance dose, either continuing on a MART regimen or changing to a fixed-dose of ICS and a LABA, with a SABA as reliever therapy
Asthma uncontrolled on a moderate maintenance ICS dose with a LABA (either as MART or fixed-dose regimen), with or without an LTRA	Consider increasing ICS to a high maintenance dose or a trial of an additional drug (e.g. a long-acting muscarinic receptor antagonist or theophylline) or refer to specialist

CHAPTER 48

Management of acute asthma

Patients with severe asthma and one or more adverse psychosocial factors are at risk of death and should be managed as a medical emergency. The reader is also directed to Chapter 68 on shortness of breath. Determining the severity of asthma can be challenging as people with severe or even life-threatening exacerbations sometimes do not appear to be distressed. Features of acute and life-threatening asthma are outlined in Table 48.2 and should prompt urgent intervention and transfer to a hospital/medical setting for further assessment and management. In the community, assessment of clinical features should include evidence of severe breathlessness (including too breathless to complete sentences in one breath), tachypnoea, tachycardia, silent chest, cyanosis, or collapse. None of these features singly or together is specific and their absence does not exclude a severe attack. Peak flow expressed as a percentage of the patient's previous best value is most useful clinically but in the absence of this, peak expiratory flow (PEF) as a percentage of predicted is a rough guide.

All patients with severe exacerbations should be admitted to hospital but the threshold for admission in patients with SMI and moderate exacerbations may be lower. Factors warranting a lower threshold for admission are outlined in Box 48.1.

Supportive treatment whilst awaiting transfer to hospital includes the following.

1 Controlled supplementary oxygen to all people with hypoxia using a face mask, Venturi mask, or nasal cannulae. Adjust flow rates as necessary to maintain an oxygen saturation of 94–98% but do not delay oxygen administration in the absence of pulse oximetry.
2 Treatment with a short-acting β_2-agonist. A nebuliser should be used, but if not available or if the attack is of moderate severity, use a pressurised metered-dose inhaler with a large-volume spacer (can give four puffs 'back to back' with a further two puffs given every two minutes up to a maximum of 10 puffs).

Table 48.2 Features of acute and life-threatening asthma.

Moderate acute asthma	Acute severe asthma	Life-threatening asthma

Increasing symptoms
PEF >50–75% best or predicted
No features of acute severe asthma
	Any one of:
	  PEF 33–50% best or predicted
	  Respiratory rate ≥25/min
	  Heart rate ≥110 bpm
	  Inability to complete sentences in
	  one breath
		In a patient with severe asthma any one of:
		  PEF <33% best or predicted
		  Spo_2 <92%
		  Pao_2 <8 kPa
		  Normal $Paco_2$ (4.6–6.0 kPa)
		  Silent chest
		  Cyanosis
		  Poor respiratory effort
		  Arrhythmia
		  Exhaustion
		  Altered consciousness

PEF, peak expiratory flow.

Box 48.1 Factors warranting lower threshold for admission with moderate acute asthma

- Age under 18 years
- Poor treatment adherence
- Living alone/social isolation
- Psychological problems such as depression, and alcohol or drug misuse
- Physical or learning disability
- Previous severe asthma attack
- Exacerbation despite an adequate dose of oral corticosteroids before presentation
- Presentation in the afternoon or at night
- Recent nocturnal symptoms
- Recent hospital admission
- Pregnancy

References

1. World Health Organization. Asthma: definition. https://www.who.int/respiratory/asthma/definition/en/ (accessed 24 July 2019).
2. Murdoch JR, Lloyd CM. Chronic inflammation and asthma. *Mutat Res* 2010;690(1–2):24–39.
3. Eder W, Ege MJ, von Mutius E. The asthma epidemic. *N Engl J Med* 2006;355(21):2226–2235.
4. Aaron SD, Vandemheen KL, FitzGerald JM, et al. Reevaluation of diagnosis in adults with physician-diagnosed asthma. *JAMA* 2017;317(3):269–279.
5. Jose BP, Camargos PA, Cruz Filho AA, Correa R de A. Diagnostic accuracy of respiratory diseases in primary health units. *Rev Assoc Med Bras* 2014;60(6):599–612.
6. Looijmans-van den Akker I, van Luijn K, Verheij T. Overdiagnosis of asthma in children in primary care: a retrospective analysis. *Br J Gen Pract* 2016;66(644):e152–157.
7. Han YY, Forno E, Holguin F, Celedon JC. Diet and asthma: an update. *Curr Opin Allergy Clin Immunol* 2015;15(4):369–374.
8. Peckham E, Brabyn S, Cook L, et al. Smoking cessation in severe mental ill health: what works? An updated systematic review and meta-analysis. *BMC Psychiatry.* 2017;17(1):252.
9. Stubbs B, Vancampfort D, Veronese N, et al. The prevalence and predictors of obstructive sleep apnea in major depressive disorder, bipolar disorder and schizophrenia: a systematic review and meta-analysis. *J Affect Disord* 2016;197:259–267.
10. Pedersen MS, Benros ME, Agerbo E, et al. Schizophrenia in patients with atopic disorders with particular emphasis on asthma: a Danish population-based study. *Schizophr Res* 2012;138(1):58–62.
11. Chen SJ, Chao YL, Chen CY, et al. Prevalence of autoimmune diseases in in-patients with schizophrenia: nationwide population-based study. *Br J Psychiatry* 2012;200(5):374–380.
12. Eaton WW, Byrne M, Ewald H, et al. Association of schizophrenia and autoimmune diseases: linkage of Danish national registers. *Am J Psychiatry* 2006;163(3):521–528.
13. Wang W-C, Lu M-L, Chen VC-H, et al. Asthma, corticosteroid use and schizophrenia: a nationwide population-based study in Taiwan. *PLoS One* 2017;12(3):e0173063.
14. Pino O, Guilera G, Gomez-Benito J, et al. Neurodevelopment or neurodegeneration: review of theories of schizophrenia. *Actas Esp Psiquiatr* 2014;42(4):185–195.
15. Khandaker GM, Cousins L, Deakin J, et al. Inflammation and immunity in schizophrenia: implications for pathophysiology and treatment. *Lancet Psychiatry* 2015;2(3):258–270.
16. Wu Q, Dalman C, Karlsson H, et al. Childhood and parental asthma, future risk of bipolar disorder and schizophrenia spectrum disorders: a population-based cohort study. *Schizophr Bull* 2019;45(2):360–368.
17. Pacheco-Galvan A, Hart SP, Morice AH. Relationship between gastro-oesophageal reflux and airway diseases: the airway reflux paradigm. *Arch Bronconeumol* 2011;47(4):195–203.
18. Marseglia L, D'Angelo G, Manti S, et al. Melatonin and atopy: role in atopic dermatitis and asthma. *Int J Mol Sci* 2014;15(8):13482–13493.
19. Keeley D. Conflicting asthma guidelines cause confusion in primary care. *BMJ* 2018;360:k29.
20. National Institute for Health and Care Excellence. *Asthma: Diagnosis, Monitoring and Chronic Asthma Management.* NICE Guideline NG80. London: NICE, 2017. Available at https://www.nice.org.uk/guidance/ng80

CHAPTER 48

Obstructive Sleep Apnoea

Nicholas Meyer, Hugh Selsick, Kai Lee

Obstructive sleep apnoea (OSA) is the most common form of sleep-disordered breathing, affecting 1–4% of the general population [1], with higher prevalence in men and with increasing age. The condition is particularly over-represented in groups with severe mental illness (SMI); for example, prevalence estimates for OSA range from 14 to 58% in schizophrenia [2] and conversely 5–63% of patients with OSA exhibit depression [3]. When considered together with reports that treating OSA improves psychiatric symptoms, this suggests that SMI is a risk factor for OSA, and that OSA may also precipitate or exacerbate psychiatric disorder.

OSA is characterised by partial or complete collapse of the upper airway during sleep, resulting in restriction or cessation of airflow and repeated fall in oxygen saturations. The most important risk factors for OSA are obesity and retrognathia (a small or posteriorly positioned lower jaw). Airway obstruction is usually more severe during REM sleep, when pharyngeal muscles are relaxed, and when lying in the supine position. Causes and exacerbating factors are outlined in Table 49.1.

Common symptoms of OSA are loud snoring, choking or gasping during sleep, restless and unrefreshing sleep, and excessive daytime sleepiness (EDS) resulting from the repeated arousals that accompany desaturation and the consequent resumption of breathing. However, up to half of individuals with OSA do not report significant snoring or EDS [4], and the disorder is likely to be under-recognised. Therefore, OSA must be considered as a differential diagnosis in patients presenting with a range of neuropsychiatric disturbances with which it is associated, including cognitive impairments (deficits in vigilance, sustained attention, memory and executive function), depression (estimated to affect 21–41% of individuals with OSA) [5], anxiety, mood instability, irritability, and insomnia. Collectively, these can lead to significant social and occupational dysfunction, diminished quality of life, and increased risk of accidents (over 20%

The Maudsley Practice Guidelines for Physical Health Conditions in Psychiatry, First Edition.
David M. Taylor, Fiona Gaughran, and Toby Pillinger.
© 2021 John Wiley & Sons Ltd. Published 2021 by John Wiley & Sons Ltd.

Table 49.1 Common causes and exacerbating factors for OSA in the general and psychiatric patient population.

Cause	General population	Individuals with serious mental illness (SMI)
Obesity	Deposition of fatty tissue around neck causing airway compression	Higher rates of obesity in SMI, particularly schizophrenia
Anatomical	Retrognathia and micrognathia	As in the general population
	Enlarged tonsils and adenoids (more common in children)	
	Chronic nasal obstruction	
	Features of acromegaly	
Medical	Hypothyroidism	As in the general population
	Neurological disease including degenerative conditions, myopathy and bulbar palsies	
Medication	Opiates	Antipsychotics can cause sedation and weight gain
	Sedative medications may exacerbate OSA, at higher doses	More frequent use of hypnotic medications
Exacerbating factors	Alcohol consumption	Higher rates of smoking and alcohol use in several psychiatric disorders
	Smoking	

of motor vehicle accidents are due to sleepiness) [6]. OSA is also an independent risk factor for hypertension, stroke, diabetes, and cardiac disease.

DIAGNOSTIC PRINCIPLES

History

1 A thorough sleep history should be elicited (see Chapter 55), preferably together with the patient's bed partner. Nursing observations may be helpful in a hospital setting.
2 Enquire about specific symptoms relating to sleep-disordered breathing.
   a The core symptom of EDS and its consequences on functioning and quality of life should be explored. Concerns about safety, including drowsiness and accidents while driving, must be discussed. Other causes of EDS should be considered, particularly insufficient sleep due to poor sleep habits; social or work pressures; primary depression and anxiety; sleep-related movement disorder including restless legs syndrome/periodic limb movement disorder; and narcolepsy.
   b Snoring interspersed with apnoeas.
   c Restlessness during sleep, characterised by frequent tossing and turning.
   d Nocturnal choking or gasping.
   e Patients may report associated features, including morning headache, nocturia, and the neuropsychiatric manifestations already described.

3 Past medical history:
   a Elicit risk factors associated with OSA, including obesity, endocrine disorders, cardiac and cerebrovascular disease, craniofacial abnormalities, and previous ENT problems.
   b Identify associated conditions, including cardiovascular and cerebrovascular disease, hypertension, pulmonary hypertension, diabetes mellitus, and obesity.
4 Medication history, including antipsychotics, hypnotic agents, and opioids.
5 Occupational history is important, particularly if the patient is sleepy. Vocational drivers should be referred urgently for assessment and treatment.
6 Alcohol and smoking history.
7 Screening tools:
   a The Epworth sleepiness scale [7] is useful for quantifying sleepiness and confirming the core symptom of EDS.
   b A score of 3 or more on the STOP-Bang questionnaire [8] has high positive predictive value in screening for moderate to severe OSA.

Physical examination

1 Measure blood pressure (about 50% of patients with OSA have coexisting hypertension).
2 Body weight and body mass index (BMI).
3 Measurement of neck circumference: a collar size of of 43 cm (17 inches) or more is associated with an increased risk of OSA.
4 Examine oropharynx for tonsillar enlargement, high tongue base, and narrow pharyngeal diameter.
5 Assess for overbite and crowding of dentition of lower jaw, suggestive of retrognathia.
6 Cardiovascular, respiratory, and neurological examination to identify previously undiagnosed associated diseases.

Investigations

The key investigation is a diagnostic sleep study, which is undertaken by a specialist sleep service.

1 Overnight home oximetry recording is sufficient to make the diagnosis in most cases.
2 A more detailed respiratory study may be necessary, where airflow, oximetry, snoring, and markers of arousal are obtained. A full polysomnography study is not usually indicated, unless another sleep disorder is suspected.

MANAGEMENT

The decision to treat is made by a sleep specialist in collaboration with the patient, where the objective findings from the sleep study are interpreted in the context of the severity of subjective symptoms, presence of associated conditions, and patient motivation and preferences.

1 Weight loss should be encouraged in those with a BMI above 25 kg/m², and advice given to avoid alcohol and sedative medications. Consideration should be given to switching or minimising the dose of psychotropic medications that cause sedation or weight gain.

2 Continuous positive airway pressure (CPAP) ventilation is the gold-standard treatment for individuals with moderate to severe OSA, or mild OSA with severe symptoms and comorbidities. CPAP splints the upper airway by delivering positive pressure via a facial or nasal mask, and has shown efficacy in improving objective sleep indices, symptomatic outcomes, and quality of life [9]. However, other than improvements in blood pressure [10], its effect on depression, cognition, and many cardiovascular outcomes remains unclear. Adequate compliance is considered to be at least four hours' use a night for at least 70% of nights. However, only approximately half of patients will continue CPAP long term, with claustrophobia, dry mouth, and nasal congestion being commonly reported.

3 Mandibular advancement devices are worn during sleep, and prevent apnoeas by pulling the tongue base forward. They are indicated in patients with mild to moderate OSA and those intolerant to CPAP, and are more likely to be successful in the presence of retrognathia. Although CPAP is a more effective treatment for OSA, mandibular devices are better tolerated and so become a more viable treatment option when CPAP compliance is low. Discomfort, hypersalivation, and dry mouth are the most commonly reported adverse effects but are usually short term [11].

4 Nasal, palatal or bariatric surgery is reserved for specific cases.

5 Any patient with EDS that may affect driving ability must be advised to stop driving until symptoms have improved. In the UK, those with confirmed moderate or severe OSA should notify the Driver and Vehicle Licensing Agency (DVLA) immediately, including those with mild OSA if symptom control cannot be achieved in three months [12].

When to refer to a specialist

OSA is associated with a range of psychiatric symptoms, particularly cognitive and affective complaints, and may play a causal role in their development. Psychiatric practitioners should therefore maintain an awareness for OSA, and screen for the disorder with a focused history and clinical examination. Patients with symptoms and associated diagnoses suggestive of OSA should be referred to a sleep or respiratory service for further assessment.

References

1. Stradling JR, Davies RJ. Sleep. 1: Obstructive sleep apnoea/hypopnoea syndrome: definitions, epidemiology, and natural history. *Thorax* 2004;59(1):73–78.

2. Myles H, Myles N, Antic NA, et al. Obstructive sleep apnea and schizophrenia: a systematic review to inform clinical practice. *Schizophr Res* 2016;170(1):222–225.

3. Ejaz SM, Khawaja IS, Bhatia S, Hurwitz TD. Obstructive sleep apnea and depression: a review. *Innov Clin Neurosci* 2011;8(8):17–25.

4. Pavlova MK, Duffy JF, Shea SA. Polysomnographic respiratory abnormalities in asymptomatic individuals. *Sleep* 2008;31(2):241–248.

5. Harris M, Glozier N, Ratnavadivel R, Grunstein RR. Obstructive sleep apnea and depression. *Sleep Med Rev* 2009;13(6):437–444.

6. Tregear S, Reston J, Schoelles K, Phillips B. Obstructive sleep apnea and risk of motor vehicle crash: systematic review and meta-analysis. *J Clin Sleep Med* 2009;5(6):573–581.

7. Johns MW. A new method for measuring daytime sleepiness: the Epworth sleepiness scale. *Sleep* 1991;14(6):540–545.

8. Boynton G, Vahabzadeh A, Hammoud S, et al. Validation of the STOP-BANG questionnaire among patients referred for suspected obstructive sleep apnea. *J Sleep Disord Treat Care* 2013;2(4). doi: 10.4172/2325-9639.1000121

9. Kuhn E, Schwarz EI, Bratton DJ, et al. Effects of CPAP and mandibular advancement devices on health-related quality of life in OSA: a systematic review and meta-analysis. *Chest* 2017;151(4):786–794.

10. Jonas DE, Amick HR, Feltner C, et al. Screening for obstructive sleep apnea in adults: evidence report and systematic review for the US Preventive Services Task Force. *JAMA* 2017;317(4):415–433.

11. Hoffstein V. Review of oral appliances for treatment of sleep-disordered breathing. *Sleep Breath* 2007;11(1):1–22.

12. Driver and Vehicle Licensing Agency. Assessing fitness to drive: a guide for medical professionals. https://www.gov.uk/government/publications/assessing-fitness-to-drive-a-guide-for-medical-professionals

Part 9

Neurology

Delirium

Luke Jelen, Sean Cross

Delirium (otherwise described as an acute confusional state) is a common clinical syndrome that is characterised by acute onset of cognitive impairment and disturbed consciousness with a fluctuating course, often accompanied by behavioural disturbances. It is a medical emergency associated with significant mortality, especially if not recognised and managed early [1,2].

Delirium is seen in a high proportion of hospital inpatients, with an estimated prevalence of 18–35% on general medical wards and seen in 11–51% of surgical patients postoperatively [3]. There are a number of risk factors associated with delirium and although a single factor may lead to delirium, it is frequently multifactorial, especially in the elderly population. Common risk factors and precipitating factors for delirium in the general population and specific considerations in individuals with serious mental illness (SMI) are outlined in Tables 50.1 and 50.2. A number of physical disorders that might contribute to delirium are more prevalent in individuals with SMI [4], and particular attention should be paid to a psychoactive medication review, as well as a drug and alcohol history.

DIAGNOSTIC PRINCIPLES (SEE BOX 50.1)

History

1 Delirium often has a sudden onset (within hours or days) with a fluctuating course thereafter. Those at risk should be assessed for clinical features that may include the following.
   a Inattention: impaired ability to direct, sustain and shift.
   b Altered cognitive function: global impairment with disorientation, memory, and language impairments.

The Maudsley Practice Guidelines for Physical Health Conditions in Psychiatry, First Edition.
David M. Taylor, Fiona Gaughran, and Toby Pillinger.
© 2021 John Wiley & Sons Ltd. Published 2021 by John Wiley & Sons Ltd.

Table 50.1 Common risk factors for delirium in general and psychiatric patient populations [3–10].

	General risk factors	Considerations in individuals with serious mental illness
Age	65 years or older	
Comorbid conditions	Severe illness Current hip fracture History of transient ischaemia/ stroke Renal or hepatic impairment Thiamine deficiency	Many physical disorders are more prevalent in individuals with SMI: Lifestyle factors (lack of exercise, poor diet, smoking) Psychotropic medication side effects Poorer access to and compliance with physical health treatments
Cognitive status	Dementia Cognitive impairment History of delirium	Depression (both active depressive illness and history of depression are risk factors for delirium)
Drugs	Polypharmacy Alcohol/recreational drug abuse and dependency	Psychoactive medications: Anxiolytics, sedatives and hypnotics Antidepressants Antipsychotics Mood stabilisers Higher rates of alcohol/recreational drug abuse and dependency
Functional impairment	Immobility Lack of activity	Reduced physical activity or immobility: Depressive or negative symptoms Sedating effects of medication
Sensory impairment	Visual impairment Hearing impairment	
Reduced oral intake	Malnutrition Dehydration	Depression Psychosis Eating disorders

   c Clouding of consciousness.

   d Disordered thinking: rambling, incoherent, or illogical flow of speech.

   e Disturbed sleep–wake cycle with nocturnal worsening ('sundowning').

   f Psychomotor agitation or retardation.

   g Emotional lability: changes in mood that may include fear, paranoia, anxiety, depression, irritability, apathy, anger, or euphoria.

   h Altered perceptions (illusions and hallucinations).

   i Delusional thinking.

2 There are three clinical subtypes of delirium that should be considered.

   a Hyperactive: psychomotor agitation, increased arousal, aggression, delusions, and hallucinations.

   b Hypoactive: psychomotor retardation, lethargy, excessive sleeping, quiet and withdrawn.

   c Mixed: a combination of these features with varying presentation over time.

Table 50.2 Common precipitating factors for delirium in general and psychiatric patient populations [1,3,4,6,7,11–13].

	General population	Considerations in individuals with serious mental illness
Environmental	Sleep deprivation Inappropriate noise/lighting Immobility/falls	
Drugs	Alcohol or sedative withdrawal Sedative hypnotics Opioids Anticholinergics Antiparkinsonian drugs Antidepressants Anticonvulsants Corticosteroids Acute recreational drug toxicity or withdrawal	Psychoactive medications: Anxiolytics, sedatives and hypnotics Antidepressants Antipsychotics Mood stabilisers Alcohol/recreational drug abuse and dependency: drug toxicity or withdrawal
Pain	Acute or acute on chronic	
Electrolyte abnormality	Dehydration Renal failure Hyponatraemia/hypernatraemia Hypercalcaemia	Hyponatraemia: Antidepressants (SSRIs, TCAs, MAOs) Antipsychotics Mood stabilisers (carbamazepine, sodium valproate, lithium, lamotrigine) Lithium: Acute or chronic renal failure Hyponatraemia Hypercalcaemia
Infective	Urinary tract infection Pneumonia Wound abscess Cellulitis Gastroenteritis	May be at increased risk for infection in the community: Homelessness/poor housing Poor nutrition and hygiene Illicit drug use: HIV, viral hepatitis Increased prevalence of diabetes mellitus increases vulnerability to infection (and severity of infection) Use of clozapine: risk of infection with neutropenia and agranulocytosis

(continued)

Table 50.2 (Continued)

	General population	Considerations in individuals with serious mental illness
Intracranial	Stroke Head injury, subdural haematoma Seizures Encephalitis Raised intracranial pressure	Higher rates of cerebrovascular disease in individuals with SMI: Lifestyle factors (smoking, diet) Psychotropic medication side effects
Respiratory/ cardiovascular	Respiratory failure (hypoxia, hypercapnia) Cardiac failure Myocardial infarction	Higher rates of respiratory and cardiovascular disease in individuals with SMI: Lifestyle factors (smoking, diet) Psychotropic medication side effects
Metabolic/endocrine	Anaemia Hepatic encephalopathy Thiamine deficiency Hypothyroidism/hyperthyroidism Hypoglycaemia/hyperglycaemia	Lithium can cause both hypothyroidism and more rarely hyperthyroidism
Bladder/bowel	Urinary retention Constipation	Medications with anticholinergic activity: Antipsychotics (especially clozapine) Antidepressants (especially TCAs) Opioids

MAO, monoamine oxidase inhibitor; SSRI, selective serotonin reuptake inhibitor; TCA, tricyclic antidepressant.

> **Box 50.1** Diagnostic summary
>
> **History**
>
> - Define symptoms
> - Acute onset and fluctuating course
> - Inattention
> - Disorganised thinking
> - Altered level of consciousness
> - Current and past medical history to identify risk and precipitating factors
> - Collateral history
> - Medication history
> - Drug and alcohol history
>
> **Examination**
>
> - Observations including level of consciousness
> - Any signs of infection
> - Any source of pain
> - Neurological examination
> - Consider rectal examination if constipated
> - AMTS or MMSE
>
> **Investigations**
>
> - Bloods
> - Infection screen
> - ECG
> - Chest X-ray
> - CT/MRI head
> - Lumbar puncture (if indicated)
> - EEG (if indicated)

3 Delirium screening tool (Confusion Assessment Method) [14]: if features (a) and (b) and either (c) or (d) are observed, a diagnosis of delirium is suggested.

a Acute onset and fluctuating course.

b Inattention.

c Disorganised thinking.

d Altered level of consciousness.

4 Collateral history to establish what is normal for the patient:

a How long have they been confused?

b What is different?

5 Medication history, specifically asking if there has been a recent change in medication.

6 Explore current diagnoses, other presenting complaints, and past medical history, considering risk and precipitating factors of delirium as outlined in Tables 50.1 and 50.2.

Examination

1 Observations: blood pressure, pulse, temperature, respiratory rate, oxygen saturation.
2 Any signs of infection (lung, urine, skin, abdomen, central nervous system).
3 Check for pressure sores and pain.
4 Neurological examination.
5 Rectal examination (if concerns regarding faecal impaction).
6 Perform Abbreviated Mental Test Score (AMTS) or Mini Mental State Examination (MMSE). Score of 7 or less on AMTS or 24 or less on MMSE indicates cognitive impairment requiring further investigation.

Investigations

1 Bloods:
  a Full blood count: evidence of infection, anaemia, or increased mean corpuscular volume (see Chapters 15 and 72).
  b Urea and electrolytes: dehydration, renal failure, or hyponatraemia/hypernatraemia (see Chapters 32, 34, and 73).
  c Liver function: hepatic failure, malnutrition, alcohol abuse (see Chapters 23–25).
  d Thyroid function tests (see Chapter 12).
  e Calcium.
  f B_{12}/folate levels.
  g Glucose: hypoglycaemia or hyperglycaemia (see Chapters 11 and 74).
  h Arterial blood gas: if evidence of respiratory distress, hypoxia, concerns regarding hypercapnia, and to obtain lactate in context of infection (see Chapter 72).
  i Blood cultures (infection screen).
2 Urine dipstick/culture: infection screen (see Chapter 41).
3 ECG: evidence of acute event, e.g. ischaemia or pulmonary embolus (see Chapters 18, 67, and 69).
4 Chest X-ray: evidence of pneumonia (see Chapter 39).
5 CT/MRI head: evidence of ischaemic stroke, intracranial bleed (see Chapter 82), or space-occupying lesion.
6 Lumbar puncture: meningitis or encephalitis (see Chapters 51, 76, and 81).
7 EEG: non-convulsive status epilepticus or encephalitis.

MANAGEMENT

The first principle of delirium management is to rapidly identify and treat any potential underlying causes, remembering these may be multifactorial. Prophylaxis with drugs is not effective [15] and management should instead focus on providing supportive and symptomatic care consistently through to recovery, even when a cause cannot be found. Often patients with delirium lack capacity for certain decisions. If this is the case, in the UK the Mental Capacity Act is utilised and, if necessary, a Deprivation of Liberty Safeguards (DoLS) authorisation should be made.

Environmental and supportive measures

1 Optimize patient's condition paying attention to hydration, hypoxia, nutrition, and pain control.
2 Make environment safe. Consider one-to-one observation of patient: those at risk of falls should always be within arm's length.
3 Orientation techniques:
   a Clear, calm communication from consistent staff member or small group of staff members with gentle and regular reorientation and reassurance.
   b Use of visible clocks, calendars and signs.
   c Regular contact with friends and family. Ensure they receive psychoeducation.
4 Optimise environmental stimulation:
   a Adequate lighting and temperature.
   b Reduce unnecessary noise.
   c Correct any sensory impairment (e.g. glasses and/or hearing aids).
   d Encourage mobilisation under supervision.
5 In distressed and agitated patient:
   a Use of non-confrontational and empathetic de-escalation techniques.
   b Consider security involvement.

Pharmacological management

1 Review need and appropriateness of all prescribed medications, paying attention to psychoactive medications. Any drugs with anticholinergic effects should ideally be withdrawn or switched (Table 50.3). A regularly updated Anticholinergic Effect on Cognition tool can be accessed at www.medichec.com.
2 Consider medications for delirium in those at risk to self/others, in distress, or to permit essential investigations/treatments when de-escalation techniques have not been effective.
3 Treatment principles:
   a Oral route preferable.
   b Aim for a single medication: start at lowest clinically appropriate dose and titrate cautiously according to symptoms.
   c Review all drugs every 24 hours.
   d There is insufficient evidence to recommend any single drug treatment over others [16,17]. As such, treatment choice should be guided by potential interactions with other medications or medical conditions [18].
4 Haloperidol [19,20]: oral 0.5–1 mg up to maximum of 5 mg in 24 hours. If the oral route is not possible, use intramuscular (i.m.) 0.5–1 mg up to maximum of 5 mg in 24 hours.

Table 50.3 Anticholinergic effect on cognition (AEC): medications commonly used in older people with capacity to impair cognitive function to varying degrees.

Medication	AEC score	Medication	AEC score	Medication	AEC score
Alimemazine (trimeprazine)	+++	Diphenhydramine	++	Perphenazine	+
Amantadine	++	Disopyramide	++	Pethidine	++
Amiodarone	+	Domperidone	+	Pimozide	++
Amitriptyline	+++	Dothiepin	+++	Prednisolone	+
Aripiprazole	+	Doxepin	+++	Prochlorperazine	++
Atropine	+++	Fentanyl	+	Procyclidine	+++
Benztropine	+++	Fluphenazine	+	Promethazine	+++
Bromocriptine	+	Hydroxyzine	+	Propantheline	++
Carbamazepine	+	Hyoscine hydrobromide	+++	Quetiapine	++
Chlorphenamine	++	Iloperidone	+	Quinidine	+
Chlorpromazine	+++	Imipramine	+++	Sertindole	+
Citalopram	+	Levomepromazine (methotrimeprazine)	++	Sertraline	+
Clemastine	+++	Lithium	+	Solifenacin	+
Clomipramine	+++	Lofepramine	+++	Temazepam	+
Clozapine	+++	Mirtazapine	+	Tolterodine	++
Cyproheptadine	+++	Nortriptyline	+++	Trifluoperazine	++
Desipramine	++	Olanzapine	++	Trihexyphenidryl (benzhexol)	+++
Diazepam	+	Orphenadrine	+++	Trimipramine	+++
Dicycloverine (dicyclomine)	++	Oxybutynin	+++		
Dimenhydrinate	++	Paroxetine	++		

+++, review and withdraw or switch; ++, review and withdraw or switch; +, caution required.
Source: adapted from Bishara et al. [28].

a ECG should be performed before and after commencing haloperidol to rule out prolonged QTc (see Chapter 3).
b Monitor sedated patients with regular observations.
c Haloperidol administration may cause acute dystonic reaction: treat with procyclidine 5 mg oral/i.m. (see Chapter 84).
d Haloperidol should not be used in patients with Parkinson's disease/parkinsonism, Lewy body dementia, seizures, alcohol or recreational drug withdrawal.
5 Olanzapine [21–23]: oral 2.5–5 mg every two hours up to a maximum of 20 mg in 24 hours (10 mg in elderly).

6 Risperidone [22,24,25]: oral 0.25–0.5 mg initially, given twice a day if needed, with maximum of 4 mg in 24 hours (2 mg in elderly).

7 Quetiapine [26,27]: initially 12.5–25 mg orally once a day, increased to twice a day if needed. Maximum 200 mg in 24 hours (50 mg in elderly). Can be used cautiously in patients with Parkinson's disease or Lewy body dementia.

8 Lorazepam [1,6]: oral/i.m. 0.5–1 mg every two to four hours up to a maximum of 4 mg in 24 hours (2 mg in elderly).

   a Used in alcohol or sedative/hypnotic withdrawal.

   b May cause respiratory depression.

   c Associated with prolongation and worsening of delirium.

When to refer to a specialist

Delirium is a medical emergency and is therefore usually initially managed within a general medical inpatient setting. It is important that the patient has input from the appropriate medical or surgical subspecialties to investigate and treat any underlying causes of delirium. Some hospitals now have specialist delirium and dementia teams that can provide support and advice in the management of delirium. For complex and challenging cases, requiring extensive pharmacological management, seek specialist advice from general or older-adult mental health liaison psychiatry services.

References

1. Fong TG, Tulebaev SR, Inouye SK. Delirium in elderly adults: diagnosis, prevention and treatment. *Nat Rev Neurol* 2009;5(4):210–220.

2. National Institute for Health and Care Excellence. *Delirium: Prevention, Diagnosis and Management.* Clinical Guideline CG103. London: NICE, 2010. Available at https://www.nice.org.uk/guidance/cg103

3. Inouye SK, Westendorp RG, Saczynski JS. Delirium in elderly people. *Lancet* 2014;383(9920):911–922.

4. De Hert M, Correll CU, Bobes J, et al. Physical illness in patients with severe mental disorders. I. Prevalence, impact of medications and disparities in health care. *World Psychiatry* 2011;10(1):52–77.

5. Leung JM, Sands LP, Mullen EA, et al. Are preoperative depressive symptoms associated with postoperative delirium in geriatric surgical patients? *J Gerontol A Biol Sci Med Sci* 2005;60(12):1563–1568.

6. Potter J, George J. The prevention, diagnosis and management of delirium in older people: concise guidelines. *Clin Med (Lond)* 2006;6(3):303–308.

7. Inouye SK. Delirium in older persons. *N Engl J Med* 2006;354(11):1157–1165.

8. De Hert M, Cohen D, Bobes J, et al. Physical illness in patients with severe mental disorders. II. Barriers to care, monitoring and treatment guidelines, plus recommendations at the system and individual level. *World Psychiatry* 2011;10(2):138–151.

9. O'Sullivan R, Inouye SK, Meagher D. Delirium and depression: inter-relationship and clinical overlap in elderly people. *Lancet Psychiatry* 2014;1(4):303–311.

10. John A, McGregor J, Jones I, et al. Premature mortality among people with severe mental illness: new evidence from linked primary care data. *Schizophr Res* 2018;199:154–162.

11. Meulendijks D, Mannesse CK, Jansen PA, et al. Antipsychotic-induced hyponatraemia: a systematic review of the published evidence. *Drug Saf* 2010;33(2):101–114.

12. De Picker L, Van Den Eede F, Dumont G, et al. Antidepressants and the risk of hyponatremia: a class-by-class review of literature. *Psychosomatics* 2014;55(6):536–547.

13. Kibirige D, Luzinda K, Ssekitoleko R. Spectrum of lithium induced thyroid abnormalities: a current perspective. *Thyroid Res* 2013;6(1):3.

14. Inouye SK, van Dyck CH, Alessi CA, et al. Clarifying confusion: the confusion assessment method. A new method for detection of delirium. *Ann Intern Med* 1990;113(12):941–948.

15. van den Boogaard M, Slooter AJC, Bruggemann RJM, et al. Effect of haloperidol on survival among critically ill adults with a high risk of delirium: the REDUCE Randomized Clinical Trial. *JAMA* 2018;319(7):680–690.

16. Neufeld KJ, Yue J, Robinson TN, et al. Antipsychotic medication for prevention and treatment of delirium in hospitalized adults: a systematic review and meta-analysis. *J Am Geriatr Soc* 2016;64(4):705–714.

17. Kishi T, Hirota T, Matsunaga S, Iwata N. Antipsychotic medications for the treatment of delirium: a systematic review and meta-analysis of randomised controlled trials. *J Neurol Neurosurg Psychiatry* 2016;87(7):767–774.

18. Taylor DM, Barnes TRE, Young AH. *The Maudsley Prescribing Guidelines in Psychiatry*, 13th edn. Chichester: Wiley Blackwell, 2018.

19. Lonergan E, Britton AM, Luxenberg J, Wyller T. Antipsychotics for delirium. *Cochrane Database Syst Rev* 2007;(2):CD005594.

20. Schrijver EJM, de Vries OJ, van de Ven PM, et al. Haloperidol versus placebo for delirium prevention in acutely hospitalised older at risk patients: a multi-centre double-blind randomised controlled clinical trial. *Age Ageing* 2018;47(1):48–55.

21. Skrobik YK, Bergeron N, Dumont M, Gottfried SB. Olanzapine vs haloperidol: treating delirium in a critical care setting. *Intensive Care Med* 2004;30(3):444–449.

22. Kim SW, Yoo JA, Lee SY, et al. Risperidone versus olanzapine for the treatment of delirium. *Hum Psychopharmacol* 2010;25(4):298–302.

23. Grover S, Kumar V, Chakrabarti S. Comparative efficacy study of haloperidol, olanzapine and risperidone in delirium. *J Psychosom Res* 2011;71(4):277–281.

24. Han CS, Kim YK. A double-blind trial of risperidone and haloperidol for the treatment of delirium. *Psychosomatics* 2004;45(4):297–301.

25. Gupta N, Sharma P, Mattoo SK. Effectiveness of risperidone in delirium. *Can J Psychiatry* 2005;50(1):75.

26. Devlin JW, Roberts RJ, Fong JJ, et al. Efficacy and safety of quetiapine in critically ill patients with delirium: a prospective, multicenter, randomized, double-blind, placebo-controlled pilot study. *Crit Care Med* 2010;38(2):419–427.

27. Hawkins SB, Bucklin M, Muzyk AJ. Quetiapine for the treatment of delirium. *J Hosp Med* 2013;8(4):215–220.

28. Bishara D, Harwood D, Sauer J, Taylor DM. Anticholinergic effect on cognition (AEC) of drugs commonly used in older people. *Int J Geriatr Psychiatry* 2017;32(6):650–656.

Autoimmune Encephalitis

Adam Al-Diwani, Julia Thompson, Sarosh Irani

Encephalitis is inflammation of the brain caused by infectious or autoimmune mechanisms. For an overview of infectious causes, the reader is directed to Chapter 81 on encephalitis and meningitis. This chapter instead focuses on the clinical approach to autoimmune encephalitis.

It used to be thought that encephalitis was largely caused by infection, with other idiopathic cases due to as yet unidentified pathogens. However, over the past 15 years, it has become apparent that autoimmune encephalitis (AE) accounts for a large portion of previously 'idiopathic' cases [1]. Indeed, multiple contemporary estimates have suggested that the incidence of AE may be at least as frequent as that of viral encephalitis (0.8 vs. 1.0 per 100,000 person-years) [2], and these data do not account for the rapidly expanding number of autoimmune syndromes being described annually.

AE is often associated with dramatic mental state changes, so many people with AE are first seen as psychiatric referrals [3]. People may initially receive a primary psychiatric diagnosis on acute presentation, only for the clinical picture to evolve or for autoantibody testing to indicate that AE is the underlying cause. Prompt identification of AE is important because of the need for immunotherapy, which has a time-dependent link with better outcomes [4–7].

AUTOIMMUNE DISEASE MECHANISMS

Immune-mediated encephalitis can be mediated by either cytotoxic T cells or pathogenic antibodies. The former is responsible for classical paraneoplastic limbic encephalitis, clinically characterised by subacute onset of confusion, amnesia, seizure, and psychiatric disturbances. It is associated with specific malignancies and onconeural antibodies against intracellular targets such as Hu, Ma2, CV2, and amphiphysin [4].

The Maudsley Practice Guidelines for Physical Health Conditions in Psychiatry, First Edition.
David M. Taylor, Fiona Gaughran, and Toby Pillinger.

These antibodies are reliable biomarkers of a paraneoplastic form of encephalitis, but are not directly pathogenic. This syndrome is rarely responsive to tumour treatment or immunotherapy, and generally has a poor prognosis [5].

In contrast, autoantibodies against the extracellular domains of neuronal surface proteins are a far more common cause of encephalitis, namely autoantibody-mediated encephalitis. Here, autoantibodies bind to and modulate specific targets on neurons that lead to symptoms consistent with the specific neuronal systems affected. Consequently, treatments that suppress the adaptive immune system often result in favourable clinical outcomes [6].

Since the early 2000s, multiple neuronal autoantibody targets have been described. It is now recognised that the most common autoantibody-mediated encephalitides are N-methyl-D-aspartate receptor (NMDAR) antibody encephalitis and leucine-rich glioma inactivated 1 (LGI1) antibody encephalitis. NMDARs are glutamate-gated ion channels with important roles in synaptic plasticity, learning, and memory. LGI1 is a trans-synaptic secreted protein that may operate through roles that include the modulation of presynaptic voltage-gated potassium channels (VGKCs) and/or postsynaptic excitatory α-amino-3-hydroxy-5-methyl-4-isoxazolepropionic acid (AMPA) receptors. NMDAR antibody encephalitis can occur throughout the lifespan but most cases occur in young adult women [7]. About 30% of such females have an underlying ovarian teratoma [7] while approximately 5% of cases follow herpes simplex virus encephalitis [8]. Conversely, LGI1 antibody encephalitis occurs almost exclusively in older adults, with a median age of onset around 65 years, who are predominantly male. These patients do not have a strong tumour association, but instead a very strong HLA association, with more than 90% of patients showing HLA-DRB1*07:01 [9,10].

CLINICAL APPROACH

Clinical identification of AE can be challenging because classic features of encephalitis such as fever and seizures may be absent. Furthermore, in contrast to infectious encephalitis, cerebrospinal fluid (CSF) analysis may show minimal pleocytosis, and brain imaging can be normal. Nonetheless, there tends to an acute/subacute cluster of behavioural disturbance, seizures, movement disorders, and cognitive dysfunction. Also, there is often electroencephalographic (EEG) evidence of an encephalopathy.

Diagnostic suspicion is aided by characteristic demographic associations, such as young adult women in NMDAR antibody encephalitis and older adult men in LGI1 antibody encephalitis (see Table 51.1). This informs the psychiatric differential diagnosis: NMDAR antibody encephalitis is typically misdiagnosed as acute psychosis, mania, or drug intoxication [11], while LGI1 antibody encephalitis should be excluded in rapidly progressive dementia syndromes.

Ideally, an approach grounded in clinical probability with paired serum and CSF testing is advised. The varying rates of negative and positive autoantibody results in either sample type across the different autoantibody-mediated conditions mean that, where possible, both should be sent for all patients in whom the diagnosis is suspected clinically. To expedite consideration of empirical immunotherapy whilst tests results are

Table 51.1 Main clinical and paraclinical abnormalities in NMDAR and LGI1 antibody encephalitis.

	NMDAR antibody encephalitis	LGI1 antibody encephalitis
Demographic	Throughout lifespan, but most commonly women of reproductive age Strongly consider if new-onset severe mental illness during pregnancy or postpartum. Phenomenology can be identical to postpartum psychosis [22]	Largely older adult men: age and sex highly unusual for autoimmune disease Modal onset 64 years (range 22–92 years) [9]
Prodrome	Flu-like symptoms (headache, malaise, mild fever, gastrointestinal) Also, consider symptoms of ovarian teratoma, e.g. abdominal discomfort/distension, abnormal menstrual cycle	Often faciobrachial dystonic seizures (FBDS): Distinctive seizure semiology early feature Brief ipsilateral hemifacial and arm (or leg) jerks; last a few seconds, multiple per day (sometimes hundreds) Pathognomonic for LGI1 type Rarely responsive to antiepileptic drugs but highly immunotherapy-responsive, which appears to prevent progression to cognitive impairment [9,23] Also, occasionally neuro-cardiac prodrome, e.g. severe bradycardia with cardiac pauses requiring pacing [24]
Time course	Usually abrupt or subacute onset Progresses from prodrome to psychiatric, neurological, and critical illness Can be highly complex often with multiple features occurring at once Psychiatric phase can be delirium-like: disorientation and fluctuation	Subacute onset and progression If not aborted in prodromal phase, then progresses to full limbic encephalopathy

(continued)

Table 51.1 (Continued)

	NMDAR antibody encephalitis	LGI1 antibody encephalitis
Psychiatric	Often absence of personal or family history of psychiatric disorder yet profoundly unwell Effect on NMDARs yields many similarities to ketamine/phencyclidine intoxication Polymorphic syndrome spanning multiple primary syndromes is typical and likely consistent between patients Multiple domains of psychopathology, with all variants possible: Sleep: insomnia and/or variant Mood: can appear depressed at start, then manic/mixed state Psychosis: often visual as well as auditory hallucinations; multiple delusions possible, e.g. persecutory, nihilistic, grandiose, religious Behaviour: agitated with anger, violence and need for restraint common. Often profoundly disorganised with dissociation Catatonia: staring, mutism, posturing, waxy flexibility; can fluctuate between excitement and stupor 'Formes fruste' possible but rare and largely in relapse [25]. Therefore, ensure good past medical/psychiatric history to screen for previously missed first episode Consider diagnosis if profound deterioration with typical antipsychotics, e.g. haloperidol precipitating movement disorder ± full NMS-like syndrome	'Personality change': incompletely characterised but can include irritability, disinhibition, emotionality and insomnia May approximate hypomania/mania Full range of psychopathology likely incompletely explored but usually less of a 'psychiatric' feel than NMDAR type
Neurological	Speech and language: ranging from incoherence and mutism to frank dysphasias Cognition and memory: usually frontotemporal pattern, i.e. dysexecutive, amnestic, reduced verbal fluency. Parietal syndromes possible, e.g. visuospatial hemi-neglect Movement disorder: can be confused for status epilepticus. Orofacial dyskinesia common. Can be multiple simultaneous phenomenologies but dominant triad of dystonia, stereotypies, and chorea [26,27] Seizures Dysautonomia: drooling, sweating, hyperpyrexia, labile heart rate/blood pressure. Can be extreme, requiring pacemaker and/or inotropic support Central hypoventilation	Seizures in 90% [28–30]: Focal more common than general Temporal lobe Autonomic preceded by sensory aura Generalised ± status epilepticus Memory impairment: Autobiographical Disorientation, frank confusion

CSF	Cell count: ± lymphocytic pleocytosis Protein: ± raised Oligoclonal bands: ± present Normal in ~20%	Cell count: ± lymphocytic pleocytosis Protein: ± raised Oligoclonal bands: ± present Normal in ~75%
EEG	EEG often abnormal (~80%) but pattern not necessarily specific [31]: Focal or diffuse slowing or disorganised activity Epileptiform activity Extreme delta brush (only usually in patients admitted to ICU)	Diffuse slowing ± focal epileptiform
Brain MRI	Often normal (~70%) Abnormalities can be non-specific and affect cortical, subcortical, or cerebellar regions. Usually seen on T2-FLAIR sequence	~50% unilateral/bilateral hyperintensities on T2/T2-FLAIR [9,28] May resolve to leave hippocampal atrophy/mesial temporal sclerosis, particularly if aggressive disease and/or late or undertreated FBDS can associate with basal ganglia changes [32]
Neuronal surface autoantibody test	Serum: may be negative with fixed cell-based assay (CBA), the only clinically available test. Under research conditions, only 86% of CSF positive were serum positive [33] CSF: positive	Serum: positive on LGI1 CBA and usually positive on VGKC radioimmunoassay. However, VGKC radioimmunoassay is less sensitive than LGI1 CBA and is less specific due to binding of non-surface target antibodies giving positive results, so should no longer be used [28,34,35] CSF: usually positive
Other		Hyponatraemia in approximately 50% of patients

ICU, intensive care unit; NMS, neuroleptic malignant syndrome; VGKC, voltage-gated potassium channel.

pending, a clinical discussion with a specialist regional service is recommended and is usually accessed via neurology.

The rate of definite AE outside of acute rapidly progressive presentations is not firmly established, and likely to be of very low yield. CSF studies in long-standing psychotic disorders have found very few consistently positive autoantibody results [12]. However, there have been case reports of what were thought to be established schizophrenia or bipolar disorder which were then proven to be AE, with good responses to immuno-therapy [13]. Nonetheless, on close inspection these isolated psychiatric presentations are largely relapses with a more typical presentation of either a mixed psychiatric dis-order or subtle neurological features that were identifiable in the history. Therefore, patients with acute or relapsing presentations and treatment resistance, or other atypi-cal features, are investigated by some clinicians. Beyond this, the benefits of treating patients with chronic psychiatric disorders with neuronal surface antibodies only in blood, without CSF positivity, and absence of a clear encephalopathy is the subject of randomised trials, and not part of routine clinical practice (Box 51.1).

Box 51.1 An evolving concept: autoimmune psychosis?

While autoimmune encephalitis (AE) has become a well-established disorder, there remains active discussion about cases of severe mental illness that may fall short of consensus definition for AE that may yet respond positively to immunotherapy [14,15]. To address this, an international panel recently published a proposed approach to characterise such patients in a concept called 'autoimmune psychosis' (AP) [16] This encompasses concepts in AE, although patients with rapid progression of psychotic symptoms (<3 months) with additional neurological features could be considered to have a possible AP and be investigated with CSF analysis, EEG, and MRI brain. Abnormalities here can then lead to categorisation of probable AP. However, it remains to be determined if patients with AP who do not satisfy criteria for AE will derive benefit from immuno-therapy. Examples of attempts to test this hypothesis include the SINAPPS2 trial, where patients with psychosis and serum-only neuronal surface antibodies are being randomised to immunother-apy or placebo in addition to their usual psychiatric care [17].

History and examination

Screen for general features of acute encephalitis syndrome [5,14]:

- fever
- acute change in mental status
- seizures.

Screen also for possible autoimmune encephalitis as per consensus criteria of Graus et al. [15], namely subacute onset (rapid progression of less than 3 months) of:

- working memory deficits (short-term memory loss)
- altered mental status (decreased or altered level of consciousness, lethargy, or person-ality change)

- psychiatric symptoms
- new focal central nervous system (CNS) findings on neurological examination
- seizures not explained by a previously known seizure disorder.

See Table 51.1 for a summary of the characteristic clinical features of the two most common AEs, NMDAR antibody encephalitis and LGI1 antibody encephalitis.

Investigations: encephalitis panel

- Lumbar puncture for CSF analysis:
  - microscopy, culture and sensitivity to screen for bacterial, viral and parasitic causes
  - cell count including differential, protein and glucose
  - oligoclonal bands paired with serum
  - viral polymerase chain reaction (PCR) and reverse-transcriptase PCR for suspected viruses (usually working through tiers of common to rare or those associated with immunocompromise if present/suspected)
  - CSF (and serum) neuronal surface autoantibody testing.
- EEG: of note, in psychiatric practice EEG results may be confounded by the effects of psychotropic medication.
- Brain MRI including a T2-FLAIR sequence looking for temporal lobe hyperintensity, a classic feature of viral and autoimmune encephalitides.
- Blood tests:
  - infectious encephalitis serology
  - urea and electrolytes for sodium (hyponatraemia is common in LGI1 antibody encephalitis
  - consider HIV testing (immunocompromise predisposing to infectious encephalitis)
  - neuronal surface antibody testing paired with CSF
  - autoimmune encephalitis is not typically associated with raised peripheral inflammatory markers (white cell count, C-reactive protein).

MANAGEMENT

As already discussed, when AE is suspected a referral should be made to a service with experience in investigating and managing these disorders. These will usually be located in regional neuroscience centres with joint neurology and psychiatry expertise. However, if the patient is unstable, then as per any emergency medical presentation on a psychiatric ward, the patient should first be transferred to acute medical/emergency services. Indeed, seizures, persistent movement disorders, autonomic instability and/or respiratory failure may require intensive care management.

There is only one randomised trial of AE treatment in patients with LGI1/CASPR2 antibody encephalitis and this shows modest seizure and cognitive benefit from intravenous immunoglobulin [18]. However, there is now also a large body of observational evidence consistent with basic science that suggests the following key cornerstones:

- use of a specialist multidisciplinary setting
- early instigation of immunotherapy (often multiple modalities with low threshold for escalation)
- tumour search and expeditious treatment if found (most relevant for NMDAR antibody encephalitis).

Treatment setting

AE challenges the safety and efficacy of split mental–physical health systems. AE is a brain disease that manifests with both neurological and psychiatric abnormalities often at the same time requiring expert medical and nursing input, such as frequent monitoring of physiology as well as access to advanced tests.

Typically, patients with AE are managed on neurology wards. However, the behavioural disturbance often caused by AE, particularly in NMDAR antibody encephalitis, can be associated with a high risk of self-injury due to unpredictable impulsive behaviours, for example charging into walls and jumping from height, which requires experienced mental health nursing [19]. Additionally, the profound transformation of the patient can place a great deal of strain on friends and family, which can lead to challenging team dynamics. Psychiatric support and leadership can anticipate and provide strategies to contain this aspect of these illnesses. Increasingly, specialist AE centres include a multidisciplinary team including neurology, neuropsychiatry and intensive care, as well as neurophysiology, neuroradiology, and neuropsychology.

Immunotherapy

Immunotherapy in AE has traditionally been broken down into first- and second-line treatments. These are summarised in Table 51.2 and are included largely for information. Of most relevance to psychiatric management is the common use of high-dose corticosteroids in AE. Because they are disease-modifying, steroids will generally

Table 51.2 Immunotherapies used in treatment of autoimmune encephalitis.

	Example of immunotherapy
First line	Corticosteroids
	Intravenous immunoglobulin (IVIG)
	Plasma exchange (PLEX)
Second line	Cyclophosphamide
	Rituximab
	Bortezomib

contribute to amelioration of mental state. Indeed, in some patients with AE, psychiatric symptoms can improve rapidly with steroids. However, in others, steroid use can precipitate disinhibition, elevated mood, and insomnia. This can often be managed with more intensive monitoring but may require a modified immunotherapeutic approach and/or short-term sedating psychotropics.

Psychotropic medication

All forms of encephalitis can cause agitated behaviour that may necessitate pharmacological approaches as per a general approach to delirium. Given the lack of controlled evidence, a reasonable approach combines clinical experience with application of likely pathophysiology. Because of prominent agitation and frequent catatonia, benzodiazepines are a rational choice. Sleep is often highly disturbed, so sedating antihistamines such as promethazine can be useful.

Even though conditions like NMDAR antibody encephalitis have prominent psychotic symptoms, antipsychotics are not the mainstay of treatment as NMDAR antibody encephalitis has a propensity to progress to neuroleptic malignant syndrome (NMS) most commonly reported with first-generation antipsychotics, but can potentially occur with all [20]. Olanzapine may have a relatively low propensity for NMS-like effects and is useful for its sedative properties. However, nutritional status should be regularly reviewed because the combination of abnormal eating patterns caused by the disease and increased appetite from steroids and olanzapine can lead to significant weight gain and metabolic disturbance. Once the underlying autoimmune brain disease is controlled and psychiatric symptoms are adequately reduced, antipsychotics are tapered.

Electroconvulsive therapy

Immunotherapy is the treatment of choice for AE. However, despite maximal immunotherapy NMDAR antibody encephalitis can cause persistent treatment-resistant psychiatric features such as mood disorder and catatonia. There are case reports of successful use of electroconvulsive therapy in this context [21].

References

1. Granerod J, Ambrose HE, Davies NWS, et al. Causes of encephalitis and differences in their clinical presentations in England: a multicentre, population-based prospective study. *Lancet Infect Dis* 2010;10(12):835–844.
2. Gable MS, Sheriff H, Dalmau J, et al. The frequency of autoimmune N-methyl-D-aspartate receptor encephalitis surpasses that of individual viral etiologies in young individuals enrolled in the California Encephalitis Project. *Clin Infect Dis* 2012;54(7):899–904.
3. Dalmau J, Gleichman AJ, Hughes EG, et al. Anti-NMDA-receptor encephalitis: case series and analysis of the effects of antibodies. *Lancet Neurol* 2008;7(12):1091–1098.
4. Gultekin SH, Rosenfeld MR, Voltz R, et al. Paraneoplastic limbic encephalitis: neurological symptoms, immunological findings and tumour association in 50 patients. *Brain* 2000;123(7):1481–1494.
5. Dalmau J, Graus F. Antibody-mediated encephalitis. *N Engl J Med* 2018;378:840–851.
6. Varley J, Taylor J, Irani SR. Autoantibody-mediated diseases of the CNS: structure, dysfunction and therapy. *Neuropharmacology* 2018;132:71–82.
7. Titulaer MJ, McCracken L, Gabilondo I, et al. Treatment and prognostic factors for long-term outcome in patients with anti-NMDA receptor encephalitis: an observational cohort study. *Lancet Neurol* 2013;12(2):157–165.

8. Armangue T, Spatola M, Vlagea A, et al. Frequency, symptoms, risk factors, and outcomes of autoimmune encephalitis after herpes simplex encephalitis: a prospective observational study and retrospective analysis. *Lancet Neurol* 2018;17(9):760–772.

9. Thompson J, Bi M, Murchison AG, et al. The importance of early immunotherapy in patients with faciobrachial dystonic seizures. *Brain* 2017;141(2):348–356.

10. Binks S, Varley J, Lee W, et al. Distinct HLA associations of LGI1 and CASPR2-antibody diseases. *Brain* 2018;141(8):2263–2271.

11. Al-Diwani A, Handel A, Townsend L, et al. The psychopathology of NMDAR-antibody encephalitis in adults: a systematic review and phenotypic analysis of individual patient data. *Lancet Psychiatry* 2019;6(3):235–246.

12. Oviedo-Salcedo T, de Witte L, Kümpfel T, et al. Absence of cerebrospinal fluid antineuronal antibodies in schizophrenia spectrum disorders. *Br J Psychiatry* 2018;212(5):318–320.

13. Simabukuro MM, de Andrade Freitas CH, Castro LHM. A patient with a long history of relapsing psychosis and mania presenting with anti-NMDA receptor encephalitis ten years after first episode. *Dement Neuropsychol* 2015;9(3):311–314.

14. Varley J, Vincent A, Irani SR. Clinical and experimental studies of potentially pathogenic brain-directed autoantibodies: current knowledge and future directions. *J Neurol* 2015;262(4):1081–1095.

15. Graus F, Titulaer MJ, Balu R, et al. A clinical approach to diagnosis of autoimmune encephalitis. *Lancet Neurol* 2016;15(4):391–404.

16. Pollak TA, Lennox BR, Müller S, et al. Autoimmune psychosis: an international consensus on an approach to the diagnosis and management of psychosis of suspected autoimmune origin. *Lancet Psychiatry* 2020;7(1):93–108.

17. Lennox BR, Yeeles K, Jones PB, et al. Intravenous immunoglobulin and rituximab versus placebo treatment of antibody- associated psychosis: study protocol of a randomised phase IIa double-blinded placebo-controlled trial (SINAPPS2). *Trials* 2019;20(1):331.

18. Dubey D, Britton J, McKeon A, et al. Randomized placebo-controlled trial of intravenous immunoglobulin in autoimmune LGI1/CASPR2 epilepsy. *Ann Neurol* 2020;87(2):313–323.

19. Moran N, Munro N, Lawson K, et al. Safe management of psychiatrically disturbed patients on non-psychiatric wards in the UK. *BMJ* 2014;348:g1466.

20. Lejuste F, Thomas L, Picard G, et al. Neuroleptic intolerance in patients with anti-NMDAR encephalitis. *Neurol Neuroimmunol Neuroinflamm* 2016;3(5):e280.

21. Warren N, Grote V, O'Gorman C, Siskind D. Electroconvulsive therapy for anti-N-methyl-D-aspartate (NMDA) receptor encephalitis: A systematic review of cases. *Brain Stimul* 2019;12(2):329–334.

22. Berginck V, Armangue T, Titulaer MJ, et al. Autoimmune encephalitis in postpartum psychosis. *Am J Psychiatry* 2015;172(9):901–908.

23. Irani SR, Stagg CJ, Schott JM, et al. Faciobrachial dystonic seizures: the influence of immunotherapy on seizure control and prevention of cognitive impairment in a broadening phenotype. *Brain* 2013;136(10):3151–3162.

24. Naasan G, Irani SR, Bettcher BM, et al. Episodic bradycardia as neurocardiac prodrome to voltage-gated potassium channel complex/leucine-rich, glioma inactivated 1 antibody encephalitis. *JAMA Neurol* 2014;71(10):1300–1304.

25. Kayser MS, Titulaer MJ, Gresa-Arribas N, Dalmau J. Frequency and characteristics of isolated psychiatric episodes in anti-N-methyl-D-aspartate receptor encephalitis. *JAMA Neurol* 2013;70(9):1133–1139.

26. Varley JA, Webb AJS, Balint B, et al. The movement disorder associated with NMDAR antibody-encephalitis is complex and characteristic: an expert video-rating study. *J Neurol Neurosurg Psychiatry* 2019;90(6):724–726.

27. Balint B, Vincent A, Meinck H-M, et al. Movement disorders with neuronal antibodies: syndromic approach, genetic parallels and pathophysiology. *Brain* 2018;141(1):13–36.

28. van Sonderen A, Schreurs MW, de Bruijn M, et al. The relevance of VGKC positivity in the absence of LGI1 and Caspr2 antibodies. *Neurology* 2016;86(18):1692–1699.

29. Aurangzeb S, Symmonds M, Knight RK, et al. LGI1-antibody encephalitis is characterised by frequent, multifocal clinical and subclinical seizures. *Seizure* 2017;50:14–17.

30. Bakpa OD, Reuber M, Irani SR. Antibody-associated epilepsies: clinical features, evidence for immunotherapies and future research questions. *Seizure* 2016;41:26–41.

31. Gillinder L, Warren N, Hartel G, et al. EEG findings in NMDA encephalitis: a systematic review. *Seizure* 2019;65:20–24.

32. Flanagan EP, Kotsenas AL, Britton JW, et al. Basal ganglia T1 hyperintensity in LGI1-autoantibody faciobrachial dystonic seizures. *Neurol Neuroimmunol Neuroinflamm* 2015;2(6):e161.

33. Gresa-Arribas N, Titulaer MJ, Torrents A, et al. Antibody titres at diagnosis and during follow-up of anti-NMDA receptor encephalitis: a retrospective study. *Lancet Neurol* 2014;13(2):167–177.

34. Lang B, Makuch M, Moloney T, et al. Intracellular and non-neuronal targets of voltage-gated potassium channel complex antibodies. *J Neurol Neurosurg Psychiatry* 2017;88(4):353–361.

35. Binks SN, Klein CJ, Waters P, et al. LGI1, CASPR2 and related antibodies: a molecular evolution of the phenotypes. *J Neurol Neurosurg Psychiatry* 2018;89(5):526–534.

CHAPTER 51

Catatonia
Jonathan P. Rogers, Ali Amad

Catatonia is a severe form of psychomotor disturbance with a heterogeneous presentation (Box 52.1). It affects approximately 10% of acute psychiatric inpatients and is frequently under-recognised [1]. It is associated with high rates of infection, pressure sores, urinary retention, rhabdomyolysis, dehydration, renal failure, deep vein thrombosis (DVT), pulmonary embolism, cardiac arrhythmia, and neuroleptic malignant syndrome (NMS; see Chapter 85), as well as increased overall mortality (odds ratio 4.8) [2,3].

Diagnosis of catatonia in the *International Classification of Diseases* (ICD)-11 or the fifth edition of the *Diagnostic and Statistical Manual of Mental Disorders* (DSM-5) requires the presence of three of the signs in Box 52.1. Other features that are not described in diagnostic criteria include ambitendence (indecisive, hesitant movements), verbigeration (repetitive speech, like a scratched record), gegenhalten (resistance proportionate to the force exerted by the examiner), mitgehen (limbs moving much further than a force applied by the examiner would indicate), and automatic obedience (exaggerated compliance with commands). Autonomic instability (pyrexia, tachycardia, hypertension, increased respiratory rate, and diaphoresis) in the presence of catatonia indicates the presence of *malignant catatonia*, a life-threatening variant of the syndrome; however, autonomic dysregulation should always prompt a search for serious non-psychiatric disease as well. The Bush–Francis Catatonia Rating Scale (BFCRS) consists of 23 items rated from 0 to 3, giving a total score out of 69. It is useful and reliable on an intra-individual level for assessing improvement and response to treatment.

Differential diagnosis includes NMS, extrapyramidal side effects, akinetic mutism, locked-in syndrome, stiff person syndrome, Parkinson's disease, delirium (see Chapter 50), akathisia, tardive dyskinesia (see Chapter 56), elective mutism, anti-*N*-methyl-D-aspartate (NMDA) receptor encephalitis (see Chapter 51), and non-convulsive status epilepticus (see Chapter 76).

The Maudsley Practice Guidelines for Physical Health Conditions in Psychiatry, First Edition.
David M. Taylor, Fiona Gaughran, and Toby Pillinger.
© 2021 John Wiley & Sons Ltd. Published 2021 by John Wiley & Sons Ltd.

> **Box 52.1** Features of catatonia in DSM-5 and ICD-11 with definitions [4–6]
>
> - Stupor: alertness with minimal responsiveness to the environment
> - Catalepsy: after positioning by the examiner, postures are maintained
> - Waxy flexibility: light and even resistance to examiner moving limbs
> - Mutism: absent or minimal speech (not applicable if pre-existing aphasia)
> - Negativism: refusal to obey commands or performance of an opposite action
> - Posturing: spontaneous assumption and maintenance of a posture for an abnormally long period of time
> - Mannerism: odd, exaggerated example of a normal action
> - Stereotypy: repetitive, non-goal-directed movement
> - Psychomotor agitation: hyperactivity unrelated to external stimuli
> - Grimacing: spontaneous contortion of the facial muscles maintained for an abnormally long period
> - Echolalia: repetition of another person's speech
> - Echopraxia: copying another person's movements

Depression, especially in the context of a bipolar disorder, is the most common cause of catatonia, but non-psychiatric causes account for 20–25% of cases and must be considered (Box 52.2) [7].

DIAGNOSTIC PRINCIPLES

The work-up in catatonia serves to:

1 rule out a wide differential diagnosis
2 establish the cause of the catatonia and
3 assess for complications of catatonia.

History

Collateral history is essential, as that from the patient is often very limited.

1 History of catatonic features.
2 Recent oral intake.
3 Screening for underlying mental disorder, especially for a mood disorder or schizophrenia (see Box 52.2).
4 Screening for underlying non-psychiatric disorder, e.g. recent infection, seizure, dizziness, visual disturbance, weakness, numbness, cold/heat intolerance, change in bowel habit.
5 Past medical history, including:
   a epilepsy
   b other neurological disorders
   c autoimmune disease.
6 Medication history, including any recent change and use of recreational drugs.
7 Sexual history (if appropriate), assessing for risk of HIV and syphilis.

> **Box 52.2** Common causes of catatonia [7–9]
>
> **Psychiatric causes**
>
> - Depression (most common, especially in the context of bipolar disorder)
> - Schizophrenia
> - Mania
> - Autism
> - Tourette's syndrome
> - Obsessive–compulsive disorder
>
> **Non-psychiatric causes**
>
> - Central nervous system (CNS) structural lesions (e.g. bilateral infarction of the parietal lobes, temporal infarcts, thalamic lesions, bilateral lesions in globus pallidus)
> - CNS infections (especially HSV, neurosyphilis)
> - Human immunodeficiency virus (HIV) infection
> - Autoimmune encephalitis (especially N-methyl-D-aspartate receptor encephalitis)
> - Dementia (frontotemporal dementia, Alzheimer's disease, Lewy body dementia, Creutzfeldt–Jakob disease)
> - Multiple sclerosis
> - Systemic lupus erythematosus
> - Thyroid disease
> - Vitamin B_{12} deficiency, nicotinic acid deficiency, pellagra
> - Wilson's disease
> - Drug toxicity (especially disulfiram, phencyclidine, steroids, and antipsychotics)
> - Drug withdrawal (especially benzodiazepines and clozapine)
> - Seizure

Examination

Catatonia examination [10]

1 Observe indirectly (stupor, posturing, mannerism, stereotypy, psychomotor agitation, grimacing, consistency).
2 Offer to shake hands (ambitendence, i.e. indecisive, hesitant movements). If no ambitendence, offer hand again instructing patient not to take it.
3 Attempt to engage in conversation (mutism, echolalia, repetitive speech).
4 Scratch head in an exaggerated manner and observe for echopraxia.
5 Assess tone, asking the patient to keep arm loose (waxy flexibility, catalepsy, gegenhalten).
6 Ask the patient to hold their arms out and to keep them in place. Attempt to raise their arms (mitgehen).
7 Check charts (autonomic abnormality and reduced oral intake).

Other systems

1 Volume status: mucous membranes, skin turgor, postural blood pressure.
2 Neurological examination.

3 Respiratory examination, if considering benzodiazepines.
4 Cardiovascular examination, if considering electroconvulsive therapy (ECT).
5 Lower limbs (for DVT).
6 Pressure sites: heels, occiput, lower back, buttocks, hips, shoulders, elbows (for pressure sores).

Investigation

The extent of investigation depends on the clinical circumstances. The high mortality in catatonia should be considered when deciding whether to act coercively to investigate and treat patients lacking capacity. Most patients should have the following work-up.

1 Frequent physical observations (at least three times daily).
2 Food and fluid chart (may require one-to-one nursing for accurate completion).
3 Bloods:
   a full blood count (evidence of infection)
   b electrolytes (particularly hyponatraemia)
   c renal function (dehydration, acute kidney injury)
   d liver function (prior to high-dose benzodiazepines)
   e bone profile (evidence of hypercalcaemia; consider parathyroid function)
   f glucose (hypoglycaemia due to poor oral intake)
   g thyroid function (dysfunction can cause catatonia)
   h B_{12}/folate and B_3 levels (deficiency can cause catatonia)
   i creatine kinase (rhabdomyolysis, NMS)
   j iron (low level may predict poor response to antipsychotics)
   k ceruloplasmin and blood copper test (Wilson's disease can be associated with catatonia)
   l antinuclear antibodies (systemic lupus erythematosus)
   m anti-NMDA receptor antibodies
   n HIV and syphilis serology.
4 Urinalysis for ketones (reduced oral intake).
5 ECG (prior to ECT).

The investigations in Table 52.1 should be considered in specific groups, or if the above diagnostic work-up is inconclusive.

MANAGEMENT

The lorazepam challenge may be considered soon after the diagnosis of catatonia. A positive result (generally 50% reduction in symptoms) predicts a good response to benzodiazepine treatment. Sometimes the lorazepam challenge can be used if the diagnosis of catatonia is in doubt, though a positive response is not diagnostic of catatonia. The procedure is as follows [11].

Table 52.1 Additional investigations for particular indications.

Additional investigation	Indication
Neuroimaging (ideally MRI, but CT often more readily available)	First episode of neuropsychiatric disease or significant change in presentation If considering ECT
EEG	History of epilepsy, episodes of duration of minutes or other features of complex partial seizures
Lumbar puncture	Suspected autoimmune encephalitis, viral encephalitis or meningitis (see encephalitis panel in Chapter 51)

1 Assess for features of catatonia (ideally using the BFCRS).
2 Administer lorazepam 1 or 2 mg i.v./i.m./p.o. A rapid alternative to oral administration is sublingual lorazepam (if possible).
3 Reassess five minutes after intravenous, 15 minutes after intramuscular, and 30 minutes after oral challenge.
4 If no response, administer further lorazepam 1 or 2 mg.
5 Reassess after a further 5, 15 or 30 minutes (as step 3).

There is some variation in practice in the lorazepam challenge (see Table 52.2 for details).
An alternative is the zolpidem challenge following the same procedure. In this test, 10 mg of zolpidem is administered orally and after 30 minutes the patient is reassessed.
Catatonia and any underlying disorder must be treated concurrently, while preventing and treating the physical consequences of catatonia.

Treatment of catatonia

Benzodiazepines are the most common initial treatment, with a remission rate of approximately 80%, regardless of the cause or the clinical manifestations. ECT should be started in a patient with catatonia that is not responding to benzodiazepines or when

Table 52.2 Lorazepam challenge protocols.

Study	Study type	Regimen
Bush et al. [12]	Original	2 mg i.m. or 1 mg i.v., repeated after 5 minutes
Sienaert et al. [11]	Review	1–2 mg p.o./i.m./i.v., reassessing after 5, 15 or 30 minutes (respectively). Give second dose after this time period
Pelzer et al. [13]	Systematic review	Discusses treatment with lorazepam, not lorazepam challenge Effective dose range 2–16 mg, mainly oral, but sometimes i.m. or i.v.
Rosebush and Mazurek [14]	Review, based on original work	1–2 mg s.l. or i.m. Repeat after 3 hours if no response Repeat again after 3 hours if no response

CHAPTER 52

CHAPTER 52

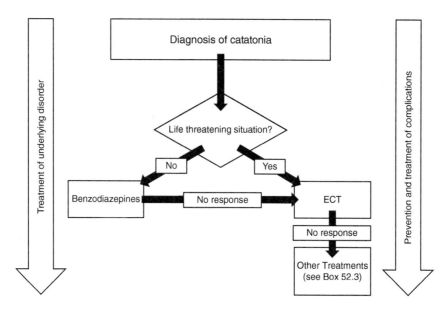

Figure 52.1 Treatment algorithm for catatonia.

a decisive and short-term improvement is required in severe cases with life-threatening conditions such as malignant catatonia.

The benzodiazepine with the largest evidence base is lorazepam. Lower doses should be used with children, the elderly and medically unwell. The lorazepam treatment protocol (Figure 52.1) is as follows [7,13,15,16].

1 Lorazepam 2 mg p.o./i.m./i.v. twice daily. Optimal route is dependent on circumstances: the oral route risks non-adherence in negativism; the intramuscular route involves painful injections; and the intravenous route requires careful monitoring with intravenous access maintained, usually in a medical ward.
2 If no response after one to two days, titrate lorazepam up, increasing dose daily until either effective treatment of catatonia or sedation is reached. Monitor carefully for respiratory depression. High doses (occasionally up to 30 mg/day) are sometimes needed.

Bitemporal ECT tends to be very effective in catatonia, especially when started early in the illness [17]. For patients on benzodiazepines, seizure threshold is likely to be raised, so higher energy stimulus may be required. Patients may need their medical state optimised prior to ECT, but long delays should be avoided [7].

In cases of treatment failure with benzodiazepines and ECT, the evidence base is poor, as summarised in Box 52.3.

Treatment of underlying disorder

Treatment should generally follow standard algorithms for the underlying disorder. There is controversy over the role of antipsychotics: they may be required for underlying psychosis, but they risk precipitating NMS (3.6% in catatonia, compared with

---

Box 52.3 Alternative treatments for catatonia [13,18]

Antipsychotics

- Several low-quality studies with variable results. Most evidence is for atypical antipsychotics in patients with a psychotic illness.
- Use of antipsychotics should be carefully considered and several authors recommend that antipsychotics should be avoided in catatonic patients.
- Note cautions in section Treatment of underlying disorder.

Carbamazepine

- A few reports have shown benefit in patients resistant to lorazepam, most in the context of mood disorders.

Valproate

- A few case reports have shown benefit, most in excited catatonia.

Topiramate

- One small study suggests benefit in patients resistant to benzodiazepines and antipsychotics.

N-methyl-D-aspartate antagonists (amantadine, memantine)

- Growing case report literature supports use.

0.07–1.8% in the general antipsychotic-treated population) [14]. If antipsychotics are used, use atypical agents, especially those with low dopamine D2 receptor blockade (quetiapine, olanzapine) or with D2 partial agonism (aripiprazole) [11], with caution and consider adjuvant treatment with benzodiazepines while catatonic features persist. There is some evidence that low serum iron in catatonia predicts NMS development, so these patients may be a group in which to avoid antipsychotics when possible [19].

Approaches to the prevention and management of complications of catatonia are documented in Box 52.4.

Box 52.4 Prevention and management of complications of catatonia [7,20]

Dehydration

- Food and fluid chart
- Prescribe oral fluids (e.g. 250 mL water four times daily)
- One-to-one nursing to frequently encourage drinking
- Intravenous fluids

Malnutrition

- Lorazepam 30–60 minutes before meals (relieves stupor to facilitate eating)
- Consider nasogastric feeding if five to seven days of inadequate intake
- If chronic, consider percutaneous endoscopic gastrostomy

Pressure sores

- Daily skin assessment
- Pressure mattress
- Bed head at ≤30°
- Repositioning (every two hours if bedbound)
- Emollients
- Keeping skin dry
- Dietician involvement for consideration of high calorie and protein diet

Muscle contractures

- Passive (± active) range of movement exercises
- Stretching for 30 minutes daily
- Physiotherapy

Venous thromboembolism

- Consider thromboembolism deterrent stockings or prophylactic subcutaneous low-molecular-weight heparin
- ECT cautioned in proximal DVT [21]

Neglect of medical comorbidities

- Monitor established comorbidities (e.g. blood sugar, blood pressure)
- Ensure medication compliance with consideration of nasogastric, intramuscular or intravenous administration

Aspiration

- In case of pneumonia, ensure antibiotic with broad spectrum to cover Gram-negative organisms

Urinary retention

- Consider catheterisation

When to refer to a specialist

Catatonia can be managed on inpatient psychiatric units or very occasionally, in milder presentations, in the community. Specialist referral to acute medicine is most commonly required for intravenous rehydration and should also take place if malignant catatonia is present. Input from physiotherapists or dieticians may be required (see Box 52.4), but this is ideally provided within the patient's current setting, so that ward staff can be appropriately advised.

References

1. Solmi M, Pigato GG, Roiter B, *et al*. Prevalence of catatonia and its moderators in clinical samples: results from a meta-analysis and meta-regression analysis. *Schizophr Bull* 2018;44:1133–1150.
2. Funayama M, Takata T, Koreki A, et al. Catatonic stupor in schizophrenic disorders and subsequent medical complications and mortality. *Psychosom Med* 2018;80(4):370–376.

3. Fricchione G, Bush G, Fozdar M, et al. Recognition and treatment of the catatonic syndrome. *J Intensive Care Med* 1997;12:135–147.

4. Denysenko L, Freudenreich O, Philbrick K, et al. *Catatonia in Medically Ill Patients: An Evidence-based Medicine (EBM) Monograph for Psychosomatic Medicine Practice.* European Association of Psychosomatic Medicine, April 2015. Available at https://www.eapm.eu.com/wp-content/uploads/2018/06/Catatonia_APM-EAPM_2015-04-17.pdf

5. American Psychiatric Association. *Diagnostic and Statistical Manual of Mental Disorders*, 5th edn. Washington, DC: APA, 2013.

6. World Health Organization. *ICD-11 for Mortality and Morbidity Statistics.* Geneva: WHO, 2018. Available at https://icd.who.int/browse11/l-m/en (accessed 4 February 2019).

7. Caroff SN, Mann SC, Francis A, Fricchione GL (eds) *Catatonia : From Psychopathology to Neurobiology.* Washington, DC: American Psychiatric Association, 2004.

8. Carroll BT, Anfinson TJ, Kennedy JC, et al. Catatonic disorder due to general medical conditions. *J. Neuropsychiatry Clin Neurosci* 1994;6:122–133.

9. Jaimes-Albornoz W, Serra-Mestres J. Catatonia in the emergency department. *Emerg Med J* 2012;29:863–867.

10. Bush G, Fink M, Petrides G, et al. Catatonia. I. Rating scale and standardized examination. *Acta Psychiatr Scand* 1996;93:129–136.

11. Sienaert P, Dhossche DM, Vancampfort D, et al. A clinical review of the treatment of catatonia. *Front Psychiatry* 2014;5:181.

12. Bush G, Fink M, Petrides G, et al. Catatonia. II. Treatment with lorazepam and electroconvulsive therapy. *Acta Psychiatr Scand* 1996;93:137–143.

13. Pelzer AC, van der Heijden FM, den Boer E. Systematic review of catatonia treatment. *Neuropsychiatr Dis Treat* 2018;14:317–326.

14. Rosebush PI, Mazurek MF. Catatonia and its treatment. *Schizophr Bull* 2010;36:239–242.

15. Fink M, Taylor MA. The catatonia syndrome: forgotten but not gone. *Arch Gen Psychiatry* 2009;66:1173–1176.

16. Fink M, Taylor MA. *Catatonia : a Clinician's Guide to Diagnosis and Treatment.* Cambridge: Cambridge University Press, 2006.

17. Leroy A, Naudet F, Vaiva G, et al. Is electroconvulsive therapy an evidence-based treatment for catatonia? A systematic review and meta-analysis. *Eur Arch Psychiatry Clin Neurosci* 2018;268:675–687.

18. Beach SR, Gomez-Bernal F, Huffman JC, Fricchione GL. Alternative treatment strategies for catatonia: a systematic review. *Gen Hosp Psychiatry* 2017;48:1–19.

19. Lee J. Serum iron in catatonia and neuroleptic malignant syndrome. *Biol Psychiatry* 1998;44:499–507.

20. Clinebell K, Azzam PN, Gopalan P, Haskett R. Guidelines for preventing common medical complications of catatonia. *J Clin Psychiatry* 2014;75:644–651.

21. Inagawa Y, Saito S, Okada T, et al. Electroconvulsive therapy for catatonia with deep venous thrombosis. *Prim Care Companion CNS Disord* 2018;20(4):18m02286.

CHAPTER 52

Seizure Disorders

Emanuele F. Osimo, Brian Sweeney

A seizure is defined as 'a transient occurrence of signs and/or symptoms due to abnormal excessive or synchronous neuronal activity in the brain' [1]. Seizures are common, with an approximate 10% lifetime prevalence in the general population [2]. Epilepsy affects about 1% of the population. Causes of seizures are summarised in Box 53.1.

There is a complex relationship between seizures and psychiatric conditions. Seizures, especially focal seizures, can be mistaken for psychiatric symptoms or presentations, such as panic attacks or dissociative experiences. Conversely, psychiatric symptoms may resemble seizure activity in the form of psychogenic non-epileptic seizures (PNES). People with true epilepsy (the definition of which is provided in Box 53.1) may also experience PNES, further complicating diagnosis [3]. Many psychiatric treatments reduce seizure threshold, and psychiatric patients present with increased risk of various conditions that can result in seizure, such as glucose dysregulation, alcohol dependence (and thus withdrawal), and recreational drug use (see Box 53.1). The relationship between epilepsy and psychiatric disorders goes beyond shared symptoms and misdiagnosis, with a 'bidirectional' association between epilepsy and psychiatric comorbidity recognised [4]. Furthermore, some antiepileptic drugs (AEDs) are associated with development of psychiatric symptoms, while the mood-stabilising and potential antipsychotic effects of various AEDs are well recognised [5].

There are thus several contexts in which a psychiatric practitioner may have to deal with seizures and epilepsy. This chapter considers an approach to acute seizure in a person attending the outpatient department or inpatient psychiatric services, psychiatric comorbidity in people with epilepsy (PwE), psychiatric drug treatment in PwE, PNES, the role of surgery in treatment-refractory epilepsy, and the relationship between epilepsy and learning disability and the challenges such comorbidity poses to epilepsy treatment.

The Maudsley Practice Guidelines for Physical Health Conditions in Psychiatry, First Edition.
David M. Taylor, Fiona Gaughran, and Toby Pillinger.

Box 53.1 Causes of seizures

- Epilepsy, current definition of which is a disease characterised by any one of the following [6]:
  - At least two unprovoked (or reflex, i.e. in response to a provocative factor such as flashing lights) seizures occurring more than 24 hours apart
  - One unprovoked (or reflex) seizure and a probability of further seizures similar to the general recurrence risk after two unprovoked seizures (at least 60%), occurring over the next 10 years
  - Diagnosis of an epilepsy syndrome
- Infection of the brain (meningitis/encephalitis/abscess; see Chapter 81), or systemic infection (see Chapter 72)
- Brain injury (see Chapter 80)
- Stroke (see Chapter 82)
- Malignancy
- Biochemical/metabolic abnormalities:
  - Hypoglycaemia/hyperglycaemia (see Chapter 74)
  - Electrolyte disturbance: hyponatraemia (see Chapter 32), hypocalcaemia, hypomagnesaemia
  - Uraemia in context of renal failure (see Chapters 34 and 73)
- Hyperthyroidism (see Chapter 12)
- Recreational drug intoxication (e.g. cocaine, amphetamines) or withdrawal (e.g. benzodiazepines, alcohol (see 'Alcohol and Physical Health' Chapter 24)
- Psychogenic non-epileptic seizures

ACUTE SEIZURE

Most seizures are self-limited. Acute care should involve an ABCDE approach with maintenance of a safe airway, supporting breathing with supplemental oxygen, recognition and treatment of reversible causes (e.g. hypoglycaemia), consideration of administration of thiamine, timely treatment and medical transfer of patients with status epilepticus (see Chapter 76), and ensuring that the patient avoids injury.

History

In patients who report a seizure-like episode now resolved, assessment includes history and determining the context of the episode and consideration of possible risk associations such as childhood febrile convulsions, previous central nervous system infection (e.g. meningitis or encephalitis), head injury, family history of epilepsy, prescribed medicines (see Box 53.2 for medicines known to lower seizure threshold), and alcohol/recreational drug use. Depending on the brain region of seizure origin, there may be psychological symptoms as part of the seizure semiology (Box 53.3). The presence of these symptoms in the right context should trigger the consideration of epilepsy as a possible cause and the consideration of neurological referral and further investigations, as described in the following section.

Examination and investigations

After general physical, cardiological, and neurological examination, investigations should include blood testing (Box 53.4), electrocardiogram (ECG), and potentially

Box 53.2 Medications associated with reduction in seizure threshold

General medical medications

- Methylxanthines: aminophylline, theophylline
- Antibiotics: isoniazid, metronidazole, penicillins
- Antimalarials: mefloquine, chloroquine
- Opioids

Psychiatric medications

Antidepressants

- High risk: tricyclic antidepressants, amoxapine, bupropion, maprotiline
- Moderate risk: trazodone, venlafaxine, vilazodone
- Low risk: selective serotonin reuptake inhibitors, mirtazapine

Antipsychotics[a]

- High risk: clozapine, zotepine, loxapine, chlorpromazine
- Moderate risk: olanzapine, quetiapine
- Low risk: amisulpride/sulpiride, aripiprazole, ziprasidone, fluphenazine, haloperidol, trifluoperazine, flupentixol, risperidone
- Lithium is associated with moderate risk

[a] Depot formulation of any antipsychotic is not recommended where there are concerns regarding risk of seizure/epilepsy, since if seizures occur the causative drug cannot immediately be removed.

Box 53.3 Symptoms of seizures that can mimic psychiatric presentations

Temporal lobe

- Visceral sensations, including nausea and palpitations
- Hallucinatory behaviour, including olfactory and gustatory, hallucinatory memories, autoscopy
- Illusions (e.g. macropsia, micropsia, movement, metamorphopsia)
- Affective symptoms (fear, anxiety, apprehension, depression, pleasure, displeasure)
- Oneiroid state, altered sense of time, derealisation, depersonalisation
- Déjà vu, déjà vécu, déjà pensé
- Absence
- Vertiginous sensations
- Transient amnesia

Frontal lobe

- Non-fluent dysphasia, impaired comprehension, vocal arrest
- Word ejaculation
- Absence

Parietal lobe

- Somatosensory: pins and needles, tingling, numbness, formication
- Visual seizures: darkness, sparks/flashes of light, momentary blindness

Temporal and frontal lobes

- Automatisms, from simple repetitive movements such as lip smacking, to complex behaviours started before seizure onset such as walking around, undressing, turning pages, driving
- Violence and aggression

> **Box 53.4** Blood tests to consider in a patient presenting with seizure
>
> - Full blood count (infection)
> - Electrolytes: sodium, calcium, magnesium
> - Renal function (chronic renal failure and uraemia)
> - Liver function tests
> - C-reactive protein (infection)
> - Glucose
> - HbA$_{1c}$
> - Thyroid function tests

more prolonged cardiac monitoring such as a 24-hour tape to screen for arrhythmia or conduction defect (see Chapters 1–4 and 70). Urine testing to screen for infection (see Chapter 41), recreational drug use, and pregnancy may be appropriate. With the increasing recognition of psychosis and seizures as manifestations of autoimmune encephalitis, consideration should also be given to checking serum and cerebrospinal fluid for any evidence of autoantibodies, such as the anti-NMDA or LGI1 receptor antibodies (see Chapter 51). Lumbar puncture will also be indicated where infective meningitis or encephalitis are suspected, as well as testing of HIV status.

Acute imaging in the emergency department is usually with CT brain, but MRI brain is the recommended modality for seizure, especially if there is a 'focal' onset. Other forms of imaging, such as CT or magnetic resonance venography of the brain, may be indicated in seizures occurring in certain situations, such as women developing seizures peripartum who are at risk of cerebral venous thrombosis. Electroencephalogram (EEG) is used to demonstrate focal and/or generalised abnormalities consistent with epilepsy but can be normal in people with epilepsy interictally, so a single normal EEG result does not exclude it. In addition, 'borderline' EEG abnormalities can sometimes be over-interpreted leading to an incorrect diagnosis of epilepsy or delay in considering other possible causes of altered consciousness. Psychotropic drugs also influence EEG waveforms, complicating interpretation [7]. Further refinements of EEG such as sleep EEG and video EEG can be helpful for diagnosing a seizure syndrome or PNES, or in those being worked up for possible epilepsy surgery.

Management

Unless there is a clear reversible cause (e.g. metabolic derangement), it is recommended that all patients be referred to neurology following their first seizure, or at least a discussion held with medical colleagues. The most important aspects of seizure management include decisions regarding whether long-term AEDs are required, possible side effects of treatment (including interactions with the oral contraceptive pill and potential teratogenic effects; see Chapter 62), informing patients of lifestyle factors that might increase seizure risk, providing counselling about not engaging in risky activities (e.g. lone swimming), and informing them about the driving regulations. PwE are at risk of sudden unexpected death in epilepsy [8], with a risk of 1.2 per 1000 patient-years in adults; discussion of this risk can be difficult but should be a part of the counselling for PwE [9].

PSYCHIATRIC COMORBIDITY IN PEOPLE WITH EPILEPSY

PwE have an increased lifetime prevalence of depression, anxiety, and suicidality compared with the general population (odds ratio, OR, 2.2–2.4) [10] and an even higher risk of psychosis (OR 7.8) [4,11]. PNES may occur in PwE [3], and there are recognised psychiatric side effects of AEDs [5]. Determining the aetiology of seizures and psychiatric symptoms where comorbidity exists can therefore be difficult. It has also been proposed that there may be personality 'types' or changes found in PwE, for example in people with temporal lobe epilepsy (TLE). Certain traits, such as hypergraphia, hyper-religiosity, atypical sexuality, circumstantiality, and intensified mental life, have been linked to TLE. Also, the term 'viscosity', defined as talking repeatedly about a limited number of topics, has been applied [12,13]. Whether these are true associations or easily defined syndromes is moot.

Post-ictal psychosis describes when psychotic symptoms develop within hours or days of a seizure/seizure cluster, often with an initial 'lucid period' immediately after the seizure. *Ictal psychosis* refers to psychotic symptoms occurring during a seizure, usually ending with seizure cessation. *Pre-ictal psychosis* is defined as psychosis occurring in the hours or days leading up to a seizure. *Inter-ictal psychosis* occurs between seizures and is not temporally related to them. Risk factors for psychosis in epilepsy include family history of psychosis or affective disorder, early onset of epilepsy, structural brain lesions, and left temporal seizure onset [14]. Differential diagnosis includes encephalitis (infective or autoimmune), delirium, AED side effects, recent drug or alcohol misuse, thiamine deficiency, non-convulsive status epilepticus, and dementia. Prescription of benzodiazepines such as lorazepam, diazepam or clobazam as well as antipsychotic drugs are helpful until the psychosis has resolved. Prevention, in those already known to be vulnerable to post-ictal psychosis, by early commencement of adjunctive benzodiazepines like clobazam during or after a seizure cluster, may also be useful.

Where the aetiology of psychiatric symptoms in PwE is unclear, one approach is to consider the following questions.

1 Are psychiatric symptoms temporally related to the occurrence of seizures (pre-ictal, ictal, or post-ictal)?
2 Did psychiatric symptoms emerge in association with the prescription or withdrawal of AEDs?
3 Did psychiatric symptoms emerge with remission of seizures in patients whose presumed epilepsy had previously failed to respond to AEDs?

An affirmative response to question 1 suggests symptoms of seizures that mimic psychiatric presentations (Box 53.3). An affirmative response to question 2 suggests psychiatric side effects of AEDs (see following section and Box 53.5). An affirmative response to question 3 points towards PNES in the context of a comorbid psychiatric disorder (see following and Box 53.6).

CHAPTER 53

Box 53.5 Potential psychiatric side effects of antiepileptic drugs [17–19]

- *Sedation:* acetazolamide, brivaracetam, carbamazepine, clobazam, clonazepam, eslicarbazepine acetate, ethosuximide, gabapentin, lacosamide, lamotrigine, levetiracetam, oxcarbazepine, pregabalin, phenobarbital, phenytoin, piracetam, pregabalin, primidone, rufinamide, sodium valproate, stiripentol, tiagabine, topiramate, zonisamide
- *Irritability or aggression:* brivaracetam, carbamazepine, clobazam, clonazepam, eslicarbazepine acetate, gabapentin, lacosamide, lamotrigine, levetiracetam, oxcarbazepine, phenobarbital, perampanel, pregabalin, sodium valproate, stiripentol, topiramate, vigabatrin, zonisamide
- *Insomnia:* brivaracetam, everolimus, ethosuximide, levetiracetam, phenytoin, rufinamide, stiripentol, topiramate, vigabatrin
- *Hyperactivity:* ethosuximide
- *Depression:* acetazolamide, brivaracetam, carbamazepine, clonazepam, clobazam, eslicarbazepine acetate, gabapentin, lacosamide, levetiracetam, oxcarbazepine, piracetam, pregabalin, tiagabine, topiramate, vigabatrin, zonisamide
- *Anxiety:* brivaracetam, clonazepam, eslicarbazepine acetate, ethosuximide, gabapentin, levetiracetam, lacosamide, oxcarbazepine, perampanel, piracetam, rufinamide, tiagabine, topiramate, vigabatrin, zonisamide
- *Emotional lability:* eslicarbazepine acetate, gabapentin, lacosamide, levetiracetam, oxcarbazepine, tiagabine, topiramate, zonisamide
- *Psychosis:* carbamazepine, clonazepam, ethosuximide, levetiracetam, brivaracetam, lacosamide, lamotrigine, phenobarbital, pregabalin, primidone, sodium valproate, tiagabine, topiramate, zonisamide
- *Confusional state:* carbamazepine, clonazepam, clobazam, eslicarbazepine acetate, lacosamide, lamotrigine, levetiracetam, oxcarbazepine, perampanel, phenobarbital, pregabalin, phenytoin, sodium valproate, tiagabine, topiramate, zonisamide
- *Suicidality:* brivaracetam, eslicarbazepine acetate, lacosamide, levetiracetam, perampanel, topiramate, vigabatrin, zonisamide

---

Box 53.6 Consensus guidelines for diagnosis of psychogenic non-epileptic seizures (PNES) [30]

Signs that favour PNES diagnosis

- Long duration seizure
- Fluctuating course
- Asynchronous movements
- Pelvic thrusting
- Side-to-side head or body movements
- Closed eyes
- Ictal crying
- Memory recall

Signs that favour epilepsy diagnosis

- Occurrence from EEG-confirmed sleep
- Post-ictal confusion
- Stertorous breathing

Levels of evidence to support diagnosis of PNES

Possible

Activity self-reported, no evidence on EEG.

Probable

Event is described by a clinician who reviewed video recording, no evidence on EEG.

Clinically established

The event is witnessed by a clinician experienced in diagnosis of seizure disorders and there is no epileptiform activity in the EEG during a typical event in which the semiology would make ictal epileptiform EEG activity expected during an equivalent epileptic seizure.

Documented

The event is witnessed by an experienced clinician in seizure disorders while there is no epileptiform activity immediately before, during, or after the event captured on ictal video EEG with typical PNES semiology.

PSYCHIATRIC SIDE EFFECTS OF ANTIEPILEPTIC DRUGS

Box 53.5 provides a list of currently available AEDs which report neuropsychological/psychiatric side effects. One current area of interest is the use of cannabinoids in the treatment of epilepsy. This is based on studies of cannabidiol (CBD) in two relatively rare forms of severe childhood epilepsy, Dravet syndrome [15] and Lennox–Gastaut syndrome [16]. In both cases, the Food and Drug Administration and European Medicines Agency have given clearance for use of CBD. However, it remains unclear if CBD is effective in all forms of refractory epilepsy and it cannot be considered to be a 'standard' AED at this time. Some AEDs (e.g. carbamazepine, lamotrigine, and valproate) have positive effects on mood, and withdrawal can be associated with deterioration in mental state.

PSYCHIATRIC DRUG THERAPY IN PEOPLE WITH EPILEPSY

As shown in Box 53.2, various psychiatric drugs lower the seizure threshold, which should be considered in psychiatric treatment of PwE, as well as potential drug interactions. For depression, selective serotonin reuptake inhibitors have low seizure propensity and are used most commonly, with other antidepressants such as trazodone, moclobemide, and mirtazapine also likely to have minimal proconvulsive effects [20].

Antipsychotic agents seem to vary regarding risk of seizures. Clozapine has a clear association with increasing risk of seizure and should be used cautiously in PwE with slow titration of dose. However, clozapine has been successfully used in patients with epilepsy who are established on antiepileptic treatment [21]. A risk–benefit decision to use clozapine should be made following a multidisciplinary discussion involving neurology and psychiatry.

Seizure prophylaxis in clozapine treatment

Clozapine increases risk of seizures in a dose-dependent manner [22]. Myoclonus can precede a full tonic–clonic seizure, although may also occur without progression to seizure. In such a circumstance, plasma level monitoring is recommended and consideration of dose reduction. Prophylactic AED treatment in patients without epilepsy may reduce risk of progression to seizures (lamotrigine recommended as first line). If supratherapeutic plasma levels of clozapine are sought, it is generally recommended to introduce seizure prophylaxis. The precise plasma level at which seizure prophylaxis should be initiated is unclear, although introduction when trough levels exceed 0.6 mg/L has traditionally been advised, regardless of seizure history.

Pharmacokinetic interactions between psychotropic and antiepileptic agents

Pharmacokinetic interactions between psychotropics and AEDs occur via their actions on cytochrome P450 enzymes. As such, psychotropics that act as enzyme inhibitors (e.g. fluoxetine and fluvoxamine) will increase AED levels. In contrast, some AEDs are potent enzyme inducers (e.g. carbamazepine and phenytoin), which can lower plasma levels of multiple psychotropics leading to treatment failure. Close monitoring of mental state is therefore recommended where there are concerns regarding drug interactions, alongside plasma drug monitoring.

PSYCHOGENIC NON-EPILEPTIC SEIZURES

Psychiatric practitioners may be consulted regarding patients presenting with PNES, also referred to as non-epileptic attack disorder or 'dissociative seizures'. PNES are characterised by sudden changes in consciousness, movements, and other behaviours similar to those seen in epilepsy, but not associated with epileptiform activity on video-EEG and with psychological underpinnings. PNES has transitioned from being classified as a dissociative disorder in the *Diagnostic and Statistical Manual of Mental Disorders* (DSM)-III-R to a conversion-type somatoform disorder in DSM-5. Of patients with PNES, 75–80% are women [23] with a mean age of onset of 30 years [24]. There is a well-established association between chronic pain, psychiatric illness, and PNES (especially depression, anxiety and personality disorders) [25,26]. PNES can also coexist with epilepsy. PNES is often diagnosed late or misdiagnosed due to lack of knowledge by physicians, stigma associated with a PNES diagnosis, and lack of necessary diagnostic facilities [27]. Many features that have historically been considered typical of PNES are now deemed non-specific as they can also be found in epileptic seizures, especially frontal epilepsies. Furthermore, many features characteristic of epileptic seizures can be present in PNES, such as tongue biting and urinary incontinence [28,29]. As such, the gold standard for diagnosing both epileptic and non-epileptic seizures is video-EEG [30]. Box 53.6 presents consensus guidelines for diagnosis of PNES [30]. There is usually certainty about the diagnosis given that video-EEG is diagnostic, but even with that degree of proof, the patient, family and friends, and even physicians can remain uncertain about the diagnosis. Management includes a clear and unambiguous discussion of the diagnosis with the patient, cognitive-behavioural therapy, and treatment of any associated mental health disorders.

EPILEPSY SURGERY

Patients with a history of seizures that have not responded to trials of two or three AEDS, and in whom factors like compliance and lifestyle are not causative of this failure of treatment, may be candidates for surgical resection of the seizure focus. Assessment for such surgery is by multidisciplinary teams, including neurology, neurophysiology, neuroradiology, neurosurgery, neuropsychiatry, neuropsychology, and neuropathology. Essential investigations include video-EEG monitoring to capture attack semiology and origin, and MRI brain by seizure protocol to look for lesions consistent with the EEG findings. Brain positron emission tomography can be helpful for localisation in 'non-lesional' focal onset seizures. Mental health disorders following surgery include depression, anxiety, and psychosis, and this does not always relate to whether there is a good outcome in terms of seizure control [31]. The idea of 'the burden of normality' with a major psychosocial adjustment to being free of seizures has been invoked in PwE who experience difficulties despite seizure control being greatly improved [32].

EPILEPSY AND LEARNING DISABILITY

There is a strong link between learning disability and epilepsy [33]. This epilepsy can be difficult to control, and individuals can have multiple seizure types. There is a trend towards polypharmacy, with consequent complexity of drug interactions. It is important to realise that complete control of seizures may not be possible and to counsel the person, family, and carers about this fact. On occasion, carers and family may report altered behaviour with trials of a new AED, which may require drug withdrawal if severely disruptive, even if seizure control has improved. Buccal midazolam as required can be helpful for acute seizure care where there is poor control of seizures with AEDs.

CHAPTER 53

References

1. Fisher RS, van Emde Boas E, Blume W, et al. Epileptic seizures and epilepsy: definitions proposed by the International League Against Epilepsy (ILAE) and the International Bureau for Epilepsy (IBE). *Aktuel Neurol* 2005;32(5):249–252.
2. Annegers JF, Hauser WA, Lee JR, Rocca WA. Incidence of acute symptomatic seizures in Rochester, Minnesota, 1935–1984. *Epilepsia* 1995;36(4):327–333.
3. Vincentiis S, Valente KD, Thome-Souza S, et al. Risk factors for psychogenic nonepileptic seizures in children and adolescents with epilepsy. *Epilepsy Behav* 2006;8(1):294–298.
4. Mula M. Bidirectional link between epilepsy and psychiatric disorders. *Nat Rev Neurol* 2012;8(5):252–253.
5. Trimble MR, Rusch N, Betts T, Crawford PM. Psychiatric symptoms after therapy with new antiepileptic drugs: psychopathological and seizure related variables. *Seizure* 2000;9(4):249–254.
6. Fisher RS, Acevedo C, Arzimanoglou A, et al. ILAE official report: a practical clinical definition of epilepsy. *Epilepsia* 2014;55(4):475–482.
7. Aiyer R, Novakovic V, Barkin RL. A systematic review on the impact of psychotropic drugs on electroencephalogram waveforms in psychiatry. *Postgrad Med* 2016;128(7):656–664.
8. Harden C, Tomson T, Gloss D, et al. Practice guideline summary: Sudden unexpected death in epilepsy incidence rates and risk factors: Report of the Guideline Development, Dissemination, and Implementation Subcommittee of the American Academy of Neurology and the American Epilepsy Society. *Neurology* 2017;88(17):1674–1680.
9. Morton B, Richardson A, Duncan S. Sudden unexpected death in epilepsy (SUDEP): don't ask, don't tell? *J Neurol Neurosurg Psychiatry* 2006;77(2):199–202.
10. Tellez-Zenteno JF, Patten SB, Jetté N, et al. Psychiatric comorbidity in epilepsy: a population-based analysis. *Epilepsia* 2007;48(12):2336–2344.

11. Clancy MJ, Clarke MC, Connor DJ, et al. The prevalence of psychosis in epilepsy; a systematic review and meta-analysis. *BMC Psychiatry* 2014;14(1):75.

12. Dodrill C, Batzel L. Interictal behavioral features of patients with epilepsy. *Epilepsia* 1986;27(Suppl 2):S64–S76. 1986.

13. Bear DM, Fedio P. Quantitative analysis of interictal behavior in temporal lobe epilepsy. *Arch Neurol* 1977;34(8):454–467.

14. Maguire M, Singh J, Marson A. Epilepsy and psychosis: a practical approach. *Pract Neurol* 2018;18(2):106–114.

15. Devinsky O, Cross JH, Laux L, et al. Trial of cannabidiol for drug-resistant seizures in the Dravet syndrome. *N Engl J Med* 2017;376(21):2011–2020.

16. Devinsky O, Patel AD, Cross JH, et al. Effect of cannabidiol on drop seizures in the Lennox–Gastaut syndrome. *N Engl J Med* 2018;378(20):1888–1897.

17. Kwan P, Brodie MJ. Neuropsychological effects of epilepsy and antiepileptic drugs. *Lancet* 2001;357(9251):216–222.

18. Vermeulen J, Aldenkamp AP. Cognitive side-effects of chronic antiepileptic drug treatment: a review of 25 years of research. *Epilepsy Res* 1995;22(2):65–95.

19. Brodie MJ. Tolerability and safety of commonly used antiepileptic drugs in adolescents and adults: a clinician's overview. *CNS Drugs* 2017;31(2):135–147.

20. Curran S, de Pauw K. Selecting an antidepressant for use in a patient with epilepsy: safety considerations. *Drug Saf* 1998;18(2):125–133.

21. Langosch JM, Trimble MR. Epilepsy, psychosis and clozapine. *Hum Psychopharm Clin* 2002;17(2):115–119.

22. Varma S, Bishara D, Besag FM, Taylor D. Clozapine-related EEG changes and seizures: dose and plasma-level relationships. *Ther Adv Psychopharmacol* 2011;1(2):47–66.

23. Bodde NM, Brooks JL, Baker GA, et al. Psychogenic non-epileptic seizures: diagnostic issues. A critical review. *Clin Neurol Neurosurg* 2009;111(1):1–9.

24. Duncan R, Graham CD, Oto M, et al. Primary and secondary care attendance, anticonvulsant and antidepressant use and psychiatric contact 5–10 years after diagnosis in 188 patients with psychogenic non-epileptic seizures. *J Neurol Neurosurg Psychiatry* 2014;85(9):954–958.

25. Benbadis SR. A spell in the epilepsy clinic and a history of 'chronic pain' or 'fibromyalgia' independently predict a diagnosis of psychogenic seizures. *Epilepsy Behav* 2005;6(2):264–265.

26. Bowman ES, Markand ON. Psychodynamics and psychiatric diagnoses of pseudoseizure subjects. *Am J Psychiatry* 1996;153(1):57–63.

27. Bodde N, Brooks J, Baker G, et al. Psychogenic non-epileptic seizures: definition, etiology, treatment and prognostic issues. A critical review. *Seizure* 2009;18(8):543–553.

28. Pillai JA, Haut SR. Patients with epilepsy and psychogenic non-epileptic seizures: an inpatient video-EEG monitoring study. *Seizure* 2012;21(1):24–27.

29. Brigo F, Ausserer H, Nardone R, et al. Clinical utility of ictal eyes closure in the differential diagnosis between epileptic seizures and psychogenic events. *Epilepsy Res* 2013;104(1–2):1–10.

30. LaFrance WC Jr, Baker GA, Duncan R, et al. Minimum requirements for the diagnosis of psychogenic nonepileptic seizures: a staged approach. A report from the International League Against Epilepsy Nonepileptic Seizures Task Force. *Epilepsia* 2013;54(11):2005–2018.

31. Macrodimitris S, Sherman EMS, Forde S, et al. Psychiatric outcomes of epilepsy surgery: a systematic review. *Epilepsia* 2011;52(5):880–890.

32. Wilson S, Bladin P, Saling M. The 'burden of normality': concepts of adjustment after surgery for seizures. *J Neurol Neurosurg Psychiatry* 2001;70(5):649–656.

33. Morgan CL, Baxter H, Kerr MP. Prevalence of epilepsy and associated health service utilization and mortality among patients with intellectual disability. *Am J Ment Retard* 2003;108(5):293–300.

Headache

Ines Carreira Figueiredo, Nazia Karsan, Peter Goadsby

Headache is one of the most common medical complaints, representing 2% of emergency department visits and 4.4% of consultations in general practice [1,2]. Worldwide, migraines are in the top 40 conditions causing disability, and in the UK are responsible for an estimated annual loss of 230,000 disability-adjusted life-years [2]. Headache disorders are more prevalent in a variety of psychiatric conditions, including depression, anxiety, and stress-related disorders [3]. The relationship between headache and psychiatric presentations is multifactorial and bidirectional. For example, chronic pain increases the likelihood of developing a mood disorder [3], while a comorbid psychiatric diagnosis increases the frequency and severity of both tension-type headache and migraine, and reduces likelihood of a satisfactory treatment response [3,4], Furthermore, some psychiatric medications (e.g. selective serotonin reuptake inhibitors and benzodiazepines) [5,6] may worsen headache disorders, as can substance and alcohol abuse [4]. However, some antidepressants (e.g. amitriptyline, mirtazapine and venlafaxine) are used in the prevention of tension-type headache [7,8].

Acute headaches are classified as either primary or secondary (Box 54.1), with up to 90% of primary headaches consisting of migraines, tension-type, and cluster headaches [9]. While episodic tension-type headache is the most frequent headache reported in population-based studies [10], migraine is the most common headache disorder that presents to primary care [11]. Cluster headache is relatively uncommon and requires management within a specialist headache service. Although most patients presenting with headache will have a disabling but not life-threatening primary headache disorder, the assessing clinician should be aware of red flag signs/symptoms that may herald more serious pathoaetiology or a secondary headache disorder (Box 54.2) [1].

The Maudsley Practice Guidelines for Physical Health Conditions in Psychiatry, First Edition.
David M. Taylor, Fiona Gaughran, and Toby Pillinger.
© 2021 John Wiley & Sons Ltd. Published 2021 by John Wiley & Sons Ltd.

Box 54.1 Classification of headache [4]

Primary headaches

- Migraine
- Tension-type headache
- Trigeminal autonomic cephalalgias (e.g. cluster headache)
- Other primary headache disorders (e.g. primary cough headache, cold-stimulus headache)

Secondary headaches

- Trauma or injury to the head and/or neck
- Cranial and/or cervical vascular disorder (e.g. intracerebral haemorrhage, central venous thrombosis, giant cell arteritis)
- Non-vascular intracranial disorder (e.g. idiopathic intracranial hypertension or malignancy)
- Substance use or withdrawal (e.g. alcohol, cocaine, opioids, ergotamine, simple analgesics)
- Infection (e.g. viral or bacterial meningitis)
- Disorder of homoeostasis (e.g. hypotension, hypoxia)
- Disorder of the cranium, neck, eyes, ears, nose, sinuses, teeth, mouth or other facial or cervical structure (e.g. acute glaucoma, sinusitis, temporomandibular disorder)
- Psychiatric disorder (e.g. somatisation)

Painful cranial neuropathies, other facial pain, and other headaches

- Painful lesions of the cranial nerves and other facial pain (e.g. trigeminal neuralgia, neck–tongue syndrome, painful optic neuritis, burning mouth syndrome)
- Other headache disorders (e.g. not elsewhere classified, unspecified)

Box 54.2 Red flag signs/symptoms that may herald more serious pathoaetiology/secondary headache disorder

Headache red flags

'SNOOP': these should prompt discussion with neurology, and consideration of brain imaging.
- **S**ystemic symptoms (e.g. fever, weight loss) or secondary risk factors (e.g. HIV or cancer).
- **N**eurological symptoms or confusion/reduced Glasgow Coma Scale.
- **O**nset: sudden, e.g. thunderclap (possible subarachnoid haemorrhage).
- **O**lder: new onset and progressive headache especially age over 50 years (possible giant cell arteritis).
- **P**revious headache history: first headache or change in headache frequency/presentation.

Other red flag presentations

Includes headache in association with the following.
- Acute neck pain with Horner syndrome and/or focal neurology (possible cervical artery dissection).
- Neurological signs/symptoms, bilateral papilloedema, nausea and vomiting (raised intracranial pressure).
- Neck stiffness (meningitis).
- Subacute head trauma (intracranial bleed).
- Pregnancy or recently postpartum (cerebral venous thrombosis).

DIAGNOSTIC PRINCIPLES

History

1 Define headache location, temporal pattern, precipitating factors, associated features, and burden (i.e. impact headaches are having on an individual's functioning). Precipitating factors may include postural change, light, alcohol, menses, stress, and disturbed sleep. Associated symptoms such as sensory sensitivities, aura, and cranial autonomic symptoms can help differentiate primary from secondary headache disorder, and between the primary headache disorders described in Table 54.1.

2 Typical migraine is characterised by unilateral head pain worsened by movement and associated with nausea and sensitivity to light and/or sound. A family history of similar symptoms supports the diagnosis [12]. In those without a clear family history of migraine, or in the absence of a clear personal history of episodic tension-type headache, the presence of migraine markers such as headache after alcohol and headache associated with menses can be useful in assisting diagnosis.

3 Take a drug history including recent changes that may indicate a drug-related headache. Medication overuse headache should be considered if headache develops or worsens while taking the following drugs for three months or more (although causality versus consequence may be difficult to disentangle) [13]:

   a triptans, opioids, ergots, analgesic combinations (≥10 days per month)

   b aspirin, paracetamol or short-acting non-steroidal anti-inflammatories, either alone or in combination (≥15 days per month).

4 Associated fever is suggestive of infection such as encephalitis, meningitis, brain abscess or otitis media (see Chapter 81).

5 Simultaneous neck pain may point towards a musculoskeletal aetiology, meningitis, subarachnoid haemorrhage (sudden 'thunderclap' headache), or cervical artery dissection. However, the clinician should be aware that neck stiffness with migraine is relatively common [14,15].

6 Suspect menstrual-related migraine if it occurs predominantly between two days before and three days after the start of menstruation in more than two out of three consecutive menstrual cycles. Use of a headache diary for at least two menstrual cycles is recommended to help diagnosis [13].

7 Past medical history should document presence of the following.

   a Hypertension (see Chapter 5): hypertension may result in headache.

   b Immunodeficiency such as HIV infection (see Chapter 45): predisposes to rare infectious causes.

   c Connective tissue disorders such as systemic lupus erythematosus (see Chapter 60): cerebral vasculitis.

   d Malignancy: possible central nervous system metastases.

8 As part of the social history, quantify alcohol intake and psychotropic drug consumption.

Table 54.1 Tension-type headache, migraine and cluster headache syndromes [13].

	Tension-type	Migraine	Cluster
Location of pain	Bilateral	In adults, unilateral in 60–70%, bifrontal or global in 30%	Unilateral (usually begins around the eye or temple)
Characteristic of pain	Pressure, tightness (waxes and wanes pattern)	Gradual onset, crescendo Pulsating Moderate to severe intensity Worsened by physical activity	Rapid onset, crescendo within minutes Explosive Deep, continuous, excruciating pain
Duration	30 minutes to 7 days	4–72 hours	15–180 minutes

Associated symptoms	None	Nausea, vomiting, photophobia, phonophobia
		May have aura (usually visual, but can involve other senses, cause speech or motor deficits)
		Aura symptoms can occur with or without headache and:
		    are fully reversible.
		    develop over ≥5 minutes
		    last 5–60 minutes
			Ipsilateral lacrimation and redness of the eye
			Stuffy nose, rhinorrhoea
			Constricted pupil and/or drooping eyelid, swollen eyelid
			Pallor
			Sweating
			Restlessness or agitation
			Focal neurological symptoms (rare)
			Sensitivity to alcohol

Impact on functioning	Patient does not need to stop activity	Patient prefers a quiet, dark room	Patient remains active

Examination

Most patients presenting with headache have a normal physical examination.

1 Measure blood pressure and heart rate. As well as hypertension being associated with headache, some treatments used to treat headache disorders can affect blood pressure.
2 Examine for bruits at the neck, eyes, and head as clinical signs of arteriovenous malformation.
3 Palpate head, neck, and shoulders, examining spine and neck muscles. Palpation over the greater occipital nerve on each side may help to decide if this is a primary headache disorder. Tenderness on palpation of the greater occipital nerve (back of head, base of skull) may indicate occipital neuralgia and a good potential therapeutic opportunity with a local anaesthetic/steroid injection [16].
4 Examination of the neck in flexion versus lateral rotation for meningeal irritation. Even a subtle limitation of neck flexion may be considered an abnormality.
5 Check temporal arteries for superficial tenderness (possible temporal arteritis).
6 Perform a neurological examination, including assessment of orientation, cranial nerve examination, plantar responses, gait assessment, and arm–leg coordination.

CHAPTER 54

Investigations

While there is no routine set of investigations that must be done in every patient presenting with headache, there are several which may be helpful, depending on the clinical context.

1 A headache diary should be considered, recording the following for a minimum of eight weeks.
   a Frequency, duration and severity of headaches.
   b Associated symptoms.
   c Medications taken to relieve clinical symptoms.
   d Potential triggers.
   e If appropriate, relationship to menstruation.
2 Laboratory tests:
   a Full blood count: anaemia/infection may be associated with headache.
   b Urea and electrolytes: renal failure can cause headache.
   c Urinalysis: pregnancy with pre-eclampsia can cause headache.
   d Erythrocyte sedimentation rate, C-reactive protein, rheumatoid factor, antinuclear antibody: evidence of systemic inflammatory conditions, infection, autoimmune disorder, giant cell arteritis.
   e HIV test: immunodeficiency predisposing to infection.
   f Coagulation profile: protein C/S deficiency, factor V Leiden, lupus anticoagulant, and antiphospholipid antibodies (cerebral venous thrombosis).
   g Thyroid-stimulating hormone: hypothyroidism.
3 Neuroimaging is indicated for patients with red flag signs/symptoms or other features suggesting a secondary headache source (see Box 54.2 and Table 54.2) and should be discussed with a neurologist [17,18].

Table 54.2 Specific neuroimaging recommendations in patients with headaches [18].

Clinical presentation of headache	Recommended imaging modality
Sudden onset or thunderclap headache	Head CT (without contrast) Head CTA (with contrast) Head MRA (with and without contrast) *or* Head MRI (without contrast)
Severe unilateral headache by possible dissection of carotid	Head MRI (with and without contrast) Head and neck MRA *or* Head and neck CTA
Suspected meningitis	Head CT or MRI (without contrast, as a prelude to lumbar puncture)[a]
Pregnancy	Head CT or MRI (without contrast)
Suspected temporal arteritis	Head MRI (with and without contrast)
Immunodeficiency	Head MRI (with and without contrast)

[a] Waiting for imaging should *not* preclude early and prompt antibiotic treatment in suspected cases (see Chapter 81).
CT, computed tomography; CTA, computed tomographic angiography; MRA, magnetic resonance angiography; MRI, magnetic resonance imaging.

MANAGEMENT

Many headaches, particularly tension-type headaches, will settle spontaneously without the need for pharmacological treatment.

Non-pharmacological therapy

For primary headaches, education and lifestyle changes are often required.

1 Stress reduction, eating and sleeping schedules, and regular aerobic exercise benefit most patients.
2 Food and alcohol triggers are only present in a small percentage of patients.
3 The overuse of acute treatment drugs may result in chronic daily headache. The use of non-steroidal anti-inflammatory drugs (NSAIDs) for nine days or more a month or aspirin for more than 15 days was thought to be associated with increased risk but growing evidence suggests the opposite, pointing to opioids, ergots, triptans, and paracetamol instead [19].
4 It should be explained that primary headaches often are not eradicated completely, although remission can be achieved.

Some non-pharmacological adjunctive treatments are used in the treatment of migraine, especially in the elderly, and include cognitive-behavioural therapy, relaxation, and biofeedback, i.e. using information (feedback) about muscle tension to ease stress and thus reduce/attenuate migraine symptoms [20].

Pharmacological therapy

The pharmacological treatment of primary headaches is traditionally divided into two categories [2,20].

1 Acute abortive treatment, targeting the individual episode with pharmacological and/or non-pharmacological therapies. It is important to provide education and set therapeutic goals to prevent avoidance and/or overuse of the medication, and to advise trigger management where appropriate.
2 Preventive treatment to reduce the frequency, duration, and severity of headache episodes. Considered when attacks significantly affect daily functioning.

Acute treatments should be given according to diagnosis (Table 54.3) and early when the pain is mild [21]. It is important to take into consideration the patient's previous experience, comorbidities, and the potential for medication overuse [2]. Pharmacological treatment of acute headache should not regularly exceed more than two days per week.

Headaches occurring during perimenopause or after menopause may respond to hormonal therapy. Women presenting with migraine associated with aura have a higher risk of stroke with the use of oestrogen-containing contraceptives compared to those without migraine [22].

CHAPTER 54

Table 54.3 Pharmacological treatment of the most common types of headache.

	Tension-type headache [2,7,8,23,24]	Migraine [2,25–30]	Cluster headache [2,31–34]

Acute treatment	Paracetamol 1000 mg
	Aspirin 500–1000 mg
	NSAIDs:
	  Ibuprofen 200–800 mg
	  Ketoprofen 25 mg
	  Naproxen 250–500 mg
		Paracetamol 1000 mg
		(+ metoclopramide 10 mg accelerates gastric absorption of paracetamol)
		Aspirin 1000 mg
		Diclofenac 50 mg
		Ibuprofen 400 mg
		Tolfenamic acid 200 mg
		Naproxen 500–825 mg
		If analgesics ineffective:
		  Triptans (if first choice ineffective, consider increasing the dose, altering the mode of delivery or trying another member of the class)
		  Single pulse transcranial magnetic stimulation (sTMS)
		  Anti-emetics
		Metoclopramide 10 mg
		Domperidone 10 mg
		Buccal prochlorperazine or cyclizine
			Triptans:
			  Subcutaneous sumatriptan 6 mg
			Intranasal zolmitriptan 10 mg
			Intranasal sumatriptan 20 mg
			High-flow 100% oxygen (12 L/min delivered by face mask)
			Prednisolone ≥40 mg daily (up to 80% recurrence as dose is tailed off)
			Non-invasive vagus nerve stimulation (nVNS)

Preventive treatment	Amitriptyline 75 mg daily (starting at 10–25 mg daily, and titrated steadily upwards until positive response)
	Mirtazapine 30 mg daily
	Venlafaxine 150 mg daily
		Candesartan 16 mg
		Beta-blocker (propranolol, nadolol, metoprolol, atenolol, timolol and bisoprolol)
		Tricyclic antidepressant:
		  Amitriptyline at 1 mg/kg as tolerated
		  Nortriptyline
		  Imipramine
		Topiramate
		Fovatriptan 2.5 mg twice daily (especially useful in perimenstrual migraine)
		sTMS
		Botulinum toxin type A (if unresponsive to three or more preventive treatments and medication overuse headache has been addressed)
		Calcitonin-gene related peptide monoclonal antibodies:
		  Erenumab
		  Fremanezumab
		  Galcanezmab
			Verapamil 360 mg daily (titration may go up to 960 mg daily, with ECG monitoring)
			  Second-line therapies:
			  nVNS
			  Topiramate
			  Lithium carbonate
			  Melatonin

When to refer

Box 54.3 details when an emergency or specialty referral may be indicated. Headache specialist clinics may offer novel therapeutic avenues not available in primary care. These may include use of human monoclonal antibody treatment that binds to the

CHAPTER 54

Box 54.3 Indications to refer to emergency services or headache specialists

Emergency department

- Secondary headache diagnosis with red flag signs
- Patient in status migrainosus (an attack lasting longer than 72 hours)

Specialty consultation

- Diagnosis unclear
- Significant impact on quality of life despite treatment
- Failure of acute therapies
- Suspicion or likely diagnosis of a trigeminal autonomic cephalalgia
- Comorbid psychiatric diagnosis (may require multidisciplinary approach involving both psychiatric practitioner and headache specialist)

---

calcitonin-gene related peptide (CGRP) receptor. CGRP is released by neurons and is implicated in different pain processes, including migraine. Inhibition of CGRP function can therefore prevent migraine attacks. Other novel treatments include non-invasive neuromodulation and botulinum toxin type A injections (see Table 54.3).

References

1. Ramirez-Lassepas M, Espinosa CE, Cicero JJ, et al. Predictors of intracranial pathologic findings in patients who seek emergency care because headache. *Arch Neurol* 1997;54(12):1506–1509.
2. Weatherall MW. Drug therapy in headache. *Clin Med* 2015;15(3):273–279.
3. Minen MT, De Dhaem OB, Van Diest AK, et al. Migraine and its psychiatric comorbidities. *J Neurol Neurosurg Psychiatry* 2016;87(7):741–749.
4. Headache Classification Committee of the International Headache Society (IHS). The International Classification of Headache Disorders, 3rd edition. Asbtracts. *Cephalalgia* 2018;38(1):1–211.
5. Ferguson JM. SSRI antidepressant medications: adverse effects and tolerability. *Prim Care Companion J Clin Psychiatry* 2001;3(1):22–27.
6. Harnod T, Wang YC, Lin CL, Tseng CH. Association between use of short-acting benzodiazepines and migraine occurrence: a nationwide population-based case-control study. *Curr Med Res Opin* 2017;33(3):511–517.
7. Bendtsen L, Jensen R, Olesen J. A non-selective (amitriptyline), but not a selective (citalopram), serotonin reuptake inhibitor is effective in the prophylactic treatment of chronic tension-type headache. *J Neurol Neurosurg Psychiatry* 1996;61(3):285–290.
8. Bendtsen L, Jensen R. Mirtazapine is effective in the prophylactic treatment of chronic tension-type headache. *Neurology* 2004;62(10):1706–1711.
9. Lynch K, Brett F. Headaches that kill: a retrospective study of incidence, etiology and clinical features in cases of sudden death. *Cephalalgia* 2012;32(13):972–978.
10. Feigin VL, Abajobir AA, Abate KH, et al. Global, regional, and national burden of neurological disorders during 1990–2015: a systematic analysis for the Global Burden of Disease Study 2015. *Lancet Neurol* 2017;16(11):877–897.
11. Tepper SJ, Dahlof CGH, Dowson A, et al. Prevalence and diagnosis of migraine in patients consulting their physician with a complaint of headache: data from the Landmark Study. *Headache* 2004;44(9):856–864.
12. Goadsby PJ, Holland PR, Martins-Oliveira M, et al. Pathophysiology of migraine: a disorder of sensory processing. *Physiol Rev* 2017;97(2):553–622.
13. National Institute for Health and Care Excellence. *Headaches in over 12s: Diagnosis and Management.* Clinical Guideline CG150. London: NICE, updated November 2015. Available at https://www.nice.org.uk/guidance/cg150
14. Giffin NJ, Ruggiero L, Lipton RB, et al. Premonitory symptoms in migraine: an electronic diary study. *Neurology* 2003;60(6):935–940.
15. Karsan N, Prabhakar P, Goadsby PJ. Characterising the premonitory stage of migraine in children: a clinic-based study of 100 patients in a specialist headache service. *J Headache Pain.* 2016;17(1):94.
16. Afridi SK, Shields KG, Bhola R, Goadsby PJ. Greater occipital nerve injection in primary headache syndromes: prolonged effects from a single injection. *Pain* 2006;122(1–2):126–129.
17. Medical Advisory Secretariat. Neuroimaging for the evaluation of chronic headaches: an evidence-based analysis. *Ont Health Technol Assess Ser* 2010;10(26):1–57.

18. Strain JD, Strife JL, Kushner DC, et al. Headache. American College of Radiology. ACR Appropriateness Criteria. *Radiology* 2000;215(Suppl):855–860.

19. Schwedt TJ, Alam A, Reed ML, et al. Factors associated with acute medication overuse in people with migraine: results from the 2017 Migraine in America Symptoms and Treatment (MAST) study. *J Headache Pain* 2018;19(1):38.

20. Berk T, Ashina S, Martin V, et al. Diagnosis and treatment of primary headache disorders in older adults. *J Am Geriatr Soc* 2018;66(12):2408–2416.

21. Goadsby P, Gobel H, Insa SD, Vila C. 'Act when mild (AwM)': Early vs. non-early intervention with almotriptan in acute migraine. *Neurology* 2007;68(12):A261.

22. Sheikh HU, Pavlovic J, Loder E, Burch R. Risk of stroke associated with use of estrogen containing contraceptives in women with migraine: a systematic review. *Headache* 2018;58(1):5–21.

23. Prior MJ, Cooper KM, May LG, Bowen DL. Efficacy and safety of acetaminophen and naproxen in the treatment of tension-type headache. A randomized, double-blind, placebo-controlled trial. *Cephalalgia* 2002;22(9):740–748.

24. Steiner TJ, Lange R, Voelker M. Aspirin in episodic tension-type headache: placebo-controlled dose-ranging comparison with paracetamol. *Cephalalgia* 2003;23(1):59–66.

25. Derry S, Moore RA. Paracetamol (acetaminophen) with or without an antiemetic for acute migraine headaches in adults. *Cochrane Database Syst Rev* 2013;(4):CD008040.

26. Orr SL, Aube M, Becker WJ, et al. Canadian Headache Society systematic review and recommendations on the treatment of migraine pain in emergency settings. *Cephalalgia* 2015;35(3):271–284.

27. Ong JJY, Wei DY, Goadsby PJ. Recent advances in pharmacotherapy for migraine prevention: from pathophysiology to new drugs. *Drugs* 2018;78(4):411–437.

28. Myllyla VV, Havanka H, Herrala L, et al. Tolfenamic acid rapid release versus sumatriptan in the acute treatment of migraine: comparable effect in a double-blind, randomized, controlled, parallel-group study. *Headache* 1998;38(3):201–207.

29. Lipton RB, Dodick DW, Silberstein SD, et al. Single-pulse transcranial magnetic stimulation for acute treatment of migraine with aura: a randomised, double-blind, parallel-group, sham-controlled trial. *Lancet Neurol* 2010;9(4):373–380.

30. Starling AJ, Tepper SJ, Marmura MJ, et al. A multicenter, prospective, single arm, open label, observational study of sTMS for migraine prevention (ESPOUSE Study). *Cephalalgia* 2018;38(6):1038–1048.

31. May A, Leone M, Afra J, et al. EFNS guidelines on the treatment of cluster headache and other trigeminal-autonomic cephalalgias. *Eur J Neurol* 2006;13(10):1066–1077.

32. Cohen AS, Burns B, Goadsby PJ. High-flow oxygen for treatment of cluster headache: a randomized trial. *JAMA* 2009;302(22):2451–2457.

33. de Coo IF, Marin JC, Silberstein SD, et al. Differential efficacy of non-invasive vagus nerve stimulation for the acute treatment of episodic and chronic cluster headache: a meta-analysis. *Cephalalgia* 2019;39(8):967–977.

34. Gaul C, Diener HC, Silver N, et al. Non-invasive vagus nerve stimulation for PREVention and Acute treatment of chronic cluster headache (PREVA): a randomised controlled study. *Cephalalgia* 2016;36(6):534–546.

CHAPTER 54

Disorders of Sleep and Circadian Rhythm

Nicholas Meyer, Hugh Selsick

Problems with sleep and its timing are strikingly over-represented in patients with psychiatric disorders, and are associated with significant distress, dysfunction, and diminished quality of life. Despite accumulating evidence that sleep pathology is a core feature of psychiatric disorder, it remains under-recognised in this patient group. Conversely, certain sleep disorders may also present to the psychiatrist after being mis-interpreted as psychiatric in nature [1]. This chapter aims to introduce the practitioner to common sleep problems presenting in psychiatry, and to encourage clinicians to routinely enquire about sleep as part of their assessment. For a more comprehensive review, the reader is directed to Selsick and O'Regan [2] and Selsick [3].

DEFINITIONS OF COMMON SLEEP DISORDERS IN PSYCHIATRIC POPULATIONS

Insomnia

Insomnia is a difficulty in initiating or maintaining sleep, or waking too early despite adequate opportunity for sleep, that is associated with significant daytime impairment (e.g. impairment in attention and concentration) [4]. It is classified as chronic insomnia when occurring on at least three days of the week, for at least three months. In addition to having an enormous impact on quality of life, insomnia is comorbid with many psychiatric disorders [5–7] and is an independent risk factor for their development [8,9]. Therefore, insomnia should not be dismissed as merely arising secondary to another diagnosis, and shoulf rather be identified and managed as a co-occurring psychiatric disorder in its own right.

The Maudsley Practice Guidelines for Physical Health Conditions in Psychiatry, First Edition.
David M. Taylor, Fiona Gaughran, and Toby Pillinger.
© 2021 John Wiley & Sons Ltd. Published 2021 by John Wiley & Sons Ltd.

Obstructive sleep apnoea

Obstructive sleep apnoea (OSA) is an important yet frequently overlooked disorder in people with serious mental illness (SMI), and is covered separately in Chapter 49. Its cardinal symptoms are breathing disturbance that interrupts sleep, and consequent excessive daytime sleepiness.

Restless leg syndrome

Restless leg syndrome (RLS) is an unpleasant and irresistible urge to move the legs, often worsening in the evening, which is transiently relieved by movement [10]. Periodic limb movements in sleep (PLMS), which co-occurs in up to 80% of people with RLS [11], are repetitive, stereotyped movements of the lower limbs that occur during sleep. Both conditions interfere with sleep, often present with insomnia and daytime fatigue, and can be caused by several psychiatric medications [12]. They are also more common in people with attention deficit hyperactivity disorder, depression, and anxiety.

Hypersomnia

Hypersomnia describes excessive daytime sleepiness, usually accompanied by excessive duration of unrefreshing nocturnal sleep and/or extended time in bed [13]. Though definitions are evolving and heterogeneously defined, in recent classification systems [4] hypersomnia can occur secondary to a medical or psychiatric disorder, or medication (Table 54.1). Other sleep disorders (including OSA, RLS/PLMS, circadian rhythm disorder) and insufficient sleep due to lifestyle habits must first be excluded as a cause. Hypersomnia is a common feature of depression, bipolar disorder, and psychosis. Narcolepsy is a relatively uncommon cause of sleepiness and is not discussed further here.

Circadian rhythm disorders

Circadian rhythm disorders arise from misalignment of the internal clock with environmental light–dark cycles, leading to difficulty in falling asleep or staying awake at conventional times, and impairments in social and occupational functioning [14]. Categories include (i) delayed sleep phase disorder (DSPD), with consistently later sleep–wake times than are socially acceptable; (ii) advanced sleep phase disorder (ASPD), distinguished by a habitually earlier sleep onset and offset than is desired; and (iii) irregular sleep–wake rhythm disorder, with disorganised sleep–wake rhythms that are not entrained to the light–dark cycle.

Parasomnias

Parasomnias are undesirable behaviours or experiences that occur during non-REM sleep (sleepwalking, sleep terrors), REM sleep (nightmare disorder, REM sleep behavioural disorder), or the boundaries of sleep and wake [15]. REM behavioural disorder

Table 55.1 Prevalence and common causes of sleep disorders in the general and psychiatric patient population.

Sleep disorder	Causes in general population	Causes in psychiatric patient population
Insomnia	Predisposing: female sex, increasing age, low socioeconomic status, unemployment Precipitating: psychosocial stressors, e.g. life transitions, occupational or interpersonal problems Maintaining: ruminative cognitive style; distorted beliefs about consequences of sleep loss; maladaptive compensatory sleep habits aimed at maximising sleep Medications: beta-blockers, diuretics, statins, corticosteroids, hypnotic withdrawal, caffeine, nicotine	Same as in the general population, with additional contribution of: Psychopathology (including depression and mania, anxiety, hallucinations or delusions) that drive increased arousal Antidepressants (particularly SSRIs), stimulants (methylphenidate) Unsuitable sleeping environment and poor sleep hygiene
Restless leg syndrome and periodic limb movements in sleep	Female sex, increasing age, family history Medical: diabetes, kidney disease and dialysis, liver disease, spinal and peripheral neuropathy, immobilisation, iron deficiency Nicotine, caffeine, alcohol, antihistamines	Antipsychotics and other dopamine depleting/blocking agents Antidepressants, especially mirtazapine, SSRIs and SNRIs Others: lithium, antihistamines, melatonin, opiate withdrawal
Circadian rhythm disorders	Loss of circadian rhythmicity often accompanies ageing Genetic predisposition to advanced sleep phase disorder (ASPD) and delayed sleep phase disorder (DSPD)	Neurodegenerative disease Psychotropic medication may cause circadian disturbances Circadian dysregulation may be an intrinsic feature of several psychiatric disorders
Hypersomnias Idiopathic hypersomnia (IH) Hypersomnia due to medication Hypersomnia associated with psychiatric disorder	Uncertain, however a deficient arousal system and viral infection have been implicated Sedative medications, antihypertensives (α_1 and α_2 receptor antagonists), beta-blockers, antiarrhythmic agents	Multifactorial aetiology in psychiatric populations: Psychotropic medication, particularly antidopaminergic, anti-adrenergic, anticholinergic and antihistaminergic drugs; withdrawal of stimulant medication. Clozapine and quetiapine are particularly sedative Psychopathology: anergia, fatigue and avolition associated with depression and negative symptoms of schizophrenia Fewer scheduled occupational activities
Parasomnias	Stress, alcohol and sleep deprivation can trigger non-REM parasomnias Hypnotics, dopamine agonists and beta-blockers are associated with nightmare disorder	Parkinson's disease and Lewy body dementia can cause REM sleep disorder Nightmares and sleep terrors are associated with past traumatic experiences, and SSRI withdrawal Parasomnias can emerge following treatment with, or withdrawal from, antidepressants and antipsychotics

SNRI, serotonin/noradrenaline reuptake inhibitor; SSRI, selective serotonin reuptake inhibitor.

CHAPTER 55

is strongly predictive of neurodegeneration, particularly Parkinson's disease and Lewy body dementia. Though often unpleasant, hypnagogic (when falling asleep) and hypnopompic (on waking) hallucinations are common in the general population and are not necessarily pathological.

DIAGNOSTIC PRINCIPLES

Sleep history

1 Obtaining a thorough and systematic sleep history is the cornerstone of diagnosis, and is essential to guiding further management [16].
   Identify which category their primary complaint falls into, its time course, potential triggers, and functional impact.
   a Problems falling or staying asleep (suggestive of insomnia, RLS/PLMS, and circadian rhythm disorder).
   b Problems staying awake during the day (key differential diagnoses are OSA, RLS/PLMS, circadian rhythm disorder, and hypersomnia).
   c Unusual or complex behaviours occurring during sleep (suggestive of a parasomnia).
2 Explore the typical 24-hour sleep–wake pattern.
   a Pre-sleep routines: people with SMI can have limited awareness of sleep hygiene (e.g. avoiding caffeine or nicotine before bed) and may live in environments that are not conducive to healthy sleep.
   b Sleep routines: bedtime, time taken to fall asleep, number and duration of nocturnal awakenings, wake time, and rise time. Explore the *regularity* of routines over a typical week, which can be highly variable in SMI.
   c Daytime: number, time and duration of daytime naps; differentiate between *fatigue* (subjective weariness and tiredness) and *sleepiness* (increased tendency to fall asleep).
3 Screen for specific sleep disorders (Box 55.1).
4 Explore psychiatric and medical problems interfering with sleep.
   a Comorbid psychiatric disorders frequently affect sleep and circadian function.
   b Assess comorbid medical disorders, which may impact sleep through pain, discomfort, and their psychological impact.
5 Review medications and substance use.
   a Prescribed and over-the-counter agents which may interfere with sleep.
   b Drugs and alcohol, which may be used to aid sleep or promote wakefulness.
6 Family history: RLS, OSA, narcolepsy, circadian rhythm disorder, and non-REM parasomnias can cluster in families.

Physical examination

1 Examination of the oropharynx and cardiorespiratory system is particularly important when OSA is suspected (see Chapter 49).
2 Neurological and cognitive examination are important for assessment of possible parasomnia and sleep-related movement disorder.

CHAPTER 55

Box 55.1 Core features and key questions of common sleep disorders

Insomnia

Insomnia is conceptualised as a disorder of physiological hyperarousal: sufferers are typically fatigued but unable to sleep ('tired but wired'), and usually find it difficult to nap during the day.
    'Do you have difficulty falling asleep, or waking up during the night and getting back to sleep, or waking up too early?'
    'How does this affect you during the day?' (Ask about energy levels, concentration, memory, mood.)

RLS/PLMD

Always ask about RLS: *'When you try to relax in the evening and sleep at night, do you have unpleasant, restless feelings in your legs that can be relieved by walking or movement?'* [17]
    PLMS: patients are usually unaware of movements; however, a bed-partner may report repetitive, stereotyped movements during sleep or sleep onset.

Circadian rhythm disorders

'When do you feel most alert, and most sleepy?'
    ASPD: inability to stay awake until desired bedtime, and remain asleep until desired awakening time.
    DSPD: inability to fall asleep at desired time, and awaken at desired time.

Hypersomnias

Long sleep periods, long duration spent in bed, sleep inertia (grogginess and reduced alertness on waking), and excessive sleepiness and napping during the day. Sleep is often unrefreshing. Explore effects on mood and functioning.

Parasomnias

Non-REM disorders tend to occur earlier in the night, during deep sleep, are usually not remembered, and can involve complex behaviours.
    REM parasomnias occur toward the latter half of the night, when REM sleep predominates. They can involve intense dreams which are remembered, and violent movements associated with acting out of dreams.

Investigations

1 A sleep diary, usually completed by the patient over two weeks, can be a very useful tool for assessing longitudinal sleep patterns, particularly where insomnia or circadian rhythm disorder is suspected [18].
2 Measure serum ferritin in RLS/PLMS, as low iron (ferritin <75 µg/L) can be a cause.
3 Actigraphy (a wrist-worn device that measures movement) can be helpful for the diagnosis of circadian rhythm disorders.
4 Magnetic resonance imaging (MRI) may be warranted for excluding structural brain lesions in adult-onset REM parasomnias.
5 Laboratory sleep studies (polysomnography) are indicated for the diagnosis of parasomnias, narcolepsy, and sleep-related movement disorders.

CHAPTER 55

MANAGEMENT

The patient should be equipped with a basic understanding of the functions and mechanisms of sleep, and healthy sleep habits promoted. Where feasible, any medications associated with the sleep disorder should be withdrawn or switched to agents that are less likely to disrupt sleep. Alcohol or substance use should also be addressed.

Insomnia

Insomnia may be treated with hypnotic medications (benzodiazepines and Z-drugs), melatonin (e.g. 2 mg taken one to two hours before bedtime, licensed for up to 13 weeks), or sedating antihistamines. Where insomnia is comorbid with depression, sedative antidepressants in low doses (e.g. trazodone 50–150 mg, or mirtazapine 15–30 mg at bedtime) may be useful. Hypnotic drugs with shorter half-lives (e.g. zolpidem 5–10 mg at bedtime, licensed for up to four weeks) are preferred for treating sleep-onset insomnia, and those with longer duration of action (e.g. zopiclone 3.75–7.5 mg at bedtime, for up to four weeks) may be useful for middle or late insomnia. However, their efficacy and safety over longer periods is uncertain, and the evidence supporting cognitive-behavioural therapy (CBT) for insomnia (CBT-I) in chronic insomnia is more robust. CBT-I has been shown to be an effective intervention in patients with psychiatric disorder [19] and treatment of insomnia may also ameliorate comorbid psychiatric symptoms.

RLS/PLMS

Where appropriate, RLS/PLMS can be treated by iron supplementation (e.g. ferrous sulfate tablets 325 mg twice daily, until ferritin reaches at least 75 µg/L; see Chapter 15). In other cases, dopamine agonists such as ropinirole or pramipexole are effective [20]; however, the induction of impulse-control disorders is a risk with these drugs, which are also contraindicated in those with a history of psychosis. Pregabalin (e.g. 50–300 mg) or gabapentin (300–1200 mg) taken at night, one to two hours before symptoms emerge, may be a useful alternative.

Circadian rhythm disorders

Circadian rhythm disorders are treated with a combination of melatonin and light exposure, both of which must be carefully timed to delay or advance circadian phase, as appropriate. For example, DSPD is treated by administering melatonin (e.g. 2 mg six hours before habitual sleep), and with exposure to bright light upon waking.

Hypersomnia

Hypersomnia may respond to behavioural strategies such as planned naps, and treatment with stimulant medication (e.g. modafinil 100–200 mg twice daily, usually taken on waking or at lunch, or extended-release methylphenidate 18–108 mg in the morning). These medications are best prescribed and monitored by sleep specialists.

Parasomnias

In all parasomnias, risks to the safety of the patient and bed-partner should be assessed. REM-sleep behaviour disorders are treated with low doses of clonazepam, melatonin, or cholinesterase inhibitors; nightmare disorder may respond to cognitive strategies for restructuring thoughts. Non-REM parasomnias are often managed conservatively or treated with relaxation strategies and low-dose clonazepam (e.g. 0.5 mg at bedtime).

When to refer to a specialist

Given the ubiquity of sleep disturbances in their patients, psychiatric practitioners should develop a secure understanding of the main categories of sleep disorder and remain alert for them in daily practice. Psychiatrists must maintain awareness of the effects of many psychotropic medications on sleep and enquire about treatment-emergent or discontinuation effects.

In most cases, insomnia can be managed by the GP or psychiatrist, although specialist services offering CBT-I are increasingly available. Where hypersomnia, sleep-related movement disorder, circadian rhythm disorder, parasomnia or OSA are suspected, referral to a multidisciplinary sleep service for further assessment and management is warranted.

References

1. Stores G. Clinical diagnosis and misdiagnosis of sleep disorders. *J Neurol Neurosurg Psychiatry* 2007;78(12):1293–1297.
2. Selsick H, O'Regan D. Sleep disorders in psychiatry. *BJPsych Advances* 2018;24(4):273–283.
3. Selsick H (ed.) *Sleep Disorders in Psychiatric Patients*. Berlin: Springer, 2018.
4. American Academy of Sleep Medicine. *International Classification of Sleep Disorders*, 3rd edn. Darien, IL: AASM, 2014.
5. Xiang YT, Weng YZ, Leung CM, et al. Prevalence and correlates of insomnia and its impact on quality of life in Chinese schizophrenia patients. *Sleep* 2009;32(1):105–109.
6. Harvey AG, Talbot LS, Gershon A. Sleep disturbance in bipolar disorder across the lifespan. *Clin Psychol (New York)* 2009;16(2):256–277.
7. Buysse DJ, Rössler W, Eich D, et al. Prevalence, course, and comorbidity of insomnia and depression in young adults. *Sleep* 2008;31(4):473–480.
8. Baglioni C, Battagliese G, Feige B, et al. Insomnia as a predictor of depression: a meta-analytic evaluation of longitudinal epidemiological studies. *J Affect Disord* 2011;135(1):10–19.
9. Talbot LS, Stone S, Gruber J, et al. A test of the bidirectional association between sleep and mood in bipolar disorder and insomnia. *J Abnorm Psychol* 2012;121(1):39–50.
10. Allen RP, Earley CJ. Restless legs syndrome: a review of clinical and pathophysiologic features. *J Clin Neurophysiol* 2001;18(2):128–147.
11. Montplaisir J, Boucher S, Poirier G, et al. Clinical, polysomnographic, and genetic characteristics of restless legs syndrome: a study of 133 patients diagnosed with new standard criteria. *Mov Disord* 1997;12(1):61–65.
12. Hening WA, Allen RP, Chaudhuri KR, et al. Clinical significance of RLS. *Mov Disord* 2007;22(Suppl 18):S395–S400.
13. Sowa NA. Idiopathic hypersomnia and hypersomnolence disorder: a systematic review of the literature. *Psychosomatics* 2016;57(2):152–164.
14. Bjorvatn B, Pallesen S. A practical approach to circadian rhythm sleep disorders. *Sleep Med Rev* 2009;13(1):47–60.
15. Markov D, Jaffe F, Doghramji K. Update on parasomnias: a review for psychiatric practice. *Psychiatry (Edgmont)* 2006;3(7):69–76.
16. Selsick H. Taking a sleep history. In: Selsick H (ed.) *Sleep Disorders in Psychiatric Patients*. Berlin: Springer, 2018:41–62.
17. Ferri R, Lanuzza B, Cosentino FI, et al. A single question for the rapid screening of restless legs syndrome in the neurological clinical practice. *Eur J Neurol* 2007;14(9):1016–1021.
18. Carney CE, Buysse DJ, Ancoli-Israel S, et al. The consensus sleep diary: standardizing prospective sleep self-monitoring. *Sleep* 2012;35(2):287–302.
19. Harvey AG, Buysse DJ. *Treating Sleep Problems: A Transdiagnostic Approach*. New York: Guilford Press, 2018.
20. Hornyak M, Scholz H, Kohnen R, et al. What treatment works best for restless legs syndrome? Meta-analyses of dopaminergic and non-dopaminergic medications. *Sleep Med Rev* 2014;18(2):153–164.

CHAPTER 55

Extrapyramidal Side Effects

Graham Blackman, R. John Dobbs, Sylvia Dobbs

Extrapyramidal tracts originate in the brainstem and carry motor fibres to the spinal cord allowing unconscious and reflexive movement of muscles that control balance, locomotion, posture, and tone. Blockade of dopamine D2 receptors interferes with the functioning of these tracts, leading to extrapyramidal side effects (EPSEs) [1]. EPSEs can be broadly subdivided into three types: akathisia, parkinsonism, and dystonia (see Chapter 84). The reader is also directed to Chapter 57 on tardive dyskinesia.

All antipsychotics have the potential to cause EPSEs, particularly so-called first-generation antipsychotics [2]. In this context it has previously been recommended that patients are monitored for emergence of EPSEs on a weekly basis following imitation of an antipsychotic, for two weeks after reaching target antipsychotic dose, and on a two-weekly basis following any subsequent dose increases [3]. However, EPSEs can occur with a range of other psychiatric treatments including sodium valproate [4], lithium [5], and various antidepressants [6–8]. Thus, a large proportion of patients with serious mental illness (SMI) are at risk of EPSEs. Furthermore, there is evidence that patients with psychotic disorder may have an intrinsic predisposition to developing EPSEs; these side effects have been reported in up to 17% of antipsychotic-naive patients with schizophrenia [9,10]. People with SMI also present with risk factors that influence risk of developing EPSEs; alcohol and broader substance misuse increase EPSE risk [11–13].

Regardless of aetiology, EPSEs are debilitating and can interfere with motor tasks, communication, and activities of daily living; they are associated with poor quality of life and contribute to patchy psychiatric medication compliance and thus relapse [14,15]. This chapter provides the psychiatric practitioner with an approach to assessing a patient with suspected EPSEs before considering specific management approaches for akathisia, parkinsonism, and dystonia.

The Maudsley Practice Guidelines for Physical Health Conditions in Psychiatry, First Edition.
David M. Taylor, Fiona Gaughran, and Toby Pillinger.
© 2021 John Wiley & Sons Ltd. Published 2021 by John Wiley & Sons Ltd.

CLINICAL APPROACH

History

- Box 56.1 describes clinical features of akathisia, dystonia, and parkinsonism. Determine the time course of emergence of presumed EPSEs (e.g. confirming that they did not start prior to medical treatment).
- Determine the impact of EPSEs on functioning, quality of life, and whether the patient has considered stopping their psychiatric medication because of these side effects.
- Scrutinise medication history for causative agents, noting any newly prescribed medications or recent dose changes. The following psychiatric and non-psychiatric agents may be causative.
  - All antipsychotics [2].
  - Some mood stabilisers: sodium valproate and lithium; in both cases, however, EPSE risk is low [5,16].
  - Various antidepressants: many have been implicated, especially selective serotonin reuptake inhibitors (SSRIs), but overall risk of EPSE with antidepressants is low [6–8].
  - Anti-emetic and prokinetic medications, e.g. metoclopramide [17].
  - Phenothiazine calcium channel blockers [18].
  - Dopamine-depleting agents, e.g. vesicular monoamine transporter type 2 (VMAT2) inhibitors (tetrabenazine, valbenazine, deutetrabenazine), which may be used in the treatment of tardive dyskinesia (see Chapter 57) [19].
- Screen for any other potential causes of movement disorder, e.g. alcohol abuse, chronic liver disease, antiphospholipid syndrome, multiple sclerosis, vasculitis, and family history of neurological disease.
- As part of a social history, quantify alcohol intake and enquire about recreational drug use.

Box 56.1 Clinical features of akathisia, dystonia, and parkinsonism

Akathisia (a subjective unpleasant state of inner restlessness)

- Foot stamping when seated
- Constantly crossing/uncrossing legs
- Rocking from foot to foot
- Constantly pacing up and down

Dystonia (uncontrolled muscle spasm)

- Can impact any muscle group, e.g. oculogyric crisis, torticollis (neck rotation), retrocollis (neck extension), opisthotonos (backward arching of the head, neck, and spine), laryngeal dystonia
- Can impact ability to speak/swallow
- See Chapter 84 for further information

Parkinsonism

- A syndrome characterised by mask-like facies, resting tremor, lead-pipe rigidity, cogwheeling, bradykinesia, and bradyphenia (slowed thinking)

Examination

Examine the patient seated

- With the patient sat on a chair with hands on knees, observe hands and other body areas at rest.
- Ask the patient to open their mouth and observe the tongue at rest within the mouth. Then ask the patient to protrude the tongue and observe any abnormalities of tongue movement.
- Ask the patient to touch their thumb with each finger on the same hand as rapidly as possible for 10–15 seconds, then repeat for other hand (examining for bradykinesia).
- Examine the patient's arms for rigidity by flexing and extending the elbow and rotating the wrist. Assess for evidence of resistance (lead-pipe rigidity), or intermittent resistance overcome by passive movement (cogwheel rigidity).
- Ask the patient to sit on an examination couch or a desk so that their feet are not touching the floor. Examine the patient's legs for rigidity by flexing and extending, then swinging the leg in a pendular motion.
- Ask the patient to stretch both arms out in front and to spread the fingers and observe for postural tremor.
- Ask the patient to extend both arms to the side, raising them to shoulder level and then allowing them to fall freely down to the sides again. Observe freeness of fall, audible contact and rebound (for evidence of bradykinesia).

Examine the patient standing

Ask the patient to turn around through 360° and view from all sides; observe for involuntary truncal movements.

Examine the patient walking

Observe for characteristics of a parkinsonian stance and gait (forward and lateral lean, flexed arms, general poverty and slowness of movement, reduced arm swing). The classical shuffling 'festinating' gait is generally a late sign of parkinsonism.

Investigations

A diagnosis of EPSE does not normally require laboratory tests or imaging. However, if examination reveals focal neurology, then an MRI head may be considered to rule out structural disease. If Parkinson's disease (or a related nigrostriatal degeneration syndrome) is a differential diagnosis, then ^{123}I-FP-CIT single photon emission computed tomography (DaTSCAN) can be used; in drug-induced parkinsonism, striatal uptake of the isotope will be normal, whereas in Parkinson's disease, uptake will be reduced.

CHAPTER 56

MANAGEMENT

Akathisia

- A suggested management algorithm for akathisia is presented in Figure 56.1. Risk of akathisia is higher with first-generation antipsychotics and partial dopamine receptor agonists (aripiprazole, brexpiprazole, cariprazine) [20].
- Where akathisia is reported or observed, first consider a cautious dose reduction of the likely causative agent. If this is ineffective and ongoing psychotropic treatment is required, consider a switch to a drug with lower propensity to cause akathisia. In the case of antipsychotics, reasonable agents are quetiapine, olanzapine, and clozapine [20].
- Where symptoms persist, there is some (if weak) evidence of beta-blockers (propranolol) [21], anticholinergics (benzatropine) [22], benzodiazepines [23], serotonergic antagonists (e.g. mirtazapine) [24], and the α_2-adrenoceptor antagonist clonidine [25] being effective in reducing symptoms of akathisia. All agents are unlicensed for this indication.

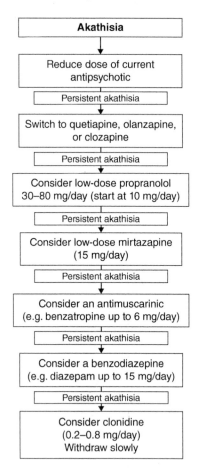

Figure 56.1 Suggested treatment algorithm for antipsychotic-induced akathisia.

Parkinsonism

- As described for akathisia, where antipsychotic-induced parkinsonism is reported or observed, first consider a cautious dose reduction of the causative agent.
- If side effects persist, consider switching to an agent with lower propensity to cause parkinsonism such as a partial dopamine receptor agonist (e.g. aripiprazole), quetiapine, olanzapine, or clozapine.
- If side effects persist, consider prescribing an anticholinergic, monitoring for side effects (e.g. dry mouth, urinary retention, constipation, and cognitive impairment). Review use of anticholinergics regularly. Example agents are:
  - procyclidine (initially 2.5 mg three times daily, increased in steps of 2.5–5 mg daily if required, increased if necessary to 30 mg daily in two to four divided doses)
  - benzatropine (initially 1–2 mg/day in divided doses, increased every three days up to a maximum of 8 mg/day).

Acute dystonia

The reader is directed to Chapter 84 for an in-depth discussion of its management. A recommended treatment algorithm is as follows.

- First-line treatment: oral/intramuscular/intravenous anticholinergic medication, depending on severity (e.g. procyclidine 5–10 mg p.o./i.m./i.v.) [26–28]. Intravenous treatment should have an effect within 5 minutes, intramuscular treatment may take 20 minutes, and oral treatment half an hour or more. Alternatively, some US sources suggest an intramuscular/intravenous antihistamine (e.g. diphenhydramine 1–2 mg/kg up to 100 mg by slow i.v. infusion) [26–28].
- Second-line treatment options:
  - Give second, and if necessary third, dose of anticholinergic at 10–30 minute intervals [26,28].
  - Diazepam 5–10 mg i.v. [26,28]. In laryngeal dystonia, parenteral benzodiazepines should be avoided because of the risk of respiratory depression [29].
- Subacute management:
  - Continue oral anticholinergic for 2–7 days [27,28].
  - Consider reducing dose of antipsychotic or switching to an agent with a lower propensity to cause dystonia (e.g. quetiapine, olanzapine, and clozapine) [26].

References

1. Marsden CD, Jenner P. The pathophysiology of extrapyramidal side-effects of neuroleptic drugs. *Psychol Med* 1980;10(1):55–72.
2. Leucht S, Wahlbeck K, Hamann J, Kissling W. New generation antipsychotics versus low-potency conventional antipsychotics: a systematic review and meta-analysis. *Lancet* 2003;361(9369):1581–1589.
3. Marder SR, Essock SM, Miller AL, et al. Physical health monitoring of patients with schizophrenia. *Am J Psychiatry* 2004; 161(8):1334–1349.
4. Lautin A, Stanley M, Angrist B, Gershon S. Extrapyramidal syndrome with sodium valproate. *BMJ* 1979;2(6197):1035–1036.
5. Kane J, Rifkin A, Quitkin F, Klein DF. Extrapyramidal side effects with lithium treatment. *Am J Psychiatry* 1978;135(7):851–853.
6. Guo MY, Etminan M, Procyshyn RM, et al. Association of antidepressant use with drug-related extrapyramidal symptoms: a pharmacoepidemiological study. *J Clin Psychopharmacol* 2018;38(4):349–356.

7. Hawthorne JM, Caley CF. Extrapyramidal reactions associated with serotonergic antidepressants. *Ann Pharmacother* 2015; 49(10):1136–1152.

8. Madhusoodanan S, Alexeenko L, Sanders R, Brenner R. Extrapyramidal symptoms associated with antidepressants: a review of the literature and an analysis of spontaneous reports. *Ann Clin Psychiatry* 2010;22(3):148–156.

9. Rybakowski JK, Vansteelandt K, Remlinger-Molenda A, et al. Extrapyramidal symptoms during treatment of first schizophrenia episode: results from EUFEST. *Eur Neuropsychopharmacol* 2014;24(9):1500–1505.

10. Pappa S, Dazzan P. Spontaneous movement disorders in antipsychotic-naive patients with first-episode psychoses: a systematic review. *Psychol Med* 2009;39(7):1065–1076.

11. Potvin S, Blanchet P, Stip E. Substance abuse is associated with increased extrapyramidal symptoms in schizophrenia: a meta-analysis. *Schizophr Res* 2009;113(2–3):181–188.

12. Hansen LK, Nausheen B, Hart D, Kingdon D. Movement disorders in patients with schizophrenia and a history of substance abuse. *Hum Psychopharmcol* 2013;28(2):192–197.

13. Duke PJ, Pantelis C, Barnes TRE. South Westminster Schizophrenia Survey: alcohol-use and its relationship to symptoms, tardive-dyskinesia and illness onset. *Br J Psychiatry* 1994;164:630–636.

14. Frances A, Weiden P. Treatment planning: promoting compliance with outpatient drug-treatment. *Hosp Community Psychiatry* 1987;38(11):1158–1160.

15. Haddad PM, Das A, Keyhani S, Chaudhry IB. Antipsychotic drugs and extrapyramidal side effects in first episode psychosis: a systematic review of head–head comparisons. *J Psychopharmacol* 2012;26(5 Suppl):15–26.

16. Brugger F, Bhatia KP, Besag FMC. Valproate-associated Parkinsonism: a critical review of the literature. *CNS Drugs* 2016;30(6):527–540.

17. Grimes JD, Hassan MH, Preston DN. Adverse neurologic effects of metoclopramide. *Can Med Assoc J* 1982;126(1):23–25.

18. Capella D, Laporte JR, Castel JM, et al. Parkinsonism, tremor, and depression induced by cinnarizine and flunarizine. *BMJ* 1988;297(6650):722–723.

19. Jankovic J, Casabona J. Coexistent tardive-dyskinesia and parkinsonism. *Clin Neuropharmacol* 1987;10(6):511–521.

20. Hirose S. The causes of underdiagnosing akathisia. *Schizophr Bull* 2003;29(3):547–558.

21. Adler L, Duncan E, Angrist B, et al. Effects of a specific beta-2-receptor blocker in neuroleptic-induced akathisia. *Psychiatry Res* 1989;27(1):1–4.

22. Adler LA, Peselow E, Rosenthal M, Angrist B. A controlled comparison of the effects of propranolol, benztropine, and placebo on akathisia: an interim analysis. *Psychopharmacol Bull* 1993;29(2):283–286.

23. Lima AR, Soares-Weiser K, Bacaltchuk J, Barnes TR. Benzodiazepines for neuroleptic-induced acute akathisia. *Cochrane Database Syst Rev* 2002;(1):CD001950.

24. Poyurovsky M, Pashinian A, Weizman R, et al. Low-dose mirtazapine: a new option in the treatment of antipsychotic-induced akathisia. A randomized, double-blind, placebo- and propranolol-controlled trial. *Biol Psychiatry* 2006;59(11):1071–1077.

25. Rose VL. APA practice guideline for the treatment of patients with schizophrenia. *Am Fam Physician* 1997;56(4):1217–1220.

26. Raja M. Managing antipsychotic-induced acute and tardive dystonia. *Drug Saf* 1998;19(1):57–72.

27. van Harten PN, Hoek HW, Kahn RS. Acute dystonia induced by drug treatment. *BMJ* 1999;319(7210):623–626.

28. Campbell D. The management of acute dystonic reactions. *Aust Prescr* 2001;24:19–20.

29. Christodoulou C, Kalaitzi C. Antipsychotic drug-induced acute laryngeal dystonia: two case reports and a mini review. *J Psychopharmacol* 2005;19(3):307–311.

Tardive Dyskinesia

Graham Blackman, Toby Pillinger, R. John Dobbs,
Sylvia Dobbs

Tardive dyskinesia (TD) is a syndrome of involuntary movements and postures (Box 57.1) that occurs after chronic use of dopamine receptor-blocking drugs, usually antipsychotics. The presence of at least mild TD has an overall global mean prevalence of 25% in patients receiving antipsychotic therapy [1]. However, there is substantial variability in prevalence between different populations of patients; 20% of patients currently receiving so-called second-generation antipsychotics have at least mild TD (although a proportion of these patients will have previously received first-generation antipsychotic treatment) compared with 30% of patients currently receiving first-generation antipsychotics [1]. Furthermore, prevalence of TD in patients who have only ever received second-generation antipsychotic therapy is much lower at 7% [1]. Risk factors for antipsychotic-induced TD include older age and longer duration of psychotic illness. There is also geographical variation in reported TD risk: TD prevalence is 17% in Asia, 22% in Europe, 31% in the USA, and 32% in the rest of the world (Australia, Africa, and Middle East) [1]. Other risk factors for TD that have been historically reported include early emergence of extrapyramidal symptoms following antipsychotic initiation (see Chapter 56); female sex; alcohol misuse; pre-existing mood, movement, or cognitive disorder; diabetes mellitus; and human immunodeficiency virus (HIV) infection [2–4]. There may be a genetic predisposition to TD: spontaneous TD has been reported in antipsychotic-naive patients with schizophrenia [5,6], siblings of patients with schizophrenia are more prone to TD than members of the general population [7], and there is evidence that a poor metaboliser phenotype of CYP2D6 is associated with increased TD risk [8]. The pathophysiology of TD is poorly understood; hypotheses include neuroleptic-induced dopamine supersensitivity, unbalanced blockade of D2 over D1 dopamine receptors, and excitotoxic loss of gamma-aminobutyric acid (GABA)-ergic striatal interneurons [9–11]. Regardless of aetiology, TD can be intolerable, painful, and physically disabling, and is associated with marked psychosocial

The Maudsley Practice Guidelines for Physical Health Conditions in Psychiatry, First Edition.
David M. Taylor, Fiona Gaughran, and Toby Pillinger.

Box 57.1 Involuntary movements characteristic of tardive dyskinesia

Oro-bucco-lingual and facial dyskinesia

- Tongue protrusion/twisting
- Smacking/pouting of lips
- Chewing movements
- Grimacing
- Blepharospasm and excessive eye blinking

Limb/trunk dyskinesia

- 'Piano playing' finger movements
- Tapping of feet
- Rocking/swaying of trunk
- Thrusting hip movements

Dystonia

- Retrocollis (neck extension)
- Torticollis (neck rotation)
- Opisthotonus (backward arching of the head, neck, and spine)
- Shoulder dystonia
- Hyperextension of limbs
- Blepharospasm
- Jaw dystonia
- Laryngeal dystonia

Tardive akathisia

Tics and tremors

---

difficulties including suicidality [12]. Orofacial dyskinesia can interfere with speech, eating, drinking, and even breathing [13].

CLINICAL APPROACH

History

TD should be suspected in any patient presenting with involuntary movements where there is a recent history of dopamine receptor blocker prescription, i.e. in patients still receiving treatment, or in patients who stopped treatment up to one month (oral) or two months (long-acting injectable depot formulation) earlier [14]. TD generally emerges after at least three months of treatment but can arise earlier. Other than antipsychotics, chronic use of the anti-emetic/promotility agent metoclopramide is associated with development of TD [15], as is use of other dopamine antagonists used as anti-emetics (e.g. prochlorperazine). There are case reports of the antidepressant amoxapine being associated with TD [16]. Anticholinergics may exacerbate TD symptoms, although this association may be an epiphenomenon since people who develop extrapyramidal side effects are both more likely to receive anticholinergic treatment and develop TD [17]. Indeed, there is some (limited) evidence that anticholinergic interventions can ameliorate TD [18,19].

'Withdrawal' TD may emerge when an antipsychotic is stopped, its dose reduced, or following switching to an agent with less potent D2 dopamine receptor antagonism [20]. This form of TD may improve when the antipsychotic is reinstated or dose increased. However, withdrawal TD may represent an early phase of neurological dysfunction ultimately leading to persistent TD [21].

If movement disorder has arisen early on in treatment, try to determine if the presentation is more in keeping with an extrapyramidal side effect (see Chapter 56). Screen for any other potential causes of movement disorder such as alcohol abuse, chronic liver disease, antiphospholipid syndrome, multiple sclerosis, vasculitis, and family history of neurological disease (including Huntington's).

Examination

With the patient at rest, screen for the involuntary movements characteristic of TD (see Box 57.1). Perform a neurological examination, checking gait, coordination, tone, and cognition. The predominance of neurological signs that do not include dyskinesia may indicate an alternative neurological diagnosis.

Investigations

A diagnosis of TD does not require any specific investigations unless an alternative cause of movement disorder is being considered.

MANAGEMENT

- A suggested algorithm for management of TD is presented in Figure 57.1. A multidisciplinary approach involving neurology is recommended where agents such as tetrabenazine and botulinum toxin are being considered.
- Where TD is suspected, review if the causative agent can be discontinued or dose reduced (first weighing up the risks and benefits of such an action). Where a first-generation antipsychotic is prescribed and ongoing treatment is indicated, consider switching to a second-generation antipsychotic. Clozapine is the antipsychotic most likely to be associated with resolution of symptoms [22]. Olanzapine and aripiprazole appear to confer the lowest risk of TD of all the non-clozapine second-generation antipsychotics [1]. Paradoxically, if withdrawal TD is suspected, resuming treatment with the antipsychotic may suppress TD.
- Evidence to support use of benzodiazepines in treatment of TD is mixed, but may be considered where first-line treatments have failed [23,24].

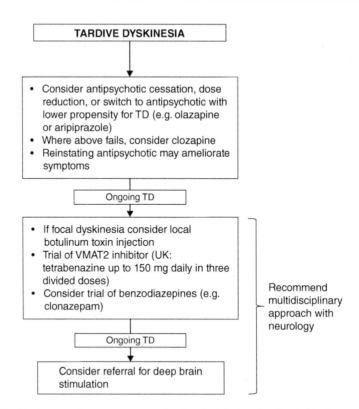

Figure 57.1 Algorithmic approach to management of antipsychotic-induced tardive dyskinesia.

- The vesicular monoamine transporter type 2 (VMAT2) inhibitor valbenazine has emerged in recent years as a novel treatment for TD (starting dose 40 mg daily increasing to 80 mg daily if necessary; monitor for QTc prolongation) [25–27]; there are also limited data from the 1970s and 1980s supporting the use of another VMAT2 inhibitor tetrabenazine (starting dose 12.5 mg daily increasing up to 150 mg daily) for the same purpose [18,28,29]. Deutetrabenazine also has evidence of efficacy of treating TD [30]. Valbenazine is not currently available in the UK.
- Other oral drug treatments with some (if mixed) evidence of efficacy in the treatment of TD include vitamin E (600–1600 units daily) [31], ginko biloba [32], and anticholinergics [18].
- Botulinum toxin may be used where there are localised/focal dyskinetic movements (e.g. laryngeal/cervical dystonia or blepharospasm) [33].
- Deep brain stimulation (to the globus pallidus) has been used successfully in a small number of patients with neuroleptic-induced TD resistant to medical management [34].

References

1. Carbon M, Hsieh CH, Kane JM, Correll CU. Tardive dyskinesia prevalence in the period of second-generation antipsychotic use: a meta-analysis. *J Clin Psychiatry* 2017;78(3):e264–e278.

2. Eberhard J, Lindstrom E, Levander S. Tardive dyskinesia and antipsychotics: a 5-year longitudinal study of frequency, correlates and course. *Int Clin Psychopharmacol* 2006;21(1):35–42.

3. Margolese HC, Chouinard G, Kolivakis TT, et al. Tardive dyskinesia in the era of typical and atypical antipsychotics. Part 2: Incidence and management strategies in patients with schizophrenia. *Can J Psychiatry* 2005;50(11):703–714.

4. Shedlack KJ, Soldatocouture C, Swanson CL. Rapidly progressive tardive-dyskinesia in Aids. *Biol Psychiatry* 1994;35(2):147–148.

5. Khot V, Wyatt RJ. Not all that moves is tardive-dyskinesia. *Am J Psychiatry* 1991;148(5):661–666.

6. McCreadie RG, Thara R, Padmavati R, et al. Structural brain differences between never-treated patients with schizophrenia, with and without dyskinesia, and normal control subjects: a magnetic resonance imaging study. *Arch Gen Psychiatry* 2002;59(4):332–336.

7. van Harten PN, Tenback DE. Tardive dyskinesia: clinical presentation and treatment. *Int Rev Neurobiol* 2011;98:187–210.

8. Andreassen OA, MacEwan T, Gulbrandsen AK, et al. Nonfunctional CYP2D6 alleles and risk for neuroleptics-induced movement disorders in schizophrenic patients. *Psychopharmacology* 1997;131(2):174–179.

9. Trugman JM. Tardive dyskinesia: diagnosis, pathogenesis, and management. *Neurologist* 1998;4(4):180–187.

10. Gerlach J, Hansen L. Clozapine and D1/D2 antagonism in extrapyramidal functions. *Br J Psychiatry* 1992;160:34–37.

11. Dekeyser J. Excitotoxic mechanisms may be involved in the pathophysiology of tardive-dyskinesia. *Clin Neuropharmacol* 1991;14(6):562–565.

12. Yassa R. Functional impairment in tardive-dyskinesia: medical and psychosocial dimensions. *Acta Psychiatr Scand* 1989;80(1):64–67.

13. Strassnig M, Rosenfeld A, Harvey PD. Tardive dyskinesia: motor system impairments, cognition and everyday functioning. *CNS Spectr* 2018;23(6):370–377.

14. Waln O, Jankovic J. An update on tardive dyskinesia: from phenomenology to treatment. *Tremor Other Hyperkinet Mov (NY)* 2013;3:tre-03-161-4138-1.

15. Ganzini L, Casey DE, Hoffman WF, McCall AL. The prevalence of metoclopramide-induced tardive-dyskinesia and acute extrapyramidal movement-disorders. *Arch Intern Med* 1993;153(12):1469–1475.

16. Madhusoodanan S, Alexeenko L, Sanders R, Brenner R. Extrapyramidal symptoms associated with antidepressants: a review of the literature and an analysis of spontaneous reports. *Ann Clin Psychiatry* 2010;22(3):148–156.

17. Bergman H, Soares-Weiser K. Anticholinergic medication for antipsychotic-induced tardive dyskinesia. *Cochrane Database Syst Rev* 2018;(1):CD000204.

18. Kang UJ, Burke RE, Fahn S. Natural-history and treatment of tardive dystonia. *Neurology* 1986;36(4):121–121.

19. Suzuki T, Hori T, Baba A, et al. Effectiveness of anticholinergics and neuroleptic dose reduction on neuroleptic induced pleurothotonus (the Pisa syndrome). *J Clin Psychopharmacol* 1999;19(3):277–280.

20. Polizos P, Engelhardt DM, Hoffman SP, Waizer J. Neurological consequences of psychotropic drug withdrawal in schizophrenic children. *J Autism Child Schizophr* 1973;3(3):247–253.

21. Schultz SK, Miller DD, Arndt S, et al. Withdrawal-emergent dyskinesia in patients with schizophrenia during antipsychotic discontinuation. *Biol Psychiatry* 1995;38(11):713–719.

22. Pardis P, Remington G, Panda R, et al. Clozapine and tardive dyskinesia in patients with schizophrenia: a systematic review. *J Psychopharmacol* 2019;33(10):1187–1198.

23. Thaker GK, Nguyen JA, Strauss ME, et al. Clonazepam treatment of tardive-dyskinesia: a practical GABA-mimetic strategy. *Am J Psychiatry* 1990;147(4):445–451.

24. Bergman H, Bhoopathi PS, Soares-Weiser K. Benzodiazepines for antipsychotic-induced tardive dyskinesia. *Cochrane Database Syst Rev* 2018;(1):CD000205.

25. Hauser RA, Factor SA, Marder SR, et al. KINECT 3: A phase 3 randomized, double-blind, placebo-controlled trial of valbenazine for tardive dyskinesia. *Am J Psychiatry* 2017;174(5):476–484.

26. O'Brien CF, Jimenez R, Hauser RA, et al. NBI-98854, a selective monoamine transport inhibitor for the treatment of tardive dyskinesia: a randomized, double-blind, placebo-controlled study. *Mov Disord* 2015;30(12):1681–1687.

27. McIntyre RS, Calabrese JR, Nierenberg AA, et al. The effects of valbenazine on tardive dyskinesia in patients with a primary mood disorder. *J Affect Disord* 2019;246:217–223.

28. Godwin-Austen RB, Clark T. Persistent phenothiazine dyskinesia treated with tetrabenazine. *BMJ* 1971;4(5778):25–26.

29. Kazamatsuri H, Chien C, Cole JO. Treatment of tardive dyskinesia. 1. Clinical efficacy of a dopamine-depleting agent, tetrabenazine. *Arch Gen Psychiatry* 1972;27(1):95–99.

30. Fernandez HH, Factor SA, Hauser RA, et al. Randomized controlled trial of deutetrabenazine for tardive dyskinesia: the ARM-TD study. *Neurology* 2017;88(21):2003–2010.

31. Soares-Weiser K, Maayan N, Bergman H. Vitamin E for antipsychotic-induced tardive dyskinesia. *Cochrane Database of Systematic Reviews.* 2018;(1):CD000209.

32. Zhang WF, Tan YL, Zhang XY, et al. Extract of *Ginkgo biloba* treatment for tardive dyskinesia in schizophrenia: a randomized, double-blind, placebo-controlled trial. *J Clin Psychiatry* 2011;72(5):615–621.

33. Bhidayasiri R, Fahn S, Weiner WJ, et al. Evidence-based guideline: Treatment of tardive syndromes. Report of the Guideline Development Subcommittee of the American Academy of Neurology. *Neurology* 2013;81(5):463–469.

34. Pouclet-Courtemanche H, Rouaud T, Thobois S, et al. Long-term efficacy and tolerability of bilateral pallidal stimulation to treat tardive dyskinesia. *Neurology* 2016;86(7):651–659.

Tremor

Graham Blackman, R. John Dobbs, Sylvia Dobbs

Tremor is defined as involuntary rhythmic oscillation of one or more body parts due to alternating contractions of reciprocally acting muscles [1]. It is the most commonly observed movement disorder [2] and usually affects the hands but can also involve the arms, legs, torso, and head/neck. In the field of psychiatry, tremor is often due to extrapyramidal side effects (EPSE) and tardive dyskinesia (TD) (see Chapters 56 and 57). However, there are several other causes of tremor (Box 58.1), some of which may be more prevalent in patients with serious mental illness, such as associated with anxiety or functional neurological disorder, recreational drug use/withdrawal (e.g. alcohol), neurological disease with psychiatric sequalae (e.g. Parkinson's disease and Lewy body dementia), and non-EPSE tremor associated with psychiatric drug use [3]. Tremor, especially in association with psychiatric comorbidity (e.g. anxiety and depression), can have a significant impact on functioning and quality of life [4]. This chapter considers causes of tremor other than EPSE/TD, detailing an approach to assessment and management.

CLINICAL APPROACH

Although tremor is a common presentation, it can also portend significant pathology such as alcohol withdrawal, hypoglycaemia, and thyrotoxicosis (see, respectively, Chapters 24, 74, and 79 for the assessment and management of these presentations).

The Maudsley Practice Guidelines for Physical Health Conditions in Psychiatry, First Edition.
David M. Taylor, Fiona Gaughran, and Toby Pillinger.
© 2021 John Wiley & Sons Ltd. Published 2021 by John Wiley & Sons Ltd.

CHAPTER 58

Box 58.1 Types of tremor

Resting tremor

- Parkinson's disease
- Parkinson's plus syndromes (multisystem atrophy, progressive supranuclear palsy, corticobasal degeneration)
- Lewy body dementia
- Parkinsonism (toxin/drug-induced; see Chapter 56)
- Wilson's disease (can cause resting, action, or mixed tremor)

Action tremor

- Essential tremor
- Enhanced physiological tremor, e.g. enhanced adrenergic activity secondary to anxiety, stimulant use (e.g. caffeine, nicotine, cocaine/amphetamines), β-adrenergic agonists (e.g. salbutamol), tricyclic antidepressants and selective serotonin reuptake inhibitors [3], alcohol withdrawal, hyperthyroidism (see Chapter 12), hypoglycaemia (see Chapter 74). Certain other medications and toxins can enhance physiological tremor via as yet undetermined mechanisms (e.g. lithium, sodium valproate, mercury, lead, and arsenic)
- Cerebellar tremor: secondary to alcoholism (see Chapter 24), stroke (see Chapter 82), multiple sclerosis
- Orthostatic tremor (tremor confined to the trunk and legs on standing)
- Neuropathic tremor (i.e. tremor in the presence of a peripheral neuropathy)
- Genetic, e.g. fragile X tremor ataxia syndrome (FXTAS)
- Wilson's disease (can cause resting, action, or mixed tremor)

Mixed tremor

- Some drug-induced tremors (e.g. EPSEs) can present with mixed tremor
- Dystonic tremor (tremor occurring in a body part affected by dystonia)
- Wilson's disease (can cause resting, action, or mixed tremor)
- Functional tremor (previously termed 'psychogenic tremor') is a tremor typically of rapid onset, complex/variable movements, and with disability out of proportion to degree of tremor

---

History

- Determine age of tremor onset: although Parkinson's disease can occur at any age, symptoms typically emerge in patients in their fifties or sixties, or older. The prevalence and incidence of essential tremor increase with age but can appear in early adulthood in familial essential tremor. Wilson's disease occurs in patients under 40 years of age and should be considered in patients presenting with an atypical tremor below this age.
- Determine speed of tremor onset: most tremors have a gradual onset and are noticed intermittently before occurring constantly. If a tremor starts abruptly, a functional (psychogenic) cause should be considered.
- Determine whether the presentation is in keeping with a resting or action tremor (or both). An action tremor occurs during voluntary movement of a muscle. A resting tremor occurs when the muscle is relaxed and is often limited to the hands or

fingers; this type of tremor is most often seen in people with Parkinson's disease or other parkinsonian syndromes and is referred to as a 'pill-rolling' tremor. Pill rolling is where the thumb and forefinger rub rhythmically against each other in a rotating movement, resembling the technique used by nineteenth-century pill rollers trained in the art of preparing and dispensing drugs.

- Determine the body region affected: parkinsonism typically affects the arms, legs and head; essential tremor typically affects the hands, head, and voice, but uncommonly the legs; isolated head tremor may suggest a dystonic tremor.
- Determine if there any associated symptoms, e.g. bradykinesia or postural instability of Parkinson's disease.
- Determine if there are any alleviating or exacerbating factors: most causes of tremor worsen with anxiety, cold, and fatigue. Improvement with alcohol and worsening with caffeine is suggestive of essential tremor.
- Assess degree of associated functional limitation, such as ability to hold a cup or write.
- Scrutinise medication lists for causative agents, including:
  - antipsychotics (all) [5]
  - antidepressants (all) [6–8]
  - mood stabilisers (lithium, sodium valproate, lamotrigine) [9,10]
  - stimulants (e.g. methylphenidate)
  - agents that deplete dopamine (e.g. vesicular monoamine transporter 2 inhibitors such as tetrabenazine, valbenazine, and deutetrabenazine)
  - metoclopramide [11]
  - phenothiazine calcium channel blockers [12]
  - amiodarone
  - immunosuppressants (e.g. ciclosporin, tacrolimus, corticosteroids)
  - asthma medications (e.g. salbutamol, theophylline)
  - hormonal treatments (e.g. thyroxine).
- Screen for comorbidity with which tremor may associated, e.g. multiple sclerosis, stroke (screen also for cardiovascular risk factors), and neuropathy.
- Screen for a family history of tremor: essential tremor is familial in approximately 50% of cases and follows an autosomal dominant pattern of inheritance.
- As part of a social history, determine alcohol intake, use of recreational drugs, and likelihood of exposure to any toxins associated with tremor (e.g. lead).

Examination

- Examine the patient at rest. Attempt to differentiate the tremor from other motor disorders such as myoclonus (shock-like jerks) or dystonia (uncontrolled muscle spasm). The patient should be observed with hands resting on the lap (resting tremor), hands held straight out in front (postural tremor), and when engaging in finger-to-nose movements (intention/action tremor). Localise the tremor, for example hands, arms, legs, trunk, or head (tremor of Parkinson's disease, but not parkinsonism, is often unilateral), and define its frequency and amplitude (e.g. fine or coarse tremor). A tremor that is distractible, of varying frequency, or demonstrates entrainment (disappears transiently or changes in rhythm when copying movements with the opposing arm or leg) is suggestive of a functional tremor.

- Perform a full neurological examination including cranial nerves. In the case of progressive supranuclear palsy there may be impaired vertical eye movement; in multiple sclerosis there may be a relative afferent pupillary defect.
- As part of an assessment for parkinsonism, check for gait disturbance (bradykinesia, decreased arm swing, festinating gait), lead-pipe rigidity, cogwheeling, and mask-like facies.
- As part of an assessment for cerebellar symptoms, test for nystagmus, dysmetria on finger-to-nose movements, dysdiadochokinesia, rebound phenomenon, and cerebellar ataxia.
- If history is suggestive, perform a thyroid examination (see Chapter 12 for full description) or an abdominal examination in the context of suspected Wilson's disease.

Investigations

- Bloods:
    - Liver, renal, and thyroid function tests.
    - If Wilson's disease is suspected, test serum ceruloplasmin alongside 24-hour urinary copper.
    - If appropriate, check serum lithium concentration. A fine tremor is a common side effect but a course tremor can be a sign of lithium toxicity.
- If history or examination is suggestive, consider neuroimaging (MRI or CT) to exclude stroke, tumour, multiple sclerosis, or structural causes of parkinsonism.
- If Parkinson's disease (or a related nigrostriatal degeneration syndrome) is a differential diagnosis, then ^{123}I-FP-CIT single photon emission computed tomography (DaTSCAN) can be used; in drug-induced parkinsonism, striatal uptake of the isotope will be normal, whereas in Parkinson's disease, uptake will be reduced.

MANAGEMENT

Please see Chapters 56 and 57 for the management of EPSE and TD. Where a psychiatric drug is suspected of causing the tremor, a risk–benefit decision regarding continuing that agent should be made. Cautious dose reduction prior to switching the agent may be trialled.

Patients with neurological conditions such as Parkinson's disease (or related syndromes), cerebellar disease, and multiple sclerosis will be managed by neurology. Where Parkinson's disease develops in the context of psychotic illness, a multidisciplinary approach involving both neurology and psychiatry is required to appropriately manage the symptoms of both disorders. Clozapine is a reasonable antipsychotic to use in such a circumstance, regardless of whether the patient has treatment-resistant psychosis (in which case clozapine use would be off-licence) [13].

Essential tremor

Essential tremor may improve with simple lifestyle interventions (e.g. reduce caffeine intake). Depending on the severity of symptoms and impact on the patient's life, medical management may be indicated; intermittent treatment may be enough in some cases such as during a stressful period. Propranolol is usually first-line medical management for essential tremor [14]. The usual starting dose is 40 mg two to three times a day, but a lower dose is indicated in elderly patients. A slow-release preparation can be used once a stable dose is achieved. A typical maintenance dose is 80–160 mg daily. Advise the patient of potential side effects that include dizziness, fatigue, and erectile dysfunction. Propranolol should not be used in patients with asthma and related respiratory disorders. Caution should be observed in patients with diabetes mellitus. If propranolol is not tolerated or contraindicated, primidone is a common alternative treatment [14]. Primidone is an anticonvulsant of the barbiturate class, which is licenced for treatment of essential tremor in the UK. The starting dose is 50 mg daily, increased as appropriate to a maximum of 750 mg daily. Warn the patient of side effects that include drowsiness, nausea, and apathy; caution should be taken when prescribing in the elderly. Primidone is a potent central nervous system depressant and prolonged administration can lead to tolerance, dependence, and a withdrawal reaction on abrupt cessation. Other treatments available for essential tremor include topiramate and gabapentin. Botulinum toxin injections may be effective for vocal tremor.

Enhanced physiological tremor

Enhanced physiological tremor is managed by treating any underlying illness (physical/mental), reducing/stopping caffeine and/or recreational drug use, and withdrawing any causative prescribed agents. Single doses of propranolol may be taken prior to any events that exacerbate tremor (e.g. public speaking).

Functional tremor

Management of functional tremor is focused on non-pharmacological approaches. There is evidence that specialist physiotherapy incorporating graded exercise and cognitive-behavioural therapy (addressing cognitive distortions and promoting behavioural changes) are effective and well tolerated [15]. There is limited evidence for the role of pharmacotherapy in functional tremor. Antidepressant medication, particularly selective serotonin reuptake inhibitors, may be helpful [16].

When to refer

Essential tremor and medication-induced causes of tremor can usually be managed in primary care. Neurological causes, such as Parkinson's disease, warrant input by a neurologist and/or geriatrician. Frequent falls, which may be a feature of postural hypotension (see Chapter 6) in the context of Parkinson's, may warrant referral to a specialist service designed to reduce falls risk (a 'falls prevention clinic'). Functional tremor is optimally managed by either a neuropsychiatry or motor disorder neurology service with access to multidisciplinary services including physiotherapy and cognitive-behavioural therapy.

References

1. Bhatia KP, Bain P, Bajaj N, et al. Consensus statement on the classification of tremors. From the Task Force on Tremor of the International Parkinson and Movement Disorder Society. *Mov Disord* 2018;33(1):75–87.
2. Wasielewski PG, Burns JM, Koller WC. Pharmacologic treatment of tremor. *Mov Disord* 1998;13:90–100.
3. Arbaizar B, Gomez-Acebo I, Llorca J. Postural induced-tremor in psychiatry. *Psychiatry Clin Neurosci* 2008;62(6):638–645.
4. Chandran V, Pal PK. Quality of life and its determinants in essential tremor. *Parkinsonism Relat Disord* 2013;19(1):62–65.
5. Leucht S, Wahlbeck K, Hamann J, Kissling W. New generation antipsychotics versus low-potency conventional antipsychotics: a systematic review and meta-analysis. *Lancet* 2003;361(9369):1581–1589.
6. Guo MY, Etminan M, Procyshyn RM, et al. Association of antidepressant use with drug-related extrapyramidal symptoms a pharmacoepidemiological study. *J Clin Psychopharmacol* 2018;38(4):349–356.
7. Hawthorne JM, Caley CF. Extrapyramidal reactions associated with serotonergic antidepressants. *Ann Pharmacother* 2015;49(10):1136–1152.
8. Madhusoodanan S, Alexeenko L, Sanders R, Brenner R. Extrapyramidal symptoms associated with antidepressants: a review of the literature and an analysis of spontaneous reports. *Ann Clin Psychiatry* 2010;22(3):148–156.
9. Brugger F, Bhatia KP, Besag FMC. Valproate-associated Parkinsonism: a critical review of the literature. *CNS Drugs* 2016;30(6):527–540.
10. Kane J, Rifkin A, Quitkin F, Klein DF. Extrapyramidal side effects with lithium treatment. *Am J Psychiatry* 1978;135(7):851–853.
11. Grimes JD, Hassan MH, Preston DN. Adverse neurologic effects of metoclopramide. *Can Med Assoc J* 1982;126(1):23–25.
12. Capella D, Laporte JR, Castel JM, et al. Parkinsonism, tremor, and depression induced by cinnarizine and flunarizine. *BMJ* 1988;297(6650):722–723.
13. Klein C, Gordon J, Pollak L, Rabey JM. Clozapine in Parkinson's disease psychosis: 5-year follow-up review. *Clin Neuropharmacol* 2003;26(1):8–11.
14. Zesiewicz TA, Sullivan KL, Ponce de Leon M, et al. Quality improvement in neurology: essential tremor quality measurement set. *Neurology* 2017;89(12):1291–1295.
15. Ricciardi L, Edwards MJ. Treatment of functional (psychogenic) movement disorders. *Neurotherapeutics* 2014;11(1):201–207.
16. Voon V, Lang AE. Antidepressant treatment outcomes of psychogenic movement disorder. *J Clin Psychiatry* 2005;66(12):1529–1534.

Part 10

Rheumatology and Musculoskeletal Health

Low Back Pain

Jennifer Ireland, Matthew Cheetham

In the general population, low back pain has a lifetime incidence of approximately 85% and represents a leading cause of disability worldwide [1]. Poor mental health is recognised as both a risk factor and a consequence of low back pain [2]. This chapter focuses on an approach to non-specific/mechanical low back pain, defined by the National Institute for Health and Care Excellence (NICE) as 'tension, soreness, and/or stiffness in the lower back region for which it is not possible to identify a specific cause' [3]. This presentation represents the overwhelming burden of back pain disease [4].

Although the aetiology of non-specific/mechanical low back pain is incompletely understood, it is considered to arise from disorders of various spinal anatomical structures, including muscles, vertebrae, facet joints, intervertebral discs, fascia, and ligaments. A combination of personal, social, and psychological factors also contribute. There is growing evidence that non-specific low back pain may be a manifestation of undiagnosed depression [2]. However, whether depression and back pain are causal, correlated, mutually exacerbating, or synergistic is unclear [5]. Major depressive disorder is the most common serious mental illness (SMI) associated with low back pain [6]. Those with anxiety, somatoform, and substance misuse disorders are also at an increased risk of developing non-specific low back pain [6]. This association is unsurprising when one considers that chronic pain, anxiety, and depression may share common underlying neural, behavioural, and cognitive patterns [7]. Both pain and depression are associated with, and exacerbated by, social isolation and reduced physical activity [8,9]. Moreover, experiencing pain can stimulate feelings of anxiety, which can in turn increase sensitivity to pain [2].

The Maudsley Practice Guidelines for Physical Health Conditions in Psychiatry, First Edition.
David M. Taylor, Fiona Gaughran, and Toby Pillinger.
© 2021 John Wiley & Sons Ltd. Published 2021 by John Wiley & Sons Ltd.

DIAGNOSTIC PRINCIPLES

Given the link between depression and chronic low back pain, traditional medical models of assessment, which see musculoskeletal pain only as a guide to underlying pathology, are inadequate. Instead, a biopsychosocial approach is recommended that considers not only the physical symptoms and examination findings but also the impact of the pain on the patient's functioning and general well-being [4].

A focused history and examination may be used to eliminate rare but serious causes of low back pain (Box 59.1), as well as referred pain from other joints or organ systems. However, it is important to remember that red flags are common, not diagnostic, and merely indicate a need for the clinician to consider further investigation and/or referral, based on the strength of clinical suspicion and the potential consequences of a delayed diagnosis.

It is also important to recognise patients' fears or avoidant behaviour so that these can be addressed specifically when formulating a management plan. Identification of

---

Box 59.1 Red flag features of back pain [11]

Cauda equina

Bowel or bladder disturbance, saddle anaesthesia, lower motor neuron weakness (these features require *emergency referral*)

Vertebral infection or discitis

New-onset fever, history or intravenous drug use or tuberculosis, immunosuppression, previous spinal procedures (these features require *emergency referral*)

Metastatic disease

History of cancer that spreads to bone (breast, lung, prostate, thyroid, renal)

Inflammatory axial spondyloarthritis

Age of onset under 45 years, insidious onset, pain on waking during the second part of the night, early morning stiffness that improves with exercise, history of psoriasis, enthesitis, uveitis, psoriasis, or family history of spondylarthritis

Vertebral fracture

History of osteoporosis, trauma, systemic steroids, age over 65 years

Spinal stenosis

Bilateral buttock, thigh or leg pain, pseudo-claudication pain, history of age-related degenerative changes

Radicular pain

Leg pain in the sciatic nerve distribution, sensory loss, myotomal weakness in spinal nerve distribution, reduced reflexes

risk factors for chronicity and high healthcare resource utilisation can be performed using a validated screening tool such as the Keele STarT Back Tool, which incorporates an assessment of psychosocial disability [10].

Examination

Examination is essential, even if a serious cause of low back pain is not suspected. Its purpose is not necessarily to arrive at a single anatomical diagnosis, as this often leads to ineffective structural-based treatments [11]. Instead, it functions as an important tool to signal to patients that their concerns have been heard and to validate their pain. A summary of a focused examination for low back pain is presented in Box 59.2.

Investigations

Imaging in lower back pain is rarely helpful unless a specific diagnosis is suspected (see Box 59.1). In fact, imaging in non-specific back pain is unlikely to result in any lasting patient reassurance and can cause harm via the following mechanisms [12].

- Misinterpretation of results by clinicians resulting in unhelpful advice, needless subsequent investigations, and invasive interventions.
- Misinterpretation of results by patients resulting in catastrophising, fear, avoidance of movement and activity, and low expectations of recovery.
- Inappropriate exposure to radiation.

Decisions to perform imaging in the context of non-specific low back pain are best made by specialist multidisciplinary teams after a trial of treatment [11].

Box 59.2 Focused examination for low back pain

- Inspect the back for scoliosis.
- Observe the patient tiptoe and heel walk as a screening test for whether a full motor examination is required (ability to perform both tiptoe/heel walking suggests motor function is intact).
- Palpate the back for tenderness of spinous processes or musculature.
- Test active spinal movements:
  - Flexion increases the pressure in the intervertebral discs, and stretches the paraspinal muscles.
  - Extension loads the facet joint and relaxes the paraspinal muscles.
  - Lateral flexion loads the discs and ipsilateral facet joint and stretches the contralateral musculature.
- Perform a hip examination to exclude referred pain from the hip joint.
- Perform a straight-leg raise test to examine for radiculopathy, often due to a herniated disc. With the patient lying supine, the examiner lifts the patient's leg while the knee is straight. The test is positive if the patient experiences pain in the distribution of the sciatic nerve (i.e. through the buttock, down the back of the thigh, and into the foot).

CHAPTER 59

MANAGEMENT

The main goals of management of low back pain are to promote a positive message, including the safety of physical activity and the efficacy of simple treatments, and to support patients to live and participate in daily life despite their pain. Strategies to manage pain can be divided into active and passive modalities. Active coping strategies are where the patient takes on a key role within their own recovery and include exercise, stretching, and meditation. Passive coping strategies are where the patient yields responsibility for pain management to an outside agent or individual and include methods such as medication, imaging, massage, mobilisation, or acupuncture [13]. Patients who utilise active coping strategies have less disability and distress due to pain compared with those patients relying on passive strategies [14]. In a condition such as non-specific low back pain which frequently relapses, it is important that the patient has a variety of both active and passive coping strategies for flares so they can self-manage with confidence. Non-pharmacological options are the preferred approach in the management of acute, subacute, and chronic back pain [11].

Symptoms of acute or subacute low back pain generally improve over time regardless of treatment [11]. Patient education is thus key to management, which should involve an honest discussion about the natural history of back pain. Making it clear that recovery is expected usually within the first two weeks but also that there is a high risk of reoccurrence over time will allow the patient to realise that she or he is faced not with a discrete illness but with a chronic vulnerability. This will allow patients to modify their activities or habits and improves engagement with active treatment strategies to prevent recurrence or shorten the severity and duration of acute episodes.

Non-pharmacological management

- Limit bed rest and move within the limits of the pain.
- Early return to work and reassurance that the patient does not need to be 'back to normal' before returning to work.
- Active physiotherapy or patient-initiated stretching/strengthening.*
- Aerobic activity.*
- Yoga, pilates, or core-strengthening exercises targeting postural muscles.*
- Superficial heat.
- There is mixed evidence for the effectiveness of massage, acupuncture, and spinal manipulation or manual therapy, but it may be pragmatic to consider these interventions in combination with exercise as a more 'active' treatment tool.
- Address poor sleep and contributing factors relating to stress.
- Treat comorbid mental illness.
- Psychological interventions such as cognitive-behavioural therapy, mindfulness-based stress reduction, or acceptance-based therapies.

---

*Exercise frequency has been shown to be more important than type, duration, or intensity of exercise [13].

Pharmacological management

- Non-steroidal anti-inflammatory drugs (NSAIDs) are first line: use at the lowest dose for the shortest duration possible, ideally less than two weeks. Before prescribing, consider risk factors for gastrointestinal bleeding and thus need for gastroprotection (e.g. advanced age, and prescription of other medications such as selective serotonin reuptake inhibitors), and the potential for liver and cardiorenal toxicity.
- Paracetamol may be considered, although its efficacy in treatment of low back pain when used alone has been questioned [15].
- Skeletal muscle relaxants (e.g. baclofen, tizanidine, and diazepam) are effective for pain relief in acute or subacute low back pain, but use with caution in those at risk of side effects (e.g. older adults) and those at risk of misuse or dependence.
- There is a growing body of evidence suggesting that opioids are harmful in the treatment of low back pain [16]. Consider weak opioids as a last resort only if NSAIDs are contraindicated or ineffective. Use only for acute presentations and flairs. Opioids should never be prescribed long term and clinicians should try to reduce and stop opioids that have been historically initiated if they are not improving functioning.
- There is no indication for gabapentinoids in low back pain or radiculopathy. A recent meta-analysis showed no improvement in pain, function, or emotional state in their use over placebo [11]. In the UK, these medications are now considered controlled drugs due to risk of dependence and misuse.
- Selective serotonin reuptake inhibitors, serotonin/noradrenaline reuptake inhibitors, and tricyclic antidepressants should not be offered specifically for managing low back pain [3]. However, as already discussed, comorbid psychiatric illness should be treated, which may involve use of these medications.

When to refer

Patients with clinical features of cauda equina or spinal infection require urgent referral to a neurosurgeon or an infectious diseases physician, respectively (see Box 59.1). In the community these patients should be sent to the accident and emergency department. A strong suspicion of metastatic disease warrants referral to oncology for a definitive diagnosis. Features of inflammatory back pain should prompt a rheumatology referral.

For patients with non-specific low back pain who do not improve with initial care or who have risk factors for persistent disability, a referral to a multidisciplinary pain management programme is indicated. Multimodal programmes, which aim to reduce the emotional component of pain and cultivate self-care techniques, are emerging as the gold-standard management of persistent non-specific lower back pain [6].

References

1. Cassidy JD, Carroll LJ, Cote P. The Saskatchewan Health and Back Pain Survey. The prevalence of low back pain and related disability in Saskatchewan adults. *Spine* 1998;23(17):1860–1866; discussion 1867.
2. Stubbs B, Koyanagi A, Thompson T, et al. The epidemiology of back pain and its relationship with depression, psychosis, anxiety, sleep disturbances, and stress sensitivity: data from 43 low- and middle-income countries. *Gen Hosp Psychiatry* 2016;43:63–70.

3. National Institute for Health and Care Excellence. *Low Back Pain and Sciatica in over 16s: Assessment and Management*. NICE Guideline NG59. London: NICE, 2016. Available at https://www.nice.org.uk/guidance/ng59

4. Croft P, Peat GM, Van der Windt DA. Primary care research and musculoskeletal medicine. *Prim Health Care Res Dev* 2009;11(1):4–16.

5. Rush AJ, Polatin P, Gatchel RJ. Depression and chronic low back pain: establishing priorities in treatment. *Spine* 2000;25(20):2566–2571.

6. Ciaramella A, Poli P. Chronic low back pain perception and coping with pain in the presence of psychiatric comorbidity. *J Nerv Ment Dis* 2015;203(8):632–640.

7. Sheng JY, Liu S, Wang YC, et al. The link between depression and chronic pain: neural mechanisms in the brain. *Neural Plast* 2017;2017:9724371.

8. Peat G, Thomas E, Handy J, Croft P. Social networks and pain interference with daily activities in middle and old age. *Pain* 2004;112(3):397–405.

9. Cacioppo JT, Hughes ME, Waite LJ, et al. Loneliness as a specific risk factor for depressive symptoms: cross-sectional and longitudinal analyses. *Psychol Aging* 2006;21(1):140–151.

10. Hill JC, Dunn KM, Lewis M, et al. A primary care back pain screening tool: identifying patient subgroups for initial treatment. *Arthritis Rheum* 2008;59(5):632–641.

11. Traeger A, Buchbinder R, Harris I, Maher C. Diagnosis and management of low-back pain in primary care. *Can Med Assoc J* 2017;189(45):E1386–E1395.

12. Darlow B, Forster BB, O'Sullivan K, O'Sullivan P. It is time to stop causing harm with inappropriate imaging for low back pain. *Br J Sport Med* 2017;51(5):414–415.

13. Carroll L, Mercado AC, Cassidy JD, Cote P. A population-based study of factors associated with combinations of active and passive coping with neck and low back pain. *J Rehabil Med* 2002;34(2):67–72.

14. Johnston V. Consequences and management of neck pain by female office workers: results of a survey and clinical assessment. *Arch Physiother* 2016;6:8.

15. Machado GC, Maher CG, Ferreira PH, et al. Efficacy and safety of paracetamol for spinal pain and osteoarthritis: systematic review and meta-analysis of randomised placebo controlled trials. *BMJ* 2015;350:h1225.

16. Deyo RA, Von Korff M, Duhrkoop D. Opioids for low back pain. *BMJ* 2015;350:g6380.

Arthritis

Sarah Griffin, Joseph Nathan, Richard Campbell

Arthritis is considered here to be any condition resulting in joint inflammation and/or pain. It affects almost 10 million people in the UK and as such represents the largest single cause of physical disability in the country [1,2], In the USA, approximately 54 million people are thought to have a diagnosis of arthritis [3].

Common causes of arthritis are detailed in Table 60.1, which also details the complex relationship between arthritic and psychiatric conditions. Some psychiatric and arthritic disorders demonstrate bidirectional and synergistic relationships; for example, people with arthritis of any form are more likely to have psychotic and affective symptoms [4]. Compared with the general population, rates of depression are higher in patients with arthritic conditions [5–11], and depression lowers pain thresholds in people with arthritis [6,12]. However, certain rheumatological conditions appear to be protective against psychotic disorders; for example, rates of schizophrenia are reduced in patients with rheumatoid arthritis and ankylosing spondylitis [13]. Some systemic rheumatological conditions such as systemic lupus erythematosus (SLE) and sarcoid have recognised neuropsychiatric sequelae [14–16], and some rheumatological treatments such as steroids and other neuromodulators can have profound effects on mental state [17,18]. The presence of psychiatric symptoms in patients with arthritis is poor prognostic marker; for example, people with arthritis and depression tend to have more functional limitations as a consequence of arthritis [6], may be less likely to adhere to rheumatological treatment regimens [19], and are more likely to develop other medical comorbidities [6,20,21].

While day-to-day management of arthritis is clearly beyond the remit of the psychiatric practitioner, there are several clinical scenarios where knowledge of appropriate history, examination, and investigation of an arthritic complaint will be of worth. For example, identifying a septic joint in a psychiatric inpatient could be life-saving, or will at least reduce the risk of long-term morbidity. Recognising the signs and symptoms of

The Maudsley Practice Guidelines for Physical Health Conditions in Psychiatry, First Edition.
David M. Taylor, Fiona Gaughran, and Toby Pillinger.
© 2021 John Wiley & Sons Ltd. Published 2021 by John Wiley & Sons Ltd.

Table 60.1 Common types of arthritis in adults, underlying pathoaetiology, typical clinical characteristics, diagnosis, common treatments, and association with psychiatric disorders.

Type of arthritis	Pathoaetiology	Typical clinical characteristics	Pattern of joint involvement	Diagnosis	Treatment	Relationship with serious mental illness
Osteoarthritis (OA)	Progressive destruction of articular cartilage, sclerosis of subchondral bone, and synovial inflammation Various biomechanical factors contribute; major risk factors are advancing age, joint injury, and obesity	Joint pain, tenderness, and stiffness with associated functional impairment. Joints commonly affected: knee, hip, interphalangeal and first metacarpophalangeal joints of the fingers, and facet joints of the cervical/lumbar spine	Mono-, oligo-, or poly-arthritis, although the latter is most common	Diagnosis is usually clinical, based on a typical presentation. X-ray of the joint may demonstrate a narrow joint space, osteophytes, subchondral sclerosis and cysts	Non-pharmacological: weight loss, exercise Pharmacological: analgesia (e.g. topical, oral NSAIDs or intra-articular joint injection) Surgical (e.g. joint replacement)	Rates of depression and anxiety increased in OA [6] Depressive symptoms worsen OA symptoms [12] Depressive symptoms worsen outcomes in OA [6]
Rheumatoid arthritis (RA)	Autoimmune-mediated synovial inflammation and joint destruction. Various genetic and environmental (e.g. smoking) causes implicated	Classically presents with stiffness (especially in the morning) of multiple joints (for >6 weeks), typically the metacarpophalangeal and proximal interphalangeal joints of the hands, the wrists, and small joints of the feet (although shoulders, elbows, knees, and ankles are often also affected) Can also present with various extra-articular manifestations affecting any organ system	Polyarthritis	On examination: symmetrical joint swelling and pain In chronic RA there may be characteristic joint deformities, e.g. ulnar deviation, boutonnière deformity X-ray of the affected joints may demonstrate erosions, joint subluxation or joint narrowing Bloods: rheumatoid factor (RF) positive in 70% [27]; anti-cyclic citrullinated peptide (anti-CCP) positive in 70% [28] (there may not be overlap in RF and anti-CCP positivity)	Disease-modifying antirheumatic drugs (DMARDs), e.g. methotrexate Adjunctive corticosteroids and/or NSAIDs Biological agents (e.g. anti-TNF-α)	Rates of depression and anxiety increased in RA [8] Rates of psychosis reduced in patients with RA [13]

Gout	Hyperuricaemia leading to crystal formation in joint space	More likely in older age, males, prescription of certain drugs (e.g. aspirin), diets rich in meat and alcohol, comorbid diseases with high cellular turnover (e.g. haemolysis) Typically, acute (onset over minutes to hours) severe monoarticular pain with associated swelling. There may be gouty tophi. Feet often affected (e.g. podagra)	Mono-, oligo- or poly-arthritis, although monoarthritis is most common	Diagnosis requires joint aspiration and observation of urate crystals. Differentiate from pseudogout (calcium pyrophosphate deposition) and septic arthritis	Acute treatment: NSAIDs, colchicine or a short course of oral steroids Prophylaxis: mainstay is allopurinol but febuxostat can be considered (but has significant cardiac risk profile)	Increased risk of depression in patients with gout; depression is also associated with poorer quality of life and functional disability in patients with gout [10]
Psoriatic arthritis (a seronegative spondyloarthritis)	A chronic inflammatory joint disease associated with or without psoriasis	A personal or family history of psoriasis, a personal history of scalp, skin or nail disorders Features can include peripheral arthritis with joint pain and stiffness, dactylitis, enthesitis, and stiffness of the spine	Mono-, oligo- or poly-arthritis	On examination, the arthritis is generally asymmetric. Joints are swollen and tender. There may be dactylitis (swelling of the whole finger) and onycholysis (nail separates from nail bed) X-ray of the pelvis may demonstrate sacroiliitis Bloods: generally, RF and anti-CCP negative Joint disease may start before, after, or in the absence of skin involvement	Non-pharmacological, e.g. physiotherapy NSAIDs, DMARDs, biological agents (e.g. anti-TNF-α)	Rates of depression and anxiety increased in psoriatic arthritis [8] Stress can make psoriasis and skin disorders worse [29]

(continued)

Table 60.1 (Continued)

Type of arthritis	Pathoaetiology	Typical clinical characteristics	Pattern of joint involvement	Diagnosis	Treatment	Relationship with serious mental illness
Ankylosing spondylitis (a seronegative spondyloarthritis)	A progressive inflammatory arthritis predominantly involving the sacroiliac joints and axial spine	More likely in men and typically presents in early 20s. Presents with back pain and stiffness that is worse in the morning and lasts for >60 minutes Associated with iritis, uveitis, and enthesitis	Polyarthritis	On examination there may be tenderness at the sacroiliac joint, kyphosis, and loss of lumbar lordosis X-ray of the pelvis or MRI may demonstrate sacroiliitis. Advanced disease may be associated with a 'bamboo spine' Individuals may complain of peripheral joint arthritis	Non-pharmacological, e.g. physiotherapy NSAIDs, biological agents (e.g. anti-TNF-α)	Rates of depression increased in people with ankylosing spondylitis [11] Rates of psychosis reduced in patients with ankylosing spondylitis [13]
Sarcoidosis	A multisystem inflammatory condition resulting in granuloma formation	Sarcoidosis can affect any organ system; acute and chronic arthritis can occur [30] Where arthritis does occur, it is often the joints of the feet that are affected	Mono-, oligo- or poly-arthritis	On examination there may be erythema nodosum, painless lymphadenopathy, uveitis, wheezing/crackles on auscultation of lung Various tests (bloods, imaging, lung function) may be used to aid a diagnosis of sarcoid. Serum angiotensin-converting-enzyme (ACE) levels may be raised [31]	NSAIDs, DMARDs biological agents (e.g. anti-TNF-α)	Neurosarcoid can be associated with mood disturbance and psychosis [22,23] High prevalence of depression in patients with sarcoid (occurring in up to 66% of patients) [5]

Systemic lupus erythematosus (SLE)	A chronic multi-system autoimmune condition [1]	Oligo- or poly-arthritis Symmetrical non-erosive polyarthritis of two or more peripheral joints with morning pain and stiffness, hand ulnar deviation, and small joint subluxations	Immunology to support diagnosis: positive antinuclear antibodies (ANA), anti-dsDNA, antiphospholipid antibodies, reduced complement (C3, C4, CH50) Urine dipstick can display renal involvement if positive for blood and or protein	Immunosuppressant treatment. Guidance varies according to staging of SLE disease [32]	Up to 75% of SLE patients have neuropsychiatric features [18] including anxiety, mood disorders, and mild cognitive impairment
Septic arthritis	Infection of the joint	Monoarthritis A hot, swollen, painful joint	Diagnosis requires joint aspiration. The synovial fluid aspirate may appear turbid. It will be sent for Gram-staining to detect the presence of bacteria and cultured to identify any microorganisms	Antibiotics or joint washout in theatre	People with serious mental illness have increased prevalence of various comorbidities that increase risk of septic arthritis, e.g. smoking, diabetes mellitus, intravenous drug use, and alcohol abuse

NSAID, non-steroidal anti-inflammatory drug; TNF, tumour necrosis factor.

a systemic rheumatological condition such as SLE and performing appropriate diagnostic tests will not only facilitate timely referral to medical colleagues but may also identify an organic cause of psychiatric symptoms, thus potentially avoiding inappropriate psychiatric treatment [18,22,23]. Finally, as part of a multidisciplinary team, the psychiatrist is in a unique position to improve outcomes for patients with arthritis; for example, treating comorbid depression improves global functioning in patients with chronic pain secondary to arthritis [24–26].

CLINICAL APPROACH

As discussed, septic arthritis (see Box 60.1 for a summary of features and risk factors) is a potentially life-threatening emergency; where such a presentation is suspected, prompt discussion with medical or surgical colleagues and transfer of care to a medical environment is necessary (see also Chapter 72).

Box 60.1 Features and risk factors for septic arthritis

- Septic arthritis typically presents as a hot, swollen, painful joint (most often the knee in adults) with a significantly restricted range of movement.
- Onset is usually over a period of two weeks or less, although onset may be more insidious in prosthetic joints or where tuberculosis is causative [33].
- Associated constitutional symptoms may include fever (although this can be absent), nausea, vomiting, reduced appetite, and malaise.
- Risk factors for septic arthritis include pre-existing joint disease (e.g. osteoarthritis and rheumatoid arthritis), smoking, diabetes mellitus, intravenous drug use, alcohol abuse, and any state of immunosuppression or a recently operated on or injected joint.

History

Presenting complaint

- A key component of the history is to determine whether the patient is presenting with single or multiple joint involvement.
- For a polyarticular presentation, ascertain which joints are involved and if they are symmetrically distributed. Determine the quality of the pain, over what time period the pain has developed and lasted, and whether there is associated stiffness (especially in the morning). Enquire about associated symptoms that may point to a rheumatological cause (e.g. shortness of breath, Raynaud phenomenon, skin rash, dry eyes or dry mouth, oral ulcers, previous blood clots, or transient temperatures).
- For a monoarticular presentation, determine which joint is involved, the quality of pain, over what time period the pain has developed, and enquire about recent trauma. As before, ask about associated symptoms (e.g. fever, rigors). Gastric and genitourinary symptomatology may point towards an infective aetiology of arthritis (either via inoculation or as a reactive arthritis).
- Assess functioning and ability to perform activities of daily living.

Past medical history

- Previous/similar arthritic presentations.
- Previous rheumatological or autoimmune diagnoses.
- Any recent tonsillitis, urinary tract infection, or sexually transmitted infections (reactive arthritis).
- Any comorbid diagnoses that may result in immunosuppression (e.g. HIV).
- Diabetes mellitus.

Drug history

- Determine drug allergy status, especially regarding antibiotics.
- Immunosuppressants (glucocorticoids, disease-modifying antirheumatic drugs, or biological agents).
- Anticoagulants (will increase risk of haemarthrosis).
- Diuretics increase risk of gout.

Family history

- Rheumatological disease.
- Autoimmune disease.
- Osteoarthritis (particularly nodular osteoarthritis that is heritable).

Social history

- Alcohol and recreational drug use.
- Smoking status.
- Travel to an area endemic for Lyme disease (e.g. northeastern North America).

Examination

- Perform a set of basic observations, including blood pressure, heart rate, temperature, respiratory rate, and oxygen saturation. Although fever may indicate a septic joint, fever can also occur in the setting of rheumatological disease (e.g. SLE) and gout.
- Examine the joints involved for evidence of tenderness (joint line tenderness), synovitis (swelling, warmth), and limitation in movement.
- Examine for nodules (rheumatoid nodules or gouty tophi). As appropriate, further examine the skin, nails, eyes, and other organ systems for evidence of a rheumatological condition, such as malar rash of SLE, onycholysis of psoriatic arthritis, wheeze/crackles of pulmonary sarcoid (see Table 60.1).
- Widespread pain, tenderness on the back of the head, elbows, shoulders, knees, and hips, and fatigue in the absence of clear joint involvement may indicate fibromyalgia.

Investigations

- Joint imaging and aspiration are not possible in a psychiatric setting, and where such investigations are indicated, the patient will require transfer to general medical services.

The urgency with which these investigations are performed should be determined following discussion with medical colleagues. Following joint aspiration, synovial fluid will be sent for microscopy, culture, and sensitivity. Polarising microscopy will show needle-shaped crystals in gout or pyrophosphate crystals in pseudogout.

■ Septic arthritis can only be ruled out completely with a negative Gram stain on joint aspiration. If there is concern for a septic joint, corticosteroid must never be injected into the joint until a Gram stain result returns.

■ In terms of blood tests, a full blood count, renal function, liver function, and inflammatory markers (C-reactive protein and erythrocyte sedimentation rate) may be requested. If there are specific concerns about a rheumatological condition, antibody tests may also be sent (as described in Table 60.1).

MANAGEMENT

As already discussed, management of arthritis (see Table 60.1) is generally beyond the remit of the psychiatric practitioner; however, treatment of comorbid psychiatric disorders such as depression and anxiety in patients with arthritic disorders should ideally involve a multidisciplinary approach involving both psychiatry and rheumatology [34]. When making a referral to general medical colleagues, ensure that the following information is included in a referral.

■ Rationale behind referral and what you are concerned about.
■ Pertinent history, family history, examination, and investigation findings (see above).
■ Brief psychiatric history, associated risk profile, and if there are any specific nursing needs.
■ Contact details of the referring psychiatric team.

References

1. Versus Arthritis. The State of Musculoskeletal Health 2019: Arthritis and Other Musculoskeletal Conditions in Numbers. https://www.versusarthritis.org/media/14594/state-of-musculoskeletal-health-2019.pdf

2. Badley EM, Tennant A. Disablement associated with rheumatic disorders in a British population: problems with activities of daily living and level of support. *Br J Rheumatol* 1993;32(7):601–608.

3. Barbour KE, Helmick CG, Boring M, Brady TJ. Vital signs: prevalence of doctor-diagnosed arthritis and arthritis-attributable activity limitation: United States, 2013–2015. *MMWR Morb Mortal Wkly Rep* 2017;66(9):246–253.

4. Stubbs B, Veronese N, Vancampfort D, et al. Lifetime self-reported arthritis is associated with elevated levels of mental health burden: a multi-national cross sectional study across 46 low- and middle-income countries. *Sci Rep* 2017;7(1):7138.

5. Chang B, Steimel J, Moller DR, et al. Depression in sarcoidosis. *Am J Respir Crit Care Med* 2001;163(2):329–334.

6. Sharma A, Kudesia P, Shi Q, Gandhi R. Anxiety and depression in patients with osteoarthritis: impact and management challenges. *Open Access Rheumatol* 2016;8:103–113.

7. Gandhi R, Zywiel MG, Mahomed NN, Perruccio AV. Depression and the overall burden of painful joints: an examination among individuals undergoing hip and knee replacement for osteoarthritis. *Arthritis* 2015;2015:327161.

8. Roubille C, Richer V, Starnino T, et al. Evidence-based recommendations for the management of comorbidities in rheumatoid arthritis, psoriasis, and psoriatic arthritis: expert opinion of the Canadian Dermatology-Rheumatology Comorbidity Initiative. *J Rheumatol* 2015;42(10):1767–1780.

9. Stubbs B, Aluko Y, Myint PK, Smith TO. Prevalence of depressive symptoms and anxiety in osteoarthritis: a systematic review and meta-analysis. *Age Ageing* 2016;45(2):228–235.

10. Fu T, Cao H, Yin R, et al. Associated factors with functional disability and health-related quality of life in Chinese patients with gout: a case-control study. *BMC Musculoskelet Disord* 2017;18(1):429.

11. Webers C, Vanhoof L, Leue C, et al. Depression in ankylosing spondylitis and the role of disease-related and contextual factors: a cross-sectional study. *Arthritis Res Ther* 2019;21(1):215.

12. Edwards RR, Calahan C, Mensing G, et al. Pain, catastrophizing, and depression in the rheumatic diseases. *Nat Rev Rheumatol* 2011;7(4):216–224.

13. Cullen AE, Holmes S, Pollak TA, et al. Associations between non-neurological autoimmune disorders and psychosis: a meta-analysis. *Biol Psychiatry* 2019;85(1):35–48.

14. Liang MH, Corzillius M, Bae SC, et al. The American College of Rheumatology nomenclature and case definitions for neuropsychiatric lupus syndromes. *Arthritis Rheum* 1999;42(4):599–608.

15. Joseph FG, Scolding NJ. Neurosarcoidosis: a study of 30 new cases. *J Neurol Neurosurg Psychiatry* 2009;80(3):297–304.

16. Zajicek JP, Scolding NJ, Foster O, et al. Central nervous system sarcoidosis: diagnosis and management. *Q J Med* 1999;92(2):103–117.

17. Dubovsky AN, Arvikar S, Stern TA, Axelrod L. The neuropsychiatric complications of glucocorticoid use: steroid psychosis revisited. *Psychosomatics* 2012;53(2):103–115.

18. Bertsias GK, Ioannidis JP, Aringer M, et al. EULAR recommendations for the management of systemic lupus erythematosus with neuropsychiatric manifestations: report of a task force of the EULAR standing committee for clinical affairs. *Ann Rheum Dis* 2010;69(12):2074–2082.

19. Vallerand IA, Patten SB, Barnabe C. Depression and the risk of rheumatoid arthritis. *Curr Opin Rheumatol* 2019;31(3):279–284.

20. Matcham F, Rayner L, Steer S, Hotopf M. The prevalence of depression in rheumatoid arthritis: a systematic review and meta-analysis. *Rheumatology* 2013;52(12):2136–2148.

21. Katon W, Lin EHB, Kroenke K. The association of depression and anxiety with medical symptom burden in patients with chronic medical illness. *Gen Hosp Psychiatry* 2007;29(2):147–155.

22. Bona JR, Fackler SM, Fendley MJ, Nemeroff CB. Neurosarcoidosis as a cause of refractory psychosis: a complicated case report. *Am J Psychiatry* 1998;155(8):1106–1108.

23. Hebel R, Dubaniewicz-Wybieralska M, Dubaniewicz A. Overview of neurosarcoidosis: recent advances. *J Neurol* 2015;262(2):258–267.

24. Teh CF, Zaslavsky AM, Reynolds CF III, Cleary PD. Effect of depression treatment on chronic pain outcomes. *Psychosom Med* 2010;72(1):61–67.

25. Lin EH, Katon W, Von Korff M, et al. Effect of improving depression care on pain and functional outcomes among older adults with arthritis: a randomized controlled trial. *JAMA* 2003;290(18):2428–2429.

26. Parker JC, Smarr KL, Slaughter JR, et al. Management of depression in rheumatoid arthritis: a combined pharmacologic and cognitive-behavioral approach. *Arthritis Rheum* 2003;49(6):766–777.

27. Aho K, Palusuo T, Kurki P. Marker antibodies of rheumatoid arthritis: diagnostic and pathogenetic implications. *Semin Arthritis Rheum* 1994;23(6):379–387.

28. Goldbach-Mansky R, Lee J, McCoy A, et al. Rheumatoid arthritis associated autoantibodies in patients with synovitis of recent onset. *Arthritis Res* 2000;2(3):236–243.

29. Seville RH. Stress and psoriasis: the importance of insight and empathy in prognosis. *J Am Acad Dermatol* 1989;20(1):97–100.

30. Kobak S, Sever F, Usluer O, et al. The clinical characteristics of sarcoid arthropathy based on a prospective cohort study. *Ther Adv Musculoskelet Dis* 2016;8(6):220–224.

31. Lieberman J. Elevation of serum angiotensin-converting-enzyme (ACE) level in sarcoidosis. *Am J Med* 1975;59(3):365–372.

32. Fanouriakis A, Kostopoulou M, Alunno A, et al. 2019 update of the EULAR recommendations for the management of systemic lupus erythematosus. *Ann Rheum Dis* 2019;78(6):736–745.

33. Coakley G, Mathews C, Field M, et al. BSR and BHPR, BOA, RCGP and BSAC guidelines for management of the hot swollen joint in adults. *Rheumatology (Oxford)* 2006;45(8):1039–1041.

34. Withers MH, Gonzalez LT, Karpouzas GA. Identification and treatment optimization of comorbid depression in rheumatoid arthritis. *Rheumatol Ther* 2017;4(2):281–291.

CHAPTER 60

Part 11

Ophthalmology

Eye Disease

Ernest Iakovlev, Radwan Almousa

People with serious mental illness (SMI) present with several risk factors for ophthalmological disease. For example, rates of type 2 diabetes mellitus, a major risk factor for visual impairment [1], are increased in psychiatric patients [2,3]. Furthermore, some psychiatric treatments are associated with specific ophthalmological disorders [4]: antipsychotics have been implicated in the development of cataracts [5]; psychotropic agents with anticholinergic activity or the potential to cause swelling of the ciliary body can induce or worsen narrow (closed)-angle glaucoma [6]; some antidepressants are associated with dry eye syndrome [4]; and electroconvulsive therapy can increase intraocular pressure and thus worsen glaucoma [7]. Refractive errors are also common in people with SMI. For example, patients with psychosis are five to six times more likely than members of the general population to have visual impairment [8]. Moreover, there is evidence of intrinsic defects in visual processing in psychotic disorders [9].

This chapter provides the psychiatric practitioner with a general approach to assessing an individual with visual disturbance and/or a disorder affecting the orbit or periorbital area. It also details specific advice for common ophthalmological disorders, including dry eye, blepharitis, hordeolum (stye), chalazion, conjunctivitis, subconjunctival haemorrhage, corneal foreign body, contact lens-associated corneal infection, and glaucoma.

CLINICAL APPROACH TO A PATIENT WITH VISUAL DISTURBANCE OR ORBITAL/PERIORBITAL DISORDERS

The extent to which a psychiatric practitioner will be able to assess visual disturbance or an orbital/periorbital disorder will depend on their previous experience and available examination equipment (recommended equipment is detailed in Box 61.1). Here

The Maudsley Practice Guidelines for Physical Health Conditions in Psychiatry, First Edition.
David M. Taylor, Fiona Gaughran, and Toby Pillinger.
© 2021 John Wiley & Sons Ltd. Published 2021 by John Wiley & Sons Ltd.

> **Box 61.1** Equipment that may be used to assess ophthalmological disease
>
> - Direct ophthalmoscope with both white and blue light sources.
> - Visual acuity chart, e.g. Snellen. Snellen results are recorded as two numbers: the first/top number indicates the distance in metres at which the test chart was presented (usually 6 m), while the second/bottom indicates the position on the chart of the smallest line read by the patient (each line is numbered). Thus, 6/60 indicates that the patient can only see the top letter when viewed at 6 m.
> - Pinhole occluder: allows one to determine if reduced visual acuity is secondary to refractive error, i.e. inability of the cornea and lens to bend light into focus on the retina. In cases of refractive error, use of the pinhole will improve visual acuity.
> - Fluorescein 0.25% drops: under blue light this allows identification of corneal defects such as ulceration or abrasion.

we detail an ideal approach, although it is recognised that abridged assessments may be unavoidable in certain settings.

History

Presenting complaint

- Was the onset sudden or gradual? How long have symptoms lasted? Sudden sight loss (seconds to minutes) almost always indicates a vascular event (e.g. occluded retinal artery or vitreous/retinal haemorrhage) and should prompt urgent referral to ophthalmology/emergency services. Gradual sight loss (months to years) usually indicates a degenerative process such as cataract or glaucoma. In young healthy patients with rapid loss of vision, consider optic neuritis as a differential.
- What was the patient doing when the symptoms occurred?
- Does the problem involve one or both eyes? If both, which is worse?
- Are there any associated symptoms? Loss of vision associated with scalp pain in an elderly person may indicate temporal arteritis. Sight loss caused by vascular disease is not usually accompanied by other symptoms, although there may be associated cardiovascular risk factors (see section Past medical history). Pain is often associated with optic neuritis. Retinal detachment occurs more frequently in people with myopia (near-sightedness) or following cataract surgery; such individuals may complain of 'floaters' prior to vision loss.
- Are there any exacerbating and/or relieving factors?
- Has this problem happened before and was it assessed/treated?
- More focused questions may be asked depending on the complaint (see later sections on specific presentations).

Past ocular history

- What is the patient's baseline vision?
- Do they wear glasses?

- Do they wear contact lenses? For any patient who wears contact lenses ask if they swim, sleep, or shower in them as these activities increase the risk of contact lens-related infection.
- Any previous eye problems including eye surgery?

Past medical history

Enquire specifically about conditions that are known to affect the eye or are associated with ophthalmological disease:

- hypertension
- high cholesterol
- atrial fibrillation
- ischaemic heart disease
- bleeding disorders
- diabetes mellitus
- hyperthyroidism
- rheumatoid arthritis
- sarcoidosis
- inflammatory bowel disease
- inflammatory arthritis.

Drug history

- Current medication including over-the-counter treatments and herbal supplements. Potential ophthalmological sequelae of common psychiatric medications are detailed in Box 61.2.
- Ask about steroid inhalers (theoretically may increase intraocular pressure and lens opacity, although note poor evidence to support this from the clinical literature) [10].

Box 61.2 Potential ophthalmological sequelae of psychiatric medications [4]

Disorders of the eyelid, cornea, and conjunctiva

- High-dose chlorpromazine can result in abnormal pigmentation of the eyelids, cornea, and lens [11]. However, this is not associated with visual disturbance and resolves on cessation of treatment. Thioridazine (now withdrawn) was also associated with pigmentary retinopathy [12].
- Corneal oedema can also (rarely) occur with chlorpromazine, leading to loss of vision if treatment is not withdrawn [13].
- Lithium can (rarely) cause irritation of the eye, particularly in the early stages of treatment [14]. The mechanism is thought to be related to increased sodium content of lacrimal fluid. However, it is a transient phenomenon and can be treated with over-the-counter tears.

Disorders of the iris, ciliary body, and choroid (uveal tract)

- Uveal tract disorders result in impaired ability to control the size of the pupil, resulting in blurred vision.
- Likely owing to their anticholinergic effects, tricyclic antidepressants (TCAs), especially early in treatment, are associated with mydriasis (dilation of the pupil) and cycloplegia (paralysis of the ciliary muscle), which can cause non-severe and transient blurred vision [15].
- Antipsychotics with strong anticholinergic and anti-α-adrenergic effects can cause mydriasis and cycloplegia and therefore blurred vision. This has been reported in treatment with chlorpromazine [16].
- Selective serotonin reuptake inhibitors (SSRIs), via their noradrenergic, anticholinergic, and serotonergic effects, can cause mydriasis [4].

Glaucoma, specifically narrow (closed)-angle glaucoma

- Glaucoma describes a heterogeneous group of conditions characterised by raised intraocular pressure (IOP) and subsequent damage to the optic nerve leading to loss of vision. IOP is maintained by a balance between aqueous humour production and drainage into the anterior chamber of the eye, and pressure increases if fluid circulation is impaired. The iridocorneal angle is the structure responsible for outflow of aqueous humour from the eye. If this angle is reduced, fluid drainage is impaired and IOP increases, i.e. narrow (closed)-angle glaucoma. Angle closure is only one type of glaucoma but is the form of glaucoma that can be induced or worsened by psychotropic medication. Other risk factors for angle closure glaucoma include hyperopia (far-sightedness), increasing age, and female sex [4].
- Because of their anticholinergic action, TCAs can cause or worsen narrow (closed)-angle glaucoma [17]. TCAs should therefore be used with caution in patients with pre-existing narrow angles.
- Theoretically, owing to their anticholinergic effects, antipsychotics should also be a risk factor for closed-angle glaucoma, although there is a paucity of evidence to support this in the literature.
- Topiramate has also been associated with the development of closed-angle glaucoma, potentially due to swelling of the lens and ciliary body [4].
- SSRIs are also associated with closed-angle glaucoma [18].

Cataracts

- Development of lens opacities has been reported in association with use of various antipsychotics, including chlorpromazine, quetiapine, risperidone, ziprasidone, olanzapine, and clozapine [4].

Dry eye

- TCAs may decrease lacrimation owing their anticholinergic effects [19].

Oculogyric crisis

- Dystonia of the extraocular muscles have been reported with not only antipsychotics but also carbamazepine, topiramate, and SSRIs [4].

Impaired eye movement

- Benzodiazepines can cause disturbances in saccadic and smooth-pursuit eye movements [4].
- Lithium, carbamazepine, lamotrigine, and topiramate can cause nystagmus [4].

- Current eye drops including strength and dose.
- Always ask about drug and preservative allergies.

Social history

- Patient's current occupation.
- Does the patient drive?
- Enquire about the patient's support at home including their ability to apply eye drops if such an intervention is indicated.

Examination

Without specialist equipment, a diagnostic eye examination is difficult. However, the following tests may enable a tentative diagnosis and facilitate appropriate referral.

Vision

- Assess distance visual acuity using an appropriate Snellen chart with the patient wearing their most up-to-date 'distance' glasses, if applicable.
- Position the patient 6 m from the chart.
- With one eye occluded, ask the patient to read the lowest line possible.
- Afterwards, put down the pinhole occluder and get the patient to repeat the test (see Box 61.1 for an explanation of why this test is performed).
- Perform the same tests on the opposite eye.
- If a patient's vision is less than Snellen 6/60, then move the patient closer to the chart and test their vision at each meter.
- If the patient is unable to see the chart at a level of Snellen 0.5/60 (i.e. inability to see the top letter 50 cm from the chart), then test for ability to detect hand movements. If they are unable to detect this, then test ability to perceive light.
- Patients with significantly reduced visual acuity should be referred to an ophthalmologist for further assessment.
- Test colour vision by showing the patient a red target (e.g. a red pin). Reduced perception of colour brightness may indicate optic neuritis, ischaemic neuropathy (i.e. occlusion of the blood vessels that supply the optic disc), or retinal artery occlusion. Disease of the optic nerve can then be confirmed by checking for a relative afferent pupillary defect (RAPD). Here, a bright light is moved between the unaffected eye and the eye with poor vision. In RAPD, shining light into the affected eye causes paradoxical pupillary dilatation because it is reliant on light detection from the unaffected eye to guide pupillary response. If disease of the optic nerve is suspected, urgent referral to ophthalmology is indicated.

Ocular examination

1 Using a white light, examine the periorbital tissue, lid margins, conjunctiva, and cornea looking for any swelling, malposition of the lens, discharge, or redness.

2 If possible, perform fundoscopy.

  a Darken the room. Ask the patient to fix their sight on the same point in the distance and over your shoulder throughout the examination. Use your right hand to hold the ophthalmoscope and right eye to examine the patient's right eye, and vice versa. Place your hand on the patient's forehead and while looking through the ophthalmoscope move in towards the patient's eye at a 45° angle until you can visualise the optic nerve. Rotate your ophthalmoscope up, down, left, and right to allow examination of the whole retina. You can ask the patient to look in these directions of gaze to aid you.

  b If available, pupils may be dilated (e.g. tropicamide 0.5% one to two drops, 15 minutes before the examination). However, this is contraindicated following head injury.

  c Examine for the following.

    i Test the red reflex prior to examining the retina: corneal scars, cataract, and vitreous haemorrhage may obscure.

    ii Optic disc: assess for cupping (glaucoma), papilloedema, new vessels on the disc (proliferative diabetic retinopathy), and colour (e.g. pallor of ischaemia).

    iii Vessels: examine for hypertensive (e.g. arteriovenous nipping) or atherosclerotic changes. Background diabetic retinopathy may be associated with microaneurysms, blot haemorrhages, and hard exudate. Cotton-wool spots appear as fluffy white patches on the retina and indicate damage to nerve fibres, most commonly due to diabetes or hypertension.

    iv Macula: this is found temporal to the optic disc. Look for haemorrhages, irregularities, and scarring.

3 Administer one drop of fluorescein into each eye and using a blue light source look for corneal staining, which could indicate a corneal defect (e.g. ulcer/abrasion).

DISORDERS OF THE EYELIDS

Dry eye syndrome [20–22]

Pathophysiology

Dry eye syndrome can be caused by the following.

- Reduced tear production: Sjögren's syndrome, lacrimal gland disease or deficiency associated with ageing, drug-related (beta-blockers, anticholinergics, antihistamines, oral contraception, eye drop preservatives), or due to reduced corneal innervation secondary to nerve dysfunction.
- Excessive tear evaporation: contact lens wear, meibomian gland dysfunction, problems with eyelid closure, reduced blinking seen during computer use or in Parkinson's disease, environmental factors (low humidity, high winds).
- A combination of both.

Symptoms

- Foreign body and/or burning sensation.
- Blurred vision which normally clears after blinking.
- Paradoxical reflex watering of the eyes.
- Heavy eyelids and eye tiredness.
- Symptoms tend to worsen with focused tasks such as reading.
- Symptoms from reduced tear production tend to be worse at the end of the day while symptoms from excessive evaporation are worse at the start of the day.

Signs

- Conjunctival redness.
- Fluorescein staining may show multiple dots known as superficial punctate erosions, indicating loss of epithelium secondary to corneal dryness.
- There may be evidence of blepharitis or meibomian gland dysfunction (see next section).

Treatment

- Mild cases can be successfully managed with over-the-counter lubricating eye drops.
- A lubricating ointment can be used as well but this is best used at night as it causes blurring of vision.
- Preservative-free drops should be given for patients requiring them more than four times a day or patients who wear contact lenses.
- Treat blepharitis and meibomian gland dysfunction if present (see next section).
- Avoid common causes of dry eye, e.g. advise patients to reduce use of contact lenses.

When to refer

- Moderate to severe cases that are not responding to regular lubricating drops after 12 weeks.
- When an underlying systemic condition is suspected (e.g. Sjögren's syndrome).

Blepharitis [21,23]

Pathophysiology

- Blepharitis is a chronic inflammatory condition of the eyelids. It can be divided into anterior and posterior blepharitis. Anterior blepharitis can be subdivided into staphylococcal and seborrhoeic. Staphylococcal blepharitis is caused by colonisation of the lash follicles by *Staphylococcus aureus* which leads to tear-film instability. Patients with seborrhoeic blepharitis have greasy scaling of the anterior eyelid and frequently have seborrhoeic dermatitis of the eyebrows and scalp as well. Blepharitis is also associated with the skin condition rosacea. Posterior blepharitis is caused by a dysfunction of the meibomian glands.

- There are multiple meibomian glands that line the posterior surface of each eyelid and release lipid-rich secretions that stabilise the tear film. As a result, any dysfunction in the meibomian glands leads to instability and excess evaporation of the tear film.
- Blepharitis can also be caused by eyelash infestation with *Demodex folliculorum*, which has been found in 30% of patients with chronic blepharitis. Cylindrical dandruff or sleeves at the eyelash base are reported to be a sign of ocular *Demodex* infestation.

Symptoms

- Symptoms of dry eye syndrome.
- Crusting, swelling, and redness of the lid margins in anterior blepharitis.
- Symptoms are worse in the morning.
- Patients experience flare-up episodes followed by periods of remission.
- Recurrent styes in anterior blepharitis and chalazia in posterior blepharitis (see section External hordeolum).

Signs

- Anterior blepharitis:
  - redness and swelling of the lids
  - crusting at the base of the lashes
  - styes.
- Posterior blepharitis:
  - lid telangiectasia
  - thickening of the meibomian gland secretions and closure of the glands by oil droplets
  - chalazia.
- Signs of dry eye syndrome.
- Fine white spots on the cornea may indicate white blood cell infiltrates at the corneal periphery.

Treatment

- Patients with meibomian gland dysfunction should perform lid hygiene in order to reduce the risk of flares.
  - Apply a warm compress to the closed eyelids for two minutes.
  - Massage the eyelids 10 times in a sweeping motion starting from the base and moving towards the eyelashes. Do this for each of the four eyelids.
  - Wipe along the eyelid margins using a wet cloth or cotton bud.
  - This should be done every day at least once a day. The benefits of lid hygiene take six weeks for full effect so patients should be encouraged to persevere.

- Patients need to be aware that meibomian gland dysfunction is a chronic condition and lid hygiene is key to preventing recurrence.
- Lid hygiene should be avoided in patients with glaucoma who should not apply pressure to the eye.
- Over-the-counter lubricating drops can be given for dry eye symptoms.
- For severe anterior blepharitis, chloramphenicol 1% ointment twice a day can be applied to the lashes for six weeks.
- For patients with blepharitis secondary to *D. folliculorum* infestation, a case series has shown that weekly 50% tea tree oil eyelid scrub and daily tea tree oil shampoo for a minimum of six weeks improved symptoms [24].
- Ensure that patients with seborrhoeic dermatitis or rosacea are adequately treated for these conditions. Patients with significant rosacea-associated blepharitis may benefit from a course of oral tetracyclines (e.g. doxycycline 100 mg once daily for four weeks, then 50 mg once daily for eight weeks). Erythromycin 500 mg twice daily for 6–12 weeks can be given to pregnant or breastfeeding women or those individuals where tetracyclines cannot be used.

When to refer

- Severe cases that are not responding to the described treatment.
- Suspected corneal infiltrates or ulceration.
- If there are irregularities in the eyelids (malignancy).

External hordeolum (stye) [21,22,25]

Pathophysiology

An acute infection within a lid lash follicle.

Signs and symptoms

Tender lump on the outer rim of the eyelid with associated erythema.

Treatment

- Chloramphenicol 1% ointment four times daily to the affected eye and lid.
- Lid hygiene (see preceding section).
- If there is evidence of spreading cellulitis, then treat with oral antibiotics (co-amoxiclav 625 mg three times daily for one week).

Internal hordeolum

This is an acute abscess within a meibomian gland. Treat the same as an external hordeolum.

Chalazion (meibomian cyst) [21,22,26]

Pathophysiology

Arises from chronic inflammation and blockage of a meibomian gland.

Signs and symptoms

- A firm, localised, immobile eyelid lump, more common on the upper eyelid.
- Usually painless but may become tender and inflamed if infected.

Treatment

- Most resolve with time, but hot compresses and lid hygiene can help.
- If there is evidence of infection or inflammation, then give chloramphenicol 1% ointment four times a day for one to two weeks.
- If there is evidence of spreading cellulitis, then treat with oral antibiotics (e.g. co-amoxiclav 625 mg three times daily for one week; however, consult local antibiotic prescribing guidelines).

When to refer

- Patients with recurrent or non-resolving chalazia.
- When there is an ulcerating lesion, eyelid deformities, or loss of lashes.

DISORDERS OF THE CONJUNCTIVA

Bacterial conjunctivitis [21,27,28]

Pathophysiology

- It is mainly spread directly from contact with contaminated individuals.
- The most common pathogens are *Staphylococcus epidermidis*, *Staphylococcus aureus*, *Streptococcus pneumoniae*, and *Haemophilus influenzae*.
- Hyperacute conjunctivitis is commonly due to *Neisseria gonorrhoeae*, a sexually transmitted disease.
- Chronic conjunctivitis is mainly due to *Chlamydia trachomatis*. Chronically unwell or immunocompromised patients may also become colonised with a variety of bacteria leading to chronic conjunctivitis.
- Isolated bacterial conjunctivitis is rare and usually affects infants, elderly patients, or patients with humeral immune or antibody deficiencies. Most patients who present with bacterial conjunctivitis have an underlying secondary ocular pathology that needs to be investigated.

Symptoms

- Gritty and foreign body sensation.
- Green/yellow mucopurulent discharge with lashes being stuck together.
- Symptoms may be bilateral or start in one eye and spread to the other.
- Incubation period is one to seven days.

Signs

- Conjunctiva are diffusely red both on the globe and inside the eyelids.
- Fluorescein may show superficial punctate erosions indicating corneal dryness.
- Fine white spots on the cornea may indicate infiltrates.
- Patients with moderate to severe conjunctivitis may develop a light-coloured membrane over the inner surface of the eyelids, which is termed a pseudomembrane. This should be removed by an ophthalmologist.

Treatment

- Mild bacterial conjunctivitis is a self-limiting condition that clears within seven days. However, the use of topical antibiotics is associated with earlier clearing and a reduction in transmissibility.
  - Chloramphenicol 1% ointment four times daily for one week, or chloramphenicol 0.5% eye drops four times daily for 10 days can be used if patients are unable to tolerate ointment.
  - Fusidic acid 1% eye drops twice daily for seven days can be used second line.
- Patients should follow steps to reduce the spread of infection to others (i.e. not sharing towels, not shaking hands, and frequent hand washing). Patients are contagious while symptoms are present and these may last up to seven days.

When to refer

- Moderate to severe conjunctivitis with copious secretions, pain, and significant conjunctival inflammation should be reviewed urgently by an ophthalmologist.
- All patients should be routinely referred to an ophthalmologist to rule out an underlying secondary ocular pathology.
- Conjunctivitis in neonates or immunocompromised individuals.
- If symptoms persist beyond 10 days.
- Recurrent episodes of conjunctivitis not responding to the treatment or chronic cases (more than four weeks).
- Suspected corneal infiltrates.
- Extensive corneal staining on fluorescein examination.
- Evidence of a pseudomembrane.
- When gonococcal conjunctivitis is suspected: hyperacute (<24 hours) development of symptoms with significant purulent discharge and marked lid/conjunctival swelling.

CHAPTER 61

Patients may have a history of unprotected sexual intercourse as well as possible urethritis, proctitis, or vaginitis (see Chapter 38).
- Patients with atypical symptoms.

Viral conjunctivitis [21,28]

Pathophysiology

The most common pathogen is adenovirus.

Signs and symptoms

- Similar to bacterial conjunctivitis, but discharge is usually clear rather than mucopurulent.
- Lid oedema.
- Tender pre-auricular lymphadenopathy.
- Incubation period is 5–12 days.

Treatment

- Simple viral conjunctivitis is a self-limiting condition and treatment is supportive. Antibiotics are not required.
- Cool compresses and artificial tears can be used to relieve symptoms.
- Viral conjunctivitis is extremely contagious (10–50% risk of transmission). Patients are normally contagious for 10–14 days and should follow steps to reduce the spread of infection to others (see section Bacterial conjunctivitis).

When to refer

- When symptoms do not resolve after 10 days.
- Suspected corneal infiltrates.
- Extensive corneal staining on fluorescein examination.

Subconjunctival haemorrhage [21,29]

Pathophysiology

- A break in the conjunctival vessels leading to blood leaking between the conjunctiva and sclera.
- Most cases are idiopathic but other causes include trauma, contact lenses, infectious conjunctivitis, Valsalva manoeuvre (vomiting, straining, or coughing), systemic diseases (bleeding disorders and hypertension), and drug-related (antiplatelet agents and anticoagulants).

Signs and symptoms

- Patients suddenly develop a flat, red haemorrhage under the conjunctiva. The haemorrhage can be localised or diffuse.

- Patients are normally asymptomatic but may experience local irritation or a foreign body sensation.
- Always check a patient's blood pressure and review their use of anticoagulants/ antiplatelet agents.

Treatment

- A simple subconjunctival haemorrhage with no history of trauma can be managed conservatively. Most resolve after 10–14 days.
- Patients with irritation can use lubricating eye drops to relieve symptoms.

When to refer

- History of trauma.
- See Chapter 5 for management of high blood pressure and when to refer in this context.
- Recurrent episodes should prompt further investigation to rule out any underlying pathological cause.
- Patients on anticoagulants/antiplatelet agents with recurrent subconjunctival haemorrhage should have their medication reviewed (see Chapter 18).

DISORDERS OF THE CORNEA

Foreign body [21]

Pathophysiology

- Patients may present with various foreign bodies in the eye, ranging from eyelashes to grit blown into the eye.
- Occasionally foreign bodies may become stuck under the upper eyelid; this is termed a subtarsal foreign body.

Symptoms

- Patients may report a history of something going into the eye with symptoms starting straight afterwards.
- Foreign body sensation.
- Watering.
- Blurred vision.
- Patients may report a scratching sensation each time they blink if they have a subtarsal foreign body.

Signs

- Redness.
- Visible foreign body on the cornea with a possible rust ring that stains on fluorescein examination.

CHAPTER 61

- There may be a linear area of fluorescein staining seen with a subtarsal foreign body corresponding to the foreign body rubbing on the cornea.
- Evert the upper lid and look for a subtarsal foreign body.
- Corneal infiltrates or haziness may indicate a corneal infection.

Treatment

- For a subtarsal foreign body, sweep it away from the cornea using a cotton bud which has been soaked in sterile 0.9% saline.
- Chloramphenicol 1% ointment four times a day for one week.
- Corneal foreign bodies (i.e. those adherent or embedded in the cornea) should be removed under magnification by someone with appropriate training. As such, these patients should be referred to an ophthalmologist.

When to refer

- Patients with a corneal foreign body.
- Patients with significant visual loss.
- Patients with organic foreign bodies.
- Patients with evidence of corneal infiltrates.

Contact lens-associated microbial keratitis (corneal infection) [21,30–32]

Pathophysiology

Most cases of contact lens-associated microbial keratitis are due to poor lens hygiene:

- swimming, sleeping, or showering in lenses
- poor storage and infrequent case replacement
- soft contact lenses
- monthly contact lenses.

The most common pathogens involved are *Pseudomonas aeruginosa*, *Staphylococcus aureus*, *Staphylococcus epidermidis*, Enterobacteriaceae, and *Streptococcus* species.

A rare but important pathogen is *Acanthamoeba*, which can be found worldwide in contaminated water and soil. It can live as active trophozoites that rapidly penetrate and destroy corneal tissue, or as dormant cysts which are extremely resistant to extreme conditions (can lie dormant within the cornea).

Symptoms

- Foreign body sensation.
- Pain.
- Reduced vision.
- Photophobia.

CHAPTER 61

- Symptoms secondary to *Acanthamoeba* typically develop gradually with only slight discomfort over a couple of weeks. Later, patients may develop significant ocular pain with very few other clinical signs.

Signs

- Corneal infiltrates.
- Epithelial defects that stain with fluorescein.
- Development of hypopyon (pus in the anterior chamber of the eye).
- Conjunctival redness.
- Eyelid swelling.

Treatment

These patients need to be urgently referred to and assessed by an ophthalmologist.

Prevention

To prevent infection, patients should be advised to follow the guidance set out here.

- Always wash and dry your hands before handling contact lenses.
- If you use a case, once you have put your lenses into your eyes, throw away the old multi-purpose solution and clean the case with fresh solution. Let the case air dry and never use tap water.
- Reusable lenses should be washed each day. Once you have taken out the lenses, place the lens in your palm with some multi-purpose solution. Rub each side of the lens for 10 seconds and rinse off with more solution.
- Store the lenses in a proper storage case using only multi-purpose solution to completely cover the lenses. Replace the case at least every three months.
- Always use approved multi-purpose solution.
- Never sleep, swim, or shower in contact lenses.
- The prescribing optometrist will set a maximum time you can wear your lenses a day. The general rule is not to wear them for more than 10–12 hours a day.
- Always replace your lenses as per your prescription.

Glaucoma [21,33]

Pathophysiology

Glaucoma describes a group of conditions characterised by damage to the optic nerve and death of retinal cells leading to visual loss. It is the second most important cause of irreversible blindness in the world, leading to significant morbidity

It can be divided into two forms, primary open angle and closed angle, relating to the anterior chamber drainage angle of the eye (see Box 61.2 for further explanation). In both types, the main risk factor for glaucoma is ocular hypertension, with most treatments aimed at reducing eye pressure

Symptoms

Primary open-angle glaucoma
- Most are asymptomatic until glaucoma becomes advanced.
- As retinal cells are irreversibly lost, patients develop visual field defects that start in the periphery and can progress over time to the whole visual field.
- Patients' symptoms are then related to their visual field defect, with advanced visual field defects giving a constricted view.

Acute closed-angle glaucoma
- Symptoms are a result of a sudden rise in intraocular pressure due to a closed anterior chamber angle.
- Sudden severe eye pain.
- Redness.
- Blurring of vision.
- Nausea and vomiting.

Signs

- Visual loss in primary open-angle glaucoma.
- Acute closed-angle glaucoma: redness, corneal oedema, fixed mid-dilated pupil.

Treatment and side effects

The mainstay of glaucoma treatment is daily eye drops. While effective, these drops do have side effects that clinicians should be aware of.

- Prostaglandin analogues such as bimatoprost (Lumigan), latanoprost (Xalatan), and travoprost (Travatan): changes in eyelid colour, eye irritation and redness, eyelash growth, and sunken eyes.
- Alpha-agonists such as apraclonidine (Iopidine) and brimonidine (Alphagan): eye irritation, fatigue and drowsiness, dry mouth, and high blood pressure.
- Beta-blockers such as timolol: hypotension, fatigue, and reduced sex drive. Contraindicated in patients with asthma and chronic obstructive pulmonary disease.
- Carbonic anhydrase inhibitors such as brinzolamide (Azopt) and dorzolamide (Trusopt): eye irritation.
- Patients may also be on combination drops: Combigan (brimonidine and timolol), Simbrinza (brinzolamide and brimonidine), Cosopt (timolol and dorzolamide).

When to refer

- Most glaucoma patients should already be under regular ophthalmology follow-up with their ophthalmology team. Where acute closed-angle glaucoma is suspected, refer as an emergency to ophthalmology. Any agents presumed to be causative should be stopped.
- Patients experiencing side effects from their eye drops should be discussed with their regular ophthalmology team.

CHAPTER 61

References

1. Buch H, Vinding T, la Cour M, et al. Prevalence and causes of visual impairment and blindness among 9980 Scandinavian adults: the Copenhagen City Eye Study. *Ophthalmology* 2004;111(1):53–61.

2. Ward M, Druss B. The epidemiology of diabetes in psychotic disorders. *Lancet Psychiatry* 2015;2(5):431–451.

3. Moulton CD, Pickup JC, Ismail K. The link between depression and diabetes: the search for shared mechanisms. *Lancet Diabetes Endocrinol* 2015;3(6):461–471.

4. Richa S, Yazbek JC. Ocular adverse effects of common psychotropic agents: a review. *CNS Drugs* 2010;24(6):501–526.

5. Ruigomez A, Garcia Rodriguez LA, Dev VJ, et al. Are schizophrenia or antipsychotic drugs a risk factor for cataracts? *Epidemiology* 2000;11(6):620–623.

6. Li J, Tripathi RC, Tripathi BJ. Drug-induced ocular disorders. *Drug Saf* 2008;31(2):127–141.

7. Edwards RM, Stoudemire A, Vela MA, Morris R. Intraocular pressure changes in nonglaucomatous patients undergoing electroconvulsive therapy. *Convuls Ther* 1990;6(3):209–213.

8. Viertio S, Laitinen A, Perälä J, et al. Visual impairment in persons with psychotic disorder. *Soc Psychiatry Psychiatr Epidemiol* 2007;42(11):902–908.

9. Brenner CA, Lysaker PH, Wilt MA, O'Donnell BF. Visual processing and neuropsychological function in schizophrenia and schizoaffective disorder. *Psychiatry Res* 2002;111(2–3):125–136.

10. Ahmadi N, Snidvongs K, Kalish L, et al. Intranasal corticosteroids do not affect intraocular pressure or lens opacity: a systematic review of controlled trials. *Rhinology* 2015;53(4):290–302.

11. Bond WS, Yee GC. Ocular and cutaneous effects of chronic phenothiazine therapy. *Am J Hosp Pharm* 1980;37(1):74–78.

12. Davidorf FH. Thioridazine pigmentary retinopathy. *Arch Ophthalmol* 1973;90(3):251–255.

13. Oshika T. Ocular adverse effects of neuropsychiatric agents. Incidence and management. *Drug Saf* 1995;12(4):256–263.

14. Pakes GE. Eye irritation and lithium carbonate. *Arch Ophthalmol* 1980;98(5):930.

15. Shur E, Checkley S. Pupil studies in depressed patients: an investigation of the mechanism of action of desipramine. *Br J Psychiatry* 1982;140:181–184.

16. Edler K, Ravn J, Gottfries CG, Haslund J. Eye changes in connection with neuroleptic treatment especially concerning phenothiazines and thioxanthenes. *Acta Psychiatr Scand* 1971;47(4):377–384.

17. Ritch R, Krupin T, Henry C, Kurata F. Oral imipramine and acute angle-closure glaucoma. *Arch Ophthalmol* 1994;112(1):67–68.

18. Costagliola C, Parmeggiani F, Sebastiani A. SSRIs and intraocular pressure modifications: evidence, therapeutic implications and possible mechanisms. *CNS Drugs* 2004;18(8):475–484.

19. Malone DA, Camara EG, Krug JH. Ophthalmologic effects of psychotropic medications. *Psychosomatics* 1992;33(3):271–277.

20. National Institute of Health and Care Excellence. Dry eye syndrome. Clinical Knowledge Summary. Last revised: August 2017. https://cks.nice.org.uk/dry-eye-syndrome

21. Denniston A, Murray P. *Oxford Handbook of Ophthalmology*, 4th edn. Oxford: Oxford University Press, 2018.

22. Sundaram V, Barsam A, Barker L, Khaw P. *Training in Ophthalmology*, 2nd edn. Oxford: Oxford University Press, 2016.

23. National Institute of Health and Care Excellence. Blepharitis. Clinical Knowledge Summary. Last revised: April 2019. https://cks.nice.org.uk/blepharitis

24. Gao YY, Di Pascuale MA, Li W, et al. In vitro and in vivo killing of ocular *Demodex* by tea tree oil. *Br J Ophthalmol* 2005; 89(11):1468–1473.

25. National Institute of Health and Care Excellence. Styes (hordeola). Clinical Knowledge Summary. Last revised: October 2019. https://cks.nice.org.uk/styes-hordeola

26. National Institute of Health and Care Excellence. Meibomian cyst (chalazion). Clinical Knowledge Summary. Last revised: March 2019. https://cks.nice.org.uk/meibomian-cyst-chalazion

27. Azari AA, Barney NP. Conjunctivitis: a systematic review of diagnosis and treatment. *JAMA* 2013;310(16):1721–1729.

28. National Institute of Health and Care Excellence. Conjunctivitis: infective. Clinical Knowledge Summary. Last revised: April 2018. https://cks.nice.org.uk/conjunctivitis-infective

29. Tarlan B, Kiratli H. Subconjunctival hemorrhage: risk factors and potential indicators. *Clin Ophthalmol* 2013;7:1163–1170.

30. Lin A, Rhee MK, Akpek EK, et al. Bacterial keratitis Preferred Practice Pattern. *Ophthalmology* 2019;126(1):P1–P55.

31. Carnt N, Hoffman JM, Verma S, et al. *Acanthamoeba* keratitis: confirmation of the UK outbreak and a prospective case-control study identifying contributing risk factors. *Br J Ophthalmol* 2018;102(12):1621–1628.

32. Association of Optometrists. Contact lens advice. https://www.aop.org.uk/advice-and-support/for-patients/contact-lenses/soft-lenses (accessed 3 February 2019).

33. Robciuc A, Witos J, Ruokonen SK, et al. Pure glaucoma drugs are toxic to immortalized human corneal epithelial cells, but they do not destabilize lipid membranes. *Cornea* 2017;36(10):1249–1255.

CHAPTER 61

Part 12

Obstetrics and Gynaecology

Pregnancy

Katherine Beck, Ruth Cochrane, Louise M. Howard

In all women of reproductive age presenting with a medical or psychiatric complaint, an important consideration for the clinician is to determine whether the patient is pregnant. Pregnancy in women with serious mental illness (SMI) is common, and this group faces significant challenges, including increased risk of psychiatric relapse [1]; increased risk of obstetric complications (including the potential risk of psychiatric medications to the physical health of the fetus) [2]; increased risk of maternal physical complications [2]; the stress of social services being involved if there are concerns for the unborn child's welfare (Children's Social Care in the UK); and the ongoing stigma of having a psychiatric diagnosis. Suicide is the third most common cause of direct maternal death [3]. The perinatal period is not a protective factor for suicide in women in contact with mental health services, unlike the general population where it is less common during this period [4]. Indeed, in women in contact with psychiatric services, suicide in the perinatal period is more likely to occur in those with depression and no active treatment [5]. This chapter covers pre-conception advice, information on routine antenatal care in the UK, and common medical illnesses in pregnancy. It also provides advice on prescribing psychiatric medication in the antenatal and postnatal periods.

Mental illness during pregnancy is associated with several obstetric complications, including restricted fetal growth, low birthweight, preterm delivery, congenital anomalies, stillbirth, and neonatal death [2,6,7]. There are a number of lifestyle factors that are more prevalent in patients with SMI that adversely affect pregnancy outcomes, including smoking, poor diet, obesity, alcohol, and recreational drug use [8]. The risks of psychiatric medication in pregnancy are hard to quantify and the evidence base weak. There is some evidence of a small association between congenital malformations and some medications such as antidepressants [2]. However, these studies are observational in nature and so are unable to determine causality. Furthermore, with the improvement in methodological quality of studies over time, the reported risk of congenital

The Maudsley Practice Guidelines for Physical Health Conditions in Psychiatry, First Edition.
David M. Taylor, Fiona Gaughran, and Toby Pillinger.
© 2021 John Wiley & Sons Ltd. Published 2021 by John Wiley & Sons Ltd.

malformations with antidepressant treatment has reduced. As with all treatments, the risk of psychiatric medication to the fetus should be balanced against the risk of untreated mental illness to both the mother and baby [5]. For example, failure to receive psychiatric treatment increases the risk of relapse in mental illness in the perinatal period [9].

Patients with SMI may need pre-conception advice and support. Asking women about their hopes and wishes for pregnancy early on and throughout their psychiatric care may increase the likelihood of women seeking and receiving pre-conception advice and appropriate support through the prenatal and postnatal periods [10]. Pregnancy can also motivate women to embrace a healthier lifestyle. This period, and ideally before with pre-conception counselling, may provide a unique opportunity to support women to moderate lifestyle factors associated with obstetric complications.

THE PRE-CONCEPTION PERIOD

All women should be offered the opportunity to discuss their mental health and associated treatment before becoming pregnant. Perinatal mental disorders often occur in the context of previous mental health problems, including illnesses in childhood and adolescence [11]. In the UK, specialist perinatal mental health services are starting to offer pre-conception counselling to all women with moderate to severe mental illness who are considering pregnancy. Early pre-conception discussion allows parents to access appropriate support and minimises risk to both mother and baby [12]. Pre-conception discussion should cover the following.

- The patient's current mental health and treatment.
- The patient's past psychiatric history, relapse indicators, and risk associated with relapse.
- The risks and benefits of psychiatric medication during pregnancy. Current evidence suggests that the risks of most psychotropic medications (other than sodium valproate and carbamazepine) are small. However, the evidence base is changing quickly, so it is always important to obtain up-to-date advice from the local perinatal team.
- Nutrition, weight management, physical exercise, smoking, alcohol and recreational drug use, and folic acid supplementation.
- Potential domestic violence and abuse.

Pre-conception medication advice

Of all the psychiatric medications prescribed, the anticonvulsant mood stabilisers sodium valproate and carbamazepine are associated with the most significant risk of teratogenicity. Therefore, sodium valproate and carbamazepine are contraindicated in pregnancy [2]. There is also a risk of developmental delay and lower IQ in children exposed to sodium valproate during pregnancy [2]. Indeed, in the UK, Medicines and Healthcare Products Regulatory Agency (MHRA) guidance states that sodium valproate should not be prescribed in women of reproductive age unless there is a 'pregnancy prevention programme' in place. This involves the patient signing a document where they acknowledge the teratogenic risk of sodium valproate, and an understanding that if sexually active they will use 'highly effective' contraception (see Chapter 36). If patients on this medication do become pregnant, the clinician should carry out the following.

- Confirm pregnancy as soon as possible.
- Obtain information on specific risks to the fetus from the medication (see UK Teratology Information Service [13]).
- Explain that stopping or switching the medication may not remove these risks but recommend doing so if the mother decides to continue the pregnancy. For information on alternative drugs and how to switch, see the position statement by the Royal College of Psychiatrists and British Association for Psychopharmacology [14].
- If the decision is to continue the pregnancy, refer for screening for fetal anomalies and offer counselling to support the woman in her decision.

For psychiatric drugs other than sodium valproate and carbamazepine, patients who become pregnant or wish to become pregnant have three options: (i) continue with treatment unchanged; (ii) switch to an agent with a lower risk of fetal complications; or (iii) stop all pharmacological treatment. Further information regarding psychiatric medication prescribing in pregnancy is provided in section Psychiatric medication in pregnancy. Decisions should be made after multidisciplinary input, with both risks and benefits of continued psychiatric treatment considered. Discontinuation of treatment should be done slowly, with careful monitoring of a woman's mental health and, where pregnancy is planned, use of effective contraception until drug washout. These changes should be done prior to pregnancy as doing this during pregnancy may increase the risk of relapse.

DURING PREGNANCY

Early antenatal care

The first antenatal appointment, which in the UK occurs at approximately 10 weeks post conception, involves a series of physical assessments including calculation of body mass index (BMI), urine dip for evidence of infection and diabetes mellitus, blood pressure assessment, and blood screening for human immunodeficiency virus (HIV), syphilis, hepatitis B, anaemia, sickle cell anaemia, and thalassaemia. Blood tests also allow assessment of rhesus status and blood grouping. In the UK, women are routinely cared for by midwives but if there are medical complications or the woman is considered obstetrically high risk, they may also be reviewed by a consultant obstetrician.

At this first meeting, women should be asked about their mental health [15] and women with SMI offered care under a specialised midwifery team trained in mental health. If a woman is not currently under a mental health team but has a history of a moderate to severe mental illness or has current symptoms of mental illness requiring further assessment, she should be referred to or discussed with the local perinatal psychiatric team. If the patient is currently under a mental health team, the team should be contacted to ensure there is good communication and information sharing between all teams involved in the patient's care. It is important to keep women involved and informed of these communications.

An assessment of the level of support available to the woman from her partner, family, and mental health services should also be made. Potential risks to the mother and safeguarding issues should be identified and the need for social services input (in the UK, Children's Social Care) considered in cases where there is a reasonable risk that mental illness or social factors will impact parenting. Referral to social services should always be discussed with the woman except in the rare circumstance where such a conversation may be associated with increased risk, for example where there is a risk of the woman absconding, thus putting the child at risk. Communication between all teams involved in the woman's care is essential.

A birth plan should be discussed with the woman early in pregnancy. This should be made in collaboration with the woman, her obstetric team, her mental health team (perinatal or community mental health team), primary care, and social services if they are providing input. The plan should be carefully documented (Box 62.1), easily accessible, and available to the woman and all teams involved in her care.

Box 62.1 Contents of a birth plan

Professionals involved in care

- Document which professionals are involved in the patient's care.
- Provide names and contact details where possible.

Description of obstetric, physical, and mental health diagnoses

Mental health relapse indicators and past risk

Hospital setting for birth (labour ward/midwifery-led unit)

Document what psychiatric services the patient has access to, e.g. 24-hour perinatal liaison services, specialist obstetric/neonatal services, access to social services.

Preferred method of delivery

- A woman's wishes should be respected while selecting the most appropriate obstetric method. This decision should be explained carefully to the woman, particularly in those with learning difficulty or with cognitive symptoms as part of a condition such as schizophrenia.
- Special consideration should be given to women with a history of sexual abuse, including careful explanation of potential procedures such as vaginal examinations and considering methods of minimising distress from these.
- Consider need for specialist mental health nurse or an advocate where appropriate.

Medication

- Document plans for psychotropic medication in pregnancy, during labour (e.g. stopping lithium when woman goes into labour; see section Psychiatric medication in pregnancy), and immediately postnatally.

- Discuss need for psychiatric drug monitoring (e.g. lithium levels) and potential risks of drugs to neonate.

Postnatal care

Document feeding choice and advice given about psychotropic medication and breast feeding

- Document plan for mental health monitoring, including frequency, by which team (community mental health team or perinatal team), by which team member (nurse, doctor and what seniority), and proposed length of time required for monitoring.
- Define psychotropic medication plan.
- Document side room requirement.
- Document specific neonatal checks required dependent on medication during pregnancy and risk of withdrawal in the neonate.

Safeguarding

Document any issues and plan.

The woman's wishes regarding breastfeeding should be considered and supported. Local sources for breastfeeding support should be identified, including support groups and cafés, websites, and local breastfeeding initiatives. Advice about the use of psychotropic medications whilst breastfeeding should be given, including risks of sedation to the newborn with certain antipsychotics (e.g. olanzapine) [16]. Most drugs are found in low concentrations in breast milk and it is worth explaining to the mother that if she has already taken the medication in pregnancy, the risk of the drug will be lower in breastfeeding as there is less exposure for most drugs. Lithium and clozapine are contraindicated in breastfeeding. The postnatal period is a risky time to switch drugs and this is not advisable unless there is a serious risk of medication non-adherence. The reader is directed to the LactMed database [16], which provides information on drugs to which breastfeeding may be exposed, including information on the levels of such substances in breast milk and infant blood and the possible adverse effects in the nursing infant. It is also worth considering the impact that lack of sleep might have on the woman with unpredictable baby feeding patterns overnight and identifying sources of support with feeding, such as friends, family, or partners (e.g. mixed feeding with breast and formula/expressing milk for bottle feeds). If a woman does not feel able to breastfeed or needs to mix feed, this should be supported, and advice given about formula feeding and bottle care (such as sterilisation).

Common medical illnesses in pregnancy

Pregnancy increases the risk of several medical complaints, and some pre-existing illnesses may worsen in the context of pregnancy. These are documented in Table 62.1. Some psychotropic medications can put women at greater risk of medical illness during pregnancy. For example, taking certain antipsychotics (the so-called second-generation antipsychotics) increases the risk of gestational diabetes [2]. Thus, women with SMI should be pre-emptively given diet and exercise advice, and antenatal services should offer all women with mental illness an oral glucose tolerance test [17,18]. Women who

Table 62.1 Medical complaints associated with pregnancy or that may pose greater risk during pregnancy.

	Symptoms	Recommended investigations	Available treatments
Morning sickness	Nausea Vomiting	Urine dip: ketones Bloods: full blood count, urea and electrolytes, liver function test, thyroid function tests, calcium, phosphate Ultrasound: multiple or molar pregnancy	Rest Ginger Anti-emetic (see Chapter 21)
Anaemia	Fatigue, pallor, weakness, headache, palpitations, dizziness, dyspnoea	Blood: full blood count, iron studies Hb <110 g/L in first trimester Hb <105 g/L in second and third trimester Hb <100 g/L postpartum	Ferrous sulfate 100–200 mg orally once daily See Chapter 15
Urinary tract infection	Often asymptomatic If symptomatic: Dysuria Polyuria Haematuria Cloudy/smelly urine Back pain Fever	Urine dip and culture If no symptoms but urine dip positive, take a second sample and send for cultures and treat based on this If Group B *Streptococcus* isolated, inform antenatal services	Nitrofurantoin 100 mg (modified release) for 7 days See local guidance and Chapter 41
Gestational diabetes	Often asymptomatic If symptomatic: Polyuria Polydipsia Fatigue	Urine dip: glycosuria 2+ or above on one occasion or 1+ on two occasions 2-hour 75-g oral glucose tolerance test (OGTT) (fasting plasma glucose 5.6 mmol/L or above, or 2-hour plasma glucose 7.8 mmol/L or above)	Refer to joint diabetes and antenatal clinic within one week Increased monitoring by antenatal team including regular blood sugar monitoring Diet and exercise, metformin, insulin if necessary
Pre-eclampsia	Severe headache Visual disturbance (blurring or flashing before the eyes) Severe pain just below the ribs Vomiting Sudden swelling (face, hands or feet)	Blood pressure (hypertension can be the only initial sign of pre-eclampsia, so refer at this point) Urine dip: protein Bloods: full blood count, urea and electrolytes, liver function tests	Increased monitoring by antenatal team including regular blood pressure, urine dip, and blood tests Oral labetalol If severe may require admission
Obstetric cholestasis	Itching Jaundice Pale stools Dark urine	Blood: liver function tests, bile acid Abdominal ultrasound to check for liver abnormalities and gallstones	Increased monitoring by antenatal team, including regular blood tests. Monitoring of baby including fetal growth scans (ultrasound) Labour is usually induced at 37–38 weeks
High body mass index (BMI)		If BMI >30 kg/m², offer OGTT at 24–28 weeks' gestation Consider need for anaesthetic review prior to delivery	Advice about low-carbohydrate diet and exercise in pregnancy

take antidepressants might be at an increased risk of hypertension [19] and pre-eclampsia [20] during pregnancy. Postnatally, selective serotonin inhibitors may increase the risk of postpartum haemorrhage [2].

Management of medical complications in pregnancy is of course beyond the remit of the psychiatrist, but if there is concern that a woman has one of the medical illnesses outlined in Table 62.1, then they should be supported to seek help from their obstetric team. The investigations and treatment described here are to ensure clinicians are aware of what the patient may be offered.

Reduced or altered food intake

This may occur in patients with eating disorders, severe depression, psychosis involving delusions about food, and alcohol misuse. Consider increased physical monitoring and growth scans from 20 weeks every four weeks.

Smoking and pregnancy

The prevalence of smoking in pregnancy is 8.1% in Europe and 1.7% globally [21]. Women with mental health problems are more likely to smoke during pregnancy [22]. Evidence suggests that women with SMI are motivated to stop smoking but require more support than women without mental illness [23]. Smoking is the single biggest modifiable risk factor for poor birth outcomes [24]. For women who smoke in pregnancy, offer the option to change to nicotine replacement therapy, which has a lower risk of adverse outcomes in pregnancy than smoking itself [25] and refer to a smoking cessation service (see Chapter 46). Smoking should ideally be identified in pre-conception discussions and smoking cessation advice and support given prior to pregnancy.

Alcohol and pregnancy

Alcohol consumption during pregnancy can be associated with harm to the fetus [2]. It is associated with fetal alcohol spectrum disorders, which include preterm birth, low birthweight, and developmental delays [26]. In the UK, National Institute for Health and Care Excellence (NICE) guidance advocates abstinence during pregnancy [27]. If a pregnant woman with alcohol dependence develops withdrawal symptoms, then pharmacological treatments such as chlordiazepoxide should be considered in an inpatient setting with specialist supervision [2,28]. Chlordiazepoxide does not appear to confer significant risk to the fetus, although there is some limited evidence for it causing developmental delay [2]. The UK Teratology Information Service provides national advice for healthcare professionals caring for pregnant patients who require alcohol detoxification [13].

PSYCHIATRIC MEDICATION IN PREGNANCY

In the UK, general guidance for healthcare professionals prescribing physical or psychiatric treatments during pregnancy can be obtained via the UK Teratology Information Service. This is a national service commissioned by Public Health England.

General prescribing principles in pregnancy and the postnatal period [2,18]

- If a patient with SMI is managed well on a certain pharmacological agent, where possible avoid making prescription changes.
- Consider the potential benefits of psychological treatment.
- Have a higher threshold for pharmacological treatment in women with mild to moderate illnesses.
- When medication is started, consider the following.
  - Choose the medication with the lowest risk profile for the woman, fetus, and baby.
  - Prescribe the lowest effective dose, especially where adverse effects are dose-related. However, take into consideration that subtherapeutic doses may expose the fetus to risks whilst not effectively treating the mother's psychiatric symptoms.
  - Use a single drug where possible.
  - Using a drug of known efficacy in a patient may be preferable to using one of unknown efficacy but with lower pregnancy risk.
  - Changes in dose may be required over the course of the pregnancy. Medications may require a dose increase in the third trimester [29]. Metabolism of drugs by the liver can also change, affecting the amount of active drug available. This is particularly true for lamotrigine where drug levels change significantly during pregnancy and so must be taken regularly [18].
  - Do not routinely offer depot antipsychotics to a woman who is planning a pregnancy, is pregnant or is considering breastfeeding unless she is already responding well to a depot or has a previous history of non-adherence with oral medication.
  - The degree of risk is uncertain for most psychotropic medications in pregnancy and it is important to explicitly acknowledge this in discussions with the woman; current evidence suggests that risks of most psychotropic medications (other than sodium valproate and carbamazepine) are small.
  - Consider detailed ultrasound scanning for mothers taking psychiatric medication with recognised risk of congenital malformations.
  - Monitor for excessive weight gain.
  - Monitor for gestational diabetes.
  - Consider high-dose folic acid 5 mg daily [30], although this may alter the efficacy of drugs such as lamotrigine [31].
  - Midwives must be made aware of any medications that should be stopped during labour, e.g. lithium.

Advice for specific psychiatric medications

Table 62.2 provides information regarding perinatal prescription of antidepressant, antipsychotic, and mood stabiliser medications [2]. This table includes the most commonly prescribed medications in pregnancy; for more information on additional psychiatric medications in pregnancy, the reader is directed to the guidelines from the British Association of Psychopharmacology [2] and NICE [18].

Table 62.2 Risks and considerations in the perinatal prescription of antidepressant, antipsychotic, and mood stabiliser medication [2,18].

	Pregnancy outcomes (neonatal)	Pregnancy outcomes (maternal)	Neonatal	Monitoring and special considerations in pregnancy/delivery	Breastfeeding
Antidepressants (SSRIs) [2]	Preterm delivery Lower birthweight Cardiac malformations (particularly for paroxetine) Persistent pulmonary hypertension of the newborn (low absolute risk)	Increased bleeding Postpartum haemorrhage	Irritability Constant crying Jitteriness Vomiting Shivering Increased tone Eating difficulties Sleeping difficulties Respiratory distress Tremors	N/A	Sertraline: low rate of reported adverse effects on breast-fed babies
Antipsychotics (second generation) [2]: most safety data for quetiapine, olanzapine and risperidone with more limited data for clozapine and aripiprazole	Risperidone: increased risk of malformations Increased birthweight Use of cariprazine in pregnancy is not currently recommended	Gestational diabetes mellitus Hypertension		Diabetes screening Monitor weight and blood pressure	Low RID for olanzapine and quetiapine Moderate RID for risperidone and aripiprazole Contraindicated for clozapine: risk of infant agranulocytosis and seizures

(continued)

Table 62.2 (Continued)

	Pregnancy outcomes (neonatal)	Pregnancy outcomes (maternal)	Neonatal	Monitoring and special considerations in pregnancy/delivery	Breastfeeding
Lithium [2,18]	Cardiac malformations including Ebstein's anomaly [32] (risk of cardiac anomaly odds ratio 1.81) [33] Dose-related risk of malformations when dose increases above 900 mg/day			Regular lithium levels (every 4 weeks in pregnancy), then weekly after the 36th week Detailed ultrasound as early as possible to detect cardiac malformations at 11–14 weeks Encourage good fluid intake Delivery in hospital Check lithium levels and fluid balance in labour as risk of lithium toxicity Stop lithium during labour and check lithium levels 12 hours after last dose for mother and baby	Significant amounts pass into the baby Contraindicated as risk of neonatal toxicity
Lamotrigine	Largest body of evidence suggests not associated with congenital abnormalities but one study found a small increase	N/A		Check blood levels of drug regularly during pregnancy and into the postnatal period because they vary substantially during these times Consider high-dose folic acid, although risk that it reduces effectiveness of lamotrigine	Significant amounts pass into breast milk. Case reports of severe apnoea and CNS depression in breast-fed neonate. Theoretical risk of dermatological problems

RID, relative infant dose (estimates infant drug exposure via breast milk); the RID uses a known milk concentration and compares it to either an infant therapeutic dose or the weight-adjusted maternal dose when an infant dose is not well established.

Advice in the postnatal period and during breastfeeding

- Be cautious when prescribing sedating medication, which can interfere with baby care and breastfeeding, as well as causing neonatal sedation. Advise all women against sleeping with their baby.
- Breastfeeding women should have rapid access to psychological therapies but if symptoms of psychiatric illness are severe, then medication may be the most effective form of treatment.
- Choose treatments with the lowest known risk and recognise there are limited long-term data on neurodevelopmental outcomes.
- A guide to the possible risk of breastfeeding to the child whilst taking medication is the relative infant dose (RID), which estimates infant drug exposure via breast milk [16].
- Monitor the infant for possible adverse side effects such as over-sedation and poor feeding.
- If the infant is premature or unwell, greater caution needs to be exercised, especially where the mother is taking more than one medication.

POSTPARTUM PSYCHOSIS

Admission to a psychiatric hospital for postpartum psychosis occurs in around 1–2 per 1000 births in the general population [34]. There is a strong association with bipolar affective disorder and women with this diagnosis have a risk of at least one in five of developing postpartum psychosis [35]. Women who have experienced previous postpartum psychosis or who have a family history of postpartum psychosis are at very high risk [35,36].

Postpartum psychosis is characterised by psychotic symptoms such as delusions and hallucinations, but women may also experience confusion. Most episodes occur within two weeks of delivery and 50% of these occur within the first one to three days [37]. It usually has a rapid onset with fluctuations in symptom intensity. It can be accompanied by notable swings in mood [37].

Where postpartum psychosis occurs in the absence of previous contact with mental health services, assessment and investigations should be as for any individual presenting with first-episode psychosis. Important differentials to consider in all patients in the postnatal period are eclampsia, delirium, thyroid disorders, and infection [38].

All women at risk of psychosis postnatally should plan to remain on the postnatal ward for five days after delivery in a side room to ensure they get as much sleep and rest as possible.

CHAPTER 62

ELECTROCONVULSIVE THERAPY IN PREGNANCY

The reader is directed to Chapter 66 on electroconvulsive therapy.

References

1. Taylor CL, Stewart RJ, Howard LM. Relapse in the first three months postpartum in women with history of serious mental illness. *Schizophr Res* 2019;204:46–54.

2. McAllister-Williams RH, Baldwin DS, Cantwell R, et al. British Association for Psychopharmacology consensus guidance on the use of psychotropic medication preconception, in pregnancy and postpartum 2017. *J Psychopharmacol* 2017;31(5):519–552.

3. Knight M, Bunch K, Tuffnell D, et al. (eds) *Saving Lives, Improving Mothers' Care. Lessons learned to inform maternity care from the UK and Ireland Confidential Enquiries into Maternal Deaths and Morbidity 2014–16*. Oxford: National Perinatal Epidemiology Unit, University of Oxford, 2018.

4. Appleby L, Mortensen PB, Faragher EB. Suicide and other causes of mortality after post-partum psychiatric admission. *Br J Psychiatry* 1998;173(3):209–211.

5. Khalifeh H, Hunt IM, Appleby L, Howard LM. Suicide in perinatal and non-perinatal women in contact with psychiatric services: 15 year findings from a UK national inquiry. *Lancet Psychiatry* 2016;3(3):233–242.

6. Stein A, Pearson RM, Goodman SH, et al. Effects of perinatal mental disorders on the fetus and child. *Lancet* 2014;384(9956):1800–1819.

7. McElhatton PR. General principles of drug use in pregnancy. *Pharm J* 2003;270:232–234.

8. Shah N, Howard L. Screening for smoking and substance misuse in pregnant women with mental illness. *Psychiatr Bull* 2006;30(8):294–297.

9. Cohen LS, Altshuler LL, Harlow BL, et al. Relapse of major depression during pregnancy in women who maintain or discontinue antidepressant treatment. *JAMA* 2006;295(5):499–507.

10. Catalao R, Mann S, Wilson C, Howard LM. Preconception care in mental health services: planning for a better future. *Br J Psychiatry* 2020;216(4):180–181.

11. Patton GC, Romaniuk H, Spry E, et al. Prediction of perinatal depression from adolescence and before conception (VIHCS): 20-year prospective cohort study. *Lancet* 2015;386(9996):875–883.

12. Dolman C, Jones I, Howard LM. Pre-conception to parenting: a systematic review and meta-synthesis of the qualitative literature on motherhood for women with severe mental illness. *Arch Womens Ment Health* 2013;16(3):173–196.

13. UK Teratology Information Service. Best use of medicines in pregnancy. www.UKTIS.org.

14. Royal College of Psychiatrists. Withdrawal of, and alternatives to, valproate-containing medicines in girls and women of childbearing potential who have a psychiatric illness. Position Statement PS04/18, December 2018. Available at https://www.bap.org.uk/pdfs/PS04-18-December2018.pdf

15. Yapp E, Howard LM, Kadicheeni M, et al. A qualitative study of women's views on the acceptability of being asked about mental health problems at antenatal booking appointments. *Midwifery* 2019;74:126–133.

16. Drugs and Lactation Database (LactMed). https://www.ncbi.nlm.nih.gov/books/NBK501922/

17. Bodén R, Lundgren M, Brandt L, et al. Antipsychotics during pregnancy. *Arch Gen Psychiatry* 2012;69(7):715–721.

18. National Institute for Health and Care Excellence. *Antenatal and Postnatal Mental Health: Clinical Management and Service Guidance*. Clinical Guideline CG192. London: NICE, 2014. Available at https://www.nice.org.uk/guidance/cg192/chapter/1-Recommendations#treatment-decisions-advice-and-monitoring-for-women-who-are-planning-a-pregnancy-pregnant-or-in-2

19. De Vera MA, Bérard A. Antidepressant use during pregnancy and the risk of pregnancy-induced hypertension. *Br J Clin Pharmacol* 2012;74(2):362–369.

20. Palmsten K, Huybrechts KF, Michels KB, et al. Antidepressant use and risk for preeclampsia. *Epidemiology* 2013;24(5):682–691.

21. Lange S, Probst C, Rehm J, Popova S. National, regional, and global prevalence of smoking during pregnancy in the general population: a systematic review and meta-analysis. *Lancet Global Health* 2018;6(7):E769–E776.

22. Goodwin RD, Keyes K, Simuro N. Mental disorders and nicotine dependence among pregnant women in the United States. *Obstet Gynecol* 2007;109(4):875–883.

23. Howard LM, Bekele D, Rowe M, et al. Smoking cessation in pregnant women with mental disorders: a cohort and nested qualitative study. *BJOG* 2013;120(3):362–370.

24. Public Health England. *Making the Case for Preconception Care. Planning and Preparation for Pregnancy to Improve Maternal and Child Health Outcomes*. London: PHE, 2018. Available at https://assets.publishing.service.gov.uk/government/uploads/system/uploads/attachment_data/file/729018/Making_the_case_for_preconception_care.pdf).

25. Cooper S, Lewis S, Thornton JG, et al. The SNAP trial: a randomised placebo-controlled trial of nicotine replacement therapy in pregnancy: clinical effectiveness and safety until 2 years after delivery, with economic evaluation. *Health Technol Assess* 2014;18(54):1–128.

26. O'Leary C, Nassar N, Kurinczuk J, Bower C. The effect of maternal alcohol consumption on fetal growth and preterm birth. *BJOG* 2009;116(3):390–400.

27. UK Departments of Health. *UK Chief Medical Officers' Low Risk Drinking Guidelines*. https://assets.publishing.service.gov.uk/government/uploads/system/uploads/attachment_data/file/545937/UK_CMOs__report.pdf

28. Lingford-Hughes A, Welch S, Peters L, Nutt D. BAP updated guidelines: evidence-based guidelines for the pharmacological management of substance abuse, harmful use, addiction and comorbidity: recommendations from BAP. *J Psychopharmacol* 2012;26(7):899–952.

29. Seeman MV. Clinical interventions for women with schizophrenia: pregnancy. *Acta Psychiatr Scand* 2013;127(1):12–22.

30. Wlodarczyk BJ, Palacios AM, George TM, Finnell RH. Antiepileptic drugs and pregnancy outcomes. *Am J Med Genet A* 2012;158A(8):2071–2090.

31. Geddes JR, Gardiner A, Rendell J, et al. Comparative evaluation of quetiapine plus lamotrigine combination versus quetiapine monotherapy (and folic acid versus placebo) in bipolar depression (CEQUEL): a 2 × 2 factorial randomised trial. *Lancet Psychiatry* 2016;3(1):31–39.

32. Patorno E, Huybrechts KF, Bateman BT, et al. Lithium use in pregnancy and the risk of cardiac malformations. *N Engl J Med* 2017;376(23):2245–2254.

33. Fornaro M, Maritan E, Ferranti R, et al. Lithium exposure during pregnancy and the postpartum period: a systematic review and meta-analysis of safety and efficacy outcomes. *Am J Psychiatry* 2020;177(1):76–92.

35. Jones I, Chandra PS, Dazzan P, Howard LM. Bipolar disorder, affective psychosis, and schizophrenia in pregnancy and the post-partum period. *Lancet* 2014;384(9956):1789–1799.

36. Robertson E, Jones I, Haque S, et al. Risk of puerperal and non-puerperal recurrence of illness following bipolar affective puerperal (post-partum) psychosis. *Br J Psychiatry* 2005;186(3):258–259.

37. Jones I, Craddock N. Familiality of the puerperal trigger in bipolar disorder: results of a family study. *Am J Psychiatry* 2001;158(6):913–917.

38. Heron J, McGuinness M, Blackmore ER, et al. Early postpartum symptoms in puerperal psychosis. *BJOG* 2008;115(3):348–353.

39. Steer P. Saving Mothers' Lives. Reviewing maternal deaths to make motherhood safer: 2006–2008. *BJOG* 2011;118(11):1404.

CHAPTER 62

Menopause

Deirdre Lundy

Menopause is defined as permanent cessation of menstrual periods; however, the term 'menopause' is often used to describe the period prior to this when ovarian function starts to decline. This symptomatic phase of sex steroid decline is in fact the perimenopause and can last months to years.

Sex steroid hormones have various neuromodulatory effects including influencing serotonergic and dopaminergic neurotransmitter systems [1]. Fluctuations in the levels of sex steroids have been implicated in psychiatric illness. For example, depressed women have lower oestrogen levels compared with non-depressed controls [2,3], and the perimenopausal period is associated with increased rates of depression [4,5]. Oestrogen is also thought to be protective against psychosis; age of onset of schizophrenia is several years later in females compared with males [6,7] and only in females is there a second peak age of onset at 40–50 years of age [8].

This chapter aims to equip the psychiatric practitioner with an understanding of the physiology and associated symptoms of the perimenopause. It also provides an overview of available treatment options with special considerations given to the patient with serious mental illness (SMI).

PHYSIOLOGY AND SYMPTOMS OF PERIMENOPAUSE

At 20 weeks of gestation a female fetus possesses approximately 7 million oocytes, which then start to decline in number so that by birth fewer than 2 million oocytes remain, dropping to 400,000 by puberty. The maturation and release of an ovum from individual oocytes is orchestrated by an array of reproductive hormones, including gonadotropin releasing hormone (GnRH), follicle stimulating hormone (FSH), oestrogens (estradiol, estriol, and estrone), inhibin, progesterone, and androgens (dehydroepiandrosterone,

The Maudsley Practice Guidelines for Physical Health Conditions in Psychiatry, First Edition.
David M. Taylor, Fiona Gaughran, and Toby Pillinger.
© 2021 John Wiley & Sons Ltd. Published 2021 by John Wiley & Sons Ltd.

Box 63.1 Symptoms of the perimenopause

- Vasomotor symptoms: hot flushes ('flashes') and night sweats
- Sleep disruption
- Mood disturbances: low mood, anxiety, irritability
- Headache
- Fatigue, anergia
- Poor memory and concentration
- Musculoskeletal symptoms: generalised aches and pains, joint stiffness
- Itchiness
- Urogenital dysfunction: urinary urgency, urge incontinence, nocturia, stress incontinence, vaginal dryness and discomfort, vaginal itching, dyspareunia
- Sexual dysfunction: loss of vaginal elasticity, loss of libido, anorgasmia, post-coital bleeding
- Menstrual irregularities: cycle variations, menorrhagia, lighter bleeds, intermenstrual bleeding, and post-coital bleeding

---

androstenedione, and testosterone). The perimenopausal symptoms described in Box 63.1 emerge as the ageing ovary struggles to maintain levels of these sex hormones. Symptoms that may exacerbate already poor mental health include disturbances in sleep, mood, and cognition [9].

CLINICAL APPROACH

History

Diagnosis of perimenopause/menopause in healthy women aged over 45 years is usually a clinical one. Thus, perimenopause in such women may simply be diagnosed based on vasomotor symptoms and irregular periods (see Box 63.1). Menopause is likely in women aged over 45 years who have not had a period for at least 12 months and who are not using hormonal contraception (with the caveat that patients with hyperprolactinaemia or eating disorders may have secondary amenorrhoea).

Once a diagnosis of perimenopause/menopause is made, history should focus on past medical history that may inform treatment decisions. Thus, enquire about history of venous thromboembolism, cardiovascular disease, sex hormone-related cancers (ovarian, cervical, uterine, breast), and previous side effects of oral contraceptives. Carbamazepine (CYP3A4 and 1A2 inducer), St John's Wort (CYP3A4 inducer), and topiramate (CYP3A4 inducer) decrease the effects of hormone replacement therapy (HRT). HRT may reduce lamotrigine levels [10].

Investigations

Few if any blood tests are required in the diagnosis of perimenopause/menopause. Some non-specific symptoms (e.g. fatigue) may warrant tests of thyroid function and measurement of haemoglobin levels. As part of a cardiovascular screen, lipids and HbA_{1c} should be checked.

CHAPTER 63

Where menopause is suspected in women aged under 45 years, blood FSH levels may be used for diagnosis. Premature ovarian insufficiency (POI) is defined as sex hormone decline and loss of fertility before the age of 40. POI is associated with increased risk of osteoporosis, cardiovascular disease, and cognitive impairment [11]. Women with suspected POI should be referred to a menopause or endocrine specialist and receive HRT.

In the UK, routine dual-energy X-ray absorptiometry (DEXA), also called bone densitometry scanning, is not recommended for women until 65 years of age. However, if a patient has osteoporosis risk factors, for example low body mass index (BMI), maternal/paternal history of hip fracture, personal history of fracture, or smokes, then a FRAX assessment (without a T-Score) can guide use of early DEXA scanning [12].

Examination

There is no need for physical examination in the assessment of perimenopause/menopause unless indicated by another presenting complaint. Blood pressure should be checked and if raised treated prior to initiation of HRT.

TREATMENT

Menopausal women, their family members, and carers (as appropriate) should be provided with information that explains the stages of menopause, the common symptoms (see Box 63.1), lifestyle changes that might help general well-being (e.g. weight loss), and long-term health implications of menopause. Broadly, there are three types of treatment available: hormonal (HRT), non-hormonal (e.g. clonidine), and non-pharmacological (e.g. cognitive-behavioural therapy, CBT).

Hormone replacement therapy

The most effective way to combat symptoms brought on by menopausal hormonal fluctuations/decline is to supplement sex steroid levels with HRT. HRT involves replacing oestrogen (which alleviates symptoms) alongside progesterone (necessary as unopposed oestrogen exposure may cause dysplastic changes in the uterine lining, increasing risk of endometrial cancers). Although not standard practice, some women also benefit from low-dose testosterone supplementation.

Concerns were raised in the early 2000s regarding the association between HRT and breast cancer [13,14]. However, this risk needs to be considered in the context of other breast cancer risk factors. For example, although HRT that contains both oestrogen and progesterone does increase risk of breast cancer, the risk is not as high as that associated with drinking 2 units of alcohol a day, and far less than the risk associated with having a BMI over 30 kg/m² [15]. Thus, in the UK, advice from the National Institute for Health and Care Excellence (NICE) is that patients should be offered HRT if clinically indicated, alongside appropriate counselling regarding risks and benefits [16].

CHAPTER 63

HRT is usually contraindicated in women with a diagnosis of either an oestrogen-sensitive cancer or established ischaemic heart disease. HRT tablets (but not patches or gels) are linked with a higher risk of venous thromboembolism (VTE). Thus, transdermal oestrogen delivery is preferred for women with VTE risk factors such as obesity, smoking, or prolonged periods of inactivity. Consultation with haematology may be indicated in patients at high risk of VTE where HRT is being considered.

Hormone replacement therapy and psychiatric disease

There is evidence (albeit cross-sectional and with a modest sample size) that HRT in postmenopausal women with schizophrenia is associated with reduced negative symptom burden and use of lower antipsychotic doses [17]. HRT may also ameliorate extrapyramidal side effects and protect against tardive dyskinesia [18,19]. Despite these potential benefits, menopausal women with schizophrenia do not use HRT as frequently as women in the general population [17].

There is mixed evidence regarding the beneficial effects of HRT on mood in the perimenopausal period. Two small randomised controlled trials have demonstrated the efficacy of short-term oestrogen therapy in improving mood in depressed menopausal women [20,21]. However, another randomised controlled trial failed to demonstrate efficacy [22]. Currently there is insufficient evidence to support the use of HRT specifically for depressive symptoms in perimenopausal women.

Local vaginal oestrogen replacement

Some women do not need systemic oestrogen therapy as their symptoms are confined to the pelvic area. Oestrogen depletion symptoms in the vagina and vulva, known as genitourinary syndrome of the menopause (see Box 63.1), do not improve over time like other menopausal symptoms. Vaginal moisturisers and lubricants may help improve the symptoms of vaginal dryness and discomfort, but nothing works as well as local oestrogen replacement in the form of local vaginal oestrogen pessaries or creams. These local oestrogen products have minimal systemic absorption so there is no need to protect the endometrium with a progestagen. They also reduce recurrent urinary tract infections in older women [23].

Non-hormonal pharmacological approaches

HRT is first-line therapy for women with perimenopausal symptoms in the absence of absolute contraindications to hormone therapy [16]. However, there are several non-hormonal treatments available.

Clonidine

Clonidine, an α-adrenergic receptor agonist, is the only non-hormonal drug with a licenced indication for control of hot flushes ('flashes') in the UK (25 mg twice daily for

CHAPTER 63

two weeks increased to a maximum of 50 mg three times daily). Although there is evidence of clonidine's efficacy over placebo in reducing menopausal hot flushes, only a few studies have been published and most have methodological deficiencies [24]. Side effects of clonidine are dose-related. It can cause sleep disturbance and caution should be taken in women with pre-existing hypotension (note potential interactions with other psychiatric drugs associated with low blood pressure such as clozapine; see Chapter 6). Clonidine must also be withdrawn gradually; abrupt discontinuation can cause rebound hypertension.

Selective serotonin reuptake inhibitors and serotonin/noradrenaline reuptake inhibitors

There is some evidence of efficacy for selective serotonin reuptake inhibitors (SSRIs) and serotonin/noradrenaline reuptake inhibitors (SNRIs) in treating hot flushes, although as with clonidine this evidence base is weak [24]. In the USA, paroxetine has Food and Drug Administration approval for treatment of menopausal hot flushes. The most effective treatments are venlafaxine 37.5 mg titrated up to 150 mg daily, paroxetine 10 mg daily, and citalopram 10–30 mg daily; the best evidence is for paroxetine 10 mg daily [24].

Isoflavones and Black Cohosh

Studies examining isoflavones (from soy/red clover) and the herb Black Cohosh (a member of the buttercup family) for treatment of menopausal hot flushes have been inconsistent and weak in design; currently there is insufficient evidence to support their use [25].

Gabapentin

Gabapentin (up to 300 mg three times daily) has been observed to be more effective than placebo in the treatment of hot flushes [26].

Non-pharmacological therapy

Cognitive-behavioural therapy

CBT appears to have some efficacy in treating menopause-associated insomnia [27], but appears less effective for hot flushes [28].

Lifestyle interventions

Any treatment discussions should cover lifestyle interventions that promote general good health, including weight loss and smoking cessation (see Chapters 14 and 46), and cancer screening (e.g. mammography and cervical smear).

When to refer to a menopause specialist

Although menopause should usually be managed in primary care, speciality advice from endocrinology or specialist menopause clinics (in the UK, a list of clinics is available at www.bms.org) may be indicated when:

- there is confusion over diagnosis
- there are contraindications to HRT (e.g. breast, ovarian or endomertrial cancer, ischaemic heart disease)
- there is a strong family history of hormone-dependent cancers and genetic testing might be appropriate
- there is suspected premature ovarian failure
- previous use of HRT has been associated with intolerable side effects.

References

1. Barth C, Villringer A, Sacher J. Sex hormones affect neurotransmitters and shape the adult female brain during hormonal transition periods. *Front Neurosci* 2015;9:37.
2. Young EA, Midgley AR, Carlson NE, Brown MB. Alteration in the hypothalamic–pituitary–ovarian axis in depressed women. *Arch Gen Psychiatry* 2000;57(12):1157–1162.
3. Harlow BL, Wise LA, Otto MW, et al. Depression and its influence on reproductive endocrine and menstrual cycle markers associated with perimenopause: the Harvard Study of Moods and Cycles. *Arch Gen Psychiatry* 2003;60(1):29–36.
4. Cohen LS, Soares CN, Vitonis AF, et al. Risk for new onset of depression during the menopausal transition: the Harvard study of Moods and Cycles. *Arch Gen Psychiatry* 2006;63(4):385–390.
5. Freeman EW, Sammel MD, Lin H, Nelson DB. Associations of hormones and menopausal status with depressed mood in women with no history of depression. *Arch Gen Psychiatry* 2006;63(4):375–382.
6. Hafner H. Gender differences in schizophrenia. *Psychoneuroendocrinology* 2003;28:17–54.
7. Eranti SV, MacCabe JH, Bundy H, Murray RM. Gender difference in age at onset of schizophrenia: a meta-analysis. *Psychol Med* 2013;43(1):155–167.
8. Hafner H, Riecher-Rossler A, An Der Heiden W, et al. Generating and testing a causal explanation of the gender difference in age at first onset of schizophrenia. *Psychol Med* 1993;23(4):925–940.
9. Brzezinski A, Brzezinski-Sinai NA, Seeman MV. Treating schizophrenia during menopause. *Menopause* 2017;24(5):582–588.
10. Harden CL, Herzog AG, Nikolov BG, et al. Hormone replacement therapy in women with epilepsy: a randomized, double-blind, placebo-controlled study. *Epilepsia* 2006;47(9):1447–1451.
11. Maclaran K, Panay N. Premature ovarian failure. *J Fam Plann Reprod Health Care* 2011;37(1):35–42.
12. Fracture Risk Assessment Tool. https://www.sheffield.ac.uk/FRAX/index.aspx (accessed 6 October 2019).
13. Chen CL, Weiss NS, Newcomb P, et al. Hormone replacement therapy in relation to breast cancer. *JAMA* 2002;287(6):734–741.
14. Rossouw JE, Anderson GL, Prentice RL, et al. Risks and benefits of estrogen plus progestin in healthy postmenopausal women: principal results from the Women's Health Initiative randomized controlled trial. *JAMA* 2002;288(3):321–333.
15. Women's Health Concern. Breask cancer: risk factors. https://www.womens-health-concern.org/help-and-advice/factsheets/breast-cancer- risk-factors/
16. National Institute for Health and Care Excellence. *Menopause: Diagnosis and Management.* NICE Guideline NG23. London: NICE, 2015. Available at https://www.nice.org.uk/guidance/ng23/chapter/recommendations
17. Lindamer LA, Buse DC, Lohr JB, Jeste DV. Hormone replacement therapy in postmenopausal women with schizophrenia: positive effect on negative symptoms? *Biol Psychiatry* 2001;49(1):47–51.
18. Akhondzadeh S, Nejatisafa AA, Amini H, et al. Adjunctive estrogen treatment in women with chronic schizophrenia: a double-blind, randomized, and placebo-controlled trial. *Prog Neuropsychopharmacol Biol Psychiatry* 2003;27(6):1007–1012.
19. Turrone P, Seeman MV, Silvestri S. Estrogen receptor activation and tardive dyskinesia. *Can J Psychiatry* 2000;45(3):288–290.
20. Schmidt PJ, Nieman L, Danaceau MA, et al. Estrogen replacement in perimenopause-related depression: a preliminary report. *Am J Obstet Gynecol* 2000;183(2):414–420.
21. Soares CN, Almeida OP, Joffe H, Cohen LS. Efficacy of estradiol for the treatment of depressive disorders in perimenopausal women: a double-blind, randomized, placebo-controlled trial. *Arch Gen Psychiatry* 2001;58(6):529–534.
22. Morrison MF, Kallan MJ, Ten Have T, et al. Lack of efficacy of estradiol for depression in postmenopausal women: a randomized, controlled trial. *Biol Psychiatry* 2004;55(4):406–412.
23. Perrotta C, Aznar M, Mejia R, et al. Oestrogens for preventing recurrent urinary tract infection in postmenopausal women. *Obstet Gynecol* 2008;112(3):689–690.

CHAPTER 63

24. Nelson HD, Vesco KK, Haney E, et al. Nonhormonal therapies for menopausal hot flashes: systematic review and meta-analysis. *JAMA* 2006;295(17):2057–2071.

25. Carroll DG. Nonhormonal therapies for hot flashes in menopause. *Am Fam Physician* 2006;73(3):457–464.

26. Loprinzi CL, Sloan J, Stearns V, et al. Newer antidepressants and gabapentin for hot flashes: an individual patient pooled analysis. *J Clin Oncol* 2009;27(17):2831–2837.

27. McCurry SM, Guthrie KA, Morin C, et al. Telephone-based cognitive behavioral therapy for insomnia in perimenopausal and postmenopausal women with vasomotor symptoms: a MsFLASH randomized clinical trial. *JAMA Intern Med* 2016;176(7):913–920.

28. Carpenter J, Gass MLS, Maki PM, et al. Nonhormonal management of menopause-associated vasomotor symptoms: 2015 position statement of the North American Menopause Society. *Menopause* 2015;22(11):1155–1174.

Part 13

Dermatology

General Dermatology

Jonathan Kentley, Ruth Taylor, Anthony Bewley

Skin disease accounts for up to 18% of presentations to primary care in the UK [1]. Patients with severe mental illness (SMI) have significantly higher rates of dermatological disease than the background population, with 71.5–77% of psychiatric patients reported to suffer from a skin condition [2,3].

Dermatology encompasses a vast amount of pathology, but we have aimed to cover some of the most commonly encountered and easily managed conditions in this chapter [2,3]. Infectious skin disease (parasitic, fungal, bacterial, or viral) are most commonly seen, particularly in patients with a diagnosis of schizophrenia [3–5]. Non-infectious skin disease is also common. Psychodermatological disease is covered in Chapter 65. Box 64.1 provides a glossary of commonly used dermatological terms, Box 64.2 describes the information one should aim to provide a dermatologist when making a referral, and Box 64.3 describes red-flag 'ABCDE' features of moles that may indicate melanoma and referral to dermatology.

INFECTIOUS SKIN DISEASE

Parasitic infection

Scabies

Scabies is an intensely itchy condition caused by the mite *Sarcoptes scabiei*; although it can affect anyone, there is evidence of higher prevalence in psychiatric inpatients and those of low socioeconomic status [8,9]. Severe pruritus is the hallmark of scabies, and there may be a history of itch in other family members or housemates. Patients may have small burrows (comma-shaped lines) in the finger or toe webs, but these may not be seen. Treat those in which you have a high index of suspicion empirically.

The Maudsley Practice Guidelines for Physical Health Conditions in Psychiatry, First Edition.
David M. Taylor, Fiona Gaughran, and Toby Pillinger.
© 2021 John Wiley & Sons Ltd. Published 2021 by John Wiley & Sons Ltd.

Box 64.1 Glossary of common dermatological descriptors [6]

Erythema	Redness
Exanthem	Rash
Desquamation	Shedding of the outermost layer of the skin (epidermis)
Hyperpigmented	Darker than normal skin
Hypopigmented	Lighter than normal skin
Macule	Circumscribed non-elevated area <5 mm
Papule	Solid raised lesion <5 mm
Patch	Circumscribed non-elevated area >5 mm
Nodule	Solid raised lesion >5 mm
Plaque	Circumscribed elevated area >5 mm
Vesicle	Fluid-filled lesion <5 mm
Bulla	Fluid-filled lesion >5 mm
Pustule	Pus-filled lesion
Petechiae/purpura	Non-blanching red/brown/purple macule
Erosion	Partial epidermal loss, heals without scarring
Ulcer	Complete loss of the epidermis, and some dermis

Box 64.2 Information to provide a dermatologist when making a referral

- Past medical and psychiatric history
- Comprehensive medication history, including over the counter and allergies
- Social history, e.g. living conditions, drug and alcohol history
- Family history of dermatological disease

Describing the lesion

1 Primary morphology (use terms from Box 64.1)
2 Size
3 Demarcation (well/poorly demarcated)
4 Colour
5 Distribution (flexor/extensor regions, generalised, or limited to certain regions, e.g. hands)
6 Systemic features (e.g. fever)

Box 64.3 British Association of Dermatologists ABCDE guide to checking moles and identifying potential melanoma [7]

Asymmetry: the two halves of the area may differ in shape
Border: the edges of the area may be irregular or blurred
Colour: this may be uneven; different shades of black, brown, and pink may be seen
Diameter: most melanomas are at least 6 mm in diameter
Evolution: the lesion changes rapidly over time

Treat with 5% permethrin cream to the whole body (from neck down) and leave on for 8–12 hours. Repeat this after seven days. All family members and close contacts should be treated whether or not they have symptoms [9].

Pediculosis (lice)

Infestation with lice may occur on the head, pubic hair, or body hair. Pruritus, if present, is due to an allergy to louse faeces. Small lice (measuring 2–4 mm) may be seen crawling, or egg cases may be seen attached to the hair shaft.

Malathion 0.5% lotion should be applied to the hair until wet and left for 8–10 hours. Repeat treatment after seven days. Launder all clothes and bedding at a high temperature [10].

Fungal infection

Pityriasis versicolor

Pityriasis versicolor (PV) is a common superficial infection caused by *Malassezia* yeasts that live in the skin and prevent the production of melanin, so leaving areas of skin unable to tan. Look for widespread brownish-red or hypopigmented macules, usually on the trunk. There may be a small amount of scale, which will become apparent when scraped. PV becomes more obvious when the patient has been in the sun and the surrounding skin has tanned.

Treatment is with 2% ketoconazole shampoo for five days, which should be left on the skin for 5 minutes. Relapses are common [11].

Dermatophyte infections

Dermatophyte fungi use keratin as a nutrient and colonise the skin, nails or hair [12].

- Tinea corporis occurs on the body and usually appears as erythematous, scaly, annular (ring-shaped) lesions with central clearing.
- Tinea cruris occurs in the groin, and appears as an erythematous, scaly annular rash with raised borders and macerated skin centrally.
- Tinea pedis occurs on the feet and can present with erythema and maceration in the toe webs, or as a scaly rash affecting the sole of the foot.
- Tinea unguium (onychomycosis) affects the nails, which appear as thickened and yellow/white with separation from the nail bed.

Treatment of cutaneous dermatophyte infections is with a topical antifungal agent such as terbinafine cream applied once or twice daily for one to two weeks, or miconazole cream applied twice daily until 10 days after lesions have healed [13,14]. Onychomycosis, if asymptomatic, need not be treated. If treatment is required, onychomycosis requires prolonged therapy (9–12 months) with amorolfine 5% nail lacquer, or a course of oral terbinafine 250 mg daily for three to six months [15].

CHAPTER 64

NON-INFECTIOUS SKIN DISEASE

Xerosis and pruritus

Generalised dry skin (xerosis) and pruritus are recognised to be the most common non-infectious dermatological complaints in patients with SMI [16]. Xerosis is common across all patients and proactive use of emollients will often prevent itch. Use of anti-histamines such as fexofenadine 180 mg daily may also be beneficial if felt to be histamine-mediated.

When bothersome itch persists secondary causes should be considered, such as eczema, scabies, allergy, and psychological disease (see Chapter 65). Systemic disease may also result in pruritus and alongside a history it may be beneficial to check full blood count, ferritin, liver function, thyroid function, and HIV status if clinically appropriate. Lymphoproliferative disease may also present with pruritus. Patients with severe pruritus of unknown cause may benefit from dermatology referral [17].

Dermatitis

Seborrhoeic dermatitis

Seborrhoeic dermatitis is a common condition that results in a greasy red rash with yellowish scale in areas rich in sebaceous glands (nasolabial folds, eyebrows, eyelids, scalp, and upper chest). It is more common in patients with underlying neurological and psychiatric disorders, and in patients receiving antipsychotics and antiepileptics [18].

Ketoconazole 2% cream (once or twice daily) can be used for at least four weeks. If the face is very inflamed, 1% hydrocortisone cream can be used as an adjunct for the same time frame.

Atopic dermatitis (eczema)

Eczema is common and affects up to 25% of children and 2–3% of adults. Patients with SMI may have pre-existing but poorly managed disease. Eczema presents as a dry, scaly, erythematous, itchy rash in the skin creases. Irritating soaps and shower gels should be avoided, and emollients should be used for both bathing and as moisturisers. In adults, a potent topical steroid such as mometasone furoate 0.1% ointment can be applied once daily to areas of eczema on the body. A moderate potency steroid such as clobetasone butyrate 0.05% cream should be used once or twice daily when treating the face or occluded areas such as the axilla and groin [6,19]. Steroids can be applied daily for six weeks, after which they should be used under medical supervision (due to risk of side effects).

Drug reactions

Cutaneous adverse drug reactions (ADRs) are the most common side effects of drug therapy and may occur in 2–5% of patients taking psychiatric medications [20]. Most drug reactions are mild and tolerable, but it is important to recognise the signs of potentially life-threatening drug reactions early. The most frequently reported cutaneous ADRs to commonly prescribed psychiatric medications are listed in Table 64.1.

Table 64.1 Frequently reported cutaneous adverse drug reactions to commonly prescribed psychiatric medications [20].

	SSRI	SNRI	TCA	Mirtazapine	Lamotrigine	Carbamazepine	Lithium	Risperidone	Olanzapine	Quetiapine	Aripiprazole	Clozapine
Pruritus	✓	✓	✓	✓	✓	✓	✓	✓	✓	✓		✓
Exanthem	✓	✓	✓	✓	✓	✓	✓	✓	✓	✓	✓	✓
Urticaria	✓	✓	✓	✓	✓	✓	✓	✓	✓		✓	✓
FDE	✓	✓	✓	✓	✓	✓	✓	✓	✓	✓		✓
Photosensitivity	✓		✓			✓		✓	✓	✓		✓
Pigmentation	✓		✓		✓	✓		✓	✓	✓		✓
Alopecia	✓	✓	✓	✓	✓	✓	✓	✓	✓		✓	
Acne	✓	✓	✓	✓	✓		✓	✓	✓	✓	✓	
Psoriasis	✓	✓	✓	✓		✓	✓	✓		✓		
Seborrhoeic dermatitis	✓	✓	✓	✓		✓	✓		✓	✓		
Hyperhydrosis			✓		✓	✓		✓	✓	✓		

SSRI, selective serotonin reuptake inhibitor; SNRI, serotonin/noradrenaline reuptake inhibitor; TCA, tricyclic antidepressant; FDE, fixed drug eruption.

The decision to stop medications following mild ADRs should be weighed up carefully by the psychiatrist. For example, acne is associated with almost all antidepressants and with some mood stabilisers; however, it can be often be managed with topical benzoyl peroxide and an oral tetracycline (doxycycline or lymecycline) antibiotic whilst continuing the drug [21]. Hair loss may also be problematic for many patients taking lithium and valproic acid and, whilst hair regrowth usually occurs after cessation of the drug, the risk of relapse must be considered [22].

An exanthem may occur with any psychiatric medication and usually appears within two weeks of starting the drug, resolving within two weeks of stopping it [20]. Painful skin, fever, lymphadenopathy, mucous membrane involvement, and Nikolsky signs (shearing of the skin on lateral pressure) should raise suspicion for a severe cutaneous ADR and prompt urgent dermatology referral or transfer to the accident and emergency department.

Stevens–Johnson syndrome (SJS) and toxic epidermal necrolysis (TEN), whilst rare, can be seen with many psychiatric medications, particularly the mood stabilisers carbamazepine, lamotrigine, and valproic acid [20]. SJS/TEN typically presents with a prodrome of fever, malaise, and upper respiratory tract involvement, which occurs several days prior to the eruption. Ocular inflammation typically occurs before skin signs become apparent. Cutaneous pain and dusky erythema then develops with progression to blistering and detachment of the skin. Mucous membranes are also involved. Mortality from SJS/TEN is high and early recognition and transfer to emergency services is critical [23].

Other serious cutaneous ADRs include drug reaction with eosinophilia and systemic symptoms (DRESS), consisting of fever, rash and internal organ dysfunction with peripheral eosinophilia; and erythroderma, in which an exanthematous rash involves more than 90% of the body surface area. Both conditions usually require hospital admission.

References

1. Kerr OA, Tidman MJ, Walker JJ, et al. The profile of dermatological problems in primary care. *Clin Exp Dermatol* 2010;35:380–383.
2. Mookhoek EJ, Van De Kerkhof PC, Hovens JE, et al. Skin disorders in chronic psychiatric illness. *J Eur Acad Dermatol Venereol* 2010;24:1151–1156.
3. Moftah NH, Kamel AM, Attia HM, et al. Skin diseases in patients with primary psychiatric conditions: a hospital based study. *J Epidemiol Glob Health* 2013;3:131–138.
4. Mercan S, Kivanc Altunay I. [Psychodermatology: a collaboration between psychiatry and dermatology]. *Turk Psikiyatri Derg* 2006;17:305–313.
5. Barrimi M, Aalouane R, Hlal H, et al. Skin disorders among psychiatric patients: a cross-sectional twelve-month study. *Inf Psychiatr* 2016;92:317–326.
6. Burge S. *Oxford Handbook of Medical Dermatology*. Oxford: Oxford University Press, 2012.
7. British Aaaociation of Dermatologists. ABCD-Easy guide to checking your moles. https://www.bad.org.uk/for-the-public/skin-cancer/melanoma-leaflets/abcd-easy-guide-to-checking-your-moles
8. Makigami K, Ohtaki N, Ishii N, Yasumura S. Risk factors of scabies in psychiatric and long-term care hospitals: a nationwide mail-in survey in Japan. *J Dermatol* 2009;36:491–498.
9. Johnston G, Sladden M. Scabies: diagnosis and treatment. *BMJ* 2005;331:619–622.
10. Sangare AK, Doumbo OK, Raoult D. Management and treatment of human lice. *Biomed Res Int* 2016;2016:8962685.
11. Gupta AK, Bluhm R, Summerbell R. Pityriasis versicolor. *J Eur Acad Dermatol Venereol* 2002;16:19–33.
12. Hainer BL. Dermatophyte infections. *Am Fam Physician* 2003;67:101–108.
13. National Institute for Health and Care Excellence. Management of fungal skin infections: body and groin. Clinical Knowledge Summary. Last revised: May 2018. https://cks.nice.org.uk/fungal-skin-infection-body-and-groin

14. Royal Pharmaceutical Society of Great Britain and British Medical Association. *British National Formulary*. London: BMJ Publishing Group, Royal Pharmaceutical Society of Great Britain, p. 1 online resource.

15. National Institute for Health and Care Excellence. Management of fungal nail infection. Clinical Knowledge Summary. Last revised: March 2018. https://cks.nice.org.uk/fungal-nail-infection

16. Qadir A, Butt G, Aamir I, Asad F. Skin disorders in patients with primary psychiatric conditions. *J Pakistan Assoc Dermatol* 2015;25:282–284.

17. Millington GWM, Collins A, Lovell CR, et al. British Association of Dermatologists' guidelines for the investigation and management of generalized pruritus in adults without an underlying dermatosis, 2018. *Br J Dermatol* 2018;178:34–60.

18. Borda LJ, Wikramanayake TC. Seborrheic dermatitis and dandruff: a comprehensive review. *J Clin Investig Dermatol* 2015;3(2):10.13188/2373-1044.1000019.

19. Eichenfield LF, Tom WL, Berger TG, et al. Guidelines of care for the management of atopic dermatitis. Section 2. Management and treatment of atopic dermatitis with topical therapies. *J Am Acad Dermatol* 2014;71:116–132.

20. Bliss SA, Warnock JK. Psychiatric medications: adverse cutaneous drug reactions. *Clin Dermatol* 2013;31:101–109.

21. Srebrnik A, Hes JP, Brenner S. Adverse cutaneous reactions to psychotropic drugs. *Acta Derm Venereol Suppl* 1991;158:1–12.

22. Mercke Y, Sheng H, Khan T, Lippmann S. Hair loss in psychopharmacology. *Ann Clin Psychiatry* 2000;12:35–42.

23. Creamer D, Walsh SA, Dziewulski P, et al. U.K. guidelines for the management of Stevens–Johnson syndrome/toxic epidermal necrolysis in adults 2016. *Br J Dermatol* 2016;174:1194–1227.

Psychodermatology

Jonathan Kentley, Ruth Taylor, Anthony Bewley

Psychodermatology is an increasingly recognised subspecialty that addresses the important link between the mind and the skin. Dermatological disease may be either the cause or the result of psychological disease, and up to one-third of dermatology patients suffer psychological comorbidity [1].

Psychodermatological conditions can be separated into four broad categories [2]:

- primary psychological disorders with cutaneous presentation
- psychophysiological conditions that are exacerbated by stress or anxiety
- secondary psychological disorders that occur due to chronic skin disease
- cutaneous sensory disorders.

PSYCHIATRIC DISORDERS WITH SKIN MANIFESTATIONS

Delusional infestation

Patients with delusional infestation (DI) hold a fixed, false belief that their skin and body are infested by pathogens, despite lack of medical evidence to support this. The infestation may be with parasites, insects, or inanimate strands of material (termed Morgellons disease) [3]. DI may be a primary delusional disorder, or may occur secondary to intoxication (amphetamines, cocaine, dopaminergic agents), medical disorders (brain injury, delirium, endocrine disease, hypovitaminosis), or other psychiatric disease (schizophrenia or major depressive disorder with psychotic symptoms) [4].

Patients with DI avoid psychiatric professionals and seek help from dermatologists and microbiologists [5]. Presentation is often with pruritus or crawling/biting sensations, and around half of patients will display the 'specimen sign' in which they bring a

The Maudsley Practice Guidelines for Physical Health Conditions in Psychiatry, First Edition.
David M. Taylor, Fiona Gaughran, and Toby Pillinger.
© 2021 John Wiley & Sons Ltd. Published 2021 by John Wiley & Sons Ltd.

container or photograph of inanimate objects that they believe to be proof of their infestation [6,7]. A thorough history should be taken, including drug use and travel. Examination for skin disease should be performed; note that patients may have extensive excoriations due to scratching, and a pruritus screen should be performed (see Chapter 64). It is important to take the patient's symptoms seriously and rule out a true infestation, as this helps build a trusting relationship [4].

In patients with secondary DI, treatment of the underlying disorder or withdrawal of the substance will be sufficient to improve symptoms. The skin should be treated concurrently with emollients, antihistamines, and antibiotics (if evidence of secondary infection). In patients with primary DI, the clinician should not try to convince the patient that they do not have an infestation. Antipsychotic therapy with low doses of risperidone 0.5–4 mg or olanzapine 1.5–10 mg is effective in reducing symptoms, although adherence can be difficult to achieve [8,9]. These patients can be challenging and specialist psychodermatology clinics are well equipped to manage their complex needs in a multidisciplinary setting.

Dermatitis artefacta

Dermatitis artefacta (DA) is a factitious disorder in which patients consciously manipulate their skin to produce a lesion and vehemently deny complicity, in order to fulfill an internal psychological need, typically to be taken care of [10,11]. DA is usually associated with underlying psychological or psychiatric disease, including adjustment disorder, depressive disorder, and personality disorder [4].

Patients may appear anxious, with 'hollow histories' regarding the onset of their lesions [12]. In some circumstances, a particular dermatosis is mimicked. However, the majority of patients will present with lesions that do not fit a pattern of disease and may display bizarre morphology. Borders are sharp and angulated with demarcation from normal skin, and friction produces irregular, linear, superficial uniform-appearing lesions [4,10]. Of course, depending on the mechanism of injury, lesions can appear in all manner of forms.

Primary skin disease should be ruled out and occasionally biopsy may be required. An open, non-judgemental relationship should be established with the patient. Skin healing is an important consideration and emollients, topical antibiotics and occlusive dressings may be beneficial. Treatment of the underlying psychological disorder is key, and will guide treatment. Cognitive-behavioural therapy (CBT) may be effective in those with an underlying depressive disorder, and selective serotonin reuptake inhibitors (SSRIs) are also useful in managing those with depressive or personality disorders. Anxiolytics and atypical antipsychotics may be required in severe cases [10,13].

Compulsive disorders

Obsessive–compulsive disorder (OCD) related to hygiene and hand washing may result in irritant or allergic contact dermatitis of the hands. This can be managed with emollients such as a soap substitute (e.g. Dermol 500) and regular use of greasy emollients to the hand. Redness and inflammation may be managed with betamethasone valerate 0.1% ointment twice daily.

Other specific compulsive disorders may present with cutaneous signs.

- Skin picking disorder (SPD) is characterised by compulsive repetitive picking, resulting in skin damage. Stress and anxiety may contribute and patients report spending a large amount of time picking their skin, resulting in social impairment [14]. Psychological comorbidity is common. Treatment of patients with SPD is with CBT (specifically habit reversal therapy) and SSRIs; N-acetylcysteine and naltrexone have been reported to be effective [15].
- Trichotillomania is a behavioural disorder in which patients pull their hair, often in response to increased stress, and report gratification afterwards. This results in patchy alopecia of the scalp, although patients may pull any of their body hair. Linear or circular patches of alopecia with irregular borders and hairs of differing length are characteristic [16]. Treatment with CBT (including stimulus control and habit reversal) has been shown to be beneficial, and whilst there is a place for the use of SSRIs, efficacy data are mixed [4,17].

Body dysmorphic disorder

Body dysmorphic disorder (BDD) is common amongst dermatology patients [18]. Patients with BDD are preoccupied by one or more perceived defects in their physical appearance, causing significant distress or social impairment [19]. Patients with BDD will often present to dermatologists or plastic surgeons long before interacting with psychiatric services. Treatment of BDD is with a choice of CBT or SSRI, or a combination of both when there is severe functional impairment [20].

PSYCHOPHYSIOLOGICAL CONDITIONS

Psychophysiological disorders are skin conditions that are not directly linked with the mind, but that are triggered or exacerbated by stress. This includes conditions such as eczema, psoriasis, lichen simplex chronicus, rosacea, and urticaria [21]. Emotional triggers are reported by up to 60% of acne patients and up to 100% of patients with hyperhidrosis [22]. CBT is helpful in this setting, and SSRIs or anxiolytics may also play a role in patient management [23].

SECONDARY PSYCHOLOGICAL DISORDERS

The skin is highly visible and whilst most cutaneous diseases are not life-threatening, many are considered 'life-ruining' by patients. Dermatological disease can be dismissed as trivial by some clinicians, but psoriasis has been reported to have a similar mental and physical effect on patients as a diagnosis of heart disease or cancer [24]. Detecting and treating underlying depression and anxiety is paramount in the management of patients with chronic dermatological conditions [25].

CUTANEOUS SENSORY DISORDERS

Cutaneous sensory disorders (CSD) encompass a heterogeneous group of disorders in which patients report skin sensations (dysaesthesia, pain or anaesthesia) in the absence of a diagnosable dermatological or medical condition [26]. Pathophysiology is poorly understood. Comprehensive history and examination should be performed, with specific enquiry into conditions that may result in dysaesthesia (shingles, peripheral neuropathy, erythromelalgia, iatrogenic nerve injury).

CSDs are typically confined to the head or perineum and include burning mouth syndrome, glossodynia, and vulvodynia/scrotodynia. Treatment with low-dose amitriptyline 5–10 mg at night is first line, and gabapentin, pregabalin, and venlafaxine may be used second line [4].

References

1. Brown GE, Malakouti M, Sorenson E, et al. Psychodermatology. *Adv Psychosom Med* 2015;34:123–134.
2. Koo JY, Do JH, Lee CS. Psychodermatology. *J Am Acad Dermatol* 2000;43:848–853.
3. Bewley AP, Lepping P, Freudenmann RW, Taylor R. Delusional parasitosis: time to call it delusional infestation. *Br J Dermatol* 2010;163:1–2.
4. Bewley A, Taylor RE, Reichenberg JS, Magid M. *Practical Psychodermatology.* Chichester: John Wiley & Sons, 2014.
5. Freudenmann RW, Lepping P. Delusional infestation. *Clin Microbiol Rev* 2009;22:690–732.
6. Freudenmann RW, Lepping P, Huber M, et al. Delusional infestation and the specimen sign: a European multicentre study in 148 consecutive cases. *Br J Dermatol* 2012;167:247–251.
7. Trabert W. 100 years of delusional parasitosis. Meta-analysis of 1,223 case reports. *Psychopathology* 1995;28:238–246.
8. Lepping P, Freudenmann RW. Delusional parasitosis: a new pathway for diagnosis and treatment. *Clin Exp Dermatol* 2008;33:113–117.
9. Freudenmann RW, Lepping P. Second-generation antipsychotics in primary and secondary delusional parasitosis: outcome and efficacy. *J Clin Psychopharmacol* 2008;28:500–508.
10. Koblenzer CS. Dermatitis artefacta. Clinical features and approaches to treatment. *Am J Clin Dermatol* 2000;1:47–55.
11. Koblenzer CS, Gupta R. Neurotic excoriations and dermatitis artefacta. *Semin Cutan Med Surg* 2013;32:95–100.
12. Krener P. Factitious disorders and the psychosomatic continuum in children. *Curr Opin Pediatr* 1994;6:418–422.
13. Winchel RM, Stanley M. Self-injurious behavior: a review of the behavior and biology of self-mutilation. *Am J Psychiatry* 1991;148:306–317.
14. Arnold LM, Auchenbach MB, McElroy SL. Psychogenic excoriation. Clinical features, proposed diagnostic criteria, epidemiology and approaches to treatment. *CNS Drugs* 2001;15:351–359.
15. Grant JE, Odlaug BL, Chamberlain SR, et al. Skin picking disorder. *Am J Psychiatry* 2012;169:1143–1149.
16. Hautmann G, Hercogova J, Lotti T. Trichotillomania. *J Am Acad Dermatol* 2002;46:807–821.
17. Duke DC, Keeley ML, Geffken GR, Storch EA. Trichotillomania: a current review. *Clin Psychol Rev* 2010;30:181–193.
18. Conrado LA, Hounie AG, Diniz JB, et al. Body dysmorphic disorder among dermatologic patients: prevalence and clinical features. *J Am Acad Dermatol* 2010;63:235–243.
19. American Psychiatric Association. *Diagnostic and Statistical Manual of Mental Disorders*, 5th edn. Washington, DC: APA, 2013.
20. National Institute for Health and Care Excellence. *Obsessive–Compulsive Disorder and Body Dysmorphic Disorder: Treatment.* Clinical Guideline CG31. London: NICE, 2005. Available at https://www.nice.org.uk/guidance/cg31
21. Wong JW, Koo JY. Psychopharmacological therapies in dermatology. *Dermatol Online J* 2013;19:18169.
22. Jafferany M. Psychodermatology: a guide to understanding common psychocutaneous disorders. *Prim Care Companion J Clin Psychiatry* 2007;9:203–213.
23. Koo J, Lebwohl A. Psycho dermatology: the mind and skin connection. *Am Fam Physician* 2001;64:1873–1878.
24. Rapp SR, Feldman SR, Exum ML, et al. Psoriasis causes as much disability as other major medical diseases. *J Am Acad Dermatol* 1999;41:401–407.
25. Connor CJ. Management of the psychological comorbidities of dermatological conditions: practitioners' guidelines. *Clin Cosmet Investig Dermatol* 2017;10:117–132.
26. Gupta MA, Gupta AK. Cutaneous sensory disorder. *Semin Cutan Med Surg* 2013;32:110–118.

CHAPTER 65

Part 14

Electroconvulsive Therapy

Electroconvulsive Therapy

James Kelly, Mariese Cooper, Mario Juruena

Electroconvulsive therapy (ECT) is used to treat a range of psychiatric conditions. Its therapeutic mechanism of action remains unclear, but most likely stems from alterations in cerebral blood flow and regional metabolism [1]. Some stigma remains regarding its use, potentially associated with the lack of anaesthesia in the early days of treatment which led to significant injuries and memory loss [2]. Now, mortality and morbidity rates are very low, and memory loss occurs in only a minority [3,4]. Furthermore, ECT can be safely used in pregnancy and the elderly, for whom the avoidance of the side effects of psychotropic medication is particularly valuable.

INDICATIONS AND CONTRAINDICATIONS

In the UK, the National Institute for Health and Care Excellence (NICE) has issued guidance on the use of ECT [5]. Currently, it is recommended for the treatment of severe depressive illness, a prolonged or severe episode of mania, and catatonia [5]. It is not currently recommended for the prevention of recurrent depressive illness or for general management of schizophrenia, except in the specific instance of catatonia. ECT is the most effective treatment of severe treatment-resistant unipolar and bipolar depression. However, ECT has also been used to treat a wide range of other psychiatric conditions, including neuroleptic malignant syndrome, neurological crises (such as extreme parkinsonism), schizophrenia if associated with abnormal motor activity or treatment resistance, schizoaffective disorder, and perinatal depressive disorders (where expediting the mother's recovery is important to allow for appropriate care of the infant) [6,7].

The Maudsley Practice Guidelines for Physical Health Conditions in Psychiatry, First Edition.
David M. Taylor, Fiona Gaughran, and Toby Pillinger.
© 2021 John Wiley & Sons Ltd. Published 2021 by John Wiley & Sons Ltd.

There are no absolute contraindications to ECT, but comorbidities should be optimised prior to treatment. Other medical conditions and contraindications to general anaesthesia are relevant. Shared decision-making should involve relevant medical specialities (e.g. cardiology), anaesthetists, and psychiatric teams regarding risks and benefits of treatment.

THE ECT PROCEDURE

ECT is most commonly performed in a dedicated suite or day surgery unit under general anaesthesia. Before induction of general anaesthesia and the procedure, electroencephalogram (EEG) probes are applied to monitor electrical activity of the brain, which allow identification of seizure activity immediately after delivery of ECT. Following venous cannulation and pre-oxygenation of the patient, general anaesthesia is induced with intravenous induction agents (e.g. propafol). Muscle relaxing drugs are given post induction (e.g. suxamethonium) and a bite-block inserted. Anticholinergic medication, such as atropine, may be given to reduce secretions and prevent bradycardia. Hyperventilation via a bag valve mask may also be performed to reduce seizure threshold.

Seizures are induced either via two electrodes placed bitemporally, or via a single electrode on the right temple. Bilateral ECT is associated with more rapid therapeutic response, while unilateral ECT is associated with a lower instance of retrograde amnesia [8]. The stimulus given can be either a brief pulse of 0.5–2 ms, which is currently the standard treatment, or an ultra-brief pulse of less than 0.5 ms, which is given when previous treatments have been poorly tolerated. Seizure threshold is established in the first treatment session by applying increasingly higher currents. For bilateral ECT, the initial treatment dose is usually 50% above threshold dose or 50–100% above threshold dose for emergency treatment. Dose increases can be substantially higher in unilateral ECT. Because ECT raises seizure thresholds, the current for subsequent treatments can rise significantly.

The number of treatments offered is dependent on clinical progress but is commonly two sessions per week for six weeks. Greater frequency of sessions is associated with increased side effects without improved treatment response. Continuation ECT can be given within six months of completion of an ECT course in order to prevent relapse. Maintenance ECT refers to treatment extending six months beyond completion of a primary course, again given to prevent relapse.

PHYSIOLOGICAL EFFECTS OF ECT

ECT can have various physiological effects throughout the body, as detailed in the following sections.

Central nervous system

ECT produces an immediate decrease in cerebral blood flow, followed a few seconds later by a prolonged increase. This is likely the result of increased cerebral oxygen demand and increased cerebral perfusion pressure [9]. Because cerebral oxygen demand increases before cerebral blood flow begins to increase, an oxygen demand and delivery mismatch may occur. These cerebral haemodynamic changes will also be provoked by systemic haemodynamic changes. A sudden increase in systemic blood pressure may overcome intracranial pressure autoregulation. ECT may also increase blood–brain barrier permeability [10]. It has been hypothesised that post-procedure cognitive dysfunction can be attributed to a combination of these factors [11,12], alongside general anaesthesia which itself can be associated with cognitive dysfunction [13].

Brain imaging studies do not support the hypothesis that ECT causes brain damage; on the contrary, ECT is associated with volume increases in fronto-limbic areas [14]. However, if prolonged seizure activity occurs, there is a risk of structural brain injury.

Cardiovascular system

ECT causes an immediate parasympathetic stimulation and a subsequent sympathetic stimulation [15]. This produces an initial bradycardia that can occasionally progress to momentary asystole (which can be opposed by anticholinergic medication on induction). This is followed by catecholamine release and a resultant transient increase in heart rate and blood pressure, which most often lasts for around five minutes after seizure induction in young and physically healthy patients. Consequently, myocardial ischaemia can be induced in patients with cardiovascular disease.

Respiratory system

ECT has few direct effects on respiratory function but can produce an increase in respiratory secretions.

Metabolic effects

ECT produces a transient increase in adrenocorticotrophic hormone, cortisol, and glucagon, and so may cause temporary insulin resistance. Indeed, in depressed patients, ECT is associated with transient increases in plasma glucose and insulin levels, peaking 15 minutes after ECT administration [16]. The degree of insulin response to ECT may be predictive of clinical response [16].

Musculoskeletal effects

ECT directly induces generalised tonic–clonic seizures. With the routine use of muscle relaxants and a bite-block, adverse effects are rare. Short-acting depolarising muscle relaxants can cause myalgia.

Other effects

ECT causes a transient increase in intragastric pressure and intraocular pressure.

PRE-ECT ASSESSMENT

The goal of the pre-ECT assessment is to identify and reduce risks to the patient from ECT and the general anaesthetic. A history should be taken for previous anaesthetic procedures, family history of complications during anaesthesia, and for any medications taken and allergies. The patient's airway and dentition should be examined alongside systemic examination. Further investigations should be organised based on history and examination findings, if relevant. An American Society of Anesthesiologists (ASA) physical status classification should be recorded [17], and a venous thromboembolism assessment and pregnancy test completed if appropriate. An ECG should be performed in all patients, alongside routine bloods checking renal and liver function, and full blood count. The anaesthetic team should be informed of any comorbidities that may increase anaesthetic risk.

A psychiatric assessment should also be conducted as close to the first treatment session as possible. A history of previous response to ECT treatments should be recorded, and mental state assessed. Severity of psychiatric symptoms should be assessed using a validated rating scale. It is also recommended that a test of baseline cognitive function is conducted and documented.

Pre-ECT optimisation

Patients should be appropriately nil by mouth for any procedure requiring general anaesthesia or sedation. This includes solid food (including milk) for six hours and no clear liquids for two hours before the procedure. In general, most medications for hypertension or cardiac disease should be continued, although angiotensin-converting enzyme inhibitors are generally stopped on the morning of the procedure. Drugs for asthma or chronic obstructive pulmonary disease should be continued and administered prophylactically before the procedure. Medications for gastro-oesophageal reflux should also be continued. Oral hypoglycaemic agents should often be withheld, but patients taking insulin should continue to take adjusted doses. When in doubt, timely discussion with the anaesthetic team due to look after the patient is recommended.

A medication history should also elicit any prescribed medications that may alter seizure threshold, interact with anaesthetic medications, or exacerbate the physiological response to ECT. Psychiatric medications are particularly relevant in this context.

- Antidepressants can decrease seizure threshold and prolong seizures. They may augment the antidepressant effect of ECT. Tricyclic antidepressants appear to be safe in combination with ECT, but caution needs to be exercised with venlafaxine and bupropion (which decrease seizure threshold) and monoamine oxidase inhibitors (which may interact with a number of anaesthetic medications). When ECT starts, low-dose stimulus should be used on first dose.
- Antipsychotics tend to decrease seizure threshold. The worst agents are chlorpromazine, zotepine, loxapine, and clozapine [18]. Clozapine should be withheld 12 hours prior to an ECT session, which in practice usually means skipping the morning dose.

- Lithium reduces seizure threshold and may prolong seizures [19]. It also potentiates the action of suxamethonium, a muscle relaxant [20]. It may also increase the risk of post-procedure confusion and delirium [21]. A low initial stimulus for ECT should be used if lithium is given concurrently.
- Benzodiazepines increase seizure threshold and shorten seizure activity [18]. They may also reduce the antidepressant effect of ECT [22]. They should be discontinued if possible, but if a patient is well established on benzodiazepines, they should be tapered to the lowest possible dose. Where possible, try to skip doses from the night before an ECT session.
- Anticonvulsants, by definition, increase seizure threshold and shorten seizure activity [18]. If they are prescribed to treat epilepsy, then they should continue without alteration. If they are prescribed as mood stabilisers, these medications are generally discontinued, although some centres continue and reduce dose if seizure induction proves problematic.

CHAPTER 66

SAFETY OF ECT

ECT remains one of the best-tolerated biological therapies, with very low risks for severe complications. The mortality rate during ECT is reported as between 1 in 25,000 and 1 in 50,000. Severe complications occur in less than 1 in 10,000 procedures [23].

ECT PRESCRIBING

- Bitemporal ECT is the recommended first-line electrode placement for severely ill patients or when a rapid response is needed. However, recent studies have observed that high-dose unilateral ECT does not differ from moderate-dose bitemporal ECT in antidepressant efficacy but with fewer cognitive side effects [24].
- Unilateral ECT should be considered in patients with underlying cognitive deficits, in patients who have previously suffered memory disturbance with bitemporal ECT, and in patients with good previous response to unilateral electrode placement.
- If no clinical improvement at all is seen after six bilateral treatments, then the prescribing physician should consider abandoning treatment. For patients who have shown definite but slight or temporary improvement with early treatments, it may be worth continuing up to 12 bilateral treatments, although decisions should be made on a case-by-case basis, alongside discussion with the patient.

GUIDANCE FOR THE DOCTOR ADMINISTERING ECT

No doctor should administer ECT without training and/or appropriate supervision. The doctor responsible for administering ECT should remain in the clinic until all patients have recovered from their treatment. The doctor administering ECT is responsible for:

- setting the dose using the stimulus dosing protocol
- applying the EEG leads to monitor seizure activity
- applying the handset electrodes correctly
- checking the patient's impedance is 100–3000 Ω, and rectifying this if necessary
- administering the treatment dose
- observing the seizure duration
- recording all relevant details of the treatment, including percentage stimulus charge given and seizure duration.

SIDE EFFECTS OF ECT

The side effects can be divided into somatic and cognitive, described in Box 66.1.

Box 66.1 Side effects of electroconvulsive therapy

Somatic

- *Headache* is a very common side effect, experienced by up to 45% of patients [25]. The vast majority can be treated with simple analgesia (e.g. paracetamol). Patients who experience regular migraines have a much higher risk of post-ictal headache and may benefit from prophylactic administration of a triptan. If severe headaches have been experienced with a prior procedure, then the responsible anaesthetist should consider an alteration to induction medications.
- *Postoperative nausea and vomiting* is now a rare occurrence following anaesthesia, and ECT does not predispose patients to an increased risk compared with other procedures. Anti-emetic prophylaxis may be given by the responsible anaesthetist.
- *Prolonged seizure activity* is rare. Seizure activity can be terminated with intravenous benzodiazepines, induction agents, or anticonvulsants.
- *Prolonged muscle relaxation* is very rare, and usually related to the use of lithium or to an inherited predisposition. Prolonged artificial ventilation may be required.
- *Cardiovascular events* such as ischaemia and arrhythmia are rare. However, risk of cardiac arrhythmias may be more common with ECT compared with other procedures performed under general anaesthesia.
- *Allergy* and other adverse reactions to anaesthetic agents may occur.

Cognitive

- *Transient confusion* on emergence from anaesthesia for ECT may be experienced by all patients. The duration and severity of this confusion is highly variable, and may depend on patient age, choice and dose of induction agents, and the administration of certain regular medications such as sedatives, anxiolytics, antipsychotics, and lithium.
- *Short-term memory disturbance (hours to days)* is experienced by approximately one-third of patients. It can be more prominent in bilateral compared with unilateral ECT, and with higher dosage of electrical stimulation.
- *Long-term memory disturbance (weeks to months to years)* is very rare. Modern techniques, such as unilateral or bifrontal pulse wave stimulation, has substantially reduced occurrence.

SPECIAL PATIENT GROUPS

There are no patient groups for whom ECT is absolutely contraindicated, but special consideration should be given to older people, young people, and pregnant women.

Older people (age 75+)

ECT is safe and well tolerated in older patients. Short-term anterograde memory impairment appears to be greater in older patients, but any additional deficits tend to disappear by six months [26]. Older people may suffer from more physical illnesses and must be thoroughly screened for problems prior to treatment. All coexisting medical or surgical conditions should be assessed and, so far as possible, stabilised or treated prior to ECT. Older people are also at greater risk of confusion post ECT, especially if suffering from pre-existing cognitive deficits. Consideration should be given as to whether bilateral or unilateral ECT should be given in these circumstances.

Young people (under the age of 18)

ECT is safe in children, although is rarely given to patients under the age of 18. It is recommended that two independent opinions are sought on the need for ECT in children. In the case of this being proposed, the referring consultant must discuss the proposed treatment with the local ECT consultant and appropriate consent procedures must be adhered to. The proposed treatment must also be discussed in depth with the patient and their family.

Pregnant women

There is no evidence that ECT is likely to jeopardise a pregnancy; ECT itself appears to carry no specific risks to the fetus, but close discussion between the referring consultant, the consultant obstetrician, and the local ECT consultant should be maintained over the duration of the treatment [7]. Nevertheless, the usual risks of general anaesthesia still apply. Hyperventilation should be avoided, as it may reduce placental blood flow and lead to fetal hypoxia.

References

1. Fosse R, Read J. Electroconvulsive treatment: hypotheses about mechanisms of action. *Front Psychiatry* 2013;4:94.
2. Ding Z, White PF. Anesthesia for electroconvulsive therapy. *Anesth Analg* 2002;94(5):1351–1364.
3. Brus O, Nordanskog P, Bave U, et al. Subjective memory immediately following electroconvulsive therapy. *J ECT* 2017;33(2):96–103.
4. Ziegelmayer C, Hajak G, Bauer A, et al. Cognitive performance under electroconvulsive therapy (ECT) in ECT-naive treatment-resistant patients with major depressive disorder. *J ECT* 2017;33(2):104–110.
5. National Institute for Health and Care Excellence. *Guidance on the Use of Electroconvulsive Therapy*. Technological Appraisal Guidance TA59. London: NICE, 2003. Last updated 1 October 2009. Available at https://www.nice.org.uk/guidance/ta59
6. Lisanby SH. Electroconvulsive therapy for depression. *N Engl J Med* 2007;357(19):1939–1945.
7. Ward H, Fromson J, Cooper J, et al. Recommendations for the use of ECT in pregnancy: literature review and proposed clinical protocol. *Eur Psychiatry* 2019;56(Suppl):S321.
8. Abrams R, Taylor MA, Faber R, et al. Bilateral versus unilateral electroconvulsive-therapy: efficacy in melancholia. *Am J Psychiatry* 1983;140(4):463–465.

9. Takano H, Motohashi N, Uema T, et al. Changes in regional cerebral blood flow during acute electroconvulsive therapy in patients with depression: positron emission tomographic study. *Br J Psychiatry* 2007;190:63–68.

10. Bolwig TG, Hertz MM, Paulson OB, et al. The permeability of the blood–brain barrier during electrically induced seizures in man. *Eur J Clin Invest* 1977;7(2):87–93.

11. Crowley K, Pickle J, Dale R, Fattal O. A critical examination of bifrontal electroconvulsive therapy: clinical efficacy, cognitive side effects, and directions for future research. *J ECT* 2008;24(4):268–271.

12. Andrade C, Bolwig TG. Electroconvulsive therapy, hypertensive surge, blood–brain barrier breach, and amnesia: exploring the evidence for a connection. *J ECT* 2014;30(2):160–164.

13. Bedford PD. Adverse cerebral effects of anaesthesia on old people. *Lancet* 1955;269(6884):259–263.

14. Gbyl K, Videbech P. Electroconvulsive therapy increases brain volume in major depression: a systematic review and meta-analysis. *Acta Psychiatr Scand* 2018;138(3):180–195.

15. Suzuki Y, Miyajima M, Ohta K, et al. A triphasic change of cardiac autonomic nervous system during electroconvulsive therapy. *J ECT* 2015;31(3):186–191.

16. Williams K, Smith J, Glue P, Nutt D. The effects of electroconvulsive therapy on plasma insulin and glucose in depression. *Br J Psychiatry* 1992;161:94–98.

17. Mayhew D, Mendonca V, Murthy BVS. A review of ASA physical status: historical perspectives and modern developments. *Anaesthesia* 2019;74(3):373–379.

18. Devinsky O, Honigfeld G, Patin J. Clozapine-related seizures. *Neurology* 1991;41(3):369–371.

19. Pisani F, Oteri G, Costa C, et al. Effects of psychotropic drugs on seizure threshold. *Drug Saf* 2002;25(2):91–110.

20. Hill GE, Wong KC, Hodges MR. Lithium carbonate and neuromuscular blocking agents. *Anesthesiology* 1977;46(2):122–126.

21. Hassamal S, Pandurangi A, Venkatachalam V, Levenson J. Delayed onset and prolonged ECT-related delirium. *Case Rep Psychiatry* 2013;2013:840425.

22. Galvez V, Loo CK, Alonzo A, et al. Do benzodiazepines moderate the effectiveness of bitemporal electroconvulsive therapy in major depression? *J Affect Disord* 2013;150(2):686–690.

23. Torring N, Sanghani SN, Petrides G, et al. The mortality rate of electroconvulsive therapy: a systematic review and pooled analysis. *Acta Psychiatr Scand* 2017;135(5):388–397.

24. Semkovska M, Landau S, Dunne R, et al. Bitemporal versus high-dose unilateral twice-weekly electroconvulsive therapy for depression (EFFECT-Dep): a pragmatic, randomized, non-inferiority trial. *Am J Psychiatry* 2016;173(4):408–417.

25. Weiner SJ, Ward TN, Ravaris CL. Headache and electroconvulsive-therapy. *Headache* 1994;34(3):155–159.

26. McClintock SM, Choi J, Deng ZD, et al. Multifactorial determinants of the neurocognitive effects of electroconvulsive therapy. *J ECT* 2014;30(2):165–176.

CHAPTER 66

Part 15

Emergencies

Chest Pain

Luke Vano, Immo Weichert

Chest pain is a common presenting complaint, accounting for approximately 1% of visits to primary care [1,2]. It has a number of different causes (Table 67.1), and therefore identifying the precise underlying pathology is often difficult. Indeed, over 70% of patients presenting with chest pain fail to receive a definitive immediate diagnosis from a general practitioner during their first clinical review [3]. While most episodes of chest pain are benign and self-limiting, it can herald life-threatening emergencies such as myocardial infarction, pulmonary embolus, and tension pneumothorax [1,2]. As such, a clinical approach should always first rule out dangerous, if rare, aetiology, before considering lower-risk causes.

Patients with serious mental illness (SMI) are at increased risk of various medical conditions that can present with chest pain, such as cardiovascular disease, venous thromboembolism (VTE), and chronic lung disease [4–6]. Certain psychiatric treatments increase the risk of ischaemic heart disease (e.g. antipsychotics), and a serious, if rare, complication of clozapine treatment is myocarditis, which may present with chest pain. Antipsychotic prescription is associated with an increased risk of both pulmonary embolism [7] and pneumonia [8]. Gastro-oesophageal reflux disease, a common gastric cause of chest pain, is more common in people with SMI and is exacerbated by some psychiatric medications (e.g. tricyclic antidepressants, anticholinergics, and some antipsychotics) [9–12]. Recreational drug use is also more prevalent in the SMI population and represents a risk factor for acute cardiac events (e.g. coronary vasospasm, atheroma formation, acute thrombosis, and dissection with cocaine) [13]. Chest pain may also be a feature of some psychiatric presentations, for example being described in up to 70% of panic attacks [14,15].

The Maudsley Practice Guidelines for Physical Health Conditions in Psychiatry, First Edition.
David M. Taylor, Fiona Gaughran, and Toby Pillinger.
© 2021 John Wiley & Sons Ltd. Published 2021 by John Wiley & Sons Ltd.

Table 67.1 Causes of chest pain in the general population presenting to primary care [2].

Cause of chest pain	Percentage
Costochondritis	46.6%
Stable angina	11.1%
Psychogenic disorders	9.5%
Upper respiratory infections	8.1%
Severe hypertension (≥180/≥110 mmHg)	4%
Acute coronary syndrome	3.6%
Gastro-oesophageal reflux disease	3.5%
Trauma	3.2%
Benign stomach problems	2.1%
Pneumonia	2.1%
Chronic obstructive pulmonary disease or asthma	1.9%
Other	4.3%

DIAGNOSTIC PRINCIPLES

Before taking a history, it is important to check that the patient is not in need of emergency care. If any immediate threats to life are present, then assessment and management of the patient using an ABCDE approach are required, alongside help from emergency services.

History

The SOCRATES mnemonic may be used as an aide-memoire to evaluate chest pain.

- Site: where is the pain?
- Onset: what were you doing when the pain started?
- Character: what does the pain feel like?
- Radiation: does the pain move anywhere?
- Associated symptoms: is the pain accompanied by other symptoms (e.g. shortness of breath, palpitations, nausea/vomiting, sweating, rigors, light-headedness, coughing, calf tenderness/swelling)?
- Timing: how long has the pain lasted for?
- Exacerbating/relieving factors: has anything made the pain better or worse?
- Severity: how bad is the pain on a scale of 0–10, with 10 being the worst pain possible and 0 being no pain at all?

The history should also document previous chest pain episodes and the results of any associated investigations; past medical history, noting any risk factors for chest pain

CHAPTER 67

(of any aetiology); drug history (noting any recent medication changes); family history (e.g. cardiovascular disease); and social history (recording smoking and alcohol status and history of substance use). Features of specific cardiac, respiratory, gastric, musculo-skeletal, and infective causes of chest pain are detailed in the following sections (although the list is not exhaustive). Psychiatric aetiology should only be considered when medical causes have been ruled out.

Cardiac causes

Acute coronary syndrome

Acute coronary syndrome (ACS) is caused by blockage of one or more of the coronary arteries resulting in myocardial ischaemia. This can be secondary to rupture of atherosclerotic plaques or arterial spasm. Angina is the name given to chest pain secondary to myocardial ischaemia. It is commonly described as a heavy/tight central crushing chest pain that may radiate to the jaw or down the arms. The use of stimulant drugs (especially cocaine) greatly increase the risk of ACS [13]. Box 67.1 outlines the symptoms that indicate ACS. The reader is also directed to Chapter 69 for further discussion regarding appropriate history, examination, investigation, and management.

Myocarditis and pericarditis

Myocarditis and pericarditis respectively describe inflammation of the heart muscle and heart-containing sac. In the general population, these conditions are most often caused by viral infections. Clozapine can cause both conditions (although myocarditis is more common), typically within the first eight weeks of starting treatment [17]. Patients may present with myalgia and flu-like symptoms. The chest pain of pericarditis is traditionally described as pleuritic and relieved on sitting forward. There may be associated shortness of breath, palpitations, or peripheral oedema (if associated with heart failure). The reader is directed to Chapter 8 for further discussion regarding appropriate history, examination, investigation, and management.

Cardiac tamponade

Cardiac tamponade occurs when fluid accumulates within the pericardial sac, impairing myocardial contraction. Onset may be gradual or acute, and as cardiac output becomes progressively impaired, the patient may develop cardiogenic shock, characterised by hypotension and tachycardia. It may be preceded by trauma, malignancy, severe renal failure, or pericarditis.

Box 67.1 Symptoms indicative of acute coronary syndrome [16]

- Pain lasting for over 15 minutes occurring in the chest, arms, back or jaw
- Chest pain associated with nausea, vomiting, marked sweating, or breathlessness
- Chest pain with haemodynamic instability
- Sudden deterioration of previously stable angina

Aortic dissection

Aortic dissection is a rare condition where the innermost layer of the aorta allows blood to flow between the layers of the aortic wall, forcing the layers apart. It is associated with a severe chest/back pain that is described as having a 'tearing' quality and is accompanied by haemodynamic instability. Advanced age, male sex, a history of arterial hypertension, and the presence of an aortic aneurysm increase the risk. However, patients with genetic connective tissue disorders such as Marfan, Loeys–Dietz, or Ehlers–Danlos syndromes, aortitis and bicuspid aortic valves can develop aortic dissection at a much younger age [18].

Respiratory causes

Pulmonary embolism

Pulmonary embolism (PE) is a blockage of one or more blood vessels that supply blood to the lungs, most commonly caused by a blood clot that has travelled from the venous system. Symptoms include shortness of breath, haemoptysis, and pleuritic chest pain. Most cases are caused by a lower limb deep vein thrombosis, and therefore the patient should be asked about recent unilateral leg swelling and/or pain. The reader is directed to Chapter 18 for further discussion regarding history (including risk factors for VTE), examination, investigation, and management.

Pneumonia

Pneumonia can be associated with pleuritic chest pain. Other signs and symptoms include fever, chills, and cough productive of purulent sputum. The reader is directed to Chapter 39.

Pneumothorax

Pneumothorax describes the collection of air in the pleural space (i.e. between a lung and its containing sac). Chest pain is typically one-sided, pleuritic, and associated with shortness of breath. A tension pneumothorax is where air enters the pleural space but cannot then escape. This medical emergency is associated with acute-onset chest pain and significant distress. Urgent treatment is indicated with needle decompression or chest drain insertion.

Gastric causes

Gastro-oesophageal reflux disease

Gastro-oesophageal reflux disease occurs when acidic stomach contents reflux back into the oesophagus. The associated chest pain is often described as a retrosternal heartburn that occurs after eating and is worse on lying flat. Associated symptoms may include cough, wheeze, and hoarseness. The reader is directed to Chapter 19.

Gastritis

Gastritis describes inflammation of the stomach lining, often caused by a bacterial or viral infection. The use of non-steroidal anti-inflammatories or high intake of alcohol can also be causative. Gastritis often presents with an aching pain that starts in the upper abdomen. It may be improved or worsened by food. There may be associated nausea and vomiting.

Oesophageal spasm

Oesophageal spasm describes painful uncoordinated contraction of the oesophagus. This rare disease causes a pain that mimics angina, though it is often associated with difficulty swallowing and may have a more 'burning' quality. It is more likely to occur in people with gastro-oesophageal reflux disease.

Psychiatric causes

Chest pain is a common complaint in patients with panic disorder. Other psychiatric presentations that may be associated with chest pain include depression and somatisation disorders.

Other causes

Costochondritis

Costochondritis describes inflammation of one or more of the costal cartilages that connect the sternum (breastbone) to the ribs. The chest pain is worse on palpation of the costochondral joints.

Herpes zoster

Herpes zoster (shingles) is a self-limiting condition caused by reactivation of the varicella zoster virus in a given ganglion (a cluster of nerve cell bodies). It is more common in those who are immunocompromised and the elderly. The chest pain experienced is neuralgic and described as having a tingling and burning quality. The pain is confined to the area demarcated by the characteristic vesicular rash. The pain can precede the rash by several days and can also recur after the rash has disappeared (post-herpetic neuralgia).

Examination and investigations

All patients should have a detailed cardiovascular, respiratory, and gastrointestinal examination along with vital sign measures and an ECG. Unstable basic observations (e.g. low oxygen saturations or hypotension) associated with chest pain, or ECG changes consistent with myocardial ischaemia, are an indication for *immediate transfer* to emergency services. Bloods may also be required. Further investigations (e.g. chest X-ray, echocardiogram, or CT-pulmonary angiogram) may be requested/performed by medical services. Specific examination and investigation findings for some cardiac, respiratory, gastric, inflammatory, and infectious causes of chest pain are detailed here.

- *Acute coronary syndrome*: see Chapter 69.
- *Myocarditis/pericarditis*: patients with pericarditis may have a pericardial friction rub on auscultation of the heart. This is described as an added squeaky sound that

CHAPTER 67

may be best heard over the left sternal border. Sinus tachycardia with non-specific ST-segment and T-waves changes are most often seen on an ECG in myocarditis. Pericarditis often produces a characteristic ST elevation that is 'saddle-shaped'. Blood tests should include C-reactive protein and troponin.

- *Cardiac tamponade*: examination may reveal tachycardia, distension of the jugular venous system, pericardial friction rub, muffled heart sounds, and hypotension. ECG may show ST-segment changes or an electrical alternans (QRS complexes vary in amplitude and/or axis from beat to beat).
- *Aortic dissection*: patients may have a pulse deficit, a murmur of aortic regurgitation, hypertension or hypotension, or neurological findings. There may be non-specific ECG changes and elevated troponin on blood tests.
- *Pulmonary embolism*: see Chapter 18.
- *Pneumonia*: see Chapter 39.
- *Pneumothorax*: may be associated with asymmetrical chest expansion on chest wall palpation, hyperresonance on percussion, and decreased breath sounds over the area of pneumothorax. In a simple spontaneous pneumothorax, the trachea may be pulled to the side of the collapsed lung, whereas in tension pneumothorax the trachea is displaced away from the affected side.
- *Gastric causes*: often no signs on examination.
- *Costochondritis*: pain on palpation of the costochondral joints.
- *Herpes zoster*: characteristic vesicular rash that is confined to one or more dermatome.

MANAGEMENT

Acute conditions such as ACS, cardiac tamponade, aortic dissection, PE, myocarditis, and pneumothorax are medical emergencies and should not be managed in a psychiatric setting: patients should be *immediately transferred* to emergency services.

The management of chest pain is dependent on the underlying cause. If ACS, myocarditis, PE, pneumonia, or gastro-oesophageal reflux disease are suspected, please refer to the relevant chapters for further information regarding immediate management. For the management of gastritis, see the peptic ulcer disease section of Chapter 19.

Patients with oesophageal spasm should be reassured that the condition is not life-threatening. Lifestyle interventions include avoiding identified triggers, dietary modification, and active stress reduction.

Costochondritis should be treated with simple analgesia, for example regular paracetamol with a short course of oral non-steroidal anti-inflammatory medication and, if there are risk factors for gastritis (e.g. old age), co-prescription of a proton-pump inhibitor for the same length of time. An example prescription is paracetamol 1 g four times daily and ibuprofen 400–800 mg orally every six to eight hours with food for three days initially, alongside omeprazole 20 mg orally once daily if gastroprotection is indicated. Avoid anti-inflammatory painkillers in the elderly, patients with poor oral intake, renal failure, heart failure, and in those with increased bleeding risk.

Herpes zoster is a self-limiting disease. Antiviral agents should be considered in those who are over the age of 50 or who are immunocompromised, including patients with diabetes mellitus. Treatment involves a seven-day course of antiviral therapy alongside simple analgesia. An example prescription is famciclovir 500 mg orally every eight hours for seven days or aciclovir 800 mg orally five times a day (less frequently in renal impairment) for seven days. It is recommended to start this within three days of the onset of rash. Calamine topical lotion should be prescribed in all patients with pain to be applied to the affected area four times daily, alongside oral analgesia.

INFORMATION TO PROVIDE IN A 'CHEST PAIN' REFERRAL TO MEDICAL SERVICES

- Rationale behind referral: chest pain, and what you are specifically concerned about.
- Pertinent history and examination findings:

- SOCRATES description of chest pain.
- Pertinent past medical history, family history, and social history.
- Current medication and any recent drug changes. Document if you are concerned that any current medications may be causative or have been stopped. If psychiatric medication has been stopped, provide rationale and interim treatment plan.
- Brief psychiatric history, associated risk profile, and if there are any specific nursing needs.
- Basic observations and examination findings.
- Any investigations performed locally, e.g. ECG (send a copy) and blood test results.
- Contact details of the referring psychiatric team.

References

1. Ruigomez A, Rodriguez LA, Wallander MA, et al. Chest pain in general practice: incidence, comorbidity and mortality. *Fam Pract* 2006;23(2):167–174.
2. Bosner S, Becker A, Haasenritter J, et al. Chest pain in primary care: epidemiology and pre-work-up probabilities. *Eur J Gen Pract* 2009;15(3):141–146.
3. Jordan KP, Timmis A, Croft P, et al. Prognosis of undiagnosed chest pain: linked electronic health record cohort study. *BMJ* 2017;357:j1194.
4. Dhar AK, Barton DA. Depression and the link with cardiovascular disease. *Front Psychiatry* 2016;7:33.
5. Hsu WY, Lane HY, Lin CL, Kao CH. A population-based cohort study on deep vein thrombosis and pulmonary embolism among schizophrenia patients. *Schizophr Res* 2015;162(1–3):248–252.
6. Correll CU, Solmi M, Veronese N, et al. Prevalence, incidence and mortality from cardiovascular disease in patients with pooled and specific severe mental illness: a large-scale meta-analysis of 3,211,768 patients and 113,383,368 controls. *World Psychiatry* 2017;16(2):163–180.
7. Allenet B, Schmidlin S, Genty C, Bosson JL. Antipsychotic drugs and risk of pulmonary embolism. *Pharmacoepidemiol Drug Saf* 2012;21(1):42–48.
8. Kuo CJ, Yang SY, Liao YT, et al. Second-generation antipsychotic medications and risk of pneumonia in schizophrenia. *Schizophr Bull* 2013;39(3):648–657.
9. van Soest EM, Dieleman JP, Siersema PD, et al. Tricyclic antidepressants and the risk of reflux esophagitis. *Am J Gastroenterol* 2007;102(9):1870–1877.
10. Koerselman J, Pursnani KG, Peghini P, et al. Different effects of an oral anticholinergic drug on gastroesophageal reflux in upright and supine position in normal, ambulant subjects: a pilot study. *Am J Gastroenterol* 1999;94(4):925–930.
11. Crouse EL, Alastanos JN, Bozymski KM, Toscano RA. Dysphagia with second-generation antipsychotics: a case report and review of the literature. *Ment Health Clin* 2017;7(2):56–64.
12. van Veggel M, Olofinjana O, Davies G, Taylor D. Clozapine and gastro-oesophageal reflux disease (GORD): an investigation of temporal association. *Acta Psychiatr Scand* 2013;127(1):69–77.
13. Schwartz BG, Rezkalla S, Kloner RA. Cardiovascular effects of cocaine. *Circulation* 2010;122(24):2558–2569.

CHAPTER 67

14. Campbell KA, Madva EN, Villegas AC, et al. Non-cardiac chest pain: a review for the consultation-liaison psychiatrist. *Psychosomatics* 2017;58(3):252–265.

15. Katon W. Panic disorder and somatization: review of 55 cases. *Am J Med* 1984;77(1):101–106.

16. Battaglia J, Houston JP, Ahl J, et al. A post hoc analysis of transitioning to oral treatment with olanzapine or haloperidol after 24-hour intramuscular treatment in acutely agitated adult patients with schizophrenia. *Clin Ther* 2005;27(10):1612–1618.

17. Wehmeier PM, Heiser P, Remschmidt H. Myocarditis, pericarditis and cardiomyopathy in patients treated with clozapine. *J Clin Pharm Ther* 2005;30(1):91–96.

18. Gawinecka J, Schönrath F, von Eckardstein A. Acute aortic dissection: pathogenesis, risk factors and diagnosis. *Swiss Med Wkly* 2017;147:w14489.

Chapter 68

Acute Shortness of Breath
Martin Osugo, Toby Pillinger, Vivek Srivastava

Acute shortness of breath (dyspnoea) is a subjective, usually distressing sensation or awareness of difficulty with breathing that develops over a period of seconds to minutes [1]. It has several different causes that can be life-threatening (Box 68.1). The most common are exacerbations of pre-existing conditions such as chronic heart failure, chronic obstructive pulmonary disease (COPD) or bronchial asthma, or acute conditions such as pneumonia, acute coronary syndrome (ACS), and pulmonary embolus (PE) [2,3]. Psychogenic breathlessness should be a diagnosis of exclusion. Patients with serious mental illness (SMI) have poorer medical outcomes where shortness of breath is a presenting complaint. For example, compared with the general population, patients with schizophrenia presenting with pneumonia have a 34% increased risk of requiring mechanical ventilation and an 81% increased risk of intensive care admission [4].

DIAGNOSTIC PRINCIPLES

The priority for any clinician assessing a patient with shortness of breath is to identify potentially life-threatening presentations and, where appropriate, instigate emergency treatment using the ABCDE approach and facilitate transfer of care to emergency services. Therefore, it is possible that history, examination, and investigations will have to be undertaken whilst simultaneously managing the patient. The goal of management may be to stabilise the patient rather than diagnose and treat the underlying condition. Respiratory rate, oxygen saturation, pulse, blood pressure, and temperature should be measured in all acutely breathless patients. Increased respiratory rate (normal rate 12–20 breaths per minute) is the single best predictor of severe illness [5].

The Maudsley Practice Guidelines for Physical Health Conditions in Psychiatry, First Edition.
David M. Taylor, Fiona Gaughran, and Toby Pillinger.
© 2021 John Wiley & Sons Ltd. Published 2021 by John Wiley & Sons Ltd.

Box 68.1 Potentially life-threatening causes of acute shortness of breath and their clinical features

Respiratory

- Infection: typical features of infection including fever, pleuritic chest pain, and potentially a productive cough (see Chapter 39).
- Pneumothorax: associated with unilateral pleuritic chest pain (see Chapter 67).
- Chronic obstructive pulmonary disease (COPD): exacerbations of COPD are associated with wheeze and cough (see Chapter 47).
- Asthma: signs of severe disease include wheeze, use of accessory muscles of respiration, and difficulty completing full sentences (see Chapter 48).
- Pulmonary embolus: may be associated with pleuritic chest pain and haemoptysis (see Chapter 18)
- Pulmonary oedema: may occur in association with heart failure or unrelated to cardiac disease, e.g. acute respiratory distress syndrome, which may arise in the context of sepsis, severe respiratory infection, and overdose (e.g. opioids, aspirin, and cocaine).

Upper airway

- Anaphylaxis: see Chapter 77.
- Angioedema: swelling of the lips, tongue, pharynx, and larynx. Can occur in association with certain medications (e.g. angiotensin-converting enzyme inhibitors or non-steroidal anti-inflammatories). Discussed further in Chapter 77.
- Foreign objects: unusual in adults, although may occur in the context of self-harm. The patient may have stridor or wheeze.

Cardiac

- Acute coronary syndrome: typically associated with heavy/tight central crushing chest pain that may radiate to the jaw or down the arms (see Chapters 67 and 69).
- Heart failure: may be associated with peripheral oedema (see Chapter 7), raised jugular venous pressure, and bibasal crackles and S3 gallop on chest auscultation. Consider myocarditis in patients who have recently started clozapine (first few weeks) who present with shortness of breath, flu-like symptoms, with or without chest pain (see Chapter 8).
- Cardiac arrhythmia: may be accompanied by palpitations, presyncope, syncope, chest pain, and other features of heart failure (see Chapters 1–3 and 70).

Other

- Toxic: for example, aspirin (salicylate) poisoning (see Chapter 83).
- Metabolic: for example, diabetic ketoacidosis (see Chapter 74).
- Sepsis: see Chapter 72.
- Anaemia: see Chapter 15.

History

Obtaining a complete history from the patient may be difficult and collateral history from carers or relatives, or in an inpatient setting ward staff, may be helpful. Aim to gather information on the following.

- History of presenting complaint: determine if there is a clear precipitant, such as infection (pneumonia), recent exposure to an allergen/new medication (anaphylaxis), recent period of prolonged immobility (PE), chest pain (ACS, pneumothorax, or PE), or chance of overdose.

- Past medical history: screen for the presentations listed in Box 68.1, and any conditions that may predispose to those presentations (e.g. immunosuppression in the case of pneumonia).
- Medication history: determine allergy status, the prescription of any recent medications, and any long-term medications that may point to aetiology (e.g. inhalers for asthma or COPD, heart failure medication such as diuretics).
- Social history: determine the patient's smoking history and any use of recreational drugs.
- Psychiatric aetiology should only be considered after exclusion of medical causes; however, where suspected, perform a mental state examination and review psychiatric history.

Examination

- An initial examination should aim to identify any serious/life-threatening presentations. Red flags for respiratory arrest include confusion, cyanosis, and fatigue/difficulty in maintaining respiration. Also note inability to complete full sentences and use of accessory muscles of respiration (sitting upright in 'tripod' position).
- If not performed already, check basic observations as described. In most patients, oxygen saturations should be over 94%. However, note that some patients with COPD may have oxygen saturations of 88–92% at baseline.
- Assess for stridor (airway obstruction), wheeze (which may occur in asthma and anaphylaxis), and crackles (infection or pulmonary oedema). Absence of breath sounds may herald severe asthma/COPD or, when unilateral, pneumothorax.
- Cardiovascular examination may demonstrate evidence of heart failure (e.g. gallop rhythm, raised jugular venous pressure, peripheral oedema).

Investigations

A psychiatric setting is an inappropriate environment in which to perform many investigations for acute shortness of breath; the priority should be to transfer an unwell patient to emergency medical services. However, where facilities allow, an ECG should be performed if cardiac aetiology is suspected.

In patients with asthma, aim to check peak expiratory flow rate (PEFR). An asthma attack is considered severe if PEFR is 33–50% of predicted, respiratory rate is 25 per minute or more, heart rate is 110 bpm or more, or if the patient is unable to complete full sentences. It is considered life-threatening if any of the following are present: PEFR less than 33%, reduced conscious level, arrhythmia, hypotension, cyanosis, silent chest, or poor respiratory effort.

MANAGEMENT

- Use an ABCDE approach.
- Sit the patient up to improve oxygenation [5].

> **Box 68.2** Features of patients with acute shortness of breath that should prompt consideration of transfer to emergency medical services [1]
>
> - Associated features:
>   - Stridor
>   - Exhaustion of respiratory effort
>   - Confusion
>   - Inability to complete sentences
>   - Elevated respiratory rate
>   - Oxygen saturation <92%
>   - Cyanosis
>   - Tachycardia
>   - Hypotension
>   - Chest pain
> - Shortness of breath during pregnancy or postnatal period
> - Significant comorbidities, e.g. immunosuppression, frailty, elderly

- If available, administer oxygen if oxygen saturations are below 94% [5]. Titrate the oxygen to achieve saturations of 94–98%. An exception to this is patients with suspected COPD, where target oxygen saturations are 88–92% (carbon dioxide 'retainers' depend on a degree of hypoxia for respiratory drive, so increasing oxygen saturations can paradoxically result in respiratory depression).
- Patients with asthma or COPD may have their own salbutamol inhaler. For suspected exacerbations of asthma or COPD, give four puffs of salbutamol 'back to back'. A further two puffs can be given every two minutes, up to a maximum of 10 puffs. Treatment can be repeated at 15–30 minute intervals if necessary [1].
- Asthma patients with severe or life-threatening attacks (described above) should be transferred to emergency services [1,6]. Other features of patients with shortness of breath that should, regardless of aetiology, prompt consideration of transfer to emergency services are presented in Box 68.2. The reader is directed to Chapters 18, 39, 69 and 72 for guidance on the acute management of venous thromboembolism, pneumonia, acute coronary syndrome, and sepsis, respectively.

References

1. National Institute for Health and Care Excellence (NICE). Breathlessness. Clinical Knowledge Summary. Last revised: April 2020. https://cks.nice.org.uk/breathlessness
2. Prekker ME, Feemster LC, Hough CL, et al. The epidemiology and outcome of prehospital respiratory distress. *Acad Emerg Med* 2014;21(5):543–550.
3. Berliner D, Schneider N, Welte T, Bauersachs J. The differential diagnosis of dyspnea. *Dtsch Arztebl Int* 2016;113(49):834–845.
4. Chen YH, Lin HC, Lin HC. Poor clinical outcomes among pneumonia patients with schizophrenia. *Schizophr Bull* 2011;37(5):1088–1094.
5. O'Driscoll BR, Howard LS, Earis J, Mak V. BTS guideline for oxygen use in adults in healthcare and emergency settings. *Thorax* 2017;72(Suppl 1):ii1–ii90.
6. British Thoracic Society and Scottish Intercollegiate Guidelines Network. *British Guideline on the Management of Asthma*. London: BTS, 2014. Available at https://www.brit-thoracic.org.uk/document-library/guidelines/asthma/btssign-asthma-guideline-2014/ (accessed 2 December 2019).

Acute Coronary Syndrome

Laura O'Sullivan, Narbeh Melikian

Acute coronary syndrome (ACS) is an umbrella term for a spectrum of conditions that occur when blood supply to the myocardium is acutely disrupted. It is a common medical emergency and an important cause of cardiovascular morbidity and mortality worldwide [1].

National Institute of Health and Care Excellence (NICE) guidance categorises ACS into three distinct conditions: (i) unstable angina (UA); (ii) non-ST-segment elevation myocardial infarction (NSTEMI); and (iii) ST-segment elevation myocardial infarction (STEMI). The three separate entities are differentiated according to well-defined 12-lead ECG criteria and the presence or absence of biochemical evidence of myocardial injury. The latter is diagnosed through measuring plasma troponin I or T level (Table 69.1).

Rates of cardiovascular disease, including ACS, are dramatically higher in patients with serious mental illness (SMI) compared with the general population and are responsible for a significant proportion of the excess mortality associated with SMI [2]. There is evidence to suggest a disparity in the treatment of patients with SMI presenting with ACS compared with the general population. Patients with SMI are less likely to be admitted to hospital following a presentation related to coronary artery disease, and even if admitted they remain less likely to undergo standard cardiac revascularisation procedures [3]. The provision of secondary prevention treatment to patients with SMI is also poorer [4]. Compared with the general population, patients with SMI have 19% increased mortality in the year following presentation with ACS [3].

The Maudsley Practice Guidelines for Physical Health Conditions in Psychiatry, First Edition.
David M. Taylor, Fiona Gaughran, and Toby Pillinger.

Table 69.1 Clinical, ECG, and biochemical features of unstable angina, non-ST-segment elevation myocardial infarction (NSTEMI), and ST-segment elevation myocardial infarction (STEMI).

	Unstable angina	NSTEMI	STEMI
Chest pain	At rest +	At rest +	At rest +++
ECG changes	Nil or T-wave inversion/ST-segment depression	Nil or T-wave inversion/ST-segment depression	ST-segment elevation
Troponin	Normal	Increased +	Increased +++

DIAGNOSTIC PRINCIPLES

Figure 69.1 provides an algorithmic approach to patients presenting with suspected ACS. Patients with ACS present with a wide spectrum of symptoms. Symptoms can be sudden in onset or develop insidiously over a period of hours to days. In the older age group and diabetic patients, ACS can be silent. Common symptoms include:

- chest discomfort typically described as a pressure or tightness (angina)
- severe chest pain
- referred discomfort to the jaw, arms, shoulders, back, neck or upper abdomen
- breathlessness
- autonomic features such as nausea/vomiting and sweating

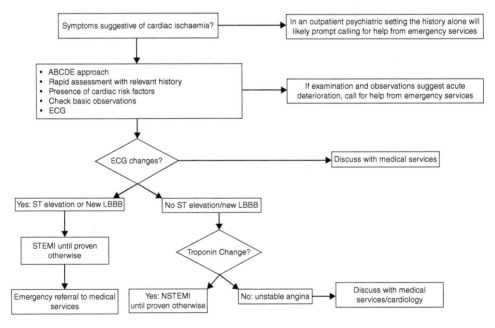

Figure 69.1 A clinical approach to a patient with suspected cardiac ischaemia. LBBB, left bundle branch block.

- palpitations
- light-headedness, dizziness, or fainting episodes
- silent ACS where the initial symptom is a complication such as heart failure.

Despite large variation in presentation, a few generalisations can be made. In almost all patients, symptoms develop without provocation at rest or on minimal activity. UA and NSTEMI commonly present with relapsing/remitting chest discomfort (pressure or tightness). In contrast, STEMI commonly presents with unremitting, progressive, severe chest pain associated with breathlessness and autonomic features.

Therefore, a careful medical history is important, including the following.

- Time course and duration of symptoms.
- Precipitants: 'What were you doing the first time the symptoms started?'
- Alleviating factors for the symptoms (if any).
- If symptoms have been going on for a while, how have they changed and what is different now?
- Risk factors, e.g. smoking, obesity, raised cholesterol, hypertension.
- Family history.
- Drug history, including any recent dose changes.

Examination and immediate investigation should include:

- emergency ABCDE assessment including pulse rate and blood pressure
- 12-lead ECG
- blood sugar (BM) level
- blood tests including high-sensitivity troponin I or T.

If history and examination is suggestive of ACS, then emergency general medical or cardiology opinion should be sought for further investigation and confirmation of diagnosis.

Unstable angina and non-ST-segment elevation myocardial infarction

Chest discomfort in UA and NSTEMI are indistinguishable from one another. Symptoms are characterised by prolonged (>20 minutes) angina at rest, new-onset severe angina, or angina that is rapidly progressive (by increasing frequency, longer duration, or lower onset threshold).

A 12-lead ECG is the first-line investigation in all patients suspected of UA and NSTEMI. In both groups the ECG may confirm myocardial ischaemia (T-wave inversion or ST-segment depression; Figure 69.2) or remain normal. ECG changes can be transient (present during symptomatic phases and improve with settling chest discomfort) or be permanent.

The prime differentiating factor between UA and NSTEMI is evidence of myocardial injury as measured by troponin levels. In UA, troponin remains negative. In contrast, in

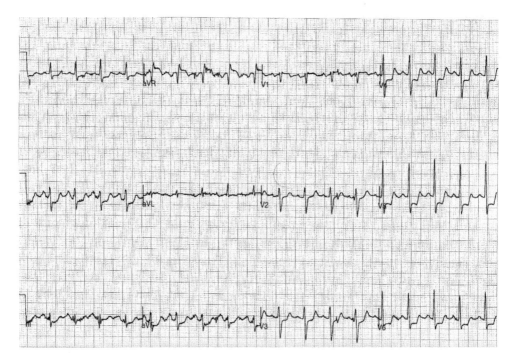

Figure 69.2 Anterolateral myocardial ischaemia as demonstrated by ST-segment depression.

NSTEMI troponin is always positive. There can be a lag of a few hours between onset of chest discomfort and elevation in troponin level. Therefore, a minimum of two troponin levels should be measured at least three to four hours apart to ensure an accurate diagnosis is reached.

ST-segment elevation myocardial infarction

Chest discomfort in STEMI is characteristically severe, unremitting, and progressive. Patients are often very unwell and without prompt treatment are at risk of life-threatening complications including cardiac arrest.

A 12-lead ECG is diagnostic of STEMI. Diagnostic changes include new ST elevation in two anatomically contiguous limb leads [0.1 mV ('one small square') ST elevation in leads I, II, III, aVR, aVL or aVF] or precordial leads [0.2 mV ('two small squares') ST elevation in leads V1–V6] (Box 69.1 and Figure 69.3), or new-onset left bundle branch block (LBBB).

Considering 12-lead ECG is diagnostic of STEMI, there is no requirement for measuring biochemical markers of myocardial injury, such as troponin, for diagnostic purposes. However, the peak troponin level can provide valuable information on the final size of the STEMI.

Box 69.1 Identifying ST-segment elevation on the 12-lead ECG

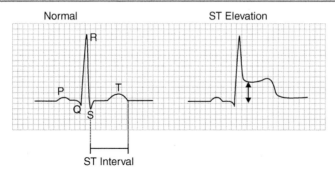

Normal   ST Elevation

ST Interval

The European Society for Cardiology (ESC) guidance defines the significant height of ST elevation as measured from the 'J point' (where the QRS complex terminates) [5].
ST-segment elevation is defined as an increase of:

- 0.1 mV in a limb lead: I, II, III, aVR, aVL and aVF ('one small square')
- 0.2 mV in a precordial lead: V1–V6 ('two small squares').

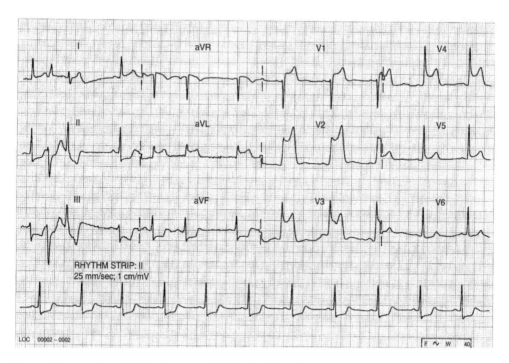

Figure 69.3 Anterolateral ST-elevation myocardial infarction (STEMI).

CHAPTER 69

Other causes of myocardial injury

Most biochemistry laboratories utilise a high-sensitivity troponin I or T assay for diagnosis of myocardial injury. High-sensitivity assays are reliably diagnostic within three hours of chest discomfort. However, it is important to note that an elevated troponin level should only be interpreted in the context of the clinical picture. In addition to ACS there are multiple other non-ischaemic causes for an elevated troponin level. Common causes encountered in a mental health setting include:

- heart failure
- myocarditis/pericarditis
- any form of prolonged tachyarrhythmia (e.g. atrial fibrillation, atrial flutter, ventricular tachycardia, or significant sinus tachycardia)
- sepsis
- chronic kidney disease
- severe anaemia
- severe hypoxaemia.

MANAGEMENT

All types of ACS are a medical emergency and immediate clinical intervention is mandated to minimise myocardial injury and to prevent long-term complications such as heart failure and life-threatening arrhythmias.

STEMI

Heart muscle starts to be lost as soon as a coronary artery becomes occluded ('time is muscle'). In the UK, current guidance is that adults with acute STEMI who present within 12 hours of onset of symptoms should be offered primary percutaneous coronary intervention (primary PCI) as the preferred coronary reperfusion strategy [6]. There is a well-established national 'hub and spoke' network of Heart Attack Centres (HAC) that oversee provision of an around-the-clock primary angioplasty service. STEMI patients are often transferred directly to the cardiac catheter laboratory in the HAC, bypassing emergency departments, to avoid delay in reperfusion. If primary PCI is due to be delayed by 120 minutes or more, then fibrinolysis (e.g. streptokinase or alteplase) should be considered [6].

NSTEMI and unstable angina

UA/NSTEMI is initially treated medically. The principles guiding medical therapy are directed towards preventing coronary thrombosis and reducing cardiac workload. This dual strategy is often sufficient to settle acute symptoms and is achieved through anticoagulation (using a low-molecular-weight heparin such as enoxaparin or fondaparinux), dual antiplatelet therapy (using aspirin and another antiplatelet agent such as clopidogrel or ticagrelor), and medication to reduce cardiac workload (using oral beta-blockade and intravenous infusion nitrates). Thereafter, every patient will require cardiac catheterisation to determine whether revascularisation (angioplasty or coronary bypass graft surgery) is required. The timing of cardiac catheterisation is determined according to the risk of adverse cardiovascular events. In practice, clinically unstable patients undergo cardiac catheterisation within 24 hours of presentation, high- and medium-risk patients who are clinically stable within 72 hours of admission, and low-risk patients on an outpatient basis.

Secondary prevention

Patients with ACS require proactive intervention to address cardiovascular risk factors. Medical intervention is needed to optimally manage high blood pressure, glycaemic control in diabetes, and lipid levels. In addition, patients benefit from enrolling on a cardiac rehabilitation programme, which provides interventions to promote smoking cessation and weight loss (dietary and aerobic exercise advice) alongside psychological support.

General consideration

All patients with ACS will require long-term cardiac medication including antiplatelet drugs (e.g. aspirin), beta-blockers, statins, and drugs for managing risk factors such as hypertension and diabetes. It is important to consider the interaction of such medication with a patient's psychiatric treatment. Because many cardiac and psychotropic agents lower blood pressure, additive hypotensive effects are not uncommon, as for example between the tricyclic antidepressants or clozapine and antihypertensives (see Chapter 6). Furthermore, additive effects may also arise from the use of psychotropic agents that slow conduction and prolong the PR, QRS, and QT intervals when they are used in conjunction with antiarrhythmic medications, resulting in heart block or the long QT syndrome (see Chapter 3) [7]. Where psychiatric–cardiac drug interactions are anticipated, a multidisciplinary discussion should take place involving cardiology, psychiatry, and the patient to discuss the most appropriate treatment regimen.

CHAPTER 69

References

1. Eisen A, Giugliano RP, Braunwald E. Updates on acute coronary syndrome. *JAMA Cardiol* 2016;1(6):718–730.
2. Correll CU, Solmi M, Veronese N, et al. Prevalence, incidence and mortality from cardiovascular disease in patients with pooled and specific severe mental illness: a large-scale meta-analysis of 3,211,768 patients and 113,383,368 controls. *World Psychiatry* 2017;16(2):163–180.
3. Mitchell AJ, Lawrence D. Revascularisation and mortality rates following acute coronary syndromes in people with severe mental illness: comparative meta-analysis. *Br J Psychiatry* 2011;198(6):434–441.
4. Mitchell AJ, Malone D, Doebbeling CC. Quality of medical care for people with and without comorbid mental illness and substance misuse: systematic review of comparative studies. *Br J Psychiatry* 2009;194(6):491–499.
5. Ibanez B, James S, Agewall S, et al. 2017 ESC Guidelines for the management of acute myocardial infarction in patients presenting with ST-segment elevation: The Task Force for the management of acute myocardial infarction in patients presenting with ST-segment elevation of the European Society of Cardiology (ESC). *Eur Heart J* 2018;39(2):119–177.
6. National Institute for Health and Care Excellence. *Myocardial Infarction with ST-Segment Elevation: Acute Management*. Clinical Guideline CG167. London: NICE, 2013. Available at https://www.nice.org.uk/guidance/cg167
7. Protty MB. Coronary artery disease and schizophrenia: the interplay of heart and mind. *Eur Heart J Qual Care Clin Outcomes* 2019;5(2):90–91.

Chapter 70

Arrhythmia

Martin Osugo, Nicholas Gall

The reader is directed to Chapters 1–3 on tachycardia, bradycardia, and prolonged QTc interval for descriptions of the aetiology, assessment, and management of non-emergency presentations of arrhythmia. Here we provide algorithmic approaches to the emergency management of arrhythmia, i.e. where cardiac arrest is either threatened or has occurred, as described by the UK Resuscitation Council [1].

It is recognised that in the psychiatric setting, certain drugs or methods of drug delivery (e.g. intravenous access) may sometimes not be readily available. As such, in the case of peri-arrest/arrest, the priority should be to manage patients according to the ABCDE approach and expedite transfer to emergency services. Where available, automated external defibrillators guide operators through the resuscitation process using verbal commands and visual prompts.

TACHYCARDIA

If the patient loses cardiac output, then manage as per the algorithm in Figure 70.1. The approach to an adult with tachycardia and a palpable pulse is shown in Figure 70.2. If the patient is unstable, synchronised cardioversion is usually the treatment of choice; however, if the patient is conscious, this will need to be carried out under sedation/anaesthesia in a medical environment.

BRADYCARDIA

Defibrillation does not play a role in the management of bradycardia, instead requiring pharmacological management (e.g. atropine) and potentially cardiac pacing (Figure 70.3). As such, in the psychiatric setting, transfer of the patient to emergency services should be the priority.

The Maudsley Practice Guidelines for Physical Health Conditions in Psychiatry, First Edition.
David M. Taylor, Fiona Gaughran, and Toby Pillinger.
© 2021 John Wiley & Sons Ltd. Published 2021 by John Wiley & Sons Ltd.

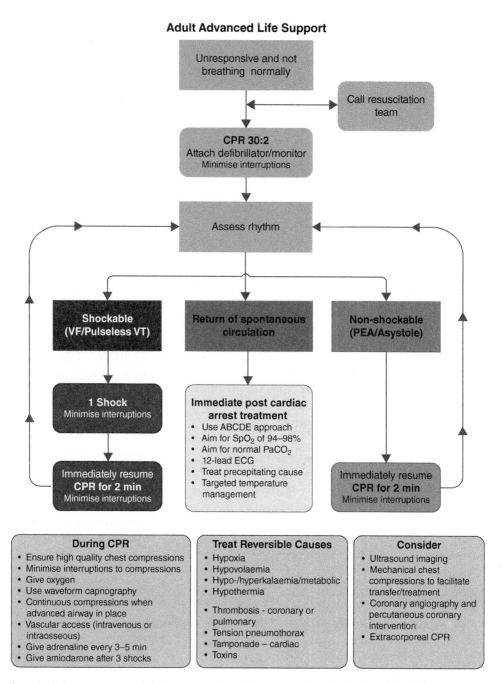

Figure 70.1 Emergency approach to the unresponsive patient. Source: Resuscitation Council (UK) [1]. Reproduced with permission of the UK Resuscitation Council.

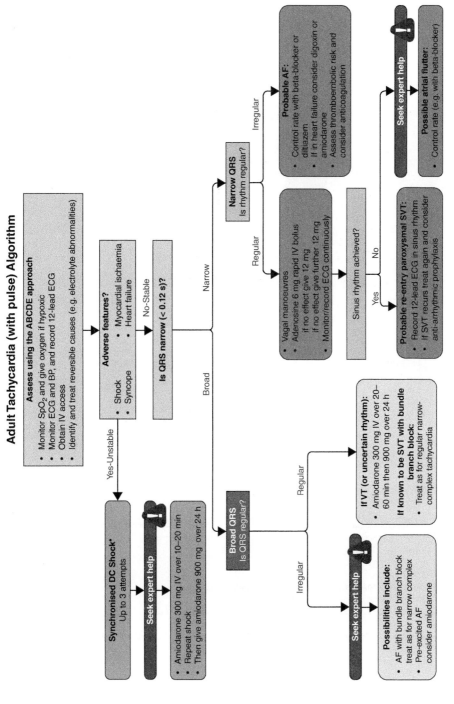

Figure 70.2 Adult tachycardia (with pulse) algorithm. Source: Resuscitation Council (UK) [1]. Reproduced with permission of the UK Resuscitation Council.

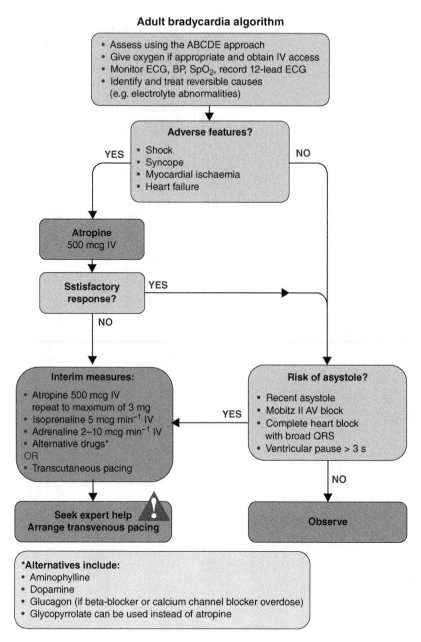

Adult bradycardia algorithm

- Assess using the ABCDE approach
- Give oxygen if appropriate and obtain IV access
- Monitor ECG, BP, SpO$_2$, record 12-lead ECG
- Identify and treat reversible causes
  (e.g. electrolyte abnormalities)

Adverse features?
- Shock
- Syncope
- Myocardial ischaemia
- Heart failure

YES   NO

Atropine
500 mcg IV

Sstisfactory response?   YES

NO

Interim measures:
- Atropine 500 mcg IV
  repeat to maximum of 3 mg
- Isoprenaline 5 mcg min^{-1} IV
- Adrenaline 2–10 mcg min^{-1} IV
- Alternative drugs*
OR
- Transcutaneous pacing

YES

Risk of asystole?
- Recent asystole
- Mobitz II AV block
- Complete heart block
  with broad QRS
- Ventricular pause > 3 s

NO

Seek expert help
Arrange transvenous pacing

Observe

*Alternatives include:
- Aminophylline
- Dopamine
- Glucagon (if beta-blocker or calcium channel blocker overdose)
- Glycopyrrolate can be used instead of atropine

Figure 70.3 Adult bradycardia algorithm. Source: Resuscitation Council (UK) [1]. Reproduced with permission of the UK Resuscitation Council.

Reference

1. Resuscitation Council (UK). *Advanced Life Support*, 7th edn. London: Resuscitation Council, 2016.

Hypertensive Crisis

Luke Vano, J. Kennedy Cruickshank

Severe hypertension is defined as a blood pressure (BP) of 180/110 mmHg or greater [1]. Severe hypertension with no evidence of acute end-organ damage is termed 'hypertensive urgency' (see Box 71.1 for signs and symptoms of end-organ damage) [2]. In the community setting, patients with hypertensive urgency may be managed with immediate treatment of an oral antihypertensive medication [1,3]. However, a severely raised BP that is accompanied by evidence of end-organ damage is considered a hypertensive crisis, and requires urgent referral to medical services. An untreated hypertensive crisis can lead to myocardial infarction, stroke, renal failure, coma and death [3–5]. We recommend that any patient with a BP of 180/110 mmHg or greater should be discussed with general medical services. Evidence of acute end-organ damage (e.g. confusion or shortness of breath) should prompt transfer of the patient to medical services as an emergency.

DIAGNOSTIC PRINCIPLES

1 History: screen for symptoms of end-organ damage (Box 71.1), history of hypertension, compliance with medications, and use of any illicit drugs (e.g. especially cocaine, amphetamines).
2 Examination should include cardiovascular (left ventricular heave of hypertrophy, raised jugular venous pressure, ankle oedema), respiratory (pulmonary oedema), and neurological (focal signs secondary to stroke) examination, including (if possible) ophthalmoscopy to examine for evidence of hypertensive retinopathy.
3 ECG: examine for acute changes suggestive of ischaemia (ST- or T-wave changes), chronic changes consistent with poorly controlled hypertension (left ventricular hypertrophy).

The Maudsley Practice Guidelines for Physical Health Conditions in Psychiatry, First Edition.
David M. Taylor, Fiona Gaughran, and Toby Pillinger.
© 2021 John Wiley & Sons Ltd. Published 2021 by John Wiley & Sons Ltd.

> **Box 71.1** Signs and symptoms of end-organ damage
>
> - *Cardiac*: shortness of breath, chest pain, palpitations, oedema, raised jugular venous pressure, orthopnoea, new murmurs, left ventricular heave of hypertrophy, acute ECG changes
> - *Neurological*: changes in mental state, blurred vision, headaches, dizziness, seizures, focal neurology
> - *Renal*: decreased or increased urine output, haematuria, proteinuria
> - *Retina*: papilloedema, retinal oedema, haemorrhages
> - *Pregnancy-related (pre-eclampsia or eclampsia)*: pitting oedema, seizures, proteinuria, new-onset hypertension, impaired liver function tests, thrombocytopenia

4 Urinalysis: examine for presence of haematuria or proteinuria.
5 Bloods: urea and electrolytes to examine for evidence of acute kidney injury and full blood count to look for signs of microangiopathic haemolytic anaemia.
6 Chest X-ray: assess for pulmonary oedema.

MANAGEMENT

Whilst severe hypertension carries a risk of acute complications, rapid reductions in BP can also result in end-organ damage owing to reduced organ perfusion (e.g. increasing risk of stroke). If in doubt, always liaise with general medical services to guide management.

Hypertensive urgency

BP should be reduced gradually over 24–48 hours with oral antihypertensive medication [2]. The National Institute for Health and Care Excellence (NICE) and British National Formulary (BNF) recommend the use of labetalol, amlodipine, or felodipine for this purpose [2]. An example treatment plan would be prescription of a stat dose of oral amlodipine 5 mg, to be prescribed once daily from the next day onwards. If the patient can self-monitor reliably, blood pressure should be measured a few hours after initial treatment. If blood pressure remains above 180 mmHg systolic or 110 mmHg diastolic, the patient should take another tablet (e.g. a second dose of 5 mg amlodipine). If the BP remains high a few hours later, the patient should seek help from an accident and emergency department (A&E). If the patient is unable to self-monitor reliably, then this process may need to be performed in a supervised medical environment (e.g. an acute medical unit following referral to A&E). If in doubt, discussion with medical services is recommended.

Patients with persistent BP above 180/110 mmHg should be discussed with medical services. In patients who respond to the antihypertensive medication, then continue treatment as per NICE guidelines (see Chapter 5).

Hypertensive crisis

This represents a medical emergency: the patient should be referred to emergency services.

A referral letter should include:

- rationale behind referral (assumed hypertensive emergency)
- comorbid psychiatric diagnosis and current treatment
- any psychosocial issues that may impact on hypertensive control, documentation of recreational drug use if relevant
- summary of potential impact of mental health on engagement with medical care
- contact details of the patients' mental healthcare team/support network who may need to be updated during treatment/discharge process.

References

1. National Institute for Health and Care Excellence. *Hypertension in Adults: Diagnosis and Management*. Clinical Guideline CG136. London: NICE, 2019. Available at https://www.nice.org.uk/guidance/ng136
2. National Institute for Health and Care Excellence. Hypertension treatment summary. https://bnf.nice.org.uk/treatment-summary/hypertension.html
3. Rodriguez MA, Kumar SK, De Caro M. Hypertensive crisis. *Cardiol Rev* 2010;18(2):102–107
4. Whelton PK, Carey RM, Aronow WS, et al. 2017 ACC/AHA/AAPA/ABC/ACPM/AGS/APhA/ASH/ASPC/NMA/PCNA guideline for the prevention, detection, evaluation, and management of high blood pressure in adults: executive summary. A Report of the American College of Cardiology/American Heart Association Task Force on Clinical Practice Guidelines. *Hypertension* 2018;71(6):1269–1324.
5. McNaughton CD, Self WH, Levy PD, Barrett TW. High-risk patients with hypertension: clinical management. *Clin Med Rev Vasc Health*. 2013;2012(4):65–71.

Chapter 72

Sepsis

Laura O'Sullivan, Immo Weichert

Sepsis, historically conceptualised as 'very severe infection', is now recognised as a clinical syndrome secondary to a dysregulated response to infection resulting in multiple organ dysfunction [1]. Sepsis can be triggered by any infection but most commonly occurs in response to bacterial infections. When promptly detected and treated, outcomes are excellent [2]. However, the consequences of unrecognised sepsis and delayed treatment (e.g. fluid resuscitation and antibiotic therapy) are dire, risking multiorgan failure, septic shock, and possibly death [3]. Every year, sepsis costs the NHS £2 billion and claims the lives of at least 52,000 people [4]. Certain factors that are more prevalent in patients with serious mental illness (SMI), such as alcohol abuse, chronic lung disease, and diabetes mellitus, may predispose people with SMI to sepsis [5].

WHEN TO THINK SEPSIS

The most recent definition of sepsis focuses on the presence of organ dysfunction. This can be assessed through use of the Quick Sequential Organ Failure Assessment (qSOFA; Table 72.1) [6]. A score of 2 out of a maximum of 3 points on the qSOFA indicates organ dysfunction. However, there is conflicting evidence regarding the prognostic accuracy of the qSOFA [7]. In most UK hospitals, a version of the National Early Warning Score (NEWS) [8] is used to assess physiological instability (Table 72.2). It is important to consider sepsis when your patient is unwell, as highlighted by their Early Warning Score, and to look for any signs of infection that will give a source and a target for antibiotic therapy. Table 72.3 describes the 'red flags' indicating organ dysfunction.

The Maudsley Practice Guidelines for Physical Health Conditions in Psychiatry, First Edition.
David M. Taylor, Fiona Gaughran, and Toby Pillinger.

Table 72.1 The Quick Sequential Organ Failure Assessment (qSOFA) score: a score of at least 2 points indicates organ dysfunction.

Parameter	Score
Respiratory rate ≥ 22/minute	1
Altered mental status	1
Systolic blood pressure ≤100 mmHg	1

Table 72.2 The NEWS2 scoring system [8].

Physiological parameter	Score						
	3	2	1	0	1	2	3
Respiration rate (per min)	≤8		9–11	12–20		21–24	≥25
Spo_2 scale 1 (%)	≤91	92–93	94—95	≥96			
Spo_2 scale 2[a] (%)	≤83	84–85	86–87	88–92 or ≥93 on air	93–94 on oxygen	95–96 on oxygen	≥97 on oxygen
Air or oxygen?			Oxygen		Air		
Systolic blood pressure (mmHg)	≤90	91–100	101–110	111–219			≥220
Pulse (bpm)	≤40		41–50	51–90	91–110	111–130	≥131
Consciousness							CVPU[b]
Temperature (°C)	≤35.0		35.1–36.0	36.1–38.0	38.1–39.0	≥39.1	

[a] Patients with hypercapnic respiratory failure (e.g. CO_2 retention due to chronic obstructive pulmonary disease) and those requiring supplemental oxygen should have a prescribed oxygen saturation target range of 88–92% and a dedicated Spo_2 scoring scale on the NEWS2 chart (scale 2).
[b] CVPU stands for new confusion, responsiveness to voice or pain only, or unconsciousness.

SEPTIC SHOCK

Septic shock is defined as sepsis with profound circulatory, cellular, and metabolic abnormalities that are associated with a greater risk of mortality than with sepsis alone [9]. Patients with septic shock can be clinically identified by the inability to maintain a mean arterial pressure of 65 mmHg or greater and serum lactate level greater than 2 mmol/L (>18 mg/dL) despite appropriate fluid resuscitation without the use of vasopressor drugs. This combination is associated with hospital mortality rates in excess of 40%.

MANAGEMENT

Figure 72.1 describes the principles of screening, assessment, and management of a septic patient. The key immediate interventions and investigations that increase survival are termed the 'Sepsis Six' [4]. This package of measures has been shown to be associated with a significant reduction in mortality when applied within the first hour

Table 72.3 ABCDE assessment of patient with suspected sepsis, and associated red flags.

	Examination	Red flags
Airway	Ask patient to speak	Conscious level so reduced that airway threatened (immediate support needed)
Breathing	Count respiratory rate Listen to breath sounds Check oxygen saturation	Respiratory rate ≥25/minute Oxygen saturation <92% (or <88% in patients with hypercapnic respiratory failure)
Circulation	Capillary refill Radial pulse (character and volume) Jugular venous pressure Heart sounds	Heart rate ≥130 bpm Systolic blood pressure ≤90 mmHg or a significant drop in systolic blood pressure from the patient's baseline
Disability	ACVPU assessment: Is the patient alert? Are they newly confused, responsive to voice, pain, or are they unresponsive? Able to move all limbs? Any localising signs?	Acute confusional state Decreased responsiveness
Exposure	Appearance: wounds, rashes Capillary blood glucose measurement Urine output Past medical history that may predispose to infection?	Non-blanching rash Not passed urine in last 18 hours Recent chemotherapy Patients that are on immunosuppressants or are immunodeficient

Source: adapted from UK Sepsis Trust [4].

[10]. The Sepsis Six consists of (i) administering oxygen; (ii) taking blood cultures and considering infective sources; (iii) giving intravenous antibiotics; (iv) giving intravenous fluids; (v) checking serial lactates (a surrogate marker of tissue perfusion); and (vi) measuring urine output.

It will almost certainly not be possible to implement fully the Sepsis Six in a mental health setting. If sepsis is suspected, it is essential that the patient is transferred promptly to emergency services.

POST-SEPSIS SYNDROME

The multiple physical, emotional, and psychological symptoms that can occur as a consequence of sepsis can be severely debilitating and are termed 'post-sepsis syndrome'. They can manifest as one or more of [2]:

- anxiety/fear of sepsis recurring
- depression
- flashbacks
- nightmares
- insomnia (due to stress or anxiety)
- post-traumatic stress disorder
- poor concentration
- short-term memory loss
- mood swings.

CHAPTER 72

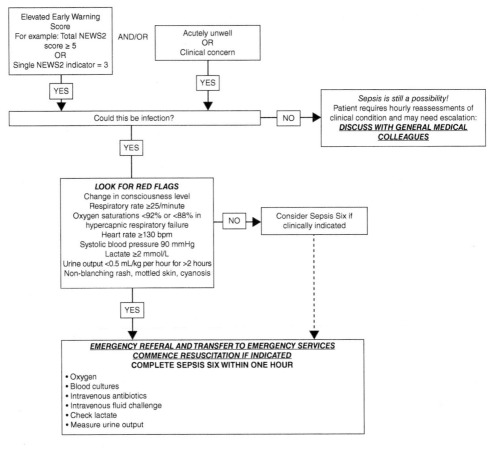

Figure 72.1 Sepsis screening and treatment.

References

1. Seymour CW, Liu VX, Iwashyna TJ, et al. Assessment of clinical criteria for sepsis: For the Third International Consensus Definitions for Sepsis and Septic Shock (Sepsis-3). *JAMA* 2016;315(8):762–774.
2. Levy MM, Evans LE, Rhodes A. The Surviving Sepsis Campaign Bundle: 2018 Update. *Crit Care Med* 2018;46(6):997–1000.
3. National Confidential Enquiry into Patient Outcome and Death. Sepsis: Just Say Sepsis! https://www.ncepod.org.uk/2015sepsis.html (accessed 22 April 2019).
4. UK Sepsis Trust. https://sepsistrust.org/ (accessed 22 April 2019).
5. O'Brien JM, Lu B, Ali NA, et al. Alcohol dependence is independently associated with sepsis, septic shock, and hospital mortality among adult intensive care unit patients. *Crit Care Med* 2006;35(2):345–350.
6. De Backer D, Dorman T. Surviving sepsis guidelines: a continuous move toward better care of patients with sepsis. *JAMA* 2017;317(8):807–808.
7. Lo RSL, Leung LY, Brabrand M, et al. qSOFA is a poor predictor of short-term mortality in all patients: a systematic review of 410,000 patients. *J Clin Med* 2019;8(1):61.
8. Royal College of Physicians. National Early Warning Score (NEWS) 2. https://www.rcplondon.ac.uk/projects/outputs/national-early-warning-score-news-2 (accessed 22 April 2019).
9. Singer M, Deutschman CS, Seymour CW, et al. The Third International Consensus Definitions for Sepsis and Septic Shock (Sepsis-3). *JAMA* 2016;315(8):801–810.
10. Rivers E, Nguyen B, Havstad S, et al. Early goal-directed therapy in the treatment of severe sepsis and septic shock. *N Engl J Med* 2001;345(19):1368–1377.

Acute Kidney Injury

Phillipa Brothwood, Toby Pillinger, Anne Connolly,
Peter Conlon

Acute kidney injury (AKI) is a rapid reduction in renal function that manifests as a rise in serum creatinine and/or a fall in urine output [1]. If untreated, AKI can have potentially life-threatening consequences, such as volume overload, hyperkalaemia, and metabolic acidosis. It is associated with prolonged general medical hospital admissions and increased social and healthcare costs [2].

It is estimated that approximately one in five adult general medical patients have AKI [3,4]. The incidence of AKI in patients with severe mental illness (SMI) is not clearly defined. However, psychiatric patients represent a vulnerable cohort for AKI by virtue of several risk factors. These include the risk of dehydration (in association with self-neglect in severe depression, catatonia, stupor, negative symptoms of schizophrenia, and reduced oral intake in eating disorders), excessive use of laxatives in eating disorders, self-harm attempts involving nephrotoxic drugs, and rhabdomyolysis secondary to restraint, neuroleptic malignant syndrome (see Chapter 85), or serotonin syndrome (see Chapter 86). Furthermore, compared with the general population, patients with SMI are more likely to have chronic kidney disease (CKD; see Chapter 34), itself a risk factor for AKI [5]. AKI can also be associated with neuropsychiatric presentations such as delirium (see Chapter 50) and, in severe cases, uraemic encephalopathy.

CATEGORISATION OF ACUTE KIDNEY INJURY

Causes of AKI can be divided into three groups (Box 73.1): pre-renal (40–80% of cases, secondary to reduced renal perfusion), renal (35–40% of cases, secondary to intrinsic renal disease), and post-renal (2–10% of cases, secondary to urinary outflow

The Maudsley Practice Guidelines for Physical Health Conditions in Psychiatry, First Edition.
David M. Taylor, Fiona Gaughran, and Toby Pillinger.
© 2021 John Wiley & Sons Ltd. Published 2021 by John Wiley & Sons Ltd.

Box 73.1 Causes of acute kidney injury

Pre-renal

Hypovolaemia

- Haemorrhage
- Gastrointestinal losses (e.g. vomiting, diarrhoea)
- Urinary losses (e.g. glycosuria, post-obstructive diuresis, diuretics)
- Cutaneous losses (e.g. burns)
- Fluid redistribution (e.g. gastrointestinal obstruction, pancreatitis)

Hypotension

- Cardiogenic shock
- Distributive shock (e.g. sepsis, anaphylaxis)

Renal hypoperfusion

- Reduced renal perfusion plus impaired autoregulation (e.g. hypovolaemia plus ACE inhibitor use)
- Renal artery stenosis or occlusion
- Hepatorenal syndrome

Oedema states

- Cardiac failure
- Hepatic cirrhosis
- Nephrotic syndrome

Renal

Glomerular disease

- Inflammatory (e.g. post-infectious glomerulonephritis, systemic lupus erythematosus, ANCA-associated glomerulonephritis, anti-GBM disease)
- Thrombotic (e.g. disseminated intravascular coagulation)

Tubular injury

- Ischaemia: prolonged renal hypoperfusion
- Toxins: drugs (e.g. aminoglycosides), radiocontrast, pigments (e.g. myoglobin), heavy metals (e.g. cisplatinum)
- Metabolic: hypercalcaemia, immunoglobulin light chains, myeloma
- Crystals (e.g. urate, oxalate)

Interstitial nephritis

- Drug-induced (e.g. NSAIDs, antibiotics, proton pump inhibitors)
- Infiltrative (e.g. lymphoma)

- Granulomatous: sarcoidosis, tuberculosis
- Infection-related (e.g. post-infective, pyelonephritis)

Vascular

- Vasculitis (usually ANCA associated)
- Cryoglobulinaemia
- Polyarteritis nodosa
- Thrombotic microangiopathy
- Cholesterol emboli
- Renal artery or renal vein thrombosis

Post-renal

Intrinsic

- Intraluminal (e.g. blood clot, stone)
- Intramural (e.g. urethral stricture, prostatic hypertrophy/malignancy, bladder tumour)
- Radiation fibrosis

Extrinsic

- Pelvic malignancy
- Retroperitoneal fibrosis

ACE, angiotensin-converting enzyme; ANCA, antineutrophil cytoplasmic antibodies; GBM, glomerular basement membrane; NSAID, non-steroidal anti-inflammatory drug.

Table 73.1 Simplified version of the Kidney Disease: Improving Global Outcomes (KDIGO) staging system for acute kidney injury [1].

Stage	Serum creatinine rise	Urine output
1	≥1.5× baseline level presumed to have occurred in the last 7 days, *or* >26 µmol/L (0.29 mg/dL) in 48 hours	<0.5 mL/kg per hour for 6–12 hours
2	≥2× baseline level	<0.5 mL/kg per hour for >12 hours
3	≥3× baseline level, *or* ≥1.5× baseline level to >354 µmol/L (4 mg/dL)	<0.3 mL/kg per hour for >24 hours or anuria for 12 hours

obstruction). Most cases of AKI are the result of infection, hypovolaemia, hypotension, or medication effects. Severity of AKI can be classified into three stages (Table 73.1) which may be used to guide management. For example, stage 3 AKI should prompt an urgent medical review.

DIAGNOSTIC PRINCIPLES

AKI is often asymptomatic and most commonly identified on routine blood tests. AKI may herald a life-threatening emergency (e.g. sepsis). Where such a presentation is suspected, the patient should be managed according to the ABCDE approach and immediate transfer to emergency medical services arranged. However, where a patient is medically stable, the following sections on history and examination will guide the investigations and management that may be performed in a psychiatric setting, according to staff experience and local facilities.

History

Promptly determining whether a blood test result represents a true acute deterioration in kidney function or is simply representative of CKD saves time and resources through avoidance of unnecessary investigations. As such, it is recommended that previous blood test results are checked early. Where AKI is suspected, a history should cover the following.

Presenting complaint

- Adequate fluid intake.
- Recent diarrhoea/vomiting or use of purging agents.
- Any recent symptoms that may suggest an underlying obstructive cause (e.g. lower urinary tract symptoms, bloating from a pelvic mass, haematuria).
- Abdominal pain (gastrointestinal obstruction, pancreatitis, aortic aneurysm).
- Possibility of rhabdomyolysis. In an inpatient, consider if there has been recent restraint, or screen for features of neuroleptic malignant syndrome/serotonin syndrome (see Chapters 85 and 86).
- Any features of drug toxicity if concerns regarding drug accumulation (e.g. tremor in context of raised plasma lithium levels).

Past medical history

- Chronic kidney disease.
- Risk factors for chronic kidney disease (see Chapter 34).
- Presence of rheumatological disease.
- History of tuberculosis infection (see Chapter 44).
- Liver disease.
- History of any pathology affecting the urinary tract (e.g. prostatic hypertrophy).

Drug history

- Scrutinise medication lists for agents associated with AKI (Box 73.2). Polypharmacy is also a risk for AKI [6].
- The reader is directed to the latest edition of the *Maudsley Prescribing Guidelines in Psychiatry* for a comprehensive description of the risk of kidney injury with individual

---

Box 73.2 Drugs commonly implicated in acute kidney injury [6]

- Antibiotics and antivirals
- Angiotensin-converting enzyme inhibitors
- Angiotensin receptor blockers
- Non-steroidal anti-inflammatory drugs
- Antineoplastic agents
- Contrast agents (used in hospital for imaging)
- Diuretics

---

psychotropic agents [7]. Some antipsychotics may be associated with AKI, potentially via their effects on blood pressure and urinary retention, although studies are conflicting [8,9]. Antidepressants are unlikely to cause AKI, with only isolated reports of AKI with certain agents. In terms of mood stabilisers, lithium is generally associated with chronic rather than acute kidney disease (see Chapter 34), while there are isolated reports of AKI with carbamazepine, lamotrigine, and sodium valproate. Any agent that has the potential to cause rhabdomyolysis (e.g. via neuroleptic malignant syndrome or serotonin syndrome) will, by association, have the potential to cause AKI.

- The reader should also be aware that many drugs and their active metabolites [10] can accumulate in renal impairment. Psychiatric medications to be particularly concerned about owing to their almost total renal excretion are lithium, amisulpride, and sulpiride.

Examination

Check basic physical observations, including blood pressure, heart rate, respiratory rate, oxygen saturation, and temperature.

A general physical examination, including cardiac, respiratory, and abdominal examination, may provide insight into the underlying cause of AKI, and will be helpful when making a referral to medical colleagues. Particular attention should be paid to the patient's volume status. Evidence of dehydration (dry mucous membranes, reduced skin turgor, low urine output, hypotension, tachycardia) may suggest a pre-renal cause of AKI requiring fluid resuscitation, while evidence of fluid overload (peripheral oedema, crackles on chest auscultation, raised jugular venous pressure) may suggest heart failure/cirrhosis/nephrotic syndrome. A typical 'drug rash' may indicate drug-induced AKI. Abdominal examination may demonstrate a palpable bladder in cases of urinary retention.

Investigations

In a psychiatric setting, and where the patient appears clinically stable, the following investigations may be performed in the context of evolving AKI:

- urea, electrolytes, and creatinine; note potassium levels (see Chapter 33)
- where appropriate, check lithium levels

- creatine kinase (if rhabdomyolysis, neuroleptic malignant syndrome, or serotonin syndrome suspected)
- full blood count (infection)
- C-reactive protein (infection)
- urine dipstick for blood and/or protein (renal inflammatory process)
- ECG (evidence of hyperkalaemia).

Investigations that may be performed by general medical colleagues may include an arterial blood gas, urine microscopy for cells, casts, and crystals, serum immunoglobulins, serum protein electrophoresis, urinary Bence Jones proteins, blood film, coagulation profile, autoimmune screen, and an ultrasound scan of the kidneys, ureters, and bladder.

MANAGEMENT

The mainstay of treatment of AKI is supportive care with management of the underlying cause and correction of any electrolyte and volume abnormalities. This will require general medical input; however, immediate general medical admission or referral to hospital from a community setting is not always needed [11] 'Red flag' features suggesting that a patient should be urgently referred to medical services are listed in Box 73.3. When in doubt, discuss the case with general medical/renal colleagues, detailing the history, examination, and investigation findings previously described.

PSYCHIATRIC MEDICATION AND ACUTE KIDNEY INJURY

Psychiatric medication may be responsible for kidney injury and/or may accumulate in the context of kidney injury. Except for lithium, amisulpride, and sulpiride, most antipsychotics, mood stabilisers, and antidepressants are well tolerated in kidney disease. Therefore, as a rule, stopping lithium, amisulpride, and sulpiride should be strongly

---

Box 73.3 Red flags that should prompt consideration of referral to medical colleagues [11]

- Stage 3 acute kidney injury (see Table 73.1)
- An underlying cause that requires urgent secondary care management, such as when an obstructed infected kidney is suspected
- No identifiable cause for acute kidney injury
- A risk of urinary tract obstruction, for example known prostate or bladder disease; abdominal or pelvic cancer; known previous hydronephrosis; recurrent urinary tract infections; or other conditions consistent with possible obstruction, for example anuria, single functioning kidney, neurogenic bladder
- Sepsis
- Evidence of hypovolaemia and need for intravenous fluid replacement and monitoring
- A deterioration in clinical condition or a need for observation or monitoring of a frequency which is impractical in primary care
- A complication of acute kidney injury requiring urgent secondary care management, such as pulmonary oedema, uraemic encephalopathy or pericarditis, or severe hyperkalaemia

considered in AKI (regardless of the aetiology), while decisions to continue other psychiatric medications should be made on a case-by-case basis. Decisions should weigh up the risks and benefits, be informed by the likely cause of AKI and drug plasma levels, and involve a multidisciplinary discussion between the psychiatrist, renal physician, and pharmacist.

References

1. Khwaja A. KDIGO clinical practice guidelines for acute kidney injury. *Nephron Clin Pract* 2012;120(4):c179–c184.
2. Silver SA, Chertow GM. The economic consequences of acute kidney injury. *Nephron* 2017;137(4):297–301.
3. Hoste EAJ, Kellum JA, Selby NM, et al. Global epidemiology and outcomes of acute kidney injury. *Nat Rev Nephrol* 2018;14(10):607–625.
4. Susantitaphong P, Cruz DN, Cerda J, et al. World incidence of AKI: a meta-analysis. *Clin J Am Soc Nephrol* 2013;8(9):1482–1493.
5. Hsu RK, Hsu CY. The role of acute kidney injury in chronic kidney disease. *Semin Nephrol* 2016;36(4):283–292.
6. Pierson-Marchandise M, Gras V, Moragny J, et al. The drugs that mostly frequently induce acute kidney injury: a case–noncase study of a pharmacovigilance database. *Br J Clin Pharmacol* 2017;83(6):1341–1349.
7. Taylor DM, Barnes TRE, Young AH. *The Maudsley Prescribing Guidelines in Psychiatry*, 13th edn. Chichester: Wiley Blackwell, 2018.
8. Jiang Y, McCombs JS, Park SH. A retrospective cohort study of acute kidney injury risk associated with antipsychotics. *CNS Drugs* 2017;31(4):319–326.
9. Ryan PB, Schuemie MJ, Ramcharran D, Stang PE. Atypical antipsychotics and the risks of acute kidney injury and related outcomes among older adults: a replication analysis and an evaluation of adapted confounding control strategies. *Drugs Aging* 2017;34(3):211–219.
10. Nagler EV, Webster AC, Vanholder R, Zoccali C. Antidepressants for depression in stage 3–5 chronic kidney disease: a systematic review of pharmacokinetics, efficacy and safety with recommendations by European Renal Best Practice (ERBP). *Nephrol Dial Transplant* 2012;27(10):3736–3745.
11. National Institute for Health and Care Excellence. Acute kidney injury. Clinical Knowledge Summary. Last revised: April 2018. https://cks.nice.org.uk/acute-kidney-injury#!topicSummary

Diabetic Emergencies

Toby Pillinger, Yuya Mizuno, Sophie Harris

Diabetic emergencies can be categorised simply into scenarios involving either very low or very high blood sugars. This chapter focuses on the acute management of hypoglycaemia, diabetic ketoacidosis, and hyperosmolar hyperglycaemic state. The guidance provided is for psychiatric practitioners, either in the outpatient or inpatient environment, who may not have immediate access to acute medical support.

HYPOGLYCAEMIA [1]

Hypoglycaemia is defined as glucose levels below 4 mmol/L (72 mg/dL). Hypoglycaemia may be accompanied by sweating, anxiety, aggression, tremor, nausea, tachycardia, blurred vision, and drowsiness. However, in people with diabetes and recurrent hypoglycaemia, these features may be absent.

In the acute setting, and if the patient is conscious, the patient should be provided with 15–20 g of oral glucose, either in liquid form or as granulated sugar/sugar lumps (approximately two to four teaspoons). If sugar is not available, consider using anything sugar-rich (e.g. jam, fruit juice, or sugar drink). On inpatient wards, proprietary products providing quick-acting carbohydrate may be available (e.g. GlucoGel, Glucotabs, Dextrosol, Dextrogel). Repeat blood glucose level after 15 minutes, and if persistently hypoglycaemic this process can be repeated up to three times. If persistently hypoglycaemic the patient will likely require transfer to a general medical setting. If initial treatment is successful, offer a snack providing sustained carbohydrate release such as a biscuit or sandwich.

Loss of consciousness in the context of hypoglycaemia is a medical emergency. The patient will require parenteral treatment that is unlikely to be available in a psychiatric setting and therefore the patient will require urgent transfer to emergency services.

Patients should be managed as per the ABCDE approach (see Chapter 78). If facilities are available, glucagon (1 mg subcutaneous or intramuscular injection) may be given. Alternatively, or if there has been no response to glucagon after 10 minutes, intravenous glucose infusion (10 or 20%) should be administered. This needs to be delivered via a large-gauge needle as the solution is an extreme irritant in the context of extravasation.

DIABETIC KETOACIDOSIS [2]

Diabetic ketoacidosis (DKA) is an acute metabolic complication of diabetes that is potentially fatal and requires prompt medical attention. It is the result of reduced insulin levels or reduced efficacy of insulin leading to hyperglycaemia, volume depletion, and electrolyte disturbance. Insulin deficiency and thence impaired glucose metabolism results in the body turning to metabolism of fat stores as a source of energy. This results in the formation of ketone bodies and acidosis. DKA may represent the first presentation of a patient with diabetes mellitus (typically but not always type 1) or may occur in patients with established diabetes mellitus who have either failed to adequately treat with insulin, or who have an intercurrent illness that disrupts insulin efficacy (e.g. infection, myocardial infarction, or stroke). Drugs can also precipitate DKA, including corticosteroids, thiazide diuretics, and some second-generation antipsychotics [3].

The main management goals in DKA are to resolve volume deficits, and normalise hyperglycaemia, acidosis, and electrolyte disturbance, e.g. hypokalaemia (as well as treating any precipitant). This will not be possible in a psychiatric setting, so the priority for psychiatric practitioners is for prompt identification of DKA and immediate transfer of the patient as an emergency to medical services.

In the general medical setting, DKA is defined by presence of diabetes with current or recent high blood glucose levels, ketosis (serum ketones >1.5 mmol/L, urine ketones >++), and acidosis (pH <7.35 +/– HCO_3^- <12 mmol/L). The tools at the psychiatric practitioner's disposal will be clinical examination, blood glucose monitoring, and potentially urinalysis to measure glucose and ketones.

Clinically, a patient with DKA may present with polyuria, polydipsia, weakness, nausea/vomiting, dry mucous membranes, tachycardia, hypotension, rapid and deep breathing (Kussmaul respiration, a response to metabolic acidosis), acetone 'pear drop' smelling breath (ketosis), and altered mental state (ranging from mild confusion to coma in severe cases). Examine for any precipitant that may also need urgent treatment, e.g. evolving sepsis or myocardial infarction (see Chapters 69 and 72).

Usually, marked hyperglycaemia is revealed by blood glucose levels in excess of 14 mmol/L (>250 mg/dL), although be aware that a small proportion (approximately 10%) of patients with DKA may present with lower blood glucose levels ('euglycaemic DKA') [4]. Be aware that in marked hyperglycaemia, blood sugar monitors may register an 'error' or 'HI': do not assume that the monitor is faulty. Urinalysis will usually test positive for both glucose and ketones (>++).

If there are concerns that a patient has developed DKA in the psychiatric setting, they should be managed according to the ABCDE approach and transferred as an emergency to medical services. In severe cases the patient may require admission to intensive care.

HYPEROSMOLAR HYPERGLYCAEMIC STATE [5]

Hyperosmolar hyperglycaemic state (HHS) is an acute metabolic complication of type 2 diabetes mellitus, typically in older people, characterised by extreme hyperglycaemia (glucose >33.3 mmol/L or >600 mg/dL), hyperosmolality, and volume depletion. Mortality is much higher than in DKA, estimated at between 5 and 20% [4]. HHS is the result of hyperglycaemia leading to diuresis and dehydration with residual low-level insulin production protecting from ketosis. Infection is most often the precipitant.

Management involves intravenous fluids, correction of electrolyte abnormalities, and insulin. This will not be possible in a psychiatric setting so, as with DKA, the priority for psychiatric practitioners is for prompt identification of HHS and immediate transfer of the patient as an emergency to medical services.

Clinically, patients are often confused (comatose in extreme cases), and may present with polyuria, polydipsia, weakness, nausea/vomiting, dry mucous membranes, tachycardia, hypotension, and seizures. Blood glucose testing will reveal extreme hyperglycaemia. Be aware that in marked hyperglycaemia, blood sugar monitors may register an 'error' or 'HI': do not assume that the monitor is faulty. Urinalysis will test positive for glucose, but usually not ketones.

If there are concerns that a patient has developed HHS in the psychiatric setting, they should be managed according to the ABCDE approach and transferred as an emergency to medical services. In severe cases the patient may require admission to intensive care.

References

1. National Institute for Health and Care Excellence. Treatment of hypoglycaemia. https://bnf.nice.org.uk/treatment-summary/hypoglycaemia.html

2. Joint British Diabetes Societies Inpatient Care Group. *The Management of Diabetic Ketoacidosis in Adults*, 2nd edn. Document JBDS 02. September 2013. Available at https://abcd.care/sites/abcd.care/files/resources/2013_09_JBDS_IP_DKA_Adults_Revised.pdf

3. Umpierrez G, Korytkowski M. Diabetic emergencies: ketoacidosis, hyperglycaemic hyperosmolar state and hypoglycaemia. *Nat Rev Endocrinol* 2016;12(4):222–232.

4. Kitabchi AE, Umpierrez GE, Murphy MB, Kreisberg RA. Hyperglycemic crises in adult patients with diabetes: a consensus statement from the American Diabetes Association. *Diabetes Care* 2006;29(12):2739–2748.

5. Joint British Diabetes Societies Inpatient Care Group. *The Management of the Hyperosmolar Hyperglycaemic State (HHS) in Adults with Diabetes*. Document JBDS 06. August 2012. Available at https://abcd.care/sites/abcd.care/files/resources/JBDS_IP_HHS_Adults.pdf

CHAPTER 74

Acute Upper Gastrointestinal Bleeding

Douglas Corrigall, David Dewar

If there is frank haematemesis and haemodynamic instability, do not delay transferring the patient to an acute medical setting with a resuscitation area. For psychiatric inpatients, this will involve calling the medical emergency team and likely an ambulance if the ward is not connected to a general medical hospital. In the outpatient department an ambulance should be called.

SIGNS OF ACUTE UPPER GASTROINTESTINAL BLEEDING

1 Haematemesis (vomiting fresh blood): frank haematemesis suggests moderate to severe bleed usually from stomach or oesophagus.
2 Coffee ground vomitus: altered blood from an upper gastrointestinal (GI) source that has been in the stomach for a period of time. Bleeding may still be ongoing.
   Melaena (blood altered by passage through the GI tract):
   a characteristic sickly-sweet smell
   b present in 70% of upper GI bleeds
   c black tarry stool indicates at least 50 mL of blood loss
   d generally means blood has been in GI tract for eight hours or more
   e oral iron supplementation causes tarry black stool, so beware.
3 Haematochezia (frank blood per rectum): can represent upper GI bleed.

WAITING FOR TRANSFER

If possible and facilities allow, carry out the following.

1 Ensure airway patent and secure.
2 Ensure regular observations.

The Maudsley Practice Guidelines for Physical Health Conditions in Psychiatry, First Edition.
David M. Taylor, Fiona Gaughran, and Toby Pillinger.
© 2021 John Wiley & Sons Ltd. Published 2021 by John Wiley & Sons Ltd.

3 Gain intravenous access with two large-bore cannulae and take bloods for full blood count, urea and electrolytes, clotting, liver function tests, blood cultures and cross-match at least four units.
4 If blood pressure is low, fluid resuscitation should be commenced (e.g. normal saline 0.9%) while rapid transfer is arranged.
5 Ensure nil by mouth.

HANDING OVER TO THE ACUTE MEDICAL TEAM

Make sure that someone stays with the patient at all times in case they deteriorate further. Salient information to pass on to the medical/gastroenterology team includes the following.

1 Immediate handover: 'This patient is having an acute upper GI bleed and requires immediate transfer as we cannot manage them safely in this environment.'
2 Current state of patient (airway, breathing, circulation), what treatments they are currently receiving, and results of any recent investigations.
3 Past medical history, in particular any history of previous gastric ulcers, gastritis, GI bleeds, or liver disease.
4 Drug history including allergies. In particular, state if the patient on non-steroidal anti-inflammatory drugs (NSAIDs) or anticoagulants such as warfarin.
5 Psychiatric history, risk assessment, and what level of psychiatric nursing may be required.
6 When the patient last ate.

Status Epilepticus

Emanuele F. Osimo, Brian Sweeney

Status epilepticus is defined as a single epileptic seizure that lasts more than five minutes, or if more than one seizure occurs in the space of five minutes without recovery. A psychiatric setting is an inappropriate environment in which to manage such patients, and therefore *immediate transfer* of the patient to emergency services should be arranged.

The following approach is recommended for management of a patient experiencing a seizure in a psychiatric setting.

1 Apply an ABCDE approach. Assess cardiorespiratory function: ensure the airway is patent and secure. If available, provide high-flow oxygen. Remove any nearby objects that could cause injury and cushion head. If possible, gain intravenous access (which will facilitate intravenous antiepileptic treatment by medical colleagues).
2 Check blood glucose and treat if low (see Chapter 74).
3 Deliver diazepam 10–20 mg rectally or midazolam 10 mg buccally, or if intravenous access is established and resuscitation facilities are available, 4 mg intravenous lorazepam (rate not critical). This may be repeated after 15 minutes.
4 Check the time of seizure onset. If the seizure lasts longer than five minutes, emergency transfer to medical services is indicated.
5 Ensure regular observations and that someone stays with the patient at all times.

Salient information to provide the medical team on handover is as follows.

1 Immediate handover: 'This patient is experiencing a seizure and requires immediate transfer as we cannot manage them safely in this environment'.
2 Current state of the patient: airway, breathing, circulation, latest set of observations, blood glucose.

The Maudsley Practice Guidelines for Physical Health Conditions in Psychiatry, First Edition.
David M. Taylor, Fiona Gaughran, and Toby Pillinger.
© 2021 John Wiley & Sons Ltd. Published 2021 by John Wiley & Sons Ltd.

3 What treatment you have instigated (e.g. rectal diazepam) and the patient's response, if any.
4 Past medical history, including if there is a history of epilepsy or other seizure activity, and if alcohol abuse or impaired nutrition is suspected.
5 Drug history including any allergies.
6 Psychiatric history, risk assessment, and the level of psychiatric nursing that will be required.

Anaphylaxis

James Kelly, Immo Weichert

An anaphylactic reaction can be considered as any allergic reaction which is rapid in onset, triggers a systemic response caused by release of immune and inflammatory mediators from basophils and mast cells, and may cause death. The onset is usually within minutes of exposure, although it may be delayed for several hours depending on route of exposure, quantity of antigen, and rate of administration. Common triggers include, but are not limited to, foods (including nuts, milk, fish, shellfish, eggs and some fruits), medications such as antibiotics and non-steroidal anti-inflammatory drugs (NSAIDs), insect stings (particularly wasp and bee stings), contrast agents, and latex. An algorithm for its emergency management is presented in Figure 77.1. A differential diagnosis for anaphylaxis is angioedema, described further in Box 77.1.

Anaphylaxis is likely when all the following criteria are met:

- sudden onset and rapid progression of symptoms
- life-threatening airway, breathing and/or circulatory problems
- skin and/or mucosal changes (rashes, angioedema).

Exposure of the patient to a known allergen supports the diagnosis.

Skin or mucosal changes alone are not a sign of an anaphylactic reaction. They can be subtle or absent in up to 20% of patients. There can also be gastrointestinal symptoms such as vomiting, abdominal pain, and incontinence.

MANAGEMENT

Call for emergency support for anyone suspected of developing anaphylaxis. Unless attached to a general medical hospital, in a psychiatric setting this will involve calling an ambulance.

The Maudsley Practice Guidelines for Physical Health Conditions in Psychiatry, First Edition.
David M. Taylor, Fiona Gaughran, and Toby Pillinger.
© 2021 John Wiley & Sons Ltd. Published 2021 by John Wiley & Sons Ltd.

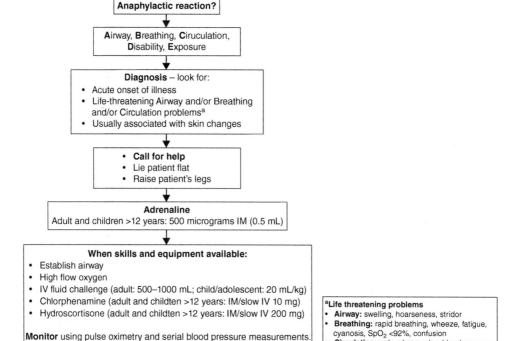

Figure 77.1 Management of anaphylaxis in adults. Source: Resuscitation Guidelines, 2015 (https://www.resus.org.uk/resuscitation-guidelines/). Reproduced with kind permission of the Resuscitation Council (UK).

Box 77.1 Angioedema: its differentiation from anaphylaxis and management

■ Angioedema describes oedema of subcutaneous and mucosal tissue (typically face, mouth, and upper airway) in the absence of urticaria or pruritis. It is an important differential diagnosis since management is different from that of anaphylaxis.
■ Angioedema should be suspected where there is an absence of multisystem involvement, where there is no known or suspected causative allergen, where there is a personal or family history of angioedema, or if the patient is prescribed an angiotensin-converting enzyme (ACE) inhibitor (a common precipitant of angioedema).
■ Emergency management of angioedema involves an ABCDE approach.
■ Causative agents such as ACE inhibitors should be discontinued (angioedema caused by these drugs should resolve within 72 hours).
■ Specific treatments that may be available in accident and emergency or general medical settings include complement C1 esterase inhibitor, icatibant, and ecallantide.

   This section details an approach to management of anaphylaxis while awaiting emergency support. The extent to which these actions may be carried out will depend on the clinician's experience and the facilities available in a given psychiatric setting.

Acute

- Stop any ongoing precipitants (e.g. disconnect intravenous infusions, remove the stinger following a bee sting).
- Secure airway and give high-flow oxygen.
- Give adrenaline 1 in 1000 0.5 mL (500 μg) intramuscularly.
  - Repeat adrenaline after five to ten minutes if there is no clinical improvement.
  - Note that patients taking tricyclic antidepressants or monoamine oxidase inhibitors may have an exaggerated response to adrenaline [1].
  - Adrenaline may be ineffective in treating anaphylaxis in patients on beta-blockers. In such cases, and where facilities allow, administration of glucagon (1–5 mg intravenously over five minutes followed by an infusion at 5–15 mg/min titrated to clinical response) may be necessary [2].
- Give chlorphenamine 10 mg intramuscularly or slowly intravenously.
- Give hydrocortisone 200 mg intramuscularly or slowly intravenously.
- If clinical manifestations of shock do not respond quickly to pharmacological treatment, give 0.5–1 L of intravenous fluids (crystalloid) rapidly.
- Salbutamol (5 mg given via oxygen-driven nebuliser) may be helpful if bronchospasm is severe and slow to respond to treatment.

Following symptomatic resolution

- All patients should be observed in a general medical setting with access to resuscitation facilities for six to eight hours. Thus, even if a patient recovers from an acute anaphylactic reaction, they should still be transported to a general medical setting, or at least discussed with general medical colleagues.
  - 'Biphasic' or late reactions occur in up to 21% of patients, typically within 12 hours after resolution of the first event (although recurrence up to 72 hours following resolution has been reported) [3].
  - Antihistamines and steroids in the initial anaphylactic phase may reduce risk of a biphasic reaction.
- Where a diagnosis of anaphylaxis is uncertain, medical colleagues may take timed blood samples for mast cell tryptase levels. Serial levels are taken as follows.
  - As soon as possible after emergency treatment.
  - Within one to two hours, and no later than four hours from the onset of symptoms.
  - Again at 24 hours or during convalescence (to obtain a 'baseline').
  - Elevated mast cell tryptase confirms an allergic reaction and will support the rationale for allergy testing where the precipitant is unclear.
- All patients presenting with anaphylaxis should be referred to an allergy clinic. In the UK, a list of specialist allergy clinics is provided by the website of the British Society for Allergy and Clinical Immunology [4]. Where angiotensin-converting enzyme (ACE) inhibitor-mediated angioedema is suspected, discontinue treatment and consider alternative treatments as part of a multidisciplinary approach (see Box 77.1).
- Patients with a risk of recurrence of anaphylaxis in future are often discharged from medical inpatient care with the recommendation to carry an adrenaline (epinephrine)

autoinjector. These patients must not be prescribed beta-blockers (e.g. propranolol, bisoprolol, atenolol).

- If a trigger for the anaphylactic reaction has been identified, ensure that this is documented in the relevant section of the patient's prescription sheet, case record, and in any transfer or discharge documentation.

References

1. McLean-Tooke AP, Bethune CA, Fay AC, Spickett GP. Adrenaline in the treatment of anaphylaxis: what is the evidence? *BMJ* 2003;327(7427):1332–1335.
2. Lieberman P, Nicklas RA, Randolph C, et al. Anaphylaxis: a practice parameter update 2015. *Ann Allergy Asthma Immunol* 2015;115(5):341–384.
3. Lee S, Bellolio MF, Hess EP, et al. Time of onset and predictors of biphasic anaphylactic reactions: a systematic review and meta-analysis. *J Allergy Clin Immunol Pract* 2015;3(3):408–416.e1-2.
4. British Society for Allergy and Clinical Immunology. https://www.bsaci.org/ (accessed 8 November 2019).

Reduced Consciousness and Coma

James Kelly, Immo Weichert

Coma is a state from which patients cannot be roused, and is defined as a Glasgow Coma Scale (GCS) [1] score of 8 or below (Table 78.1), or as U on the AVPU scale (Box 78.1) [2]. Any patient presenting with a decreased level of consciousness (GCS <15) mandates further assessment. A psychiatric setting is almost always an inappropriate environment in which to manage a patient with significantly reduced consciousness. Pragmatic management should aim to (i) maintain a patient's airway and support breathing; (ii) identify reversible causes that may be treated acutely and in a psychiatric setting (e.g. hypoglycaemia or opiate overdose); (iii) facilitate transfer to emergency medical services; and (iv) gather evidence that may aid emergency services in determining the underlying cause.

CLINICAL APPROACH

An algorithm for managing a patient with reduced consciousness in a psychiatric setting is presented in Figure 78.1. The priority should be emergency assessment and management using an ABCDE approach and seeking help from emergency medical services.

History

There is a myriad of causes of reduced consciousness and coma (Box 78.2). Collateral history to determine the aetiology of reduced consciousness should be sought from as wide a range of sources as are available, e.g. carers, family members, or ward nurses if occurring in an inpatient setting. If available, patient notes should be reviewed. History should aim to cover details of any predisposing event (e.g. recent head trauma, pyrexia

The Maudsley Practice Guidelines for Physical Health Conditions in Psychiatry, First Edition.
David M. Taylor, Fiona Gaughran, and Toby Pillinger.
© 2021 John Wiley & Sons Ltd. Published 2021 by John Wiley & Sons Ltd.

Table 78.1 Glasgow Coma Scale [1].

Eye opening	Spontaneous	4
	To sound	3
	To pressure	2
	None	1
Verbal response	Orientated	5
	Confused	4
	Words	3
	Sounds	2
	None	1
Motor response	Obeys commands	6
	Localises to pain	5
	Normal flexion	4
	Abnormal flexion	3
	Extension	2
	None	1

Box 78.1 AVPU scale [3]

A Alert
V Responds to voice
P Responds to painful stimulus
U Unresponsive

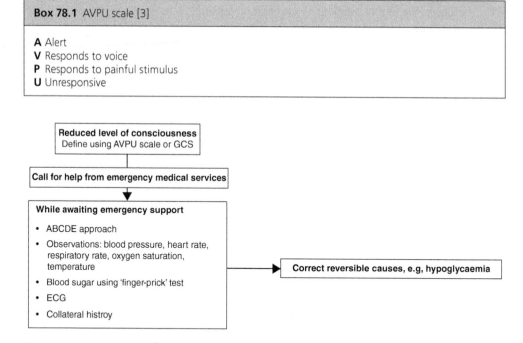

Figure 78.1 Algorithm for approach to a patient with reduced level of consciousness in the psychiatric setting.

or other features of infection), the presence of any prodromal symptoms (e.g. headache, neck stiffness, seizure), a history of previous similar episodes, and past medical history (e.g. diabetes mellitus, epilepsy, known cardiovascular disease), medication history, and psychiatric history.

> **Box 78.2** Common causes of reduced consciousness and coma
>
> - Toxins/drugs in overdose, e.g. alcohol, hypnotics, psychotropics, anticholinergics, lithium, salicylate
> - Metabolic, e.g. hypoglycaemia/hyperglycaemia, hypoxia, hypercapnia, acidosis, electrolyte disturbance, hypothyroidism, Addisonian crisis
> - Infection, e.g. sepsis, meningitis, encephalitis
> - Neurological, e.g. head trauma, status epilepticus, stroke
> - Cardiac, e.g. arrhythmia, acute coronary syndrome

Assessment

- Assess level of consciousness using the AVPU scale or GCS. To assess motor response using the GCS, apply a painful stimulus to a central part of the body, for instance trapezius squeezing or a sternal rub.
- A set of observations should be performed as part of the ABCDE approach, including blood pressure, heart rate, oxygen saturations, respiratory rate, and temperature. Also check for Medic Alert-type jewellery that may detail a patient's primary health risk (e.g. diabetes mellitus, anaphylaxis, Addison's disease).
- Check blood glucose early using a finger-prick test. Correct hypoglycaemia (see Chapter 74).
- Any patient with a decreased level of consciousness should be assumed to have a compromised airway. The airway should be opened with a chin lift or jaw thrust and any vomit cleared from the mouth, either by tilting the head or if equipment is available using suction. A nasopharyngeal airway may be useful in unconscious patients to prevent further airway obstruction.
- High-flow oxygen should be administered, and saturations monitored by pulse oximetry, as well as respiratory rate. In the context of opioid overdose and a resultant respiratory rate below 10 breaths per minute, administer naloxone. Advice regarding dosing of naloxone is provided in Chapter 83, which also addresses the circumstance where flumazenil may be considered, noting that in most cases of reduced consciousness the risks of flumazenil outweigh the benefits.
- If hypotension is noted, elevate the legs of the patient and, if facilities allow, gain intravenous access and administer fluids (500–1000 mL crystalloid). As part of circulatory assessment, aim to perform an ECG to assess for acute coronary syndrome or arrhythmia and treat as appropriate (see Chapters 69 andd 70 respectively).
- Basic examination may provide further insight into the underlying aetiology. As such, aim to examine the following.

- Evidence of head injury (see Chapter 80).
- If no risk of recent cervical spine injury, assess for neck stiffness (see Chapter 81).
- Assess pupils by holding both eyelids open and shining a light into the eyes: evidence of pinpoint pupils (see Chapter 83), pupils equal and reactive to light.
- Assess for evidence of lateralising signs on neurological examination (i.e. asymmetrical motor signs) that may point towards a structural brain lesion (e.g. stroke; see Chapter 82). Metabolic or toxic lesions will usually result in a drop in GCS score

> **Box 78.3** Indications for brain imaging in patients with a suspected head injury
>
> - GCS <13 on initial assessment
> - Suspected open or depressed skull fracture
> - Suspicion of basal skull fracture
> - Post-traumatic seizure
> - Focal neurological deficit
> - More than one episode of vomiting
> - Coagulopathy and any amnesia/loss of consciousness

without lateralising signs and are more likely in the presence of involuntary limb movements and a fluctuation in level of consciousness.
- Assess for evidence of ongoing seizure activity (see Chapter 76). This may be as subtle as eyelid flickering.

Information to provide emergency services

- Immediate handover: 'This patient is unconscious/has a reduced level of consciousness and we cannot manage them safely in this environment'.
- Current state of the patient (GCS, airway, breathing, circulation, latest set of observations, blood glucose).
- What treatment you have instigated and the patient's response, if any.
- Past medical history.
- Drug history including any allergies.
- Psychiatric history, risk assessment, and the level of psychiatric nursing that may be required. Is the patient detained under the Mental Health Act?

Ongoing care by emergency services

- Once under the care of emergency services, further investigations and management will depend on the underlying aetiology.
- Additional tests that may be performed include an arterial blood gas and brain imaging (indications for CT head in patients with a suspected head injury are documented in Box 78.3).
- Blood tests should include, but are not limited to, full blood count, coagulation screen, urea and electrolytes, liver function tests, C-reactive protein, serum toxicology, and a pregnancy test.
- If alcoholism or malnutrition are suspected, thiamine should be administered to prevent development of Wernicke's encephalopathy (see Chapter 24).
- Endotracheal intubation may be considered if GCS score is below 8.

References

1. Teasdale G, Jennett B. Assessment of coma and impaired consciousness. A practical scale. *Lancet* 1974;2(7872):81–84.
2. McNarry AF, Goldhill DR. Simple bedside assessment of level of consciousness: comparison of two simple assessment scales with the Glasgow Coma scale. *Anaesthesia* 2004;59(1):34–37.
3. Romanelli D, Farrell MW. AVPU (Alert, Voice, Pain, Unresponsive). *StatPearls*. Treasure Island, FL: StatPearls Publishing, 2019.

Thyroid Emergencies

Harriet Quigley, Jackie Gilbert

Thyroid emergencies may arise from either extreme deficiency (myxoedema coma or hypothyroid crisis) or excess (thyroid storm) of thyroid hormones, resulting in decompensation and multiorgan dysfunction.

HYPOTHYROID CRISIS/MYXOEDEMA COMA

Myxoedema coma is a manifestation of severe, long-standing, life-threatening and decompensated hypothyroidism. However, most patients with decompensated hypothyroidism are not comatose and therefore 'hypothyroid crisis' may be a more appropriate descriptor. Hypothyroid crisis occurs almost exclusively in patients over 60 years of age and is associated with a mortality rate of 25–60% [1]. Causative factors include precipitating comorbidity (such as stroke, infection, heart failure), prolonged non-compliance with thyroid hormone replacement medication, hypothermia, and use of medications such as sedatives, tranquillisers, and diuretics [2].

Diagnostic principles

The three key clinical features are altered mental status, hypothermia, and evidence of a precipitating event. Physical examination may reveal hypothermia, hypoventilation, hypotension, bradycardia, dry coarse skin, macroglossia, and delayed deep-tendon reflexes. Biochemical profile will usually demonstrate a low serum free T4 and elevated serum thyroid stimulating hormone (TSH). However, TSH may be normal in the context of central hypothyroidism or non-thyroidal illness. Patients may progress to stupor or coma and develop symptoms of multiple end-organ dysfunction.

The Maudsley Practice Guidelines for Physical Health Conditions in Psychiatry, First Edition.
David M. Taylor, Fiona Gaughran, and Toby Pillinger.
© 2021 John Wiley & Sons Ltd. Published 2021 by John Wiley & Sons Ltd.

Management

Myxoedema coma is a medical emergency and requires a multifaceted treatment approach in an intensive care unit (ICU) setting. Central to management is thyroid hormone replacement; intravenous levothyroxine is commonly used as gastrointestinal absorption may be impaired. Liothyronine (T3) may also be considered (as T4 to T3 conversion may be impaired), although this can cause cardiac arrhythmias. Supportive care includes correction of metabolic disturbances, patient warming if hypothermic, multiorgan support, and treatment of precipitating factors. Upon clinical improvement, T3 is discontinued and a daily oral T4 replacement dose is maintained. Intravenous hydrocortisone may also be required if there is concomitant adrenal insufficiency, which can be present in extreme hypothyroidism.

HYPERTHYROID CRISIS/THYROID STORM

Hyperthyroid crisis or thyroid storm is a severe manifestation of thyrotoxicosis due to over-production of thyroid hormones. The incidence of thyroid storm in Japan is 0.22% of all thyrotoxic patients [3]. It has a mortality rate of 10–20% if left untreated [4]. Hyperthyroid crises are most commonly seen in Graves' disease, though can occur in patients with a toxic adenoma or multinodular toxic goitre. Precipitants include infection or other intercurrent illness, non-compliance with antithyroid medication or overdose of thyroid hormone medication, trauma or emergency surgery, myocardial infarction, pulmonary embolism, and stroke [5].

Diagnostic principles

Thyrotoxicosis is a prerequisite for the diagnosis, with elevated levels of free T4 or free T3 and suppressed serum TSH. Clinical manifestations of thyroid storm include fever, tachycardia, tachyarrhythmias, congestive cardiac failure, nausea and vomiting, and impaired mental status. The clinical picture may overlap with signs of cocaine intoxication. Other features of decompensated homeostasis may include renal dysfunction, elevated creatine kinase, anaemia, thrombocytopenia, raised white cell count, abnormal liver function tests, hypercalcaemia, and hyperglycaemia.

Management

Early recognition of thyroid storm is essential to initiate treatment, and should be performed in an ICU setting (before the results of thyroid function tests if high index of suspicion). Immediate interventions include resuscitative measures. Antithyroid treatment takes the form of carbimazole or propylthiouracil orally. Inorganic iodide (Lugol's aqueous iodine oral solution) may be administered concurrently to inhibit the organification of iodide. Beta-blockers may be used to treat tachycardia. Hydrocortisone administration is also recommended to treat relative adrenal insufficiency, while also decreasing T4 to T3 conversion. Other measures include treating precipitating cause (e.g. infection), cooling with tepid sponging and paracetamol, and sedation for severe agitation. Patients who fail to respond to medical therapy may require therapeutic plasmapheresis or thyroidectomy.

References

1. Mathew V, Misgar RA, Ghosh S, et al. Myxedema coma: a new look into an old crisis. *J Thyroid Res* 2011;2011:493462.
2. Leung AM. Thyroid emergencies. *J Infus Nurs* 2016;39(5):281–286.
3. Akamizu T. Thyroid storm: a Japanese perspective. *Thyroid* 2018;28(1):32–40.
4. Carroll R, Matfin G. Endocrine and metabolic emergencies: thyroid storm. *Ther Adv Endocrinol Metab* 2010;1(3):139–145.
5. Chiha M, Samarasinghe S, Kabaker AS. Thyroid storm: an updated review. *J Intensive Care Med* 2013;30(3):131–140.

Head Injury

Susie Bradwell, Sophie Williams, Joanna Manson

Head injury is defined as any trauma (external force) to the head other than superficial facial injuries [1]. Traumatic brain injury is where the external force is sufficient to cause structural injury and/or physiological disruption of brain function, potentially resulting in one or more of the signs and symptoms described in Box 80.1 [1]. Head injury is the most common cause of disability and death among children and young adults in both the UK and the USA [1,2]. Each year, 1.4 million people present to UK emergency services with a head injury, of which 200,000 are admitted to hospital [1]. One-fifth of those admitted have a significant injury such as skull fracture or brain damage [1]. Psychiatric patients are vulnerable to falls and autokabalesis [3,4]. Falls are the third most commonly reported clinical incident in UK psychiatric hospitals and the most frequent cause of traumatic brain injury in the UK [2,3,5]. Psychiatric patients have poorer outcomes following traumatic brain injury compared with the general population [6].

Psychiatric practitioners are frequently asked to assess patients following head injury. This can be challenging, especially in the context of the patient presenting with already poor mental health or learning difficulties. Gaining collateral history from family members, friends, and carers can be helpful for clarifying the patient's baseline mental state and level of functioning.

CLINICAL APPROACH

When presented with a patient with a head injury, the clinician's initial assessment should aim to establish the following.

- Has there been a significant transfer of energy to the head?
- Is the patient displaying signs or symptoms consistent with an acute head injury?
- Should they be transferred to the emergency department for a CT head (Figure 80.1)?

The Maudsley Practice Guidelines for Physical Health Conditions in Psychiatry, First Edition.
David M. Taylor, Fiona Gaughran, and Toby Pillinger.
© 2021 John Wiley & Sons Ltd. Published 2021 by John Wiley & Sons Ltd.

Box 80.1 Signs and symptoms that may accompany traumatic brain injury

- Headache
- Double vision
- Amnesia
- Altered mental state (e.g. confusion or a change in behaviour)
- Loss of consciousness (any period of unresponsiveness)
- Neurological deficit (e.g. visual disturbance, speech disturbance, hemiparesis, motor deficit)
- Nausea
- Vomiting
- Seizures
- Blood or fluid from the ears or nose
- Bruising around the eyes or ears ('Panda' eyes or Battle's sign)
- Unequal pupils

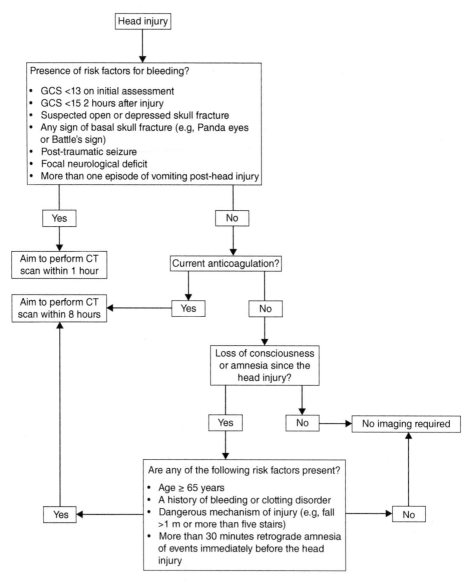

Figure 80.1 An algorithm for determining need for CT imaging post head injury. Source: adapted from National Institute for Health and Care Excellence [1].

- Are there any other injuries?
- Should the emergency services be called?

All patients who experience a traumatic injury should be assessed using the ABCDE approach.

- Assess the airway is clear and patent; if necessary try a jaw thrust, but avoid head tilt and chin lift.
- Ensure the patient is breathing comfortably, has good air entry, and adequate oxygen saturation.
- Assess for signs of active or occult haemorrhage. Stop active blood loss using pressure.
- Establish level of consciousness using the Glasgow Coma Scale (GCS) or AVPU (Table 80.1 and Box 80.2) [7–9].
- Check finger-prick blood glucose.
- Determine if the patient can move all four limbs and if movement and sensation are normal.
- Consider immobilising the patient to avoid moving the spine. However, note that placement of a neck collar may cause unnecessary distress; furthermore, such an intervention may not be immediately available in a psychiatric setting. Use your

Table 80.1 Glasgow Coma Scale [7].

Eye opening	Spontaneous	4
	To sound	3
	To pressure	2
	None	1
Verbal response	Orientated	5
	Confused	4
	Words	3
	Sounds	2
	None	1
Motor response	Obeys commands	6
	Localises to pain	5
	Normal flexion	4
	Abnormal flexion	3
	Extension	2
	None	1

Box 80.2 AVPU scale [9]

A Alert
V Responds to voice
P Responds to painful stimulus
U Unresponsive

CHAPTER 80

judgement: three-point fixation or simply holding the head still may be better tolerated. Talk to the patient, keeping them informed and calm.

- Assume the patient has a spinal injury if any of the following factors apply:
    - a significant distracting injury (e.g. an obvious fracture of a bone)
    - recreational drug or alcohol use
    - confusion
    - reduced level of consciousness
    - a motor or sensory deficit.

Gather more information about the events surrounding the injury:

- Establish the mechanism of injury. A 'high-energy' head injury includes a fall from a height (>1 m), a fall down more than five stairs, a pedestrian/cyclist hit by a car, or ejection from a motor vehicle [1].
- Assess for features consistent with a traumatic brain injury (see Box 80.1).
- Review the patient's medications, note use of anticoagulants.
- Determine past medical history.

Transfer the patient to the emergency department of a trauma centre if:

- the patient fulfils criteria for CT head (see Figure 80.1)
- there has been a significant mechanism of injury (i.e. a high-energy injury)
- the patient has reduced level of consciousness
- you are concerned about injury to any other body region
- the patient is anticoagulated
- you are concerned and believe the patient requires further assessment.

Management of the patient who appears well post head injury

Most patients with minor or moderate head injury do not require a CT scan and can be managed conservatively. However, these patients may develop a headache, concussion, reduced concentration, and reduced appetite. They should be observed carefully for 24 hours by a sensible adult who can monitor for a deterioration in neurological status and GCS. Follow the guidance in Box 80.3 if neurological observations are recommended for a period of time in a patient with a GCS of 15/15 on a psychiatric ward.

Box 80.3 Neurological observations for patients with head injury

- Glasgow Coma Scale (see Table 80.1)
- Pupil size
- Pupil reaction to light
- Motor and sensory assessment of all four limbs
- Vital signs: heart rate, blood pressure, respiratory rate, temperature, and oxygen saturation

Neurological observations should be performed every 30 minutes for two hours, then every hour for four hours, then every two hours thereafter. Stop observations after 24 hours if the patient has recorded a GCS of 15/15 throughout and there are no new clinical concerns.

Changes in conscious level or development of neurology will require reassessment and consideration of CT scan.

TYPES OF INTRACRANIAL HAEMORRHAGE

There are several areas within the head where bleeding can occur (Figure 80.2).

Extradural haematoma

These are high-pressure arterial bleeds in the temporal region that are frequently associated with a skull fracture. Blood collects in a tight space causing a characteristic convex appearance on CT. These patients can initially appear well, but suddenly deteriorate as intracranial pressure increases rapidly. They require urgent neurosurgical assessment and intervention.

Subdural haematoma

These are low-pressure venous bleeds that traverse the outer edge of the brain, giving a concave appearance on CT; they can be acute or chronic and can develop several days after the traumatic event. People at risk include the elderly, alcoholics, and patients on anticoagulation. Symptoms of subdural haematoma can be psychiatric rather than neurological [10].

Subarachnoid haemorrhage

These are bleeds into the layer between the arachnoid and the pia mater which covers the brain parenchyma.

Intraparenchymal haematoma

Bleeding within the brain parenchyma itself.

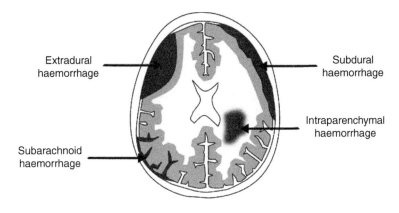

Figure 80.2 Types of intracranial haemorrhage.

Intraventricular haemorrhage

Bleeding into the ventricles.

References

1. National Institute for Health and Care Excellence. *Head Injury: Assessment and Early Management.* Clinical Guideline CG176. London: NICE, 2014. Available at https://www.nice.org.uk/guidance/cg176/chapter/Introduction

2. Centers for Disease Control and Prevention. *Surveillance Report of Traumatic Brain Injury-related Emergency Department Visits, Hospitalizations, and Deaths: United States, 2014.* Atlanta, GA: CDC, 2014. Available at https://www.cdc.gov/traumaticbraininjury/pdf/TBI-Surveillance-Report-FINAL_508.pdf

3. NHS Improvement. *The incidence and costs of inpatient falls in hospitals.* London: NHS, 2017. Available at https://improvement.nhs.uk/documents/1471/Falls_report_July2017.v2.pdf

4. Allen DE, de Nesnera A, Robinson DA. Psychiatric patients are at increased risk of falling and choking. *J Am Psychiatr Nurses* 2012;18(2):91–95.

5. Hawley C, Sakr M, Scapinello S, et al. Traumatic brain injuries in older adults: 6 years of data for one UK trauma centre. Retrospective analysis of prospectively collected data. *Emerg Med J* 2017;34(8):509–516.

6. Mooney G, Speed J. The association between mild traumatic brain injury and psychiatric conditions. *Brain Injury* 2001;15(10):865–877.

7. Teasdale G, Jennett B. Assessment of coma and impaired consciousness. A practical scale. *Lancet* 1974;2(7872):81–84.

8. McNarry AF, Goldhill DR. Simple bedside assessment of level of consciousness: comparison of two simple assessment scales with the Glasgow Coma scale. *Anaesthesia* 2004;59(1):34–37.

9. Romanelli D, Farrell MW. AVPU (Alert, Voice, Pain, Unresponsive). *StatPearls.* Treasure Island, FL: StatPearls Publishing, 2019.

10. Kar SK, Kumar D, Singh P, Upadhyay PK. Psychiatric manifestation of chronic subdural hematoma: the unfolding of mystery in a homeless patient. *Indian J Psychol Med* 2015;37(2):239–242.

Acute Meningitis and Infective Encephalitis

Hina Khan, Brian Sweeney

MENINGITIS

Meningitis is infection or inflammation of the tissue surrounding the surface of the brain and spinal cord, called the meninges. The presentation of meningitis can be acute or chronic, the former developing over hours to days, the latter over weeks. Here, the focus is on acute meningitis, considering causes and emergency management.

Bacterial meningitis is associated with case-fatality rates of up to 30%, rising to 50% in resource-poor settings [1]. Neurological sequelae (e.g. hearing loss) and neuropsychological impairment occur in up to half of disease survivors [1]. As such, patients with suspected bacterial meningitis require urgent assessment and management. The pathogens most commonly responsible are *Neisseria meningitidis* (meningococcus), *Streptococcus pneumoniae* (pneumococcus), and *Haemophilus influenzae* type b (Hib). *Neisseria meningitidis* is the leading cause of bacterial meningitis in children and young adults, with the organism causing bacterial meningitis (meningococcal meningitis, 15%), septicaemia (meningococcal septicaemia, 25%), or a combination of both (60%). Since the introduction of vaccinations for Hib, serogroup C meningococcus, and some pneumococci, the incidence of bacterial meningitis has markedly reduced in the UK [2].

Viral meningitis is usually self-limiting. Causes include enteroviruses (85% of cases), arboviruses, mumps, herpes viruses, lymphocytic choriomeningitis, mammarenavirus, adenoviruses, measles, and human immunodeficiency virus (HIV).

Initial assessment and emergency management

Meningitis has a characteristic clinical presentation, detailed in Box 81.1. Also be aware of risk factors for central nervous system (CNS) infection, including immunosuppression (including HIV diagnosis and alcohol abuse), pregnancy (*Listeria*), intravenous

---

Box 81.1 Clinical presentation of meningitis

Typical clinical presentation

- Severe headache, worsened by sudden head movements
- Fever
- Photophobia
- Nausea and vomiting
- Meningism: neck stiffness (caused by spinal muscle spasms) and Kernig's sign (pain on attempting to extend the knee with the hip flexed due to hamstring spasm)

Clinical features that may not always be present

- Cranial nerve involvement
- Focal neurological deficit
- Seizures (usually in *S. pneumoniae* and *H. influenzae* type b infection)
- Raised intracranial pressure:
  - consciousness level being affected
  - raised blood pressure
  - heart rate <60 bpm
  - abnormal breathing
  - papilloedema which can occur late in presentation
- Non-blanching purpuric or petechial rash: *N. meningitidis*
- Septic shock: *N. meningitidis*

---

drug use, and recent neurosurgery/presence of a ventriculoperitoneal shunt or another medical device that may provide a route of infection to the CNS. Note any recent travel history which may point towards atypical infection.

If bacterial meningitis is suspected, but in the absence of a purpuric/petechial non-blanching rash, UK guidance states that the patient should be transferred urgently to a general medical hospital as an emergency but without giving antibiotics, unless there is a delay. If there is a delay, antibiotics should be given: intramuscular or intravenous benzylpenicillin 1200 mg. Alternatives are cefotaxime or chloramphenicol [3].

If meningococcal disease is suspected (meningitis with purpuric/petechial non-blanching rash or meningococcal septicaemia) then give intramuscular or intravenous benzylpenicillin 1200 mg as soon as possible (although do not delay transfer to the general medical hospital to give antibiotics). If there is a history of anaphylaxis to penicillin, then antibiotics should not be given and the patient simply transferred to a general medical hospital as an emergency [3].

Patients should be managed according to the ABCDE approach. Perform a set of observations, checking heart rate, blood pressure, respiratory rate, oxygen saturations, and temperature. Provide high-flow oxygen and, if possible, insert two large-bore cannulae. If shock develops, indicated by a precipitous drop in blood pressure, intravenous fluid challenge is indicated (in adults 500–1000 mL crystalloid given rapidly). Glucose levels should be checked using a finger-prick test and treated if low (see Chapter 74). If seizures develop, treat as per the guidance provided in Chapter 76.

Once in a general medical hospital, further investigations will include the following.

- Bloods: full blood count, urea and electrolytes, liver function tests, C-reactive protein, glucose, clotting, and blood cultures.
- CT scan of the head followed by a lumbar puncture (LP). 'Coning' of the brainstem may occur in the setting of raised intracranial pressure, hence the need for a CT scan prior to LP.
- Cerebrospinal fluid (CSF) will be sent for protein, microscopy and sensitivity, and for viral polymerase chain reaction (PCR). Paired CSF and serum glucose will be measured, as well as the opening pressure.
- Note that performing a CT scan and LP should not delay antimicrobial treatment.

If there are features of septic shock or raised intracranial pressure, the patient may be transferred to an intensive care unit (ICU) [4]. Choice of antibiotic is dependent on the causative organism, and is usually made in consultation with a microbiologist. As previously mentioned, viral meningitis is often self-limiting, is diagnosed by LP, and treatment is supportive.

In cases of bacterial meningitis, prophylactic antibiotics should be issued to people who were in prolonged close contact with the patient in the same accommodation within a week before the start of the illness, and to people who have been in direct contact with droplets or secretions from the respiratory tract of the patient [5].

INFECTIVE ENCEPHALITIS

Encephalitis is inflammation of the brain parenchyma and can complicate meningitis (meningo-encephalitis). Here, focus is on the infective causes of encephalitis; auto-immune encephalitis is discussed in Chapter 51. The clinical definition of encephalitis, as stated by the International Encephalitis Consortium, states that there should be evidence of inflammation along with encephalopathy (Box 81.2) [6]. The main infective causes of encephalitis are listed in Table 81.1. Like meningitis, acute infective encephalitis is a neurological emergency; untreated, it is associated with extremely high mortality rates, for example 70% mortality in untreated herpes simplex encephalitis [7].

The underlying aetiology of infective encephalitis can often be identified by taking a careful history and examination. Details about recent travel, mosquito/tick/animal bites, preceding illnesses, or immunisations may provide clues. In immunocompetent people in the UK, the most common causes of infective encephalitis are herpes simplex virus (HSV) types 1 and 2, varicella zoster, and enteroviruses. HSV and rabies cause encephalitis via direct invasion of brain cells, while other acute infections are caused by an immune-mediated process after the acute infection. This is known as post-infectious or para-infectious encephalitis [1].

If the clinical presentation of a patient is suggestive of encephalitis, then emergency ABCDE care should be provided and the patient transferred urgently to a general medical

---

Box 81.2 Diagnosis of encephalitis requires the presence of encephalopathy accompanied by two features of inflammation [8,9]

Encephalopathy

1 An altered state of consciousness for >24 hours
2 Personality or behavioural change
3 Lethargy

Inflammation

Fever within 72 hours of presentation

1 Seizures that cannot be attributed to other seizure disorders
2 New neurological deficit
3 Cerebrospinal fluid containing raised inflammatory cells (five or more cells)
4 EEG changes suggestive of encephalitis
5 Neuroimaging with features of inflammation

Table 81.1 Main infectious causes of encephalitis listed in order of frequency [6].

Organism	Example
Virus	Herpes simplex virus (HSV)-1 and HSV-2, varicella zoster virus
	Enterovirus, Epstein–Barr virus, measles, mumps, rubella
	Arboviruses: West Nile Virus, Zika virus, dengue virus
	Mosquito-borne, e.g. Japanese encephalitis virus
Parasites	*Toxoplasma gondii*
Mycobacteria	*Mycobacterium tuberculosis* (TB)
Bacteria	Usually if encephalitic component, then combined with meningitis as meningo-encephalitis

---

hospital, as previously described. As with meningitis, routine bloods and cultures, neuroimaging, and LP (for culture and virology) should be performed. An electroencephalogram (EEG) may also be performed.

Care should be provided in a hospital where there are ICU facilities as patients with encephalitis can develop autonomic instability that needs airway support; they also require cardiovascular monitoring due to risks of arrhythmias and resultant cardiovascular compromise. In addition, patients are at high risk of developing status epilepticus, which may also require treatment in ICU.

Treatment of infective encephalitis is dependent on the aetiology, although aciclovir is typically initiated in patients with suspected encephalitis, pending results of diagnostic studies. Many causes, such as arbovirus, do not have specific treatments. In such cases, patients are managed supportively.

References

1. van de Beek D, de Gans J, Spanjaard L, et al. Clinical features and prognostic factors in adults with bacterial meningitis. *N Engl J Med* 2004;351(18):1849–1859.
2. National Institute for Health and Care Excellence. *Meningitis (Bacterial) and Meningococcal Septicaemia in Under 16s: Recognition, Diagnosis and Management.* Clinical guideline CG102. London: NICE, 2010. Available at https://www.nice.org.uk/guidance/CG102. 2010.
3. National Institute for Health and Care Excellence. Pre-hospital assessment and management of bacterial meningitis and meningococcal septicaemia. NICE Pathway, last updated November 2019. http://pathways.nice.org.uk/pathways/bacterial-meningitis-and-meningococcal-septicaemia-in-under-16s
4. Manji H, Connolly S, Kitchen N, et al. *Oxford Handbook of Neurology*, 2nd edn. Oxford: Oxford University Press, 2014.
5. Tyler KL. Acute viral encephalitis. *N Engl J Med* 2018;379(6):557–566.
6. Venkatesan A, Tunkel AR, Bloch KC, et al. Case definitions, diagnostic algorithms, and priorities in encephalitis: consensus statement of the International Encephalitis Consortium. *Clin Infect Dis* 2013;57(8):1114–1128.
7. Whitley RJ, Soong SJ, Dolin R, et al. Adenine arabinoside therapy of biopsy-proved herpes simplex encephalitis. National Institute of Allergy and Infectious Diseases collaborative antiviral study. *N Engl J Med* 1977;297(6):289–294.
8. Ellul M, Solomon T. Acute encephalitis: diagnosis and management. *Clin Med* 2018;18(2):155–159.
9. Piquet AL, Lyons JL. Infectious meningitis and encephalitis. *Semin Neurol* 2016;36(4):367–372.

Stroke and Transient Ischaemic Attack

Toby Pillinger, James Teo

Stroke occurs when there is interruption of blood supply to the brain, either because a blood vessel bursts (15% of strokes) or is blocked by a clot ('thrombus') (85% of strokes). The former is called a haemorrhagic stroke, while the latter is called an ischaemic stroke. This interruption of blood flow cuts off the supply of oxygen and nutrients to an area of brain tissue, causing damage to that region. A transient ischaemic attack (TIA) describes a similar transiently symptomatic event due to either short-lasting ischaemia that does not cause any lasting brain injury or a very small focal ischaemia which is rapidly compensated for. TIAs can be a precursor for a subsequent stroke. 'Cerebrovascular accident' is an obsolete term that is synonymous with 'stroke' and may be seen in older texts.

Compared with the general population, people with serious mental illness are approximately twice as likely to have a stroke [1]. This chapter aims to provide the reader with the necessary information to identify and provide emergency management to an individual experiencing a stroke or TIA.

STROKE

The most common symptom of a stroke is sudden weakness or numbness of the face, arm or leg, most often on one side of the body. Other symptoms include confusion and difficulty speaking or understanding speech; difficulty seeing with one or both eyes; difficulty walking, dizziness, and loss of balance or coordination; severe headache with no known cause; and fainting or unconsciousness. The effects of a stroke depend on which part of the brain is injured and how severely it is affected. A very severe stroke can cause sudden death.

The Maudsley Practice Guidelines for Physical Health Conditions in Psychiatry, First Edition.
David M. Taylor, Fiona Gaughran, and Toby Pillinger.

Box 82.1 The FAST test[a] to screen for a person having a stroke [2]

- **F**acial drooping: a section of the face, usually only on one side, that is drooping and hard to move. This can be recognised by a crooked smile
- **A**rm weakness: the inability to raise one's arm fully
- **S**peech difficulties: an inability or difficulty to understand or produce speech
- **T**ime: if any of these symptoms are showing, time is of the essence; call emergency services or go to the hospital[a]

[a] This test is highly sensitive for identifying an anterior circulation stroke. Acute-onset neurology that does not conform to FAST criteria may indicate a posterior circulation stroke.

The FAST test can help detect and enhance the speed with which care is provided to patients suffering a stroke (Box 82.1) [2]. The FAST test is widely used for screening of acute stroke by members of both the general public and clinicians [3]. However, it has some weaknesses: it has a high false-positive rate (considered acceptable for an emergency triage tool for the general public) and is designed to identify strokes that arise from the anterior portion of the brain (anterior circulation stroke), which account for approximately 70% of all ischaemic strokes [4]. As such, it is an insensitive test for identifying strokes of the posterior portion of the brain (posterior circulation strokes) or secondary to small blood vessel occlusion (lacunar stroke) [5]. Common symptoms seen in posterior circulation strokes include motor deficits (e.g. weakness), sensory deficits (e.g. numbness), visual disturbances (loss of vision or double vision), imbalance/ataxia, vertigo, difficulty swallowing, and slurred speech. Haemorrhagic strokes may also present with acute drowsiness, severe headache, and meningism (neck stiffness and photophobia).

DIAGNOSTIC PRINCIPLES

Patients who may have recently suffered a stroke should be *transferred immediately* to emergency medical services: time from onset of stroke is the main factor that determines eligibility for thrombolysis in the context of an ischaemic event.

History

Beyond eliciting the presence of neurological symptoms, the most important information to gather from the history is time of onset of symptoms. It is critical that this is not interpreted to mean 'time that symptoms were noticed'. As it is often not possible to report time of onset of symptoms if the onset was not directly witnessed, it is convention to instead state the 'time last seen well'. Some treatments can be harmful if given based on wrong timing information, so it is important to establish correct timings.

Key risk factors for stroke include older age, family history of stroke, personal history of TIA/stroke, cardiovascular risk factors (hypertension, smoking, diabetes mellitus, hypercholesterolaemia), and atrial fibrillation. Other relevant past medical history should include history of bleeding. A full drug history should be sought, including the prescription of any anticoagulants.

Examination and investigations

Patients are assessed by a standardised validated neurological examination called the National Institute of Health Stroke Scale (NIHSS) [6]. This scale has good reproducibility between clinicians and allows a quantitative measure of impairment for acute decision-making.

CHAPTER 82

MANAGEMENT

Urgent treatment in specialist facilities reduces morbidity and mortality. In an acute medical setting, initial management will involve stabilising the patient before rapidly obtaining brain imaging to differentiate between a haemorrhagic and ischaemic stroke (typically using CT scan of the brain). Often history is obtained and examination performed en route to the CT scan. If the stroke is ischaemic and if the damage to the brain is not already irreversible, then treatments can be provided to try to recanalise the blood vessel by mechanically removing the thrombus (thrombectomy) or dissolving the thrombus (thrombolysis). Conventionally, brain damage is considered reversible if the scan shows no damage and symptoms started less than 4.5 hours before [7]. However, in the last few years, more advanced brain imaging (CT perfusion and diffusion-weighted MRI) can extend this time window to evaluate the degree of irreversibility such that some strokes are suitable for thrombectomy or thrombolysis up to 24 hours after symptom onset [8,9]. The risk with the treatments (particularly thrombolysis) is that it can cause haemorrhage into the brain or anywhere in the body and this can be fatal. This risk increases the later the thrombolysis is given and if there are any risk factors, such as recent surgery or injuries. If thrombolysis or thrombectomy is not suitable, then antiplatelet medication (aspirin or clopidogrel) is given to reduce the risk of further strokes.

Patients are typically then managed in a hyperacute stroke unit (in the USA termed a 'comprehensive stroke center') where they receive multidisciplinary input from physicians, speech and language therapists, occupational therapists, and physiotherapists. Here, patients are medically stabilised (with appropriate interventions to prevent secondary complications of stroke such as aspiration pneumonia), and undergo investigations to determine the aetiology of the stroke (see Table 82.1). Neurological rehabilitation will encompass physical recovery, cognitive rehabilitation, and overlapping mental health factors. In the patient with serious mental illness, the psychiatrist will play a key role in ensuring ongoing psychiatric needs are met, for example providing advice regarding appropriate psychiatric medication for ongoing mental health needs and in the case of agitation or delirium (see Chapter 50).

Table 82.1 Adapted TOAST classification: subtypes of acute ischaemic stroke.

Type of stroke	Description
Atherosclerosis of large vessel	Includes carotid and intracranial artery stenosis
Lacunar (small-vessel occlusion)	Lacunar strokes from small-vessel disease
Cardio-embolism	Embolism from atrial fibrillation, left ventricular aneurysm, patent foramen ovale
Dissection of cervical artery	Carotid artery or vertebral dissections
Other causes	Rarer causes such as venous stroke, vasculitis, cerebral autosomal dominant arteriopathy with subcortical infarcts and leukoencephalopathy (CADASIL) syndrome
Cryptogenic (stroke of undetermined aetology)	Includes cases of multiple causes as well as embolic stroke of unknown source (ESUS)

Source: from Gordon et al. [11].

TRANSIENT ISCHAEMIC ATTACK

A TIA is a transient neurological deficit caused by ischaemia of the brain, spinal cord, or retina [10]. Conventionally this is defined as symptoms lasting for less than 24 hours, although neuroimaging now shows that even 30 minutes of symptoms can result in permanent injury to the brain. The approach to a patient with a previous TIA (i.e. where reported neurological deficits have resolved) will mirror many of those recommended for diagnostic work-up of stroke. Persistent neurological deficits should of course be treated as a stroke.

DIAGNOSTIC PRINCIPLES

History

By definition, symptoms and signs of TIA are brief, with the majority resolving within an hour. Clarify the nature of the neurological deficit and any risk factors for cerebrovascular events, as described for stroke. Collateral history may be useful. Also screen for differential diagnoses, including seizure with post-seizure (Todd's) paralysis, migraine, dystonia, labyrinthine disorders (e.g. benign positional vertigo), hypoglycaemia (usually in patients receiving anti-glycaemic agents), and conversion disorder (deficits may not fit a singular vascular territory, with inconsistencies during physical examination).

Examination and investigations

The purpose of examination and investigations is to support the diagnosis of TIA rather than alternative diagnoses (i.e. TIA mimics). Examples of alternative diagnoses are syncope, seizure, transient global amnesia, or migraine.

Once the TIA diagnosis is confirmed, the investigations are aimed at evaluating the aetiology of the TIA, which allows management of the risk of subsequent stroke. The cause is defined using an aetiological classification system such as TOAST (Trial of ORG 10172 in Acute Stroke Treatment) [11] (Table 82.1) or ASCO (Atherosclerosis, Small vessel disease, Cardiac source, Other cause) [12,13], which then determines the appropriate management strategy.

A set of basic observations and a neurological and cardiac examination should be performed. Neurological examination screens for persistent focal neurological deficits, and cardiac examination for risk factors for embolic disease such as atrial fibrillation (AF) or valvular heart disease. Auscultation of the carotid arteries for bruits may indicate atheromatous disease. Basic investigations may be performed that screen for cardiovascular risk factors (blood sugar, HbA_{1c}, cholesterol) and assess clotting, full blood count, and renal/liver function. An ECG may be requested to assess for arrhythmia that may predispose the individual to thromboembolic disease. Specialist investigations may include brain imaging (CT/MRI), CT/MR angiography, carotid Doppler ultrasound, and cardiac telemetry to detect paroxysmal AF.

MANAGEMENT

Management of TIA and ongoing cardiovascular risk is beyond the immediate remit of the psychiatrist, but recognition of the standard of care a patient with serious mental illness should be receiving is valuable if a patient is engaging poorly with medical services owing to symptoms of poor mental health. Once a transient thrombotic event has been identified in a patient, patients need to be started on aspirin 300 mg once daily and be referred immediately to a specialist stroke service within 24 hours [14].

Secondary prevention of further ischaemic events will involve antiplatelet agents (e.g. aspirin or clopidogrel) for atherosclerotic disease, and anticoagulation for cardioembolic events such as AF (e.g. warfarin or a direct oral anticoagulant). Cardiovascular risk management is of primary importance, including lifestyle modification (diet, exercise, smoking cessation, reduced alcohol intake), and where appropriate introduction of statins or antihypertensives. If a psychiatric medication is thought to be contributing to metabolic risk, then switching to an alternative agent may be considered, weighing up the risks of changing treatment (deterioration in mental state) versus increased risk of metabolic disease and stroke. Any patients with suspected TIA and their family/carers should receive information about the recognition of stroke symptoms and the action to be taken if they occur.

References

1. Lin HC, Hsiao FH, Pfeiffer S, et al. An increased risk of stroke among young schizophrenia patients. *Schizophr Res* 2008;101(1–3):234–241.
2. American Stroke Association. Stroke symptoms. https://www.strokeassociation.org/en/about-stroke/stroke-symptoms (accessed 27 May 2019).
3. Harbison J, Hossain O, Jenkinson D, et al. Diagnostic accuracy of stroke referrals from primary care, emergency room physicians, and ambulance staff using the face arm speech test. *Stroke* 2003;34(1):71–76.
4. Tao WD, Liu M, Fisher M, et al. Posterior versus anterior circulation infarction: how different are the neurological deficits? *Stroke* 2012;43(8):2060–2065.

5. Gulli G, Markus HS. The use of FAST and ABCD2 scores in posterior circulation, compared with anterior circulation, stroke and transient ischemic attack. *J Neurol Neurosurg Psychiatry* 2012;83(2):228–229.

6. National Institutes of Health. NIH Stroke Scale. https://www.stroke.nih.gov/resources/scale.htm (accessed 27 May 2019).

7. Hacke W, Kaste M, Bluhmki E, et al. Thrombolysis with alteplase 3 to 4.5 hours after acute ischemic stroke. *N Engl J Med* 2008;359(13):1317–1329.

8. Nogueira RG, Jadhav AP, Haussen DC, et al. Thrombectomy 6 to 24 hours after stroke with a mismatch between deficit and infarct. *N Engl J Med* 2018;378(1):11–21.

9. Albers GW, Marks MP, Kemp S, et al. Thrombectomy for stroke at 6 to 16 hours with selection by perfusion imaging. *N Engl J Med* 2018;378(8):708–718.

10. Easton JD, Saver JL, Albers GW, et al. Definition and evaluation of transient ischemic attack: a scientific statement for healthcare professionals from the American Heart Association/American Stroke Association Stroke Council; Council on Cardiovascular Surgery and Anesthesia; Council on Cardiovascular Radiology and Intervention; Council on Cardiovascular Nursing; and the Interdisciplinary Council on Peripheral Vascular Disease. *Stroke* 2009;40(6):2276–2293.

11. Gordon DL, Bendixen BH, Adams HP Jr, et al. Interphysician agreement in the diagnosis of subtypes of acute ischemic stroke: implications for clinical trials. The TOAST Investigators. *Neurology* 1993;43(5):1021–1027.

12. Ay H, Furie KL, Singhal A, et al. An evidence-based causative classification system for acute ischemic stroke. *Ann Neurol* 2005;58(5):688–697.

13. Marnane M, Duggan CA, Sheehan OC, et al. Stroke subtype classification to mechanism-specific and undetermined categories by TOAST, A-S-C-O, and causative classification system: direct comparison in the North Dublin population stroke study. *Stroke* 2010;41(8):1579–1586.

14. National Institiute for Health and Care Excellence. *Stroke and Transient Ischaemic Attack in Over 16s: Diagnosis and Initial Management*. NICE Guideline NG128. London: NICE, 2019. Available at https://www.nice.org.uk/guidance/ng128

CHAPTER 82

Overdose

Stephen Kaar, Immo Weichert

In the UK, suicide by injury or poisoning accounts for the highest proportion of deaths in those aged 5–19 years [1]. The UK's National Confidential Inquiry into Suicide and Safety in Mental Health published in 2018 [2] found that self-poisoning accounts for one-quarter of psychiatric patient suicides, most often involving an opiate. The inquiry also found that one-third of female patients who commit suicide do so by self-poisoning, the most common substances being opiates, antidepressants, and antipsychotics. The 2018 UK mortality statistics reported that fatal drug-related poisonings are most likely to involve opiates (mainly heroin, morphine, and methadone), then cocaine, antidepressants, benzodiazepines, paracetamol, and antipsychotics [1]. A recent national (UK) linked-database study observed that the most common substances used in overdose in those aged 10–24 years were paracetamol, alcohol, non-steroidal anti-inflammatory drugs, antidepressants, and opioids [3]. In the USA there has been a significant increase in drug overdose deaths in recent years, driven primarily by synthetic opioids; overall, opioids were responsible for 68% of drug overdose deaths [4]. Clinicians should also be mindful of the potential for poisoning with newer recreational substances such as gamma-hydroxybutyrate and its analogues. Polypharmacy is common in overdose, especially where recreational substances are involved; overdose of multiple different drugs can complicate the clinical presentation. For example, cocaine use should be suspected in patients presenting with acute coronary syndrome in the context of poisoning [5].

GENERAL PRINCIPLES [6]

Patients with features of poisoning should be managed as medical emergencies and admitted to a general medical hospital, as should patients who have taken modified-release

The Maudsley Practice Guidelines for Physical Health Conditions in Psychiatry, First Edition.
David M. Taylor, Fiona Gaughran, and Toby Pillinger.
© 2021 John Wiley & Sons Ltd. Published 2021 by John Wiley & Sons Ltd.

preparations/drugs with delayed action or a staggered overdose (defined as ingestion of multiple doses of a drug over a period of more than an hour) even if they appear well. Delayed-action drugs include aspirin, iron, paracetamol, tricyclic antidepressants, and co-phenotrope. Staggered paracetamol overdose is associated with particularly high mortality rates [7], and in such cases consider early discussion with a specialist liver centre.

In the UK, TOXBASE is the primary clinical toxicology database run by the National Poisons Information Service, accessible by NHS professional staff at www.toxbase.org or via a phone/tablet application and 24-hour phone line: 0344 892 0111. In the Republic of Ireland, the National Poisons Information Centre provides information to doctors and healthcare professionals 24 hours per day at 01 837 9964 or 01 809 2566. In the USA, clinicians can use the American Association of Poison Control Centers helpline on 1-800-222-1222.

INFORMATION GATHERING

Identifying the type, quantity, and timing of poisoning may guide early management since certain substances have antidotes (see Table 83.1). As appropriate, information should be gathered from friends, relatives, and carers. Search for empty medication boxes or medication strips, new prescriptions and receipts, or in the UK access the patient's primary care prescription records via SystmOne. In the UK, tablets may be identified through repositories such as www.tictac.org.uk or other prescribing guides such as the Monthly Index of Medical Specialities (MIMS). In the USA, pill identification services such as Pill ID can be used (https://pill-id. webpoisoncontrol.org).

A review of the patient's past medication history may provide useful information if stockpiling of old medication is suspected. Also consider that the patient may have taken medication prescribed for partners, friends, or family members. Determine the patient's past medical history to assess the effect poisoning may have on comorbid conditions (e.g. chronic liver disease). Other clues as to the aetiology of poisoning may be found on physical examination, such as pinpoint pupils in opioid overdose.

EMERGENCY ASSESSMENT AND MANAGEMENT [6]

In psychiatric practice one may be presented with a patient in the immediate aftermath of an overdose. All patients should be managed according to the ABCDE approach while emergency support from medical colleagues is sought; a psychiatric setting is an inappropriate environment in which to manage overdose.

Airway

If a person is unconscious due to an overdose, airway obstruction may occur. The airway should be opened with a chin lift or jaw thrust and any vomitus cleared from the

Table 83.1 Specific antidotes for opioid and paracetamol overdose.

Substance	Antidote	Mode of action	Mode of administration	Dose	Notes
Opioids	Naloxone (Narcan, Evzio, Prenoxad)	μ, κ, σ opioid receptor antagonist	Intramuscular: 2–5 minute onset of action Intravenous: 1–2 minute onset of action	See Figure 83.1	Naloxone has a short half-life and its duration of action is approximately 60 minutes [22] so may need repeating
Paracetamol (acetaminophen)	N-acetylcysteine	Provides cysteine for glutathione (antioxidant) synthesis	Intravenous	150 mg/kg i.v. infusion over 1 hour, followed by 50 mg/kg infusion over 4 hours, then 100 mg/kg infusion over 16 hours. May be continued afterwards	Most effective when given within 8 hours of ingestion. May offer some protection even if given 24 hours after ingestion

mouth, either by tilting the head or if equipment is available using suction. A nasopharyngeal airway may be useful in unconscious patients to prevent further airway obstruction (see Chapter 78).

Breathing

Respiratory drive may be reduced. If available, high-flow oxygen should be administered and pulse oximetry monitored, as well as respiratory rate. In the context of opioid overdose and resultant respiratory rate below 10 per minute, administer naloxone (see Figure 83.1 and Table 83.1).

Circulation

Hypotension is common in poisoning with central nervous system (CNS) depressants such as opiates. Antipsychotics may also induce hypotension through adrenoceptor blockade [8]. Elevate the feet of the patient and, if available, administer intravenous fluids. Tricyclic antidepressants, antipsychotics, and some antihistamines may induce QT prolongation, tachycardia, and arrhythmia. Thus, while awaiting emergency medical support perform an ECG.

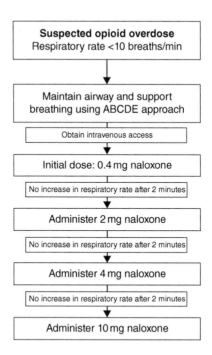

Figure 83.1 Ascending dosing of naloxone for opioid overdose in adults. Patients who do not have a response to an initial dose of naloxone should receive escalating doses until respiratory effort is restored. Source: adapted from Boyer [10].

Other observations

Check temperature, since hypothermia can develop in patients who have been unconscious for extended periods of time. Conversely, cocaine, amphetamines, monoamine oxidase inhibitors, and sympathomimetics can cause pyrexia. Blood glucose should be checked in patients who are confused, unconscious, or suffering fits. Correct hypoglycaemia (see Chapter 74).

SPECIFIC SCENARIOS

Paracetamol (acetaminophen)

Even if asymptomatic, patients who have taken an overdose of paracetamol should be transferred to emergency or acute medical services urgently. Patients with chronic alcoholism and those taking liver enzyme inducers (e.g. carbamazepine and St John's Wort) are at higher risk of toxicity owing to the liver's enhanced ability to produce the toxic metabolite of paracetamol, N-acetyl-p-benzoquinone imine (NAPQI). NAPQI binds to glutathione in the liver, and exhaustion of glutathione stores results in hepatic necrosis [9]. Malnourishment (e.g. in patients with anorexia nervosa) and fasting results in reduced levels of glutathione in the liver and therefore also predisposes to paracetamol toxicity.

Patients with paracetamol poisoning, at least early on, are often asymptomatic. However, clinical manifestations can include:

- nausea and vomiting
- right subcostal pain and tenderness (a sign of hepatic injury after two to three days)
- haemorrhage
- hypoglycaemia
- encephalopathy
- cerebral oedema
- reduced level of consciousness and respiratory depression if a combined paracetamol/opioid preparation has been taken.

Hepatotoxicity can occur after a single ingestion of 150 mg/kg of paracetamol taken in less than one hour but has been reported in single ingestions of 75 mg/kg in an hour. Activated charcoal can be used if the ingestion occurred within the last hour, although techniques to reduce absorption of any poison (e.g. activated charcoal, gastric lavage) may cause significant iatrogenic harm with little evidence that they improve outcomes.

Intravenous Parvolex (N-acetylcysteine) is used to reduce the risk of hepatic damage. The need for N-acetylcysteine can be determined by measuring plasma paracetamol concentration at four hours or more post ingestion. The Rumack–Matthew nomogram is used to predict risk of hepatotoxicity in non-alcoholic patients who have taken a non-staggered overdose and who are not malnourished/fasting and not prescribed enzyme inducers. In staggered overdoses, patients who have taken more than 150 mg/kg in a 24-hour period are at risk of toxicity so should start N-acetylcysteine immediately.

Aspirin (and other salicylates)

Symptoms of salicylate poisoning include vomiting, tinnitus, deafness, sweating, vaso-dilation, and hyperventilation. In severe cases, confusion and coma can follow. There is no specific antidote for aspirin or salicylate overdose, but patients may require intravenous fluids to correct dehydration and enhance salicylate elimination. Sodium bicarbonate may also be used to reduce transfer into the CNS and to alkalinise urine and enhance salicylate excretion.

Opioids

Clinical manifestations of opioid overdose include respiratory depression, pinpoint pupils, hypotension, and reduced levels of consciousness/coma (see Chapter 78) [10]. Obtundation may also result in rhabdomyolysis. Beyond an ABCDE approach, where the patient is unconscious and/or bradypnoeic (respiratory rate <10 breaths per minute) naloxone hydrochloride should be administered (Figure 83.1 and Table 83.1).

Naloxone may be given via intravenous, intramuscular, subcutaneous, and intranasal routes. Non-intravenous routes may be quicker because time is saved in not having to establish access, which may be difficult in patients who regularly use intravenous recreational drugs. The initial doses of naloxone are 400 µg i.v., 800 µg i.m., or 2 mg intranasally [11]. While ensuring that the airway is protected and supporting breathing, give increments of naloxone every two minutes until the victim is breathing adequately and has protective airway reflexes (see Figure 83.1 for intravenous dose escalation). For intranasal naloxone, if the patient responds to first dose but relapses rapidly into respiratory depression, give the second dose immediately. Large opioid overdoses may require titration to 10 mg naloxone. In patients who are dependent on opioids, naloxone may provoke withdrawal symptoms, such as abdominal cramps and bowel disturbance, agitation, and aggressive behaviour.

Tricyclic antidepressants

Clinical manifestations of overdose with tricyclic antidepressants and similar compounds are a result of their anticholinergic effects and sodium-channel blockade and include dry mouth, dialted pupils, urinary retention, reduced consciousness/coma, hypotension, hypothermia, hyperreflexia, extensor plantar responses, convulsions, respiratory failure, metabolic acidosis, and QRS prolongation potentially leading to life-threatening arrhythmias. Management is supportive in an acute medical or intensive care environment. Intravenous sodium bicarbonate is given to treat the metabolic acidosis.

Antipsychotics

CNS depression is common in antipsychotic overdose and may progress to coma (see Chapter 78). Anticholinergic effects may be observed, including altered mental status, urinary retention, tachycardia, dry mucosal membranes, and hyperpyrexia. Acute dystonic reactions can occur. Hypotension and QTc prolongation may also be observed. All antipsychotics lower the seizure threshold, particularly clozapine.

Treatment for antipsychotic overdose is supportive in an acute medical environment. Patients with CNS depression may require intubation. Patients should be monitored for QTc prolongation (see Chapter 3). Prophylactic anticonvulsants may be considered if not contraindicated and where seizures are threatened (e.g. if myoclonus is observed). See Chapter 84 for management of dystonic reactions.

Stimulants

Amphetamines such as ecstasy (3,4-methylenedioxymethamphetamine) produce release of serotonin and catecholamines. They cause euphoria, wakefulness, and excessive activity, but can lead to delirium, coma, convulsions, arrhythmias, hyperthermia, rhabdomyolysis, acute renal failure, acute hepatitis, disseminated intravascular coagulation, adult respiratory distress syndrome, and intracerebral haemorrhage. Inappropriate antidiuretic hormone secretion leads to thirst, and excessive water intake can result in hyponatraemia (see Chapter 32) and cerebral oedema. Severe poisoning is associated with hyperpyrexia and such patients should be transferred as an emergency to a general medical hospital. Patients with core body temperature above 38°C may require active cooling [12]. Benzodiazepines such as diazepam or lorazepam may also help.

Cocaine can cause agitation, dilated pupils, tachycardia, acute coronary syndrome (owing to coronary artery spasm, dissection, or thrombosis; see Chapters 67 and 69), mesenteric ischaemia (see Chapter 88), cerebral haemorrhage, rhabdomyolysis and renal failure (see Chapter 73), and serotonin syndrome (see Chapter 86). Diazepam may help; expert advice and treatment should be sought.

Benzodiazepines

Patients who overdose using benzodiazepines may present with drowsiness, ataxia, dysarthria, nystagmus, and sometimes respiratory depression and coma. Respiratory depression with oral benzodiazepines alone is rare and more commonly occurs when co-ingested with other substances (e.g. alcohol or opiates) which potentiate depressive effects on the respiratory system [13]. If a patient is within one hour of ingestion, then use of activated charcoal can be considered, but note the cautions raised previously regarding this intervention. Otherwise, management should follow an ABCDE approach.

Flumazenil is a competitive antagonist at the benzodiazepine-binding site on the gamma-aminobutyric acid (GABA)-A receptor and can be used as a specific antidote for benzodiazepine overdose (initial intravenous dose 200 µg over 15 seconds, further 100 µg can be given every minute to a maximum of 1 mg) [14]. However, its use can be hazardous because it risks precipitating seizures and ventricular arrhythmias [15–17]. It is contraindicated in mixed overdose and in those with benzodiazepine tolerance, seizure disorders, or prolonged QTc. It should only be used by people with previous experience of its use (or in the presence of people with experience) and in rare cases of severe isolated benzodiazepine or 'Z' drug toxicity with no other contraindications to its use (e.g. in the case of iatrogenic benzodiazepine overdose where the past medical history of the patient is known). In the UK, it is only licenced for reversal of sedative effects of benzodiazepines in anaesthesia, other clinical procedures, or in intensive care

[13]. The main focus of managing suspected benzodiazepine overdose should be to resuscitate according to the ABCDE approach and transfer care to emergency services.

Lithium

The early clinical manifestations of lithium overdose include apathy and restlessness followed by vomiting, diarrhoea, ataxia, weakness, dysarthria, and tremor. There can be a delay of up to 24 hours in the emergence of symptoms in lithium-naive patients and where modified-release preparations have been taken. In severe poisoning, confusion, coma, dehydration, and renal failure may occur. Lithium toxicity is more common in patients on chronic lithium treatment [18]. Beyond an ABCDE approach, treatment should include increasing fluid intake and intravenous fluids to aid clearance, although forced diuresis is contraindicated. Haemodialysis may be required in severe cases.

MANAGEMENT OF A PERSON WHO REFUSES ADMISSION TO HOSPITAL AFTER AN OVERDOSE

If a person refuses to go to hospital following an overdose, try to determine the reasons why. It is important to provide information about the potential consequences of not receiving hospital treatment and assessment. Attempt to gather corroborative information from family and friends. If the person continues to refuse and it is felt in their best interests to have an urgent assessment in hospital, then assess their capacity. In the UK, consider whether compulsory admission under the Mental Health Act 1983 (amended 2007) or the Mental Health (Care and Treatment) (Scotland) Act 2003 is appropriate. Also in the UK, if the person lacks capacity and further urgent assessment is felt to be in their best interests, the person may be taken to hospital against their wishes under the Mental Capacity Act 2005 or the Adults with Incapacity Act 2000 in Scotland. The Mental Health Act can be used for the treatment of a mental health disorder but only for treatment of a physical disorder (i.e. the overdose) if this is deemed to be a symptom or consequence of a mental disorder [19]. In the USA, decisional capacity should be assessed to determine if the patient possesses appropriate capacity to refuse treatment [20]. In patients with signs of active psychiatric illness, an emergency psychiatric consultation should be sought, which could include assessment for an emergency hold [21].

References

1. Office of National Statistics. Deaths registered in England and Wales – 21st century mortality: 2018. https://www.ons.gov.uk/peoplepopulationandcommunity/birthsdeathsandmarriages/deaths/datasets/the21stcenturymortalityfilesdeathsdataset

2. University Of Manchester. National Confidential Inquiry into Suicide and Safety in Mental Health. https://www.research.manchester.ac.uk/portal/en/projects/national-confidential-inquiry-into-suicide-and-safety-in-mental-health(788f9475-cadb-4697-bb82-817638044b7b).html

3. Tyrrell EG, Kendrick D, Sayal K, Orton E. Poisoning substances taken by young people: a population-based cohort study. Br J Gen Pract 2018;68(675):e703.

4. Centers for Disease Control. Drug and opioid-involved overdose deaths: United States, 2013–2017. *MMWR Morb Mortal Wkly Rep* 2018;67(5152):1419–1427.

5. Jones AL, Dargan PI. Advances, challenges, and controversies in poisoning. *Emerg Med J* 2002;19(3):190–192.

CHAPTER 83

6. National Institute for Health and Care Excellence. Poisoning, emergency treatment. https://bnf.nice.org.uk/treatment-summary/poisoning-emergency-treatment.html

7. Craig DGN, Bates CM, Davidson JS, et al. Staggered overdose pattern and delay to hospital presentation are associated with adverse outcomes following paracetamol-induced hepatotoxicity. *Br J Clin Pharmacol* 2012;73(2):285–294.

8. Gugger JJ. Antipsychotic pharmacotherapy and orthostatic hypotension. *CNS Drugs* 2011;25(8):659–671.

9. Kalsi SS, Dargan PI, Waring WS, Wood DM. A review of the evidence concerning hepatic glutathione depletion and susceptibility to hepatotoxicity after paracetamol overdose. *Open Access Emerg Med* 2011;3:87–96.

10. Boyer EW. Management of opioid analgesic overdose. *N Engl J Med* 2012;367(2):146–155.

11. Resuscitation Council UK. Cardiac arrest in special circumstances. In: *Advanced Life Support*, 7th edn. London: Resuscitation Council, 2016, chapter 12.

12. BMJ Best Practice. Amfetamine overdose. https://bestpractice.bmj.com/topics/en-gb/341

13. An H, Godwin J. Flumazenil in benzodiazepine overdose. *Can Med Assoc J* 2016;188(17–18):E537.

14. British National Formulary. Flumazenil: indications and dose. https://bnf.nice.org.uk/drug/flumazenil.html

15. Penninga EI, Graudal N, Ladekarl MB, Jurgens G. Adverse events associated with flumazenil treatment for the management of suspected benzodiazepine intoxication: a systematic review with meta-analyses of randomised trials. *Basic Clin Pharmacol Toxicol* 2016;118(1):37–44.

16. Gueye PN, Hoffman JR, Taboulet P, et al. Empiric use of flumazenil in comatose patients: limited applicability of criteria to define low risk. *Ann Emerg Med* 1996;27(6):730–735.

17. Hojer J, Baehrendtz S, Matell G, Gustafsson LL. Diagnostic utility of flumazenil in coma with suspected poisoning: a double-blind, randomized controlled study. *BMJ* 1990;301(6764):1308–1311.

18. Davis J, Desmond M, Berk M. Lithium and nephrotoxicity: a literature review of approaches to clinical management and risk stratification. *BMC Nephrol* 2018;19(1):305.

19. National Insitute for Health and Care Excellence. Poisoning or overdose. Clinical Knowledge Summary. Last revised: June 2017. https://cks.nice.org.uk/poisoning-or-overdose

20. Marco CA, Brenner JM, Kraus CK, et al. Refusal of emergency medical treatment: case studies and ethical foundations. *Ann Emerg Med* 2017;70(5):696–703.

21. Hedman LC, Petrila J, Fisher WH, et al. State laws on emergency holds for mental health stabilization. *Psychiatr Serv* 2016;67(5):529–535.

22. Lynn RR, Galinkin JL. Naloxone dosage for opioid reversal: current evidence and clinical implications. *Ther Adv Drug Saf.* 2018;9(1):63–88.

Acute Dystonia

Jonathan P. Rogers, R. John Dobbs, Sylvia Dobbs

Acute dystonia is an involuntary, intermittent or sustained muscular contraction, causing slow, often twisting movements or fixed postures.

In a psychiatric context, it is most commonly caused by treatment with antipsychotic medications and appears to be a result of dopaminergic blockade in the nigrostriatal pathway. So-called typical antipsychotics more commonly cause dystonia than atypicals, even when low doses are used [1]. After intramuscular injection, dystonia occurs in 4.7% of patients administered haloperidol and in 0.6% where an atypical antipsychotic is used [2]. The risk of acute dystonia appears to be dose-dependent [3].

Other pharmacological triggers for acute dystonia include the use of antidopaminergic anti-emetics (metoclopramide and prochloperazine), serotonergic antidepressants (occasionally), and withdrawal of anticholinergic drugs used as treatment for dystonia.

Acute dystonia is usually painful, although the intensity can vary considerably. Laryngeal dystonia is uncommon and hard to diagnose, sometimes occurring in the absence of other evidence of dystonia, yet it can be fatal [4]. Even if symptoms are mild, dystonia is important to identify because a failure to recognise and treat it may reduce long-term medication compliance.

DIAGNOSTIC PRINCIPLES

History

1 History of symptoms, including onset, pain, and difficulty breathing. Anxiety commonly accompanies acute dystonia and should be interpreted as an effect, rather than necessarily being indicative of a psychogenic cause.

The Maudsley Practice Guidelines for Physical Health Conditions in Psychiatry, First Edition.
David M. Taylor, Fiona Gaughran, and Toby Pillinger.
© 2021 John Wiley & Sons Ltd. Published 2021 by John Wiley & Sons Ltd.

2 History of timing: acute dystonia may last between seconds and hours. Cases are more common in the afternoon and evening [5].
3 History suggestive of other extrapyramidal side effects, including akathisia, parkinsonism, and tardive dyskinesia.
4 Detailed medication history with timings of antipsychotic initiation, dose changes, and prescription of anticholinergics. An estimated 95% of cases of acute dystonia occur within four days of initiation or increased dose of an antipsychotic [6]. Remember to consider the role of long-acting injectable antipsychotics.
5 Known risk factors for dystonia [5–8]:
   a male sex
   b younger age (especially children and young adults)
   c recent alcohol use
   d recent cocaine use
   e prior dystonia
   f dehydration
   g hypocalcaemia.

Examination

Acute dystonia is usually focal rather than generalised. Examine for the following specific presentations.

Core muscles

- Pisa syndrome (leaning to one side).
- Opisthotonus (arching back of head and neck).
- Tortipelvis (twisting of the pelvis).
- Torticollis (twisting of the neck).
- Retrocollis (neck extension).

Eyes

- Oculogyric crisis (fixed deviation of the eyes in one direction): check eye movements.
- Blepharospasm (forced closure of eyelids).

Mouth (buccolingual crisis)

- Trismus (lockjaw, a limited range of jaw motion): can occasionally be so severe as to cause temporomandibular dislocation.
- Risus sardonicus (fixed grimace).
- Dysarthria (difficulty articulating words).
- Dysphagia (difficulty swallowing).

Larynx

- Laryngeal dystonia: look for stridor, dyspnoea and, classically, the hands grasping at the throat [4].

Sometimes a voluntary movement may temporarily reduce or abolish dystonia; this is known as a *geste antagoniste* and does not indicate a psychogenic disorder.
  Also check physical observations.

Differential diagnosis [4,5]

- Muscle contractures: gradual onset; fixed rather than intermittent often with muscle wasting.
- Catatonia: more bizarre postures; stupor (see Chapter 52).
- Hypocalcaemia: Trousseau's sign (inflating a blood pressure cuff reproduces carpopedal spasm); Chvostek's sign (tapping the facial nerve causes twitching of ipsilateral facial muscles).
- Hyperventilation-induced muscle spasm: anxiety precedes muscle contraction.
- Neuroleptic malignant syndrome: generalised rigidity (see Chapter 85).
- Focal seizure.
- Meningism.
- Functional movement disorder.
- Simulated illness (in order to obtain the euphoric effects of anticholinergic drugs).

  Specific differentials for laryngeal dystonia include the following.

- Anaphylaxis: check for rash and angioedema.
- Airway obstruction: history of foreign body ingestion, asthma, or chronic obstructive pulmonary disease.
- Laryngeal or respiratory tardive dyskinesia: much longer history of antipsychotic exposure and tardive dyskinesia almost always evident elsewhere in the body. Does not respond dramatically to anticholinergic therapy.

Investigations

In most cases, urgent treatment is required before investigations can be undertaken. Furthermore, the most helpful 'investigation' may be a therapeutic trial of an anticholinergic drug. Possible investigations include serum calcium (for hypocalcaemia) and laryngoscopy, which can confirm laryngeal dystonia.

MANAGEMENT

If there is evidence of airway compromise, patients should be managed according to the ABCDE approach and transferred to emergency services.

CHAPTER 84

First-line treatment

- Oral, intramuscular, or intravenous anticholinergic medication, depending on severity (e.g. procyclidine 5–10 mg p.o./i.m./i.v.) [5,6,9]. Intravenous treatment should have an effect within five minutes; intramuscular treatment may take 20 minutes, while oral treatment half an hour or more.
- Alternatively, some US sources suggest an intramuscular or intravenous antihistamine (e.g. diphenhydramine 1–2 mg/kg up to 100 mg by slow intravenous infusion) [5,6,9].

Second-line treatment

- Give second and, if necessary, third dose of anticholinergic at 10–30 minute intervals [5,9].
- Diazepam 5–10 mg i.v. [5,9]. (Note that parenteral benzodiazepines should be avoided in laryngeal dystonia because of the risk of respiratory depression [4].)

Subacute management

- Continue oral anticholinergic for two to seven days [6,9].
- Consider reducing dose of antipsychotic or switching to an agent with a lower propensity to cause dystonia [5].

Adverse effects of treatment

All treatments for dystonia have occasionally been reported to *cause* dystonia [9]. Anticholinergic therapy can affect mental state by worsening confusion, psychosis, and mania. Other anticholinergic side effects include tachycardia, constipation, blurred vision, dry mouth, urinary retention (see Chapter 29), and worsening of tardive dyskinesia. They are also potentially toxic in overdose.

Special patient groups

Data to support the safe use of procyclidine in pregnancy are lacking [10]. There are some limited data suggesting that promethazine (a sedative antihistamine with anticholinergic properties) is safe in this group (it is widely used for hyperemesis gravidarum), and should therefore be used first line in this group, if cautiously [11].

In lactation, the use of anticholinergics is cautioned against, but they may be given if they are considered essential and the infant monitored for anticholinergic side effects. Long-term use may interfere with lactation.

Prevention of acute dystonia

- If high-potency antipsychotics are used, start at a low dose and titrate cautiously.
- However, if prescribing haloperidol for rapid tranquillisation, give it combined with promethazine. There is evidence that this substantially reduces the risk of extrapyramidal side effects, owing to its anticholinergic properties [12–14].
- Avoid dopamine antagonist anti-emetics in patients with current antipsychotic prescriptions or in those with prior dystonia (see Chapter 21 for alternatives) [9].

References

1. Haddad PM, Das A, Keyhani S, Chaudhry IB. Antipsychotic drugs and extrapyramidal side effects in first episode psychosis: a systematic review of head-head comparisons. *J Psychopharmacol* 2012;26(5 Suppl):15–26.

2. Satterthwaite TD, Wolf DH, Rosenheck RA, et al. A meta-analysis of the risk of acute extrapyramidal symptoms with intramuscular antipsychotics for the treatment of agitation. *J Clin Psychiatry* 2008;69(12):1869–1879.

3. Dudley K, Liu X, De Haan S. Chlorpromazine dose for people with schizophrenia. *Cochrane Database Syst Rev* 2017;(4):CD007778.

4. Christodoulou C, Kalaitzi C. Antipsychotic drug-induced acute laryngeal dystonia: two case reports and a mini review. *J Psychopharmacol* 2005;19(3):307–311.

5. Raja M. Managing antipsychotic-induced acute and tardive dystonia. *Drug Saf* 1998;19(1):57–72.

6. van Harten PN, Hoek HW, Kahn RS. Acute dystonia induced by drug treatment. *BMJ* 1999;319(7210):623–626.

7. van Harten PN, van Trier JCAM, Horwitz EH, et al. Cocaine as a risk factor for neuroleptic-induced acute dystonia. *J Clin Psychiatry* 1998;59(3):128–130.

8. Keepers GA, Casey DE. Use of neuroleptic-induced extrapyramidal symptoms to predict future vulnerability to side-effects. *Am J Psychiatry* 1991;148(1):85–89.

9. Campbell D. The management of acute dystonic reactions. *Austr Prescr* 2001;24:19–20.

10. UK Teratology Information Service. Use of procyclidine in pregnancy. http://www.medicinesinpregnancy.org/bumps/monographs/USE-OF-PROCYCLIDINE-IN-PREGNANCY/

11. UK Teratology Information Service. Use of promethazine in pregnancy. http://www.medicinesinpregnancy.org/bumps/monographs/USE-OF-PROMETHAZINE-IN-PREGNANCY/

12. Barnes TRE, Schizophrenia Consensus Group of British Association for Psychopharmacology. Evidence-based guidelines for the pharmacological treatment of schizophrenia: recommendations from the British Association for Psychopharmacology. *J Psychopharmacol* 2011;25(5):567–620.

13. Ostinelli EG, Brooke-Powney MJ, Li X, Adams CE. Haloperidol for psychosis-induced aggression or agitation (rapid tranquillisation). *Cochrane Database Syst Rev* 2017;(7):CD009377.

14. Huf G, Coutinho ES, Adams CE. Rapid tranquillisation in psychiatric emergency settings in Brazil: pragmatic randomised controlled trial of intramuscular haloperidol versus intramuscular haloperidol plus promethazine. *BMJ* 2007;335(7625):869.

Neuroleptic Malignant Syndrome

Robert A. McCutcheon, James Kelly, Toby Pillinger

Neuroleptic malignant syndrome (NMS) is characterised by muscular rigidity, hyperthermia, altered consciousness, and autonomic dysfunction following exposure to an antipsychotic, and may be life-threatening. It is rare, occurring in approximately 1% of those treated with first-generation antipsychotics [1,2] but also in those treated with second-generation drugs [3]. In addition, there have been reports of NMS following treatment with other medications, including valproate, lithium, and antidepressants [4–6]. Although typically considered to be an acute syndrome, the presentation of NMS is heterogeneous, with the acute syndrome likely presenting as the 'tip of the iceberg' of a range of non-malignant-related symptoms [7].

DIAGNOSTIC PRINCIPLES

History

- Risk factors: male gender [8], comorbid organic brain disease, alcoholism, Parkinson's disease, hyperthyroidism. While younger age is a risk factor for NMS, older age is associated with increased mortality [8].
- Has the patient had a recent increase [9] or decrease [10] in antipsychotic dose? Has a high-potency first-generation antipsychotic been used? Is there antipsychotic polypharmacy?
- Determine if anticholinergics have recently been stopped [11].
- The combination of antipsychotics and selective serotonin reuptake inhibitors (SSRIs) has been linked to an increased risk of NMS [12].

The Maudsley Practice Guidelines for Physical Health Conditions in Psychiatry, First Edition.
David M. Taylor, Fiona Gaughran, and Toby Pillinger.
© 2021 John Wiley & Sons Ltd. Published 2021 by John Wiley & Sons Ltd.

■ NMS also occurs more frequently in those who are confused, agitated, or exhausted [9,13]. It is also more common in those who are dehydrated, although whether this is a cause or consequence of the syndrome is unclear [14].

Examination

■ Basic observations: signs suggestive of NMS include tachycardia, fluctuating blood pressure, and fever.
■ Other physical signs may include rigidity, tremor, dysphagia, profuse sweating, and incontinence.
■ The patient may be confused, or have a fluctuating level of consciousness.

Investigations

Blood tests may demonstrate raised plasma creatine kinase, leucocytosis, and deranged liver function.

Differential diagnoses

■ Catatonia (see Chapter 52).
■ Serotonin syndrome (see Chapter 86): not typically associated with altered white cell count or elevated plasma creatine kinase.
■ Anticholinergic syndrome: typically secondary to accidental/deliberate overdose of medication with anticholinergic action, characterised by fever, flushed skin, mydriasis (dilated pupils), dry mouth and eyes, decreased sweating, delirium, and urinary retention.
■ Heat stroke: headache, dizziness/confusion, loss of appetite, excessive sweating, abdominal cramps, tachycardia, fever, thirst.

MANAGEMENT

NMS is a medical emergency: referral to a general medical hospital should be made *immediately* if suspected.

Acute

In psychiatric unit

Arrange transfer to general hospital immediately, and continue to monitor physical observations while awaiting transfer. Cease all dopamine antagonists. Consider benzodiazepines (intramuscular lorazepam has been used) [15].

In general-medical/emergency setting

Initiate aggressive supportive therapy, focusing on immediately stopping the offending agent, giving intravenous fluids targeted to normotension and normal heart rate, and cooling via forced air and circulating water initially, and via ice packs, cooled fluids or peritoneal lavage if needed. Early consideration should be given to an intensive care referral for intensive monitoring with regard to hyperthermia greater than 41.1°C, severe acidosis, rhabdomyolysis causing acute renal failure not responding to forced diuresis and urinary alkalinisation, and acute respiratory failure requiring ventilatory support. Specific therapies should be initiated in a stepwise manner, depending on severity. Mild cases can be treated with benzodiazepines alone, with more severe cases treated with dopamine agonists such as bromocriptine, amantadine, and levodopa. Dantrolene monotherapy is no longer advocated due to an association with higher mortality rates, but can be added as an adjunct to dopamine agonists. Electroconvulsive therapy has a role in severe cases, where antipsychotics cannot be withdrawn, and where it is difficult to distinguish between malignant catatonia and NMS.

Following symptomatic resolution

- Antipsychotics should be stopped for a minimum of five days and all symptoms of NMS should have resolved prior to attempting to restart antipsychotic treatment.
- Initial doses should be very small with concomitant close monitoring of physical observations. It remains unclear whether close monitoring of creatine kinase during re-titration is of benefit [16].
- It may be that drugs with low affinity for the D2 dopamine receptor, such as quetiapine and clozapine, are of lower risk.
- Long-acting injectable and high-potency first-generation antipsychotics should be avoided.

References

1. Keck PE, Pope HG, McElroy SL. Frequency and presentation of neuroleptic malignant syndrome: a prospective study. *Am J Psychiatry* 1987;144:1344–1346.
2. Pope HG, Keck PE, McElroy SL. Frequency and presentation of neuroleptic malignant syndrome in a large psychiatric hospital. *Am J Psychiatry* 1986;143:1227–1233.
3. Belvederi Murri M, Guaglianone A, Bugliani M, et al. Second-generation antipsychotics and neuroleptic malignant syndrome: systematic review and case report analysis. *Drugs R D* 2015;15:45–62.
4. Verma R, Junewar V, Rathaur BPS. An atypical case of neuroleptic malignant syndrome precipitated by valproate. *BMJ Case Rep* ss;2014:bcr2013202578.
5. Halman M, Goldbloom DS. Fluoxetine and neuroleptic malignant syndrome. *Biol Psychiatry* 1990;28:518–521.
6. Gill J, Singh H, Nugent K. Acute lithium intoxication and neuroleptic malignant syndrome. *Pharmacotherapy* 2003;23:811–815.
7. Bristow MF, Kohen D. How 'malignant' is the neuroleptic malignant syndrome? *BMJ* 1993;307:1223–1224.
8. Gurrera RJ. A systematic review of sex and age factors in neuroleptic malignant syndrome diagnosis frequency. *Acta Psychiatr Scand* 2017;135:398–408.
9. Viejo LF, Morales V, Puñal P, et al. Risk factors in neuroleptic malignant syndrome. A case-control study. *Acta Psychiatr Scand* 2003;107:45–49.
10. Spivak B, Weizman A, Wolovick L, et al. Neuroleptic malignant syndrome during abrupt reduction of neuroleptic treatment. *Acta Psychiatr Scand* 1990;81:168–169.
11. Spivak B, Gonen N, Averbuch E, et al. Neuroleptic malignant syndrome associated with abrupt withdrawal of anticholinergic agents. *Int Clin Psychopharmacol* 1996;11:207–209.
12. Stevens DL. Association between selective serotonin-reuptake inhibitors, second-generation antipsychotics, and neuroleptic malignant syndrome. *Ann Pharmacother* 2008;42:1290–1297.
13. Berardi D, Amore M, Keck PE, et al. Clinical and pharmacologic risk factors for neuroleptic malignant syndrome: a case-control study. *Biol Psychiatry* 1998;44:748–754.
14. Gurrera RJ. Diaphoresis and dehydration during neuroleptic malignant syndrome: preliminary findings. *Psychiatry Res* 1996;64:137–145.
15. Francis A, Chandragiri S, Rizvi S, et al. Is lorazepam a treatment for neuroleptic malignant syndrome? *CNS Spectr* 2000;5:54–57.
16. Hermesh H, Manor I, Shiloh R, et al. High serum creatinine kinase level: possible risk factor for neuroleptic malignant syndrome. *J Clin Psychopharmacol* 2002;22:252–256.

CHAPTER 85

Serotonin Syndrome

Robert A. McCutcheon, James Kelly, Toby Pillinger

Serotonin syndrome (SS), a life-threatening acute reaction to serotonergic drugs, is most frequently observed in cases of antidepressant overdose and in cases where individuals are prescribed multiple medications with serotonergic actions. Monoamine oxidase inhibitor (MAOIs) have been associated with the condition, particularly in cases where they are used in combination with other serotonergic medication. However, cases have been observed after a single dose of a selective serotonin reuptake inhibitor (SSRI) [1]. Most cases present within six hours of initial use, following overdose, or after a change in dosing of medication [2].

The onset of the syndrome is normally rapid. SS shares a number of signs and symptoms with neuroleptic malignant syndrome (NMS), and as such differentiating from NMS may be difficult. However, in contrast to NMS, SS can present with hyperreflexia and mydriasis (dilated pupils), and on blood testing white cell counts and creatine kinase levels are typically within the normal range.

DIAGNOSTIC PRINCIPLES

History

- Has the patient commenced any new medications or switched antidepressants? Combination antidepressant treatment, particularly with an MAOI, is a potential cause of serotonin syndrome.
- Recent insomnia, anxiety, agitation, or confusion.

Examination

- Tremor, clonus, and agitation in the absence of extrapyramidal signs should make the clinician consider serotonin syndrome. The diagnosis can be complicated by the fact that rigidity can occur and mask clonus and hyperreflexia.
- Mild signs and symptoms: insomnia, anxiety, hypertension, tachycardia, hyperactive reflexes (greater in lower compared to upper limbs), diarrhoea, hyperactive bowel sounds, mild fever (<38.5°C).
- Moderate signs and symptoms: clonus (spontaneous, ocular or inducible), tremor, flushing, dilated pupils, profuse sweating, increasing fever (<40°C).
- Severe signs and symptoms: severe hyperthermia (fever of 41°C or above), severe hypertension (≥180/≥110 mmHg; see Chapter 71), rigidity, respiratory failure [3].

Investigations

Creatine kinase and white cell counts may be normal in early stages, although creatine kinase may ultimately increase secondary to hyperthermia.

Differential diagnoses

- Catatonia (see Chapter 52).
- Neuroleptic malignant syndrome (see Chapter 85): more likely to be associated with leucocytosis or elevated plasma creatine kinase.
- Anticholinergic syndrome: typically secondary to accidental/deliberate overdose of medication with anticholinergic action, and characterised by fever, flushed skin, mydriasis (dilated pupils), dry mouth and eyes, decreased sweating, delirium, and urinary retention.
- Heat stroke: headache, dizziness/confusion, loss of appetite, excessive sweating, abdominal cramps, tachycardia, fever, thirst.

CHAPTER 86

MANAGEMENT

Serotonin syndrome is a medical emergency: referral to a general medical hospital should be made *immediately* if suspected.

Acute

In psychiatric unit

Arrange transfer to general hospital immediately, and continue to monitor physical observations while awaiting transfer. Stop all serotonergic agonists. Consider benzo-diazepines (e.g. lorazepam) for the treatment of agitation and to reduce muscular rigidity.

In general-medical/emergency setting

Initiate aggressive supportive therapy, focusing on immediately stopping the offending agent, giving intravenous fluids targeted to normotension and normal heart rate, and cooling via ice packs, cooled fluids, or peritoneal lavage if needed. Early consideration should be given to an intensive care referral for intensive monitoring of hyperthermia greater than 41.1°C, severe acidosis, rhabdomyolysis causing acute renal failure not responding to forced diuresis and urinary alkalinisation, and acute respiratory failure requiring ventilatory support. Benzodiazepines may be used for agitation/muscular rigidity. The serotonergic antagonist cyproheptadine, or an antipsychotic with antagonist properties (e.g. olanzapine), may be considered though evidence is weak [4,5]. Moreover, prescribing an antipsychotic for presumed SS when in fact NMS is causative will have inevitable negative clinical consequences. Dantrolene, a skeletal muscle relaxant used for treatment of NMS, has been reported to improve symptoms of SS in a case series [6], but it has also been implicated in the development of serotonin toxicity and is generally not recommended [3]. In severe cases anaesthesia and artificial ventilation may be required.

Following symptomatic resolution

Following resolution of symptoms, a careful medication review should be undertaken to identify what caused the development of SS and how this can be avoided in future.

References

1. Gill M, LoVecchio F, Selden B. Serotonin syndrome in a child after a single dose of fluvoxamine. *Ann Emerg Med* 1999;33:457–459.
2. Mason PJ, Morris VA, Balcezak TJ. Serotonin syndrome. Presentation of 2 cases and review of the literature. *Medicine (Baltimore)* 2000;79:201–209.
3. Boyer EEW, Shannon M. The serotonin syndrome. *N Engl J Med* 1991;352:1112–1120.
4. Graudins A, Stearman A, Chan B. Treatment of the serotonin syndrome with cyproheptadine. *J Emerg Med* 1998;16:615–619.
5. Boddy R, Ali R, Dowsett R. Use of sublingual olanzapine in serotonin syndrome. *J Toxicol Clin Toxicol* 2004;42:725.
6. Nisijima K, Ishiguro T. Does dantrolene influence central dopamine and serotonin metabolism in the neuroleptic malignant syndrome? A retrospective study. *Biol Psychiatry* 1993;33:45–48.

Emergencies in Obstetrics and Gynaecology

Hanine Fourie, Ruth Cochrane

Emergencies in obstetrics and gynaecology are clinical situations where urgent treatment is necessary to save the life of the woman, the life of her fetus, or the woman's future fertility. In the UK, 9 in 100,000 pregnant women die from conditions directly related to pregnancy, such as suicide, pre-eclampsia, genitourinary sepsis, and haemorrhage, or indirect conditions such as cardiac disease [1]. In sub-Saharan Africa, a woman's life-time risk of dying as a result of pregnancy and childbirth is 100 times higher [2]. Poor-quality and inaccessible pregnancy care are universal barriers to ensuring maternal safety. In regular reports on maternal and perinatal mortality, MBRRACE-UK (Mothers and Babies: Reducing Risk through Audits and Confidential Enquiries across the UK) has identified that early and forward planning of maternity care in vulnerable women may reduce the risk of complications. This sentiment is shared globally, with the UN Sustainable Development Goal 3 aiming to reduce maternal mortality through better access to healthcare [3].

Women with serious mental illness are vulnerable and at greater risk of an emergency in obstetrics and gynaecology for many complex reasons, including poor access to healthcare and increased medical comorbidity. One of the reasons for delayed access to healthcare in these patients is due to higher rates of unplanned and unwanted pregnancy. This associates with unsafe abortion practices, single parenthood, drug and/or alcohol dependence, and omission of antenatal supplements such as folic acid [4,5]. Medical comorbidity in women with serious mental illness also increases the risk of these emergencies. For example, there is a strong association between sexually trans-mitted infections, which women with significant mental illness are at greater risk of [6], and ectopic pregnancy and pelvic inflammatory disease. Therefore, it is important for psychiatrists to be aware of emergencies in obstetrics and gynaecology as they can be prevented through multidisciplinary planning, and early recognition of these condi-tions. This chapter focuses on the following emergencies: maternal collapse, pre-eclampsia,

The Maudsley Practice Guidelines for Physical Health Conditions in Psychiatry, First Edition.
David M. Taylor, Fiona Gaughran, and Toby Pillinger.
© 2021 John Wiley & Sons Ltd. Published 2021 by John Wiley & Sons Ltd.

major obstetric haemorrhage, ectopic pregnancy, miscarriage, hyperemesis gravidarum, ovarian cyst accidents, and pelvic inflammatory disease (Box 87.1).

Specialists in obstetrics and gynaecology have dual training but hospital services often separate the two. As such, non-pregnant women with problems related to their reproductive organs, and women in the early stages of pregnancy are generally managed by gynaecology services, while women in the later stages of pregnancy are generally managed by obstetric services. When making referrals, it is recommended to check with your local obstetrics and gynaecology service to determine to which subspecialty a referral should be directed.

Box 87.1 Important emergencies in obstetrics and gynaecology

Obstetrics

Maternal collapse

Non-pregnancy-specific causes
- Venous thromboembolism
- Acute coronary syndrome
- Sepsis

Pregnancy-specific causes
- Complications from pre-eclampsia
- Major obstetric haemorrhage
- Amniotic fluid embolism

Emergencies related to the fetus (beyond scope of this chapter)

- For example, intrauterine death, cord prolapse, and shoulder dystocia

Gynaecology

Early pregnancy

- Ectopic pregnancy
- Miscarriage
- Hyperemesis gravidarum

Ovarian cyst accidents

- Torsion
- Rupture

Pelvic inflammatory disease

Bleeding secondary to

- Malignancy
- Structural abnormality of genital tract
- Dysfunctional uterine bleeding

MATERNAL COLLAPSE

Maternal collapse describes when a pregnant woman, or a mother within six weeks of delivery, loses consciousness due to an acute cardiac, pulmonary, or neurological event. As shown in Box 87.1, causes of maternal collapse are often non-specific to pregnancy. For example, venous thromboembolism is the leading cause of maternal mortality [1]. Cardiac disease and sepsis are other common causes of maternal collapse. The reader is directed to Chapters 18, 69 and 72, respectively, for more information on venous thromboembolism and anticoagulation, acute coronary syndrome, and sepsis. Pregnancy-specific causes of maternal collapse include pre-eclampsia, major obstetric haemorrhage, and amniotic fluid embolism.

The mother should always remain the priority in the management of collapse: the fetus is, after all, dependent on maternal placental perfusion. Nonetheless, consideration needs to be given to the unborn child. The threshold of fetal viability is 24 weeks of gestation, or 'six months' as is often reported by the patient. Babies born prior to 24 weeks will (almost) never be resuscitated; if a baby is born dead before 24 weeks, this unfortunate event is considered a miscarriage. Maternal cardiac arrest after 20 weeks will require urgent delivery of the baby to facilitate maternal resuscitation, since the gravid uterus impacts resuscitation efforts through vascular compression. The obstetrician will carry out what is known as a peri-mortem Caesarean section. Pregnant women should be resuscitated according to the ABCDE approach. However, the physiological and physical changes of pregnancy require adaptations to standard resuscitation, as shown in Table 87.1.

PRE-ECLAMPSIA

Pre-eclampsia is a condition that develops after 20 weeks of pregnancy in about 5% of pregnant women [7]. It is characterised by proteinuria ($\geq$1+ protein on urine dipstick, quantified with a protein/creatinine ratio >30 mg/mmol), and hypertension. The condition carries maternal risks such as eclampsia, HELLP (haemolysis, elevated liver enzymes, low platelets) syndrome , stroke, pulmonary oedema, and fetal risks such as fetal growth restriction and placental abruption.

Progression to eclampsia, pulmonary oedema, and stroke can cause maternal collapse. Eclampsia is defined as convulsions in pregnancy or within 10 days post-partum, with two out of four of the following features: hypertension, proteinuria, low platelets ($<100 \times 10^9$/L), and raised alanine aminotransferase (ALT) levels (>42 IU/L) [8].

Administration of intravenous magnesium sulfate ($MgSO_4$) to women with severe pre-eclampsia can halve the incidence of eclampsia [8]. Therefore, early recognition of pre-eclampsia is important. Most women diagnosed with pre-eclampsia are managed as inpatients until delivery to allow for strict blood pressure monitoring, fetal monitoring, and pre-emptive treatment with $MgSO_4$ as appropriate.

CHAPTER 87

Table 87.1 Adaptations to resuscitation techniques in the context of pregnancy.

Feature of pregnancy	Adaptation
Airway	
Pregnant women are at high risk of aspiration due to: ■ Decreased gastric motility ■ Relaxed lower oesophageal sphincter ■ Increased weight	Early involvement of the anaesthetic team in resuscitation of a pregnant woman is crucial. Early intubation with a tracheal tube avoids aspiration and facilitates efficient ventilation. In a psychiatric setting this will often simply involve ensuring that emergency services are contacted early
Breathing	
Pregnant women are at high risk of hypoxia as: ■ The gravid uterus splints the diaphragm and reduces residual lung capacity ■ The fetoplacental unit increases oxygen demand by 20%	Supplemental oxygen should always be administered in the event of maternal collapse to mitigate the risk of hypoxia
Circulation	
Aorto-caval compression: ■ Uterine blood flow accounts for 10% of cardiac output ■ The gravid uterus, after 20 weeks' gestation, compresses the inferior vena cava and the abdominal aorta when the woman is supine ■ This reduces cardiac output, mainly by limiting venous return to the heart	The patient should be positioned tilted to the left. This may be achieved in hospital with a wedge, or outside of hospital by manual displacement of the uterus, or by a person kneeling under the patient's thorax In the event of cardiopulmonary arrest, chest compressions should be commenced without delay, prior to checking for a pulse. If no response after four minutes of CPR, preparation should be made for a peri-mortem Caesarean section to improve venous return, cardiac output, and ventilation

Risk factors

- Previous pre-eclampsia.
- Chronic hypertension or a high blood pressure at first clinical review after becoming pregnant (women tend to have low blood pressure in the first trimester due to vasodilatation).
- Chronic kidney disease.
- More subtle risk factors include nulliparity, maternal age over 40 years, interpregnancy interval of 10 years or more, body mass index over 35, family history of pre-eclampsia, and twin pregnancies.

Symptoms and signs

- Headaches and visual disturbance can be symptomatic of the hypertension associated with pre-eclampsia.
- Oedema due to proteinuria and increased vascular permeability. Most pregnant women report increased swelling of the hands and feet, especially in the third trimester, and therefore oedema is a sensitive but not specific symptom. Facial and periorbital oedema is characteristic.

- Right upper quadrant pain can be present and is suggestive of liver oedema or a subcapsular haematoma.
- Brisk patellar reflexes and clonus are signs of neuromuscular irritability.

Management

- Pre-eclampsia is a disease thought to originate from the placenta, and therefore delivery of the baby and placenta marks the start of convalescence (not cure, as characteristically patients will have a spike in blood pressure on day 4 after birth). The onset is commonly around term (37–42 weeks of pregnancy) and therefore the threshold to deliver as part of treatment is low. However, early-onset pre-eclampsia is difficult to manage and often results in iatrogenic premature delivery.
- Stringent blood pressure control improves maternal and fetal outcomes.
- Intravenous $MgSO_4$ reduces risk of progression to eclampsia.
- Fetal monitoring is important as pre-eclampsia is associated with fetal growth restriction. Fetal distress or growth restriction may necessitate delivery of the baby.

MAJOR OBSTETRIC HAEMORRHAGE

There is no universally agreed definition of major obstetric haemorrhage (MOH), but blood loss over 1500 mL is a common cut-off. Pregnant women are good at compensating for blood loss, for example the pregnant blood volume increases by almost 50%. Early recognition, although difficult due to these compensatory mechanisms, is key to preventing catastrophe. Causes of MOH include abnormally invasive placenta or placenta accreta where the placenta grows into the uterine wall, placenta praevia (low-lying placenta), placental abruption, and uterine rupture. Early identification of women at risk of MOH facilitates antenatal optimisation and safe delivery on a labour ward. A multidisciplinary approach is central to management, involving senior midwives, anaesthetists, obstetricians, haematologists, blood bank staff, and porters. Early identification of bleeding is also key. Since MOH occurs in the context of delivery it is unlikely to occur in a psychiatric setting, and therefore specific management is not discussed in this chapter.

AMNIOTIC FLUID EMBOLISM

Amniotic fluid embolism is a rare catastrophic obstetric emergency where amniotic fluid or fetal tissue enters the maternal circulation. Since it occurs in the context of delivery it is unlikely to occur in a psychiatric setting, and therefore specific management is not discussed in this chapter.

ECTOPIC PREGNANCY

Ectopic pregnancy is any pregnancy that has implanted outside of the uterine cavity, and occurs in about 1 in 100 pregnancies [9]. It is the most important pathology to exclude in women presenting with abdominal pain, abnormal vaginal bleeding, or syncope when between six and ten weeks of pregnancy, as tubal ectopic pregnancy may rupture the fallopian tube, resulting in significant intra-abdominal bleeding. Although rare, it remains the leading cause of mortality of pregnant women in the first trimester [9]. Therefore, there is an emphasis on early recognition of these pregnancies. It is important to assume that all women are pregnant until proved otherwise, so any woman between the ages of 12 and 55 presenting with pain or bleeding should have a pregnancy test.

Risk factors

- Previous ectopic pregnancy (10-fold increase in risk) [10].
- Fallopian tube damage:
  - smoking
  - history of *Chlamydia* or pelvic inflammatory disease (PID)
  - endometriosis
  - previous tubal or pelvic surgery.
- Contraceptive failure, e.g. intrauterine contraceptive device.
- Increasing age.

Signs and symptoms

Women with an ectopic pregnancy may be asymptomatic, but the following symptoms, in conjunction with a positive pregnancy test, should raise suspicion.

- Pain:
  - lower abdomen, often unilateral
  - in tubal rupture, referred pain to the shoulder tip due to diaphragmatic irritation.
- Vaginal bleeding: usually light persistent bleeding.
- Diarrhoea.
- Change in basic observations: young women can compensate for blood loss, and therefore subtle changes in basic observations, such as tachycardia, should be taken seriously.
- Syncope, and evidence of haemodynamic shock, in the event of tubal rupture.

Investigations

In a psychiatric inpatient setting where the patient is haemodynamically stable but ectopic pregnancy is a differential diagnosis, a urine pregnancy test or serum β-human chorionic gonadotrophin (β-hCG) should be performed. If this is test is not available, the patient will require assessment in the emergency department. In an emergency setting and once under the care of gynaecology services, transvaginal ultrasound scan may be used to identify ectopic or intrauterine pregnancy.

Management

A ruptured ectopic pregnancy requires immediate and urgent fluid resuscitation. The patient should be transferred to an environment where this can be achieved. In a psychiatric setting, this may simply involve providing ABC emergency care and ensuring the patient is transferred as an emergency to an acute hospital with on-site gynaecology and anaesthetic services to facilitate surgical management.

Surgical management of ectopic pregnancy usually involves laparoscopic salpingectomy where the tubal ectopic pregnancy is removed with the fallopian tube. The contralateral tube will still support future fertility, and conception may occur with oocytes from either ovary.

Medical and conservative management of ectopic pregnancy requires a motivated patient who is willing and able to attend an early pregnancy unit for follow-up, as it may take weeks for resolution. A single dose of intramuscular methotrexate is administered as medical management of the ectopic pregnancy. Methotrexate stops the pregnancy from developing any further, which is gradually reabsorbed by the body. The success of treatment is determined by a falling β-hCG on day 7 following administration, and patients often have ongoing weekly follow-up until the β-hCG is negative.

If the β-hCG trend is downward and the patient is clinically well, they can be offered expectant ('watchful waiting') management. They will require follow-up until β-hCG levels are undetectable.

MISCARRIAGE

Miscarriage is the most common complication of pregnancy, with a commonly quoted incidence of one in four pregnancies, but with a significant age-related increase to one in two pregnancies in women over the age of 40 [11].

Types of miscarriage

- Missed miscarriage: an ultrasound diagnosis where an empty large gestational sac, or fetal pole with no heartbeat, is located in the uterine cavity.
- Threatened miscarriage: vaginal bleeding and/or abdominal pain, where clinically the cervix is closed, and on ultrasound scan a fetal heartbeat is still visualised.
- Inevitable miscarriage: vaginal bleeding and/or abdominal pain, where the cervix is open on clinical examination, but the gestational sac remains present in the uterus.
- Incomplete miscarriage: the cervix is open, but only part of the pregnancy has passed.
- Complete miscarriage: a diagnosis based on ultrasound findings, where the uterine cavity is empty following a pregnancy loss.

Risk factors

- Increasing age.
- Being underweight or overweight.
- Alcohol consumption [12].
- Infection, such as malaria, cytomegalovirus, and bacterial vaginosis [13].
- Use of teratogenic drugs such as sodium valproate.
- Cervical incompetence in second-trimester miscarriages.

CHAPTER 87

Symptoms and diagnosis

Miscarriage may be asymptomatic (missed miscarriage), with diagnosis only made at the time of ultrasound surveillance. In the developed world, this only routinely happens at 11–14 weeks of gestation, during the routine first-trimester ultrasound scan. When symptomatic, patients may present with bleeding, lower abdominal pain, or loss of previously recognised pregnancy symptoms (e.g. nausea or breast tenderness). Definitive diagnosis is then made via ultrasound.

Management

If the patient is haemodynamically stable, and no signs of infection are present, the patient may opt to manage the pregnancy loss expectantly. Pelvic ultrasound is usually offered after 10–14 days to ensure completion. In the event of a missed miscarriage, medical management with per vaginal misoprostol, a prostaglandin analogue, can be offered. In the second trimester, this is preceded with a single dose of mifepristone, a progesterone antagonist. Medical and surgical management for first-trimester miscarriage are comparable in terms of effectiveness and their side-effect profile [14]. Surgical management involves dilatation of the cervix and suction evacuation. Although usually performed under general anaesthesia, it can also be performed under local anaesthesia.

Pregnancy loss is known to have a significant emotional impact on patients and their partners. Symptoms of depression and anxiety are common following pregnancy loss [15]. The Miscarriage Association is a valuable resource for patients (www.miscarriageassociation. org.uk.).

HYPEREMESIS GRAVIDARUM

Although nausea and vomiting affects a large proportion of pregnant women, hyperemesis gravidarum only affects about 1% of pregnancies, and is associated with protracted vomiting, electrolyte disturbance, and dehydration [16]. These women require hospital admission for rehydration, and anti-emetics. They also require vitamin B_1 replacement to prevent the rare complication of Wernicke's encephalopathy. Hospital protocols differ, but an inpatient prescription will usually include the following.

- Intravenous fluids.
- Thiamine supplementation.
- Anti-emetics (women need reassurance that these are safe in pregnancy):
  - intravenous cyclizine/metoclopramide
  - plus or minus intravenous ondansetron
  - promethazine may be considered in patients already receiving treatment with a dopamine antagonist.
- Steroids can be considered for refractory vomiting.
- Low-molecular-weight heparin prophylaxis for venous thromboembolism.

OVARIAN CYST ACCIDENTS

Most ovarian cysts are benign, especially in premenopausal women. Benign ovarian cysts include cystadenomas (simple cysts), mature teratomas (dermoid cysts), endometriomas (chocolate cysts), and functional cysts such as a corpus luteum. Ovarian cyst accidents occur in about 0.2% of women with cysts, and include cyst rupture and ovarian torsion [17]. Both of these accidents present with severe lower abdominal pain. It is important to distinguish between the two, as in cyst rupture conservative management with analgesia may suffice, whereas in the event of ovarian torsion urgent surgical management is required to preserve the ovary. When in doubt, referral for emergency obstetric and gynaecology review is recommended.

Ovarian cyst rupture

Risk factors

- Known ovarian cyst: simple cysts are more likely to rupture but dermoid cysts can also rupture, causing chemical peritonitis with the release of intraperitoneal sebaceous content.
- Strenuous activity, sexual intercourse, and exercise.

Symptoms

Abdominal/pelvic pain that is unilateral, severe, sudden in onset, and sometimes provoked by strenuous activity.

Investigations

- Transvaginal ultrasound may demonstrate free fluid and collapsed ovarian cyst. It is also useful for excluding other pathologies such as ectopic pregnancy, tubo-ovarian abscess, and appendicitis.
- Urinary pregnancy test to exclude ectopic pregnancy.

Management

- May only require conservative management with analgesia.
- In the event of rupture of a mature teratoma/dermoid cyst, chemical peritonitis ensues that requires emergency surgery to perform peritoneal irrigation and ovarian cystectomy.
- Ovarian cyst rupture may be associated with haemorrhage, which may be significant. If there is a significant volume of free fluid on transvaginal ultrasound and/or if the patient is haemodynamically unstable, ovarian cystectomy may be required to control the bleeding.

CHAPTER 87

Ovarian torsion

Ovarian torsion is when the ovary twists on its pedicle, which contains the ovarian vessels. The interruption of the arterial supply means the ovary becomes ischaemic and eventually necrotic if not untwisted (sometimes spontaneously, but more commonly surgically). The interruption of venous return means the ovary becomes swollen, a diagnostic feature on ultrasound.

Risk factors

- Enlarged ovary secondary to:
  - ovarian cysts greater than 5 cm (except endometriomas, which are often adherent to the pelvic side wall and therefore relatively immobilised)
  - ovarian hyperstimulation syndrome in the context of *in vitro* fertilisation (IVF).
- Pregnancy.

Symptoms

- Acute lower abdominal or lumbar pain of less than eight hours in duration. The pain is usually unilateral. Pain can also be intermittent, which may represent spontaneous untwisting of an enlarged ovary.
- Nausea and vomiting are present in up to 85% of cases [18].

Investigations

- Ultrasound:
  - Enlarged ovary with peripherally located follicles and an ill-defined border suggests oedema and central necrosis.
  - Absence of Doppler flow to the ovary is a late sign but specific for torsion.
  - The twisted ovarian pedicle can appear as a vascular mass with venous and arterial flow, described as the 'whirlpool' sign.
- MRI in pregnant women in the second or third trimester.
- Blood markers are non-specific, but C-reactive protein or white blood cell count may be raised.
- Direct visualisation through diagnostic laparoscopy.

Management

- Urgent surgical management is indicated in cases of suspected torsion as delayed action can lead to necrosis of the ovary and reduced ovarian function.
- Detorsion of the ovary via a laparoscopic approach is now the preferred surgical procedure and reperfusion of the ovary is achievable even when it appears ischaemic on initial views. Previous surgical practice of oophorectomy is now rarely needed.
- If an ovarian cyst is present, the recommendation is to perform an interval ovarian cystectomy at least two weeks after the detorsion to prevent recurrence.

PELVIC INFLAMMATORY DISEASE

Pelvic inflammatory disease (PID) is an ascending infection through the endocervix, causing inflammation of the endometrium, fallopian tubes, and/or ovaries. Mostly sexually transmitted, *Chlamydia trachomatis* and *Neisseria gonorrhoeae* are common pathogens, although anaerobes and *Mycoplasma genitalium* are also implicated (see Chapter 38). PID can also be caused by insertion of an intrauterine contraceptive device or following surgery such as termination of pregnancy. Prompt recognition and treatment of PID is important as it carries potentially devastating sequelae if left untreated, including infertility, ectopic pregnancy, and chronic pelvic pain.

Symptoms

PID typically presents with lower abdominal pain, and there may also be vaginal, often purulent, discharge and abnormal vaginal bleeding. The patient may be feverish, and on examination there may be diffuse abdominal tenderness and cervical motion tenderness on bimanual examination.

Investigations

Management will be by either the gynaecology or genitourinary medicine team, dictated by local hospital policy.

- Speculum examination and vaginal swabs:
  - high vaginal swab
  - endocervical swab for *Chlamydia* and gonococcus nucleic acid amplification test
  - endocervical swab for gonococcal culture.
- Transvaginal ultrasound: screen for presence of a tubo-ovarian abscess (a sign of severe disease).
- Venous blood tests for inflammatory markers.
- Urine/serum β-hCG to rule out ectopic pregnancy.

Management

Inpatient management should be offered if the patient is systemically unwell (e.g. febrile with evidence of peritonitis). Antibiotic agents should cover common causative pathogens: chlamydia, gonorrhoea, and anaerobes. A typical outpatient antibiotic regimen may include a single dose of intramuscular ceftriaxone 500 mg followed by 14 days of oral doxycycline 10 mg twice daily and metronidazole 400 mg three times daily.

References

1. Knight M, Bunch K, Tuffnell D, et al. (eds) *Saving Lives, Improving Mothers' Care. Lessons learned to inform maternity care from the UK and Ireland Confidential Enquiries into Maternal Deaths and Morbidity* 2014–16. Oxford: National Perinatal Epidemiology Unit, University of Oxford, 2018.
2. Koblinsky M, Moyer CA, Calvert C, et al. Quality maternity care for every woman, everywhere: a call to action. *Lancet* 2016;388(10057):2307–2320.

CHAPTER 87

3. UN General Assembly. Transforming our world: the 2030 Agenda for Sustainable Development, 21 October 2015, A/RES/70/1. https://www.refworld.org/docid/57b6e3e44.html (accessed 5 December 2019).

4. Goossens J, Van Den Branden Y, Van der Sluys L, et al. The prevalence of unplanned pregnancy ending in birth, associated factors, and health outcomes. *Hum Reprod* 2016;31(12):2821–2833.

5. Hall JA, Barrett G, Phiri T, et al. Prevalence and determinants of unintended pregnancy in Mchinji District, Malawi; using a conceptual hierarchy to inform analysis. *PLoS One* 2016;11(10):e0165621.

6. Huang SY, Hung JH, Hu LY, et al. Risk of sexually transmitted infections following depressive disorder: a nationwide population-based cohort study. *Medicine* 2018;97(43):e12539.

7. Abalos E, Cuesta C, Grosso AL, et al. Global and regional estimates of preeclampsia and eclampsia: a systematic review. *Eur J Obstet Gynecol Reprod Biol* 2013;170(1):1–7.

8. Knight M. Eclampsia in the United Kingdom 2005. *BJOG* 2007;114(9):1072–1078.

9. Cantwell R, Clutton-Brock T, Cooper G, et al. Saving Mothers' Lives: Reviewing maternal deaths to make motherhood safer: 2006–2008. The Eighth Report of the Confidential Enquiries into Maternal Deaths in the United Kingdom. *BJOG* 2011;118(Suppl 1):1–203.

10. Barnhart KT, Sammel MD, Gracia CR, et al. Risk factors for ectopic pregnancy in women with symptomatic first-trimester pregnancies. *Fert Steril* 2006;86(1):36–43.

11. Magnus MC, Wilcox AJ, Morken N-H, et al. Role of maternal age and pregnancy history in risk of miscarriage: prospective register based study. *BMJ* 2019;364:l869.

12. Feodor Nilsson S, Andersen PK, Strandberg-Larsen K, Nybo Andersen AM. Risk factors for miscarriage from a prevention perspective: a nationwide follow-up study. *BJOG* 2014;121(11):1375–1385.

13. Giakoumelou S, Wheelhouse N, Cuschieri K, et al. The role of infection in miscarriage. *Hum Reprod Update* 2016;22(1):116–133.

14. Al-Wattar BH, Murugesu N, Tobias A, et al. Management of first-trimester miscarriage: a systematic review and network meta-analysis. *Hum Reprod Update* 2019;25(3):362–374.

15. Farren J, Jalmbrant M, Ameye L, et al. Post-traumatic stress, anxiety and depression following miscarriage or ectopic pregnancy: a prospective cohort study. *BMJ Open* 2016;6(11):e011864.

16. Jarvis S, Nelson-Piercy C. Management of nausea and vomiting in pregnancy. *BMJ* 2011;342:d3606.

17. Froyman W, Landolfo C, De Cock B, et al. Risk of complications in patients with conservatively managed ovarian tumours (IOTA5): a 2-year interim analysis of a multicentre, prospective, cohort study. *Lancet Oncol* 2019;20(3):448–458.

18. Damigos E, Johns J, Ross J. An update on the diagnosis and management of ovarian torsion. *Obstet Gynaecol* 2012;14(4):229–236.

The Acute Abdomen

Sophie Williams, Joanna Manson

The term 'acute abdomen' is defined as abdominal pain which is severe in nature, rapid in onset, and usually less than five days in duration [1]. It does not incorporate pain due to traumatic injury. Abdominal pain is a common presentation (approximately 300,000 general surgical admissions per year in the UK) and there are a myriad of causes (Box 88.1) [2]. Many patients with abdominal pain are managed medically or investigated as an outpatient, but about 10% require an emergency laparotomy, which still carries at least a 15% mortality [3]. When assessing a patient with abdominal pain, it is important to consider whether the patient is well or unwell and whether they need treatment urgently (within 24 hours) or non-urgently (>24 hours).

Evaluation of abdominal pain in patients with serious mental illness can be challenging. Some patients experience functional abdominal symptoms that accompany mental illness or experience gastrointestinal side effects from medication [4,5]. Non-specific abdominal pain and irritable bowel syndrome are diagnoses of exclusion; they are made only after specialist assessment and often also imaging or endoscopy. Late presentation of severe intra-abdominal pathology is usually associated with poorer outcomes and so timely identification and treatment of patients with serious pathology is important. This chapter provides the psychiatric practitioner with a comprehensive clinical approach to the patient with an acute abdomen which should guide initial management and facilitate onward referral.

HISTORY

A good pain history is key to guiding diagnosis. Where the patient is unable to provide a reliable history, a collateral history from relatives, friends, or carers may be useful. If no history can be obtained, then imaging is usually necessary.

The Maudsley Practice Guidelines for Physical Health Conditions in Psychiatry, First Edition.
David M. Taylor, Fiona Gaughran, and Toby Pillinger.
© 2021 John Wiley & Sons Ltd. Published 2021 by John Wiley & Sons Ltd.

Box 88.1 Causes of the acute abdomen

Common presentations

- Non-specific abdominal pain
- Acute appendicitis
- Intestinal obstruction
- Gallstone disease
- Diverticular disease
- Incarcerated hernia
- Peptic ulcer disease
- Acute pancreatitis
- Inflammatory bowel disease
- Abdominal wall haematoma
- Gastroenteritis
- Gynaecological pathology:
  - Ectopic pregnancy
  - Pelvic inflammatory disease
- Urological causes:
  - Ureteric calculus
  - Pyelonephritis
  - Testicular torsion

Uncommon presentations

- Volvulus
- Intussusception
- Duodenal ulcer
- Abdominal aortic aneurysm
- Mesenteric ischaemia
- Meckel's diverticulitis
- Psoas abscess
- Ischaemic colitis
- Diabetic ketoacidosis
- Hypercalcaemia
- Oesophageal perforation
- Gynaecological pathology:
  - Ovarian torsion
  - Ruptured ovarian cyst

Presenting complaint

Pay attention to the speed of onset, quality, character, and duration of abdominal pain. For example, the pain associated with appendicitis tends to be gradual in onset, initially central, and classically increases in intensity over one to two days; it becomes constant in the right iliac fossa once the inflammation involves the peritoneum. By contrast, pain associated with gallstones tends to be rapid in onset and colicky, usually with a food precipitant. Determine if the abdominal pain is a new symptom or one that has previously been experienced. Establishing the location of pain can narrow down the

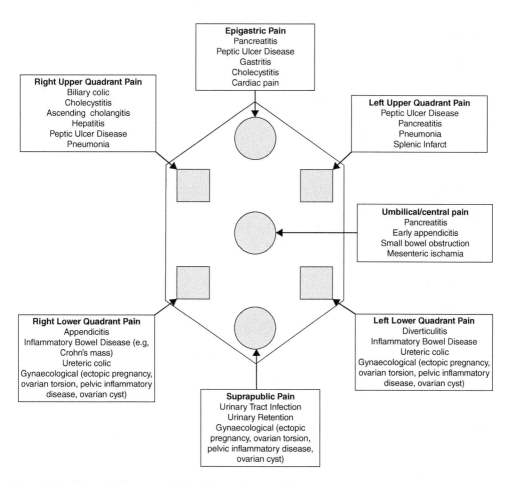

Epigastric Pain
Pancreatitis
Peptic Ulcer Disease
Gastritis
Cholecystitis
Cardiac pain

Right Upper Quadrant Pain
Biliary colic
Cholecystitis
Ascending cholangitis
Hepatitis
Peptic Ulcer Disease
Pneumonia

Left Upper Quadrant Pain
Peptic Ulcer Disease
Pancreatitis
Pneumonia
Splenic Infarct

Umbilical/central pain
Pancreatitis
Early appendicitis
Small bowel obstruction
Mesenteric ischamia

Right Lower Quadrant Pain
Appendicitis
Inflammatory Bowel Disease (e.g,
Crohn's mass)
Ureteric colic
Gynaecological (ectopic pregnancy,
ovarian torsion, pelvic inflammatory
disease, ovarian cyst)

Left Lower Quadrant Pain
Diverticulitis
Inflammatory Bowel Disease
Ureteric colic
Gynaecological (ectopic pregnancy,
ovarian torsion, pelvic inflammatory
disease, ovarian cyst)

Suprapublic Pain
Urinary Tract Infection
Urinary Retention
Gynaecological (ectopic
pregnancy, ovarian torsion,
pelvic inflammatory disease,
ovarian cyst)

Figure 88.1 Differential diagnoses of abdominal pain based on its location.

differential diagnoses (Figure 88.1). Enquire about associated symptoms such as fever, nausea/vomiting, gastro-oesophageal reflux, change in bowel habit, gastrointestinal bleeding, and urinary tract symptoms. Beware of conditions which mimic abdominal pain such as lower lobe pneumonia and acute coronary syndrome. Always ask female patients about their menstrual cycle and possible pregnancy. Ask about food intake, diet, weight loss, and bowel habit. Screen for risk factors for malignancy and ask about their family history. Consider sexually transmitted infections, HIV, and viral hepatitis.

Past medical history

- Have they had any abdominal surgery? What was the indication and when was it performed?
- Do they have any medical conditions? Consider gastro-oesophageal disease, pancreatitis, appendicitis, cholecystitis, ischaemic heart disease, inflammatory bowel disease (Crohn's disease or ulcerative colitis), or recurrent urinary tract infection.

Drug history

Screen for use of non-steroidal anti-inflammatory drugs (peptic ulcer disease), anticoagulants (abdominal wall haematoma), and any drugs that may cause diarrhoea or constipation (see Chapter 28). If history is suggestive of pancreatitis, screen for causative agents, such as angiotensin-converting enzyme inhibitors, statins, oral contraceptives/hormone replacement therapy, diuretics, some antibiotics, diabetic medications, and antiretroviral therapy. Drug-induced pancreatitis has also been associated with antipsychotic [6] and mood-stabiliser use, in particular sodium valproate [7].

Social history

- Quantify alcohol intake.
- Enquire about recreational drug use: cocaine can precipitate mesenteric ischaemia; intravenous drug use is a risk factor for viral hepatitis.
- Determine if there has been any recent travel history or animal exposure (parasitic liver abscess).

CAUSES OF THE ACUTE ABDOMEN BASED ON PAIN LOCATION

Left upper quadrant pain

The left upper quadrant (LUQ) is an unusual location for pain associated with the acute abdomen. Possible causes of LUQ pain include peptic ulcer disease, pancreatitis, left lower lobe pneumonia, and urological conditions such as ureteric stones or pyelonephritis. Less commonly, LUQ pain may herald splenic infarct (consider in clotting disorders) or a ruptured splenic artery aneurysm. In the latter there may be evidence of haemorrhagic shock and a tender mass or local peritonism (pain, tenderness and guarding; see Box 88.2).

Epigastric pain

- Epigastric pain owing to peptic ulcer disease is usually chronic and associated with gastro-oesophageal reflux (see Chapters 19, 20, and 75). Perforation of the gut as a complication of peptic ulcer disease may present with sudden-onset severe epigastric pain. On examination there will be peritonism.
- Pancreatitis presents as sudden and severe epigastric pain that radiates to the back and is often associated with bilious vomiting. Patients may have generalised peritonism. Systemic inflammation results in temperature spikes and patients can rapidly lose intravascular volume requiring aggressive fluid resuscitation. The most common causes are gallstones and alcohol, although remember the drug causes.
- Gallstone disease is discussed in the following section.
- Oesophageal perforation may be considered in the context of excessive vomiting and/or haematemesis.
- Other:
  - Acute coronary syndrome (see Chapters 67 and 69).
  - Pneumonia (see Chapter 39).

CHAPTER 88

Right upper quadrant pain

Gallstone disease

- Biliary colic classically presents with intermittent right upper quadrant (RUQ) pain following a fatty meal. The pain is severe, sudden in onset, can radiate to the back/right shoulder blade, lasts for minutes to hours, and may be associated with vomiting.
- Cholecystitis has a similar presentation to biliary colic but the associated pain usually lasts for over 24 hours and pain is accompanied by fever and tachycardia. On examination, patients will have RUQ tenderness with guarding and Murphy's sign may be positive (see Box 88.2). Mild jaundice is present in approximately 10% of patients.
- Ascending cholangitis typically presents with Charcot's triad: RUQ pain, fever (and potentially rigors), and jaundice. Patients have dark stool and pale urine. Patients are at high risk of sepsis and need early intravenous antibiotics.

Hepatic disease

- Hepatitis can be associated with constant RUQ pain in association with fever, myalgia, fatigue, and vomiting (see Chapters 23 and 43).
- Hepatic abscess is associated with RUQ pain and fever (and potentially rigors). Other symptoms/signs include malaise, vomiting, and weight loss. Abscesses may be parasitic, bacterial, or fungal in origin. Risk factors include immunosuppression, biliary tract disease, underlying malignancy, and history of foreign travel.

Other

- Urological disease, e.g. ureteric stones or pyelonephritis. Check for renal angle tenderness where urological disease is suspected.
- Consider Fitz-Hugh–Curtis syndrome in females with a history of pelvic inflammatory disease and RUQ pain. Here, pain is caused by adhesions over the liver.
- Right lower lobe pneumonia.

Left lower quadrant pain

- Diverticulitis generally presents with gradual-onset left lower quadrant (LLQ) pain increasing over one or more days. The pain is associated with fever, nausea, and

---

Box 88.2 Examination signs that provide insight into the aetiology of abdominal pain

- *Murphy's sign:* while pressing firmly in the right upper quadrant, ask the patient to take a deep breath in. The patient 'catching their breath' (ceasing inspiration) indicates cholecystitis.
- *Rovsing's sign:* palpation in the left iliac fossa causes tenderness in the right iliac fossa. This is suggestive of peritoneal inflammation secondary to appendicitis.
- *Rebound tenderness:* pain on removal of deep abdominal pressure indicates local peritonism.
- *Shifting dullness:* when examining the distended abdomen, presence of shifting dullness suggests ascites rather than obstruction.

diarrhoea (and sometimes also gastrointestinal bleeding). Patients may report a history of constipation. Diagnosis is confirmed with CT scan.

- Colitis may be related to inflammatory bowel disease, infection, or ischaemia. Ischaemic colitis usually presents with bloody diarrhoea and patients may be pyrexial. Diagnosis usually involves a CT scan and flexible sigmoidoscopy.
- Bowel obstruction with a change in bowel habit or absolute constipation can be caused by strictures, malignancy, volvulus, or inflammatory masses.
- Sigmoid volvulus (where floppy colonic mesentery leads to the bowel twisting) is usually seen in the elderly or patients with poor mobility. Patients usually present with marked abdominal distension and absolute constipation. Severe pain may herald bowel ischaemia.
- All women of childbearing age must have a pregnancy test to rule out ectopic pregnancy. Other gynaecological causes include ovarian cysts, torsion, and pelvic inflammatory disease.
- Other:
  - Ureteric stones.
  - Psoas abscess.
  - Incarcerated (stuck) or strangulated (ischaemic) hernia.

Right lower quadrant pain

- The pain of acute appendicitis is usually gradual in onset and constant, increasing over one to two days. The pain classically migrates over time from the central abdomen to the right iliac fossa. It is commonly associated with nausea, diarrhoea, and fever. On examination, there may be rebound tenderness and Rovsing's sign may be elicited (see Box 88.2).
- Gynaecological causes are as for LLQ pain.
- Other:
  - Ureteric stones.
  - Psoas abscess.
  - Incarcerated (stuck) or strangulated (ischaemic) hernia.

Central abdominal pain

- The pain of bowel obstruction is associated with abdominal distension, vomiting, and absolute constipation (i.e. no bowel movements and no flatus). The most common cause in the 'virgin' abdomen is a hernia and the most common cause in a patient with previous abdominal surgery is adhesions. Change in bowel habit, rectal bleeding, and weight loss may indicate malignancy.
- Early appendicitis is associated with central abdominal pain, which then moves to the right iliac fossa.
- In acute mesenteric ischaemia, the pain experienced by the patient is often out of proportion to the findings of the examination. The abdomen may be tender but is not peritonitic.
- A leaking/ruptured abdominal aortic aneurysm is associated with central or upper abdominal pain that radiates to the back and/or flanks and collapse. On examination

there may be a tender, pulsatile abdominal mass. Lower extremities may be pale and cold. The patient may have haemorrhagic shock.
- Other:
  - Gastroenteritis.
  - Diabetic ketoacidosis.
  - Severe constipation (see Chapter 28).
  - Abdominal wall haematoma (seen in patients on anticoagulation who have experienced physical trauma or recent cough).
  - Irritable bowel syndrome (a diagnosis of exclusion).

Groin pain

- Inguinal hernias need to be considered in all patients with abdominal pain. Groin lumps with overlying hot and erythematous skin suggest a strangulated hernia, which needs urgent surgical review.
- Pain may radiate into the groin in patients with ureteric colic or testicular pathology.
- Other:
  - Osteoarthritis.
  - Musculoskeletal injury.

EXAMINATION

Perform a set of basic observations, including a finger-prick glucose. If there is evidence of shock (profound hypotension in the context of tachycardia), manage the patient as per the ABCDE approach and transfer care to the emergency department.

The following features of the abdominal examination should be covered.

Inspect

- How is the patient walking or moving? Peritonitis is unlikely if the patient moves easily.
- *Tip*: A cough replicates rebound tenderness. Asking the patient to cough will localise an area of intra-abdominal inflammation or 'peritonism'. Don't hurt the patient, it is unnecessary.
- Does the patient's abdomen look distended?
- Look for scars (which may mean underlying adhesions).
- Look for lumps in the groin (evidence of hernia).

Palpate

- Pay attention to specific area(s) of tenderness.
- *Tip*: Don't forget the groins; hernias are easily missed.
- Try to determine where any lumps are located, i.e. skin, subcutaneous tissue, muscle, or intra-abdominal.

CHAPTER 88

Percuss

- Percussion can replicate rebound tenderness and identify organomegaly.

Auscultate

- Reduced or absent bowel sounds are serious but often misheard, and thus misleading.

Useful additional examination signs that provide insight into the aetiology of abdominal pain are described in Box 88.2. Digital rectal examination (DRE) has been shown to have low utility in the diagnosis of undifferentiated abdominal pain [8]. However, consider performing DRE in patients with rectal bleeding, obstructive symptoms, or where there are concerns regarding faecal impaction (see Chapter 28).

INVESTIGATIONS

- All females of childbearing age must have a urinary/blood beta-human chorionic gonadotrophin (β-HCG) to rule out pregnancy.
- Where urinary tract infection is suspected, perform urinalysis and send mid-stream urine for culture (see Chapter 41).
- Perform blood tests, including full blood count, urea and electrolytes, liver function tests, amylase, C-reactive protein, clotting, glucose, HbA$_{1c}$.

Investigations that may be performed by medical or surgical colleagues may include the following.

- Additional bloods: lactate (marker of tissue ischaemia), group and save.
- Abdominal X-ray (obstruction), erect chest X-ray (perforation and air under the diaphragm).
- Pelvic/abdominal ultrasound, examining for gallstones, gynaecological (e.g. ovarian) disease, free fluid in context of inflamed or perforated appendix.
- CT abdomen/CT kidney ureter bladder (in cases of suspected ureteric colic).

ONWARD REFERRAL

For patients who do not require immediate transfer to specialist services, management will depend on your diagnosis. Consider judicious analgesia. Be careful with laxatives if you are not clear about the cause for constipation (see Chapter 28).

All unwell patients with severe abdominal pain should be referred directly to surgical colleagues. If they show signs of sepsis, adhere to sepsis guidelines (see Chapter 72). If the diagnosis is less clear, then the emergency department may be a better choice initially. Women of childbearing age with right iliac fossa pain may require both a gynaecological and surgical review. As a rule, patients presenting with an acute abdomen do not usually want to eat or drink. We would recommend allowing patients to have only water to drink once a referral to general medical hospital has been instigated. This reduces dehydration and the need for intravenous fluids. Prior to surgery, patients are starved of solids for six hours and water for two hours. Regular medication should still be given (except for oral hypoglycaemics and anticoagulation).

In your telephone referral, you should detail your suspected diagnosis and the findings to support this conclusion, what treatment you have instigated, and the reason for the referral to the specialist team. A urine dip, pregnancy test, and a blood glucose reading are helpful.

The most important factor is to establish whether your patient is well or unwell and whether they need treatment urgently (within 24 hours) or non-urgently (>24 hours). Unwell patients with severe abdominal pain (with or without sepsis) require rapid surgical management, so do not delay your referral.

References

1. Gans SL, Pols MA, Stoker J, Boermeester MA. Guideline for the diagnostic pathway in patients with acute abdominal pain. *Dig Surg* 2015;32(1):23–31.
2. Royal College of Surgeons of England. Emergency General Surgery: Commissioning Guide. https://www.rcseng.ac.uk/library-and-publications/rcs-publications/docs/emergency-general-guide/
3. Saunders DI, Murray D, Pichel AC, et al. Variations in mortality after emergency laparotomy: the first report of the UK Emergency Laparotomy Network. *Br J Anaesth* 2012;109(3):368–375.
4. Clouse RE, Mayer EA, Aziz Q, et al. Functional abdominal pain syndrome. *Gastroenterology* 2006;130(5):1492–1497.
5. Ohayon MM, Schatzberg AF. Using chronic pain to predict depressive morbidity in the general population. *Arch Gen Psychiatry* 2003;60(1):39–47.
6. Koller EA, Cross JT, Doraiswamy PM, Malozowski SN. Pancreatitis associated with atypical antipsychotics: from the Food and Drug Administration's MedWatch surveillance system and published reports. *Pharmacotherapy* 2003;23(9):1123–1130.
7. Pellock JM, Wilder BJ, Deaton R, Sommerville KW. Acute pancreatitis coincident with valproate use: a critical review. *Epilepsia* 2002;43(11):1421–1424.
8. Kessler C, Bauer SJ. Utility of the digital rectal examination in the emergency department: a review. *J Emerg Med* 2012;43(6):1196–1204.

The ABCDE Approach

Toby Pillinger, Immo Weichert

The Airway, Breathing, Circulation, Disability, Exposure (ABCDE) approach provides a template for the immediate assessment and treatment of all clinical emergencies, be they within or outside a psychiatric setting [1]. This approach is described in all the chapters in Part 15 of this book.

FIRST STEPS

- Always consider your safety first. Where appropriate, wear protective equipment such as apron, gloves, face shield, and mask depending on the possible risk that you may be exposed to.
- If the patient is unconscious, try to elicit a response by asking 'How are you?' If there is no response, shake the patient. If there is still no response, look listen and feel for normal breathing, and feel for a carotid pulse. If a pulse is absent, initiate cardiopulmonary resuscitation as per the Advanced Life Support algorithm shown in Figure 89.1.
- Call for help early. In an outpatient setting, this may be from colleagues (e.g. the emergency 'Arrest' team if the outpatient department is attached to a hospital) or will involve calling the emergency services. In an inpatient setting this will involve calling the emergency 'Arrest' team.
- Monitor vital signs early on: attach a pulse oximeter, ECG monitor, and blood pressure monitor.
- If possible, gain venous access and take bloods for investigation when inserting the intravenous cannula. Check (finger-prick) capillary blood glucose.

The Maudsley Practice Guidelines for Physical Health Conditions in Psychiatry, First Edition.
David M. Taylor, Fiona Gaughran, and Toby Pillinger.
© 2021 John Wiley & Sons Ltd. Published 2021 by John Wiley & Sons Ltd.

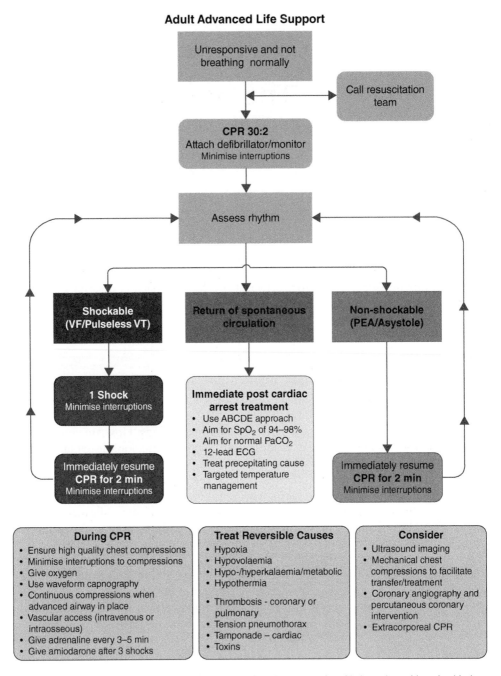

Figure 89.1 Adult Advanced Life Support algorithm. The algorithm is reproduced in its entirety although with the understanding that some procedures or investigations may not be available in a psychiatric setting, e.g. waveform capnography. Source: Resuscitation Council (UK) [1]. Reproduced with permission of the UK Resuscitation Council.

AIRWAY (A)

- Airway obstruction is an emergency: call for help.
- Look and listen for signs of airway obstruction: paradoxical chest and abdominal movements ('see-saw' respirations) and use of the accessory muscles. In partial obstruction, air entry is diminished and often noisy. In complete obstruction, no breath sounds will be heard. Remove any obvious obstructive objects (e.g. dentures or food bolus).
- If facilities allow, perform suction under direct vision if there are secretions.
- Perform a jaw thrust or head tilt/chin lift.
- Insert an oropharyngeal or nasopharyngeal airway, as appropriate.
- Provide oxygen using a mask with oxygen reservoir. Ensure that the oxygen flow is sufficient (usually 15 L/min). In acute respiratory failure, aim to maintain an oxygen saturation of 94–98%. In patients at risk of hypercapnic respiratory failure, aim for an oxygen saturation of 88–92%.

BREATHING (B)

- Look, listen, and feel for signs of respiratory distress, which include sweating, central cyanosis, and use of accessory muscles of respiration. Count respiratory rate (normal is 12–20 breaths per minute) and monitor oxygen saturation.
- If poor or absent respiratory effort, call for help.
- Assess chest expansion: is it equal between the left and right sides of the chest?
- Auscultate: is there equal air entry to both left and right lungs? Are breath sounds normal? Assess for presence of wheeze, stridor, and crackles.
- If there are concerns regarding air entry, percuss the chest wall. Is there an even percussion note between left and right lungs? Evidence of pneumothorax?

CIRCULATION (C)

- As described above, if there is no pulse initiate cardiopulmonary resuscitation as per the Advanced Life Support algorithm shown in Figure 89.1.
- Examine for evidence of poor perfusion, e.g. blue/pale/mottled hands or digits or cool peripheries. Measure capillary refill time (more than two seconds is prolonged).
- Check heart rate and measure blood pressure.
- Obtain venous access. Low blood pressure or high pulse should prompt the delivery of a fluid challenge (500 mL Hartmann's solution or, if not available, normal saline stat or 250 mL for patients with known heart failure) [1].

DISABILITY (D)

- Assess level of consciousness using the ACVPU scale (Box 89.1) [2].
- If not already performed, check finger-prick glucose and correct in the setting of hypoglycaemia (see Chapter 74).

> **Box 89.1** The ACVPU scale [2]
>
> **A** Alert
> **C** Confused
> **V** Responds to voice
> **P** Responds to painful stimulus
> **U** Unresponsive

- Check drug chart for reversible drug-induced causes of depressed consciousness (see Chapters 78 and 83).
- Nurse patients in the lateral position if the airway is not protected.

EXPOSURE (E)

Check temperature. To examine the body properly, full exposure of the body may be necessary (e.g. to examine for rash/injuries). Respect the patient's dignity and minimise heat loss.

References

1. Resuscitation Council (UK). *Advanced Life Support*, 7th edn . London: Resuscitation Council, 2016.
2. Royal College of Physicians. *National Early Warning Score (NEWS) 2. Standardising the assessment of acute-illness severity in the NHS. Updated report of a working party December 2017.* London: RCP, 2017. Available at https://www.rcplondon.ac.uk/national-early-warning-score

Index